Voice Disorders

Scope of Theory and Practice

Carole T. Ferrand
Hofstra University

PEARSON

Boston Columbus Indianapolis New York San Francisco Upper Saddle River
Amsterdam Cape Town Dubai London Madrid Milan Munich Paris Montreal Toronto
Delhi Mexico City São Paulo Sydney Hong Kong Seoul Singapore Taipei Tokyo

Vice President and Editorial Director: Jeffery W. Johnston
Executive Editor and Publisher: Stephen D. Dragin
Editorial Assistant: Jamie Bushell
Vice President, Director of Marketing: Margaret Waples
Marketing Manager: Weslie Sellinger
Senior Managing Editor: Pamela D. Bennett
Senior Project Manager: Linda Hillis Bayma
Senior Operations Supervisor: Matthew Ottenweller
Senior Art Director: Diane C. Lorenzo
Cover Designer: Ali Mohrman
Cover Image: Ted Ferrand
Full-Service Project Management: Thistle Hill Publishing Services, LLC
Composition: S4Carlisle Publishing Services
Printer/Binder: Edwards Brothers
Cover Printer: Lehigh Phoenix/ Hagerstown
Text Font: Minion

Credits and acknowledgments for materials borrowed from other sources and reproduced, with permission, in this textbook appear on appropriate page within text.

Every effort has been made to provide accurate and current Internet information in this book. However, the Internet and information posted on it are constantly changing, so it is inevitable that some of the Internet addresses listed in this textbook will change.

Photo Credits: All color insert photos courtesy of Lucian Sulica, MD—www.voicemedicine.com.

Library of Congress Cataloging-in-Publication Data
Ferrand, Carole T.
Voice disorders: scope of theory and practice / Carole T. Ferrand.
p. ; cm.
Includes bibliographical references and indexes.
ISBN-13: 978-0-205-54053-2 (casebound)
ISBN-10: 0-205-54053-8 (casebound)
1. Voice disorders. I. Title.
[DNLM: 1. Voice Disorders. 2. Respiration. 3. Respiratory Tract Diseases. WV 500]
RF510.F49 2012
616.85'56—dc23

2011021054

10 9 8 7 6 5 4 3 2 1

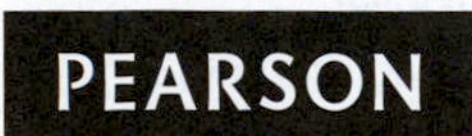

ISBN-13: 978-0-205-54053-2
ISBN-10: 0-205-54053-8

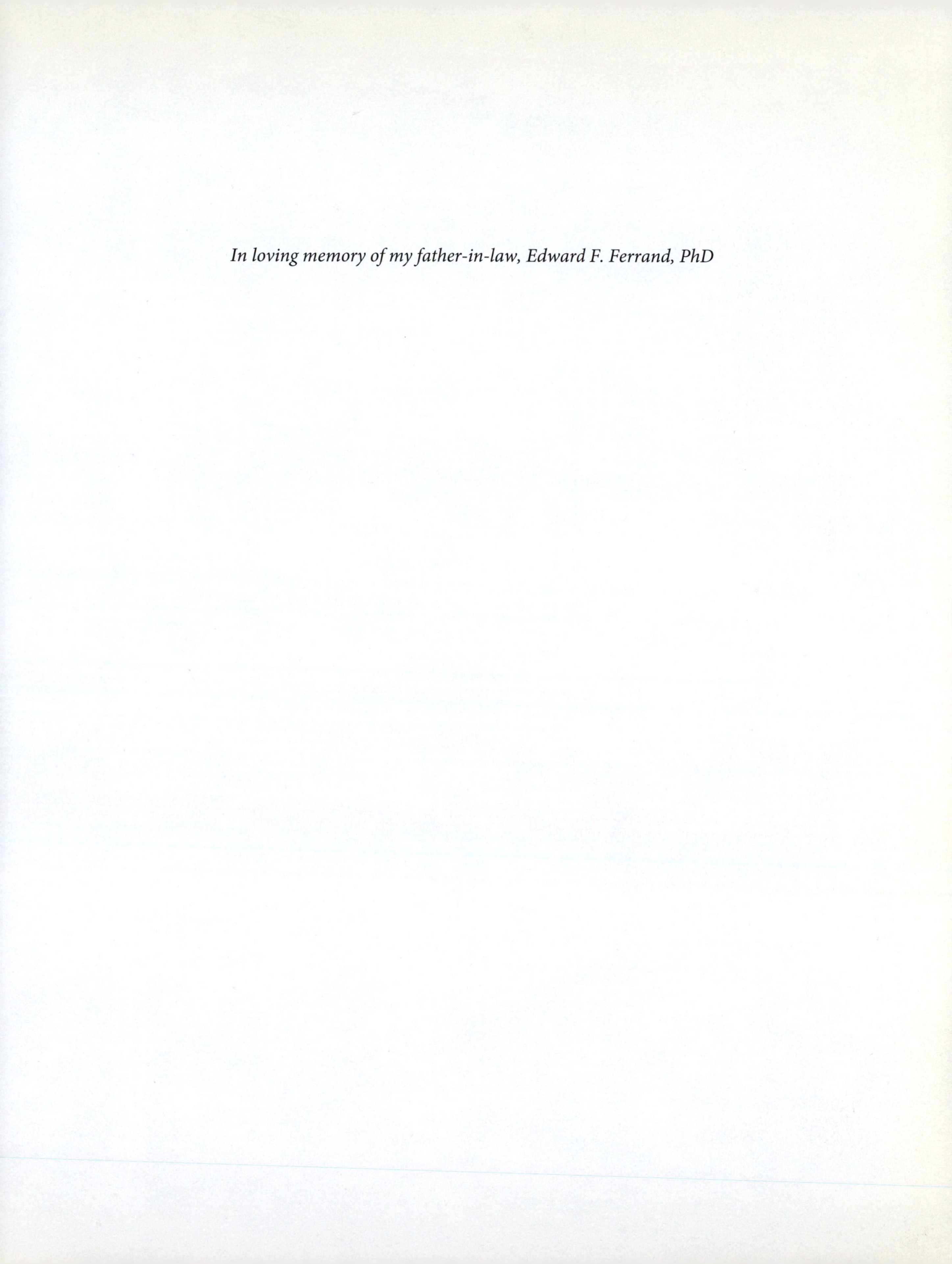

In loving memory of my father-in-law, Edward F. Ferrand, PhD

Brief Contents

List of Illustrations xvii

Preface xxi

Introduction 1

Chapter 1
Anatomy and Physiology of the Respiratory and Laryngeal Systems 5

Chapter 2
Lifespan Changes in the Respiratory and Phonatory Systems 63

Chapter 3
Considerations in Voice Treatment 85

Chapter 4
Diagnosis and Evaluation of Voice Disorders 115

Chapter 5
Clinical Management 169

Chapter 6
Inflammatory Conditions of the Larynx 215

Chapter 7
Structural Lesions of the Larynx 245

Chapter 8
Benign Lesions of the Vocal Fold Mucosa and Vocal Fatigue Associated with Lifestyle, Personality, and Occupational Factors 279

Chapter 9
Movement Disorders 303

Chapter 10
Voice Disorders Related to Self and Identity 351

Chapter 11
Disorders Related to Airway Problems and Respiration 383

Chapter 12
Laryngeal Cancer 421

Glossary 463

References 475

Name Index 529

Subject Index 543

Contents

List of Illustrations xvii
Preface xxi

Introduction 1

Expansion of Knowledge in the Field of Voice 1
Goal of the Book 2
Organization of the Book 3

1 *Anatomy and Physiology of the Respiratory and Laryngeal Systems* 5

Respiratory System 6
- Tracheobronchial Tree 6
- Nervous System Control of Respiration 15

Phonatory System 16
- Functions of the Larynx 16
- Anatomy and Physiology of the Laryngeal System 17
- True Vocal Folds 28
- Layers of the Vocal Folds 28
- Cover-Body Model of the Vocal Folds 35
- Glottis 35
- Muscles of the Larynx 37
- Myoelastic-Aerodynamic Theory 45
- Resonance 52

Nervous System Control of the Larynx 52
- Pyramidal and Extrapyramidal Pathways 53
- Cerebellum 56
- Cranial Nerves 57
- Reflexes 57

Vocal Registers 59
Modal Register 60
Pulse Register 60
Loft Register 60
Chapter Summary 61
Review Questions 62

2 *Lifespan Changes in the Respiratory and Phonatory Systems* 63

Development and Maturation of Speech Breathing 63
Structure and Function of the Larynx in Infancy and Childhood 67
Position in Neck 67
Cartilages 67
Vocal Folds 68
Acoustic Characteristics of Infant Vocalizations 70
Childhood 72
Puberty 74
The Adult Voice 75
The Aging Voice 76
Structural Changes 78
Acoustic Effects 79
Perceptual Findings 81
Health Status and Age-Related Vocal Diseases 82
Presbyphonia 83
Clinical Implications 83
Chapter Summary 83
Review Questions 84

3 *Considerations in Voice Treatment* 85

Normal Voice 86
Terminology 87
Perceptual Terms 87
Acoustic Terms 88
Causes of Voice Disorders 90
Team Approach to Diagnosis and Treatment of Voice Disorders 90
Prevention of Voice Disorders 93
Primary Prevention 93
Secondary Prevention 95
Tertiary Prevention 95

International Classification of Functioning, Disability, and Health (ICF) 96
Effects of Medications on the Voice 98
Multicultural Factors in Clinical Management of Voice Disorders 102
Evidence-Based Practice 107
Treatment Efficacy 111
Chapter Summary 112
Review Questions 123

4 *Diagnosis and Evaluation of Voice Disorders* 115

Components of the Evaluation Process 116
Case History 116
Auditory-Perceptual Evaluation 129
Instrumental Measures 134
Acoustic Analysis 145
Electroglottography 153
Aerodynamic Measures 157
Laryngeal Electromyography 158
The Diagnostic Report 158
Chapter Summary 163
Review Questions 164
Appendix 1: Preferred Practice Patterns for the Profession of Speech-Language Pathology 165

5 *Clinical Management* 169

Behavioral Voice Therapy Techniques 170
Indirect Approaches 171
Direct Approaches 179
Holistic Approaches 183
Patient Compliance 188
Motivational Interviewing 190
Transtheoretical Model of Behavior Change 192
Treatment of Children 193
Phonosurgery 195
Thyroplasty 195
Arytenoid Adduction/Arytenopexy 199
Airway Widening Procedures 199
Laser Microsurgery 203
Injection Laryngoplasty/Vocal Fold Augmentation 204
Botox Injection 210
Laryngeal Reinnervation 210

Chapter Summary 211
Review Questions 212
Appendix 1: The Use of Voice Therapy in the Treatment of Dysphonia 213

6 *Inflammatory Conditions of the Larynx* 215

Wound Healing 216
Inflammation 216
Extracellular Matrix Proliferation 216
Remodeling 218
Vocal Fold Scar 218
Sulcus Vocalis 220
Symptoms and Signs of Vocal Fold Scar and Sulcus Vocalis 221
Treatment 222
Laryngitis 225
Acute Laryngitis 226
Chronic Laryngitis 226
Gastroesophageal Reflux Disease and Laryngopharyngeal Reflux 227
Inflammatory Autoimmune Diseases 239
Systemic Lupus Erythematosus 239
Relapsing Polychondritis 240
Rheumatoid Arthritis 240
Chapter Summary 242
Review Questions 243

7 *Structural Lesions of the Larynx* 245

Laryngomalacia 246
Cause 247
Symptoms 247
Evaluation and Treatment 247
Subglottic Stenosis 248
Symptoms 250
Congenital Subglottic Stenosis 250
Acquired Subglottic Stenosis 251
Evaluation 252
Surgical Treatment 253
Laryngeal Web/Glottic Stenosis 258
Congenital Webs 258
Acquired Laryngeal Webs 259
Posterior Glottic Stenosis 260
Treatment 261

Laryngoceles and Laryngeal Cysts 262
- Laryngoceles 262
- Laryngeal Cysts 263

Recurrent Respiratory Papillomatosis 265
- Cause 266
- HPV Subtypes Associated with RRP 266
- Juvenile Onset Recurrent Respiratory Papillomatosis 267
- Adult Onset Recurrent Respiratory Papillomatosis 267
- Symptoms 268
- Diagnosis and Evaluation 268
- Treatment 268

Chapter Summary 275

Review Questions 276

Preparing for the Praxis 276
- Case Study 7.1 276

8 *Benign Lesions of the Vocal Fold Mucosa and Vocal Fatigue Associated with Lifestyle, Personality, and Occupational Factors* 279

Nodules 280
- Histology 280
- Age and Personality Factors 281
- Symptoms 282
- Evaluation and Treatment 282

Polyps 283
- Histology 284
- Reinke's Edema 285
- Symptoms 285
- Treatment 285

Leukoplakia 286
- Treatment 287

Contact Ulcers and Granulomas 288
- Causes 289
- Symptoms 289
- Evaluation and Treatment 289

Vascular Lesions of the Vocal Folds 290
- Causes 291
- Symptoms 291
- Evaluation and Treatment 291

Vocal Fatigue 292
- Central Fatigue 292
- Peripheral Fatigue 293

Recovery 293
Fatigue and Phonation Threshold Pressure 293
Occupational Voice Users 294
Occupational Risk Factors 294
Symptoms 296
Student Teachers 297
Vocational and Social Effects 298
Prevention and Treatment 298
Chapter Summary 299
Review Questions 300
Preparing for the Praxis 300
Case Study 8.1 300
Case Study 8.2 302

9 *Movement Disorders* 303

Flaccid Dysarthria 304
Vocal Fold Paresis 304
Vocal Fold Paralysis 306
Myasthenia Gravis 313
Spastic Dysarthria 316
Symptoms 316
Treatment 317
Ataxic Dysarthria 317
Symptoms 317
Treatment 318
Hypokinetic Dysarthria 318
Symptoms 319
Staging of PD 319
Treatment 320
Hyperkinetic Dysarthria 326
Chorea 326
Dystonia 327
Spasmodic Dysphonia 328
Essential Tremor 337
Mixed Dysarthrias 338
Amyotrophic Lateral Sclerosis 338
Multiple Sclerosis 340
Chapter Summary 342
Review Questions 345
Preparing for the Praxis 345
Case Study 9.1 345

Case Study 9.2 347
Case Study 9.3 348

10 *Voice Disorders Related to Self and Identity* 351

Symptoms and Features of Voice Disorders Related to Self and Identity 352
Psychiatric Caseness in Patients with Voice Disorders 353
Stress 353
Muscle Tension Dysphonia 355
Symptoms 356
Diagnosis and Evaluation 357
Voice Therapy 359
Conversion Disorders 360
Characteristics of Conversion Disorders 360
Diagnosis and Evaluation 361
Voice Therapy 362
Functional Dysphonia 362
Evaluation and Treatment 363
Mutational Falsetto 363
Evaluation 364
Treatment 364
Transgender Voice 365
Sex Reassignment Surgery 367
Evaluation 368
Treatment 370
Client Satisfaction 376
Chapter Summary 377
Review Questions 378
Preparing for the Praxis 379
Case Study 10.1 379
Case Study 10.2 380

11 *Disorders Related to Airway Problems and Respiration* 383

Dyspnea 384
Evaluation of Dyspnea 385
Stridor 385
Causes 386
Evaluation 387
Pulmonary Function Testing 387

Asthma 391
Evaluation and Treatment 392
Paradoxical Vocal Fold Motion 395
Symptoms 395
Causes 398
Links between PVFM, Asthma, and GERD 400
Diagnosis and Evaluation 401
Treatment 403
Chronic Cough 407
Causes of Chronic Cough 408
Symptoms and Associated Findings 410
Complications of CC 410
Diagnosis and Evaluation 410
Quantifying Cough 413
Treatment 413
Chapter Summary 416
Review Questions 418
Preparing for the Praxis 418
Case Study 11.1 418

12 *Laryngeal Cancer* 421

Laryngeal Cancer Evaluation and Staging 423
Risk Factors for Laryngeal Cancer 426
Symptoms 426
Diagnosis 427
Multidisciplinary Approach 427
Medical Treatment 428
Radiation Therapy 428
Chemotherapy 429
Surgical Options for Laryngeal Cancer 431
Resection 432
Vertical Partial Laryngectomy 433
Supraglottic Laryngectomy 434
Supracricoid Laryngectomy 435
Near Total Laryngectomy 436
Total Laryngectomy 436
Problems Related to Surgery 439
Voice Restoration 442
Artificial Larynx 444
Esophageal Speech 447
Tracheoesophageal Speech 450
General Considerations for Voice Restoration 456

Chapter Summary 460
Review Questions 461
Preparing for the Praxis 461
Case Study 12.1 461

Glossary 463

References 475

Name Index 529

Subject Index 543

Illustrations

Text Figures

1.1 The Tracheobronchial Tree 7
1.2 Trachea 8
1.3 Pleural Linkage 9
1.4 Diaphragm 10
1.5 Accessory Muscles of Respiration 11
1.6 Location of the Larynx in Relation to the Pharynx and Trachea 16
1.7 Hyoid Bone, Thyroid, and Cricoid Cartilages 18
1.8 Cartilages of the Larynx 19
1.9 Sectional and Posterior Views of the Larynx 20
1.10 Articular Facets of the Cricoid Cartilage 22
1.11 Cricoarytenoid Joint 23
1.12 Cricothyroid Joint 24
1.13 Effect of Thyroid Cartilage Tilting 24
1.14 Extrinsic Membranes 26
1.15 Superior View of the Folds of the Larynx 27
1.16 True and False Vocal Folds and Laryngeal Ventricle 29
1.17 Epithelial Cells 30
1.18 Extracellular Matrix 32
1.19 Layers of the Vocal Folds 34
1.20 Cover-Body Model of the Vocal Folds 35
1.21 Glottal Shapes 36
1.22 Skeletal Muscle 37
1.23 Extrinsic Muscles 39
1.24 Posterior View of Intrinsic Muscles 41

1.25 Adductor and Abductor Muscles 43
1.26 Cricothyroid Muscle 44
1.27 Thyroarytenoid Muscle 45
1.28 Myoelastic-Aerodynamic Theory of Phonation 46
1.29 Convergent and Divergent Glottal Shapes 48
1.30 Cycle of Vocal Fold Vibration 48
1.31 Phonation Threshold Pressure 49
1.32 Contributors to Pitch 51
1.33 Cortical Areas Involved in Phonation 54
1.34 Cerebellum and Subcortical Areas Involved in Phonation 55
1.35 Vagus Nerve 58
2.1 Immature and Mature Larynx 69
2.2 Infant versus Adult Vocal Folds 70
4.1 Different Points of Vocal Fold Vibration Illuminated by Stroboscopy 137
4.2 Voice Range Profile 150
4.3 Lx Waveform 153
4.4 Lx Waveforms of Vocal Registers and Qualities 154
4.5 EGG Quotients 156
4.6 Portion of a Diagnostic Report and Related Questions 159
5.1 Medialization Thyroplasty 196
5.2 Additional Types of Vocal Fold Medialization Implants 197
5.3 Arytenoid Adduction 200
5.4 Arytenoidectomy 201
5.5 Transverse Cordotomy 202
5.6 Vocal Fold Injection 205
6.1 Wound Healing 217
6.2 Sulcus Vocalis 220
6.3 Superficial and Deep Vocal Fold Injections for Scarring 223
6.4 Fat Graft for Sulcus Vocalis and Vocal Fold Scar 224
6.5 pH Monitoring 231
6.6 Fundoplication 238
7.1 Laryngomalacia 246
7.2 Subglottic Stenosis 249
7.3 Laser Treatment for Subglottic Stenosis 254
7.4 Cricotracheal Resection 257
7.5 Laryngeal Web 259
7.6 Laryngeal Cyst and Removal 263
7.7 Recurrent Respiratory Papillomatosis 265

8.1 Nodules 281
8.2 Polyp 283
8.3 Leukoplakia 287
8.4 Granuloma 288
11.1 Examples of Normal and Disordered Flow-Volume Loops 390
11.2 Normal versus Asthmatic Airway 392
11.3 Flow-Volume Loops for PVFM 404
12.1 Glottal Cancer 422
12.2 Total Laryngectomy 437
12.3 Trachea Sutured to Stoma 438
12.4 Voice Prosthesis 453

Insert Figures

1 Normal Vocal Folds
2 Aging
3 Scar 1
4 Scar 2
5 Sulcus
6 Laryngitis 1
7 Laryngitis 2
8 Reflux 1
9 Reflux 2
10 Papilloma 1
11 Papilloma 2
12 Papilloma 3
13 Nodules 1
14 Nodules 2
15 Polyp 1
16 Polyp 2
17 Polyp 3
18 Polyp 4
19 Reinke's Edema 1
20 Reinke's Edema 2
21 Reinke's Edema 3
22 Granuloma 1
23 Granuloma 2

24 Granuloma 3
25 Cyst 1
26 Cyst 2
27 Cyst 3
28 Hemorrhage 1
29 Hemorrhage 2
30 Hemorrhage 3
31 Unilateral Paralysis 1
32 Unilateral Paralysis 2
33 Bilateral Paralysis 1
34 Bilateral Paralysis 2
35 Cancer 1
36 Cancer 2

Preface

The idea for this book developed gradually over some years as I experimented with different organizational formats for my graduate course in voice disorders. It seemed logical to begin the course with a detailed discussion of respiratory and laryngeal anatomy and physiology in order to build a solid foundation of knowledge of normal structure and function. And following the initial discussion with information regarding changes in structure and function over the lifespan was also an obvious step. At what point to cover clinical management domains (i.e., diagnosis, evaluation, therapeutic approaches, treatment issues) was more difficult. I tried numerous different approaches, for example, presenting information on voice disorders (etiologies, symptoms, etc.) followed by sections on diagnosis and evaluation, and finishing up the course with treatment. However, by the end of the semester there was typically very little time (usually just one session) to cover treatment. Next I tried infusing treatment techniques into the disorders sections and leaving diagnosis and evaluation until the end of the course. But it made more clinical sense to present material on diagnosis prior to discussing specific intervention approaches. Finally, I settled on the current organization of the course, which also forms the organization of this book. The first section of the book (Chapters 1 and 2) presents the necessary anatomical information that forms the basis for rational clinical decision making. The next section (Chapters 3 to 5) provides a thorough grounding in clinical methodology in the assessment and treatment of voice disorders. Students are introduced to important diagnostic and therapeutic principles and methods that underlie many different types of voice disorders. These include the multifactorial nature of voice disorders, the necessity of an interdisciplinary team approach to provide an integrated treatment plan for the patient, the effect of different types of drugs on voice production, the role of evidence-based practice in providing effective clinical services, and multicultural considerations that may be important in assessment and treatment of voice disorders. Also included is discussion of the role of prevention in the development of voice pathologies and the World Health Organization's latest version of the International Classification of Functioning, Disability and Health. Discussion of general diagnostic and assessment issues and methods follows, with emphasis on auditory-perceptual and instrumental evaluation techniques. Material on treatment issues (e.g., patient compliance) and commonly used behavioral and medical/surgical techniques are reviewed in detail. The final section of the book (Chapters 6 to 12) is devoted to an in-depth discussion of specific voice disorders, with focused clinical management techniques elaborated on as appropriate. For example, by the time students learn about working with transgender clients, they are already familiar with many of the therapeutic approaches covered in the treatment chapter, such as vocal hygiene and various relaxation techniques. Because this is a specific type of population, extensive coverage is also provided of techniques specific to transgender individuals, such as pitch-raising techniques to feminize the voice. Similarly, medical/surgical and behavioral treatment approaches that are specific to Parkinson's disease are discussed in the chapter on movement disorders, and therapeutic strategies specific to paradoxical vocal fold motion are presented in the chapter on disorders related to respiration.

This is an exciting time to be studying and working in the field of voice disorders. Thanks to advances in technology as well as the use of sophisticated modeling techniques, we now have a vastly increased understanding of the anatomy and physiology of normal and abnormal voice production. This has resulted in refinements in behavioral and medical/surgical evaluation and treatment procedures that have benefited patients and their families. Hand-in-hand with increased knowledge is the current emphasis on treatment outcomes and therapeutic efficacy, systematized in a process called evidence-based practice (EBP). EBP places the individual seeking treatment at the center of the clinical process and integrates client preferences and values within a framework of research evidence and clinical expertise. The integration of research evidence, clinical expertise, and client input results in a higher level of accountability to the client, the family, and third-party payers.

Writing this book has been a wonderful learning experience, and it is my hope that readers will find the vast topic of voice disorders to be as fascinating and challenging as I do.

Carole Ferrand

New! CourseSmart eTextbook Available

CourseSmart is an exciting new choice for students looking to save money. As an alternative to purchasing the printed textbook, students can purchase an electronic version of the same content. With a CourseSmart eTextbook, students can search the text, make notes online, print out reading assignments that incorporate lecture notes, and bookmark important passages for later review. For more information, or to purchase access to the CourseSmart eTextbook, visit www.coursemart.com.

Supplementary Materials: Resources for Professors and Students

INSTRUCTOR'S RESOURCE MANUAL AND TEST BANK

Instructors will find a wealth of resources to support their course within the text itself. Each chapter in the Instructor's Resource Manual contains chapter-by-chapter teaching aids. The Test Bank for each chapter includes various types of test questions, including multiple choice, true/false, and essay questions. The supplement is available online or you can contact your Pearson representative. To download and print the Instructor's Resource Manual and Test Bank, go to www.pearsonhighered.com and then click on "Educators."

POWERPOINTS

In addition to the Instructor's Resource Manual and Test Bank, we have provided the instructor with PowerPoints. This supplement is also available online or you can contact your Pearson sales representative. To download and print the supplement files, go to www.pearsonhighered.com and then click on "Educators."

COMPANION WEBSITE

Located at www.pearsonhighered.com/ferrand, the Companion Website for this text includes a wealth of resources such as Learning Objectives, Practice Questions, Flash Cards, and Useful Websites that will help ensure student mastery.

Acknowledgments

I would like to thank my husband, Ted Ferrand, for his wonderful illustrations; Dr. L. Sulica for permission to use his excellent photographs; and my students, Brooke Adler, Monika Dziemianczuk, Michelle Frankino, Alyssa Maultasch, and Krishona Weller, for their help with the diagnostic case report. I appreciate the constructive feedback from the reviewers: Moya Andrews, Indiana University; Marylou Pausewang Gelfer, University of Wisconsin; Mary Hawkshaw, Drexel University College of Medicine; E. Charles Healy, University of Nebraska–Lincoln; Gary Jones, Buffalo State College; Sid Khosla, University of Cincinnati; David Kuehn, University of Illinois; Gary McCullough, University of Central Arkansas; Michael Moran, Auburn University; Richard Morris, Florida State University; Rebekah Pindzola, Auburn University; David Sorensen, Idaho State University; Celia Stewart, New York University; and Michael Trudeau, The Ohio State University. Their suggestions throughout the preparation of the manuscript helped to make this a better book. Thanks, as always, to Steve Dragin and his able assistant Jamie Bushell for their editorial help and gentle pushing when needed.

Carole Ferrand

Introduction

V*oice Disorders: Scope of Theory and Practice* presents a comprehensive account of the field of voice in the early years of the new millennium. The book is meant for graduate students in speech-language pathology as well as practicing professionals who would appreciate an up-to-date yet easy-to-read reference. The book is based on 20 years of teaching a graduate-level voice disorders course, integrated into a framework of classic and current research.

Expansion of Knowledge in the Field of Voice

The field of voice science and voice disorders has grown hugely over the past two decades. Thanks to advances in technology as well as the use of sophisticated modeling techniques we now have a vastly increased understanding of the complex histology of the vocal folds, the mucosal wave and its importance to normal voice production, the vital role of the extracellular matrix of the lamina propria, water and ion transport in the vocal folds, and the role of inflammation and wound healing in vocal fold function.

Voice-related research and clinical practice have traditionally drawn from many other disciplines such as psychology, education, physics, and chemistry. Recent research has further been enriched by incorporating techniques from engineering, cellular and molecular biology, mathematics, genetics, and neuroscience (Branski & Sivasankar, 2006). Developments such as application of growth factors to the vocal folds to reduce scarring, using collagen matrices to replace vocal fold tissue (Branski & Sivasankar, 2006), new synthetic materials for vocal fold injections and implants, and use of EMG signals to control artificial larynges have resulted in new treatments with enormous potential for helping individuals with a variety of voice disorders.

An important result of the expansion of knowledge regarding laryngeal structure and vocal fold biomechanics is that the effectiveness of clinical management strategies can be examined in light of new theoretical frameworks. For example, laryngeal hydration treatments are often advocated as a component of vocal hygiene programs. However, research by Roy et al. (2003) focusing on the cellular mechanisms responsible for water transportation in the vocal folds has shown that methods such as drinking six to eight glasses of water daily, using over-the-counter lubricants, and using steam inhalation may not be effective (Branski & Sivasankar, 2006). Another traditional therapeutic strategy that is often recommended after vocal fold injury is voice rest. However, an increased understanding of the mechanisms of wound healing and wound repair has led to a realization that voice treatment exercises may help, rather than hinder, the recovery process in certain cases (Verdolini, Rosen, Branski, & Hebda, 2003).

The push for evidence to support clinical management strategies is systematized in a process called evidence-based practice (EBP). EBP has become widely accepted in many fields of medicine and allied health sciences over the past decade. EBP calls for a three-pronged approach toward clinical decision making that contextualizes client preferences and values within a framework of research evidence and clinical expertise. Evidence-based practice is rapidly becoming integrated into the fabric of research and practice in all aspects of normal and disordered speech and voice production. The focus on evidence to support assessment and intervention choices encourages the discipline to become more grounded in objective data, with testable theories and hypotheses that provide a framework for intelligent clinical decision making. The integration of research evidence, clinical expertise, and client input results in a higher level of accountability to the client, the family, and third-party payers.

The emphasis on patient preferences and values leads naturally into a focus on multicultural issues that can affect the diagnosis and treatment of voice disorders. Individual preferences and values are strongly influenced by cultural attitudes and beliefs about the nature of disabilities, including communicative disabilities. As well, the increasingly diverse makeup of the United States demands a less restricted basis of normative voice data. Most voice-related normative data have been obtained from predominantly mainstream speakers, that is, White middle-class speakers of General American English. Over the past few years, more researchers have focused their attention on speakers from different groups and cultures, primarily African American, but also Hispanic, Russian, Cantonese, and others. It is essential that linguistically and culturally diverse individuals be included in normative sampling, and that culturally sensitive assessment and treatment procedures be developed (Duff, Proctor, & Yairi, 2004).

Goal of the Book

The goal of this book is to present a detailed picture of current theory and practice in the field of voice in a way that is both comprehensive and readily accessible to the reader. Understanding of the material is facilitated by the organization of the information. Chapters 1 and 2 present the anatomical and physiological material that is fundamental to understanding the nature of voice and breakdowns in voice production. Chapters 3, 4, and 5 focus on considerations in voice treatment, diagnosis and evaluation, and clinical management. Introducing clinical management approaches early in the sequence highlights the importance of behavioral voice therapy and phonosurgical techniques in the treatment of voice disorders. Chapters 6–12 focus on specific voice disorders. In addition to the information presented in Chapters 3–5, diagnostic and treatment techniques specific to particular voice problems are described in each disorders chapter.

Each chapter is followed by review questions that help the reader to summarize and internalize the information. The book includes 10 case studies, which are designed to help readers integrate theoretical information and evidence-based practice into the diagnosis and treatment of voice disorders.

Organization of the Book

Chapter 1 presents the anatomy and physiology of the respiratory system, including descriptions of lung volumes and capacities important for voice production. A detailed discussion of the laryngeal mechanism follows, including current information on the vital role of extracellular matrix, the importance of the mucosal wave, and the role of phonation threshold pressure in the vibratory cycle. The neurology of laryngeal motor control is discussed, including cortical, subcortical, and peripheral structures. Also included is a discussion of modal, pulse, and falsetto registers. Chapter 2 is devoted to a discussion of lifespan changes in the voice from infancy to old age. Structural and functional changes in the laryngeal system are presented along with the perceptual and acoustic effects of such changes, focusing particular attention on the aging voice. Knowledge of these changes and their effects on voice production is of crucial importance, given the dramatic and continuing increase in the elderly population in the United States. Understanding what constitutes normal aging forms the basis for differentiating between expected and pathological vocal change.

Chapter 3 presents important considerations to take into account in the assessment and treatment of voice disorders. These include the multifactorial nature of voice disorders, the necessity of an interdisciplinary team approach to provide an integrated treatment plan for the patient, the effect of different types of drugs on voice production, the role of evidence-based practice in providing effective clinical services, and multicultural considerations that may be important in assessment and treatment of voice disorders. Also included is a discussion of the role of prevention in the development of voice pathologies and the World Health Organization's latest version of the International Classification of Functioning, Disability, and Health.

Chapter 4 presents a comprehensive discussion of diagnostic and evaluation procedures. The importance of obtaining a thorough case history is emphasized, and examples of case history protocols are provided. The current emphasis on quality of life and outcomes assessment is stressed, and several examples of quality-of-life questionnaires are presented. The chapter discusses important components of the voice evaluation including auditory-perceptual assessment, endoscopic measures, acoustic analysis, aerodynamic measures, and laryngeal electromyography. The chapter concludes with a detailed case history illustrating many of the concepts, with related questions pertaining to the diagnostic process.

Chapter 5 presents a comprehensive discussion of clinical management issues. Attention focuses on behavioral voice therapy techniques including the most commonly used indirect and direct approaches. Where available, outcomes studies and efficacy research are presented for each approach. Specific techniques such as vocal hygiene, hydration, biofeedback, yawn-sigh, respiratory support, and so on are described. Additionally, holistic approaches including accent method, resonant voice therapy, vocal function exercises, and others are discussed. The important issue of patient compliance with behavioral voice therapy techniques is highlighted, and a psychotherapeutic program to increase patient compliance is presented. Discussion then turns to phonosurgical procedures such as thyroplasty, airway widening procedures, vocal fold augmentation injection, and the use of Botox.

Chapter 6 focuses on the wound healing process following injury to the vocal folds and the development of vocal fold scar. The central role of inflammation in conditions such as acute and chronic laryngitis, gastroesophageal reflux disease and laryngopharyngeal reflux, and rheumatoid arthritis is underscored. Behavioral and medical/surgical treatment options are presented for each disorder.

Chapter 7 focuses on structural lesions of the larynx including laryngomalacia, subglottic stenosis, laryngeal web, laryngeal cysts, and recurrent respiratory papillomatosis. Each disorder is presented in terms of its cause(s) and symptoms, followed immediately by discussion of assessment and treatment options. Chapter 8 addresses other benign lesions of the vocal fold mucosa such as nodules, polyps, leukoplakia, ulcers/granuloma, and vascular lesions. These pathologies are often associated with lifestyle, personality, and occupational factors. The topic of vocal fatigue is addressed with explanation of central and peripheral factors as well as the importance of recovery after heavy vocal use. Attention focuses on teachers, who form a large group of occupational voice users who are prone to vocal fatigue and benign mucosal lesions.

Chapter 9 focuses on neurological movement disorders, which are presented in terms of the classic Darley, Aronson, and Brown (1969) classification scheme of dysarthrias (flaccid, spastic, ataxic, hypokinetic, hyperkinetic, mixed). Examples and in-depth discussion of diseases resulting in movement disorders are provided along with diagnostic and treatment procedures specific to each disorder. For example, the Lee Silverman Voice Treatment used widely for treatment of hypokinetic dysarthria resulting from Parkinson's disease is discussed in depth. The chapter also includes discussion of spasmodic dysphonia as an example of a focal dystonia.

Chapter 10 focuses on voice disorders related to self and identity, usually called by a myriad of names such as psychogenic dysphonia, nonorganic dysphonia, functional dysphonia, and so on. The central role of stress in many of these disorders is emphasized. Particular attention is paid to muscle tension dysphonia, conversion disorders, functional dysphonia as a distinct clinical entity, mutational falsetto, and transgender voice. Treatment of transsexual voice following sex reassignment surgery is described.

Chapter 11 describes disorders related to airway problems and respiration. The major symptoms of airway disorders, dyspnea and stridor, are explained and several methods of evaluating dyspnea are provided. The importance of pulmonary function testing is emphasized with particular reference to distinguishing between asthma and paradoxical vocal fold motion. A laryngeal condition related to inhaled steroid use for asthma is identified, called steroid inhaler laryngitis. The disorders of paradoxical vocal fold motion and chronic cough are described, and the links between these two conditions are pointed out. Evaluation and treatment protocols specific to each disorder are presented.

Chapter 12 focuses on laryngeal cancer. The TMN classification system developed by the American Joint Committee for Cancer Staging is presented. Risk factors for laryngeal cancer are identified, and the importance of a multidisciplinary approach is emphasized. Discussion then shifts to medical treatments for removal of the cancer including radiation therapy and chemotherapy and the resulting voice and swallowing function. Surgical options for removal of the cancer are presented, including various partial laryngectomy procedures. Voice and swallowing function after each type of procedure is described. A description of total laryngectomy is provided. Physical, psychoemotional, and communicative problems related to the surgery are identified. Attention then focuses on methods of voice restoration including artificial larynx, esophageal speech, and tracheoesophageal speech. Advantages and disadvantages of each method are explored. The chapter concludes with general considerations for voice restoration including quality-of-life issues.

Chapter 1

Anatomy and Physiology of the Respiratory and Laryngeal Systems

LEARNING OBJECTIVES

1. Identify the structures and understand the mechanics of respiration.
2. List the lung volumes and capacities in reference to resting expiratory level.
3. Understand the differences between breathing for life and breathing for speech.
4. Appreciate the role of the laryngeal structures and their functions, including the cover-body model of the vocal folds.
5. Understand the myoelastic aerodynamic theory of vocal fold vibration.
6. Describe the factors involved in changing pitch and loudness.
7. Identify the structures involved in nervous system control of phonation.
8. Compare the different vocal registers and their perceptual and acoustic characteristics.

Voice production depends on the integrated coordination of the respiratory, phonatory, and resonatory systems. Voice is also influenced by the digestive and endocrine systems, and voice production is controlled and regulated by the central and peripheral nervous systems. This chapter focuses on the respiratory, laryngeal, and nervous system involvement in voice production.

The chapter begins with a discussion of the structure of the lower respiratory system and the mechanics of breathing, followed by a description of lung volumes and capacities. Differences between breathing for life and breathing for speech are identified, and nervous system control of respiration is described. Discussion then turns to the laryngeal system with a review of laryngeal structure and function, the expanded myoelastic-aerodynamic theory of phonation, and mechanisms involved in changing pitch and loudness levels. The major functional components of the central and peripheral nervous systems subserving voice production are presented followed by a description of the three primary vocal registers used in speech.

Respiratory System

The respiratory system provides the airstream that forms the basis of all voice and speech production. The respiratory system encompasses the oral and nasal cavities, pharynx, larynx, trachea, bronchi, bronchioles, alveolar sacs, and the lungs. The oral and nasal cavities and pharynx form the upper respiratory tract; the trachea and bronchial structures comprise the lower respiratory tract. The larynx is located at the junction of the upper and lower tracts. The lungs are located within the **thoracic cavity**, which is bounded laterally by the rib cage, anteriorly by the sternum, and posteriorly by the spinal vertebrae. The diaphragm muscle forms the floor of the thoracic cavity, separating it from the abdominal cavity. The chest wall forms an integral part of the respiratory system and is made up of the rib cage, the diaphragm, the abdominal wall, and the abdominal contents. The following discussion focuses on the lower respiratory system.

TRACHEOBRONCHIAL TREE

The **tracheobronchial tree** is an air conducting system formed by the trachea, bronchi, bronchioles, and alveolar sacs (Figure 1.1).

The **trachea** is a hollow tube formed by 16–20 C-shaped rings of cartilage that are closed anteriorly and open posteriorly (Figure 1.2). The cartilage is covered by layers of smooth muscle and mucous membrane, which serve to close the tube posteriorly, and are also present between the cartilages. The inside of the tube (**lumen**) is lined with pseudostratified ciliated columnar epithelium. The epithelium contains goblet cells that secrete mucus. The mucus traps particles of dust and bacteria, and the cilia move in a wavelike fashion to sweep this matter upward and out of the airways. Air traveling to the lungs is thereby cleaned and filtered.

The trachea measures approximately 19 mm in diameter in adult males and approximately 16 mm in diameter in adult females, although there is a great deal of variability between individuals (Breatnach, Abbott, & Fraser, 1984).

The trachea divides into a series of bronchi. The two primary (mainstem) bronchi each enter a lung, and then further divide into secondary and tertiary bronchi. The secondary bronchi supply the lobes of the lungs (two lobes in the left lung, three in the right); the tertiary bronchi supply the segments of the lungs (eight segments in the left lung, 10 in the right). Structurally the bronchi are similar to the trachea but smaller in diameter. Each primary bronchus is slightly less than one half the diameter of the trachea, and the secondary and tertiary bronchi become increasingly smaller and narrower. The tertiary bronchi continue to branch and divide into smaller and smaller tubes, and eventually branch into microscopic bronchioles. Bronchioles are composed solely of smooth muscle and mucous membrane. The bronchioles continue to branch and eventually terminate in respiratory bronchioles. The respiratory bronchioles open into alveolar ducts, which terminate in alveolar sacs. Each alveolar sac is a microscopic, thin-walled, air-filled structure surrounded by a network of microscopic blood capillaries. There are on average around 480 million alveoli in the human lung (Ochs et al., 2004). The alveolar sacs form the location of gas exchange between oxygen and carbon dioxide. Each inhalation of air brings fresh oxygen through the tracheobronchial tree to the alveolar sacs. The oxygen diffuses into the surrounding blood capillaries and is transported to every cell in the body via the circulatory system. The waste product of breathing, carbon dioxide, is brought by the circulatory system back to the capillary network around the alveolar sacs, where it diffuses into the alveoli and is exhaled.

The interior of the lungs is composed of the branching bronchi, bronchioles, and alveoli, in addition to blood vessels and nerves. The lungs are cone-shaped structures housed within

FIGURE 1.1 The Tracheobronchial Tree

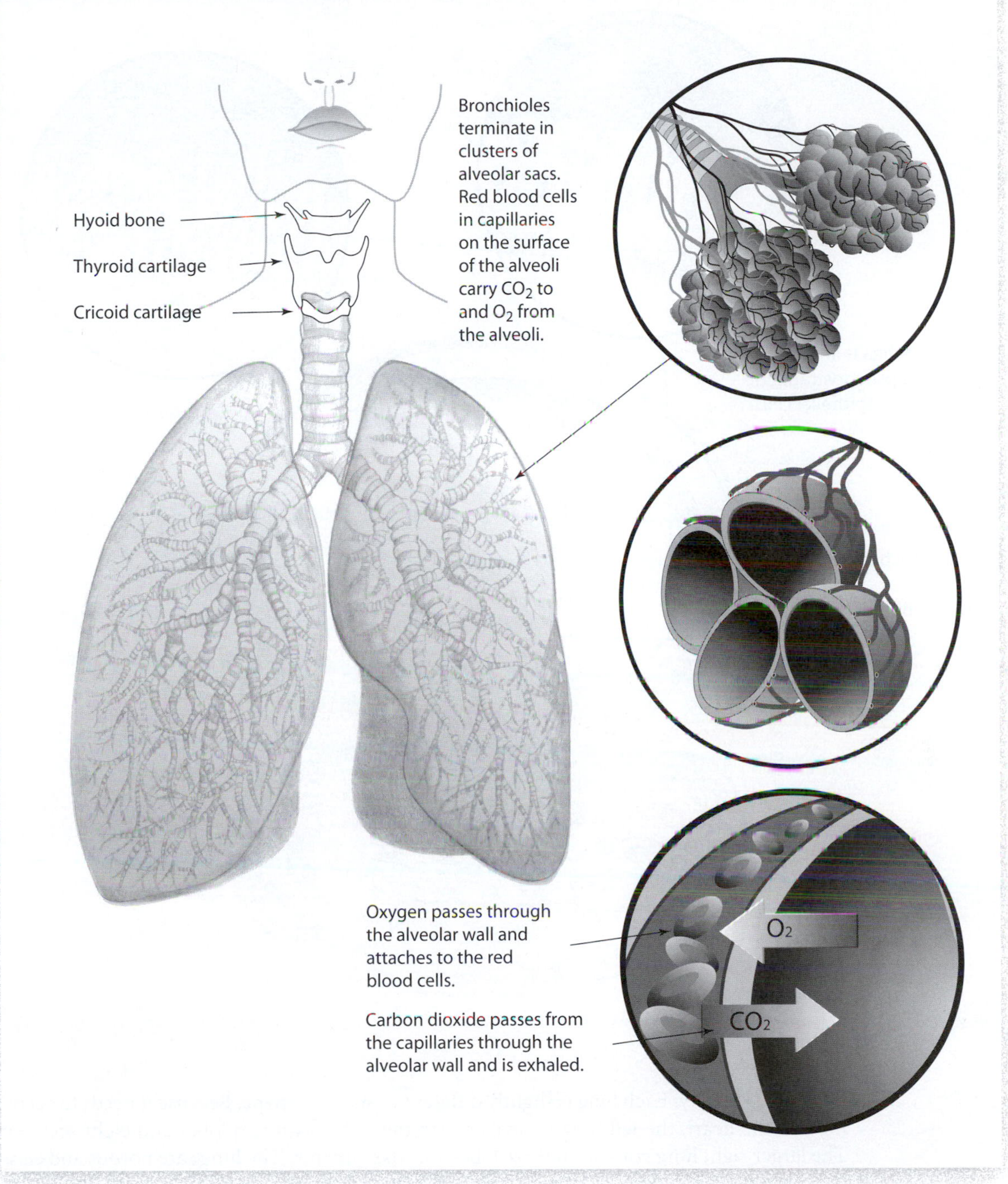

FIGURE 1.2 The Trachea

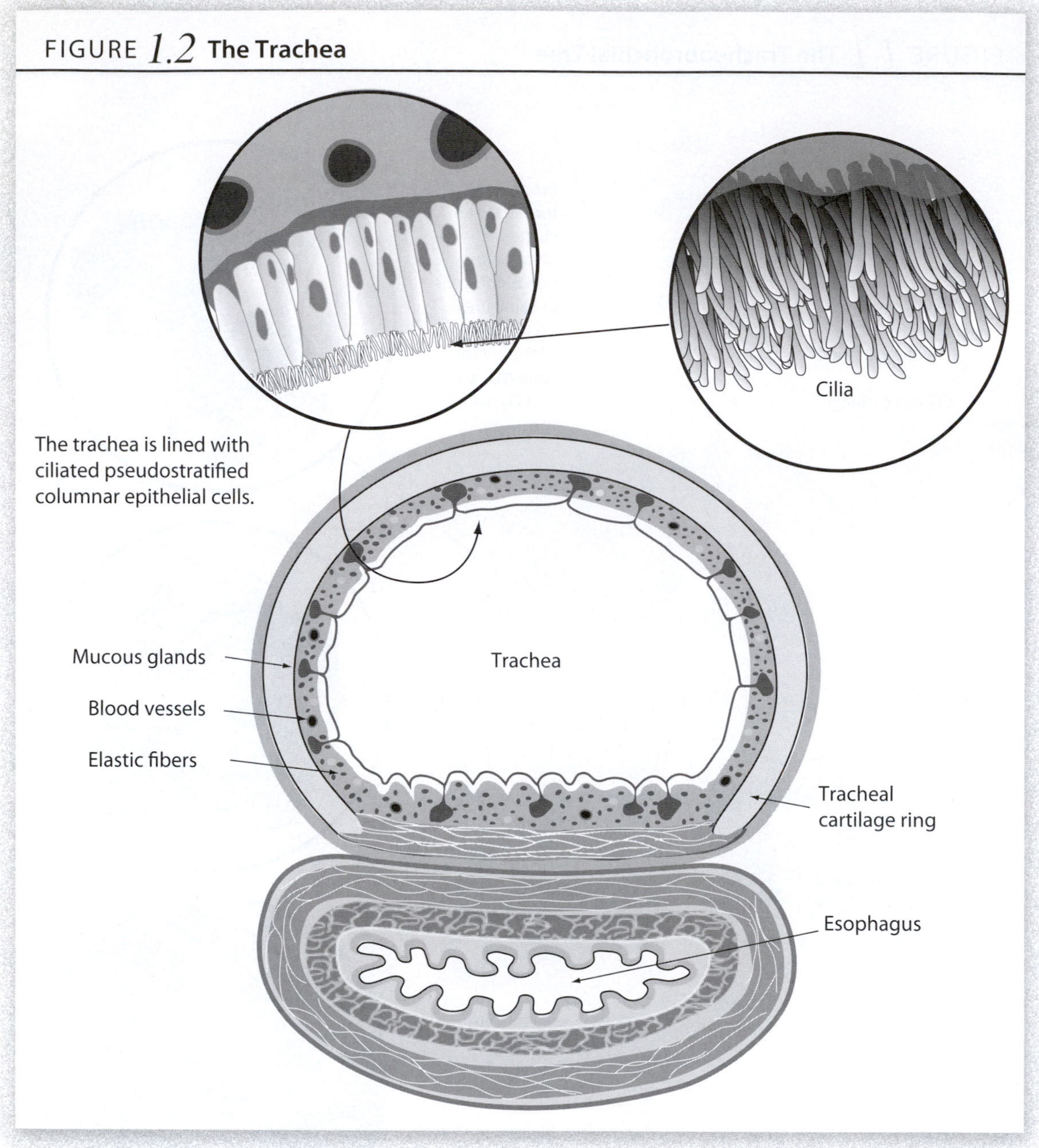

the thoracic cavity. Each lung is slightly different in size and shape. Because it needs to accommodate the heart, the left lung is smaller than the right, with two lobes and eight segments. The larger right lung consists of three lobes and 10 segments. The lungs are porous and elastic structures enabling them to be easily and expanded and contracted.

Pleural Linkage. The lungs contain very little muscle tissue and are unable to spontaneously generate movement. They are, however, highly compliant and can be easily moved by an external source. Each lung is encased in an airtight membrane called the **visceral pleura**. The inside surface of the thoracic cavity is lined by a membrane called the **parietal pleura**. Between these pleurae is a potential space known as the **pleural space**, containing **pleural fluid**. This fluid has a permanent negative pressure, which acts to hold the visceral and parietal pleurae in close approximation. Because of **pleural linkage** the thorax and lungs act as an integrated unit (Figure 1.3). Thus, whenever the thoracic cavity is moved by active or passive forces, the lungs are moved as well. This mechanism is vital to inhalation and exhalation.

FIGURE *1.3* **Pleural Linkage**

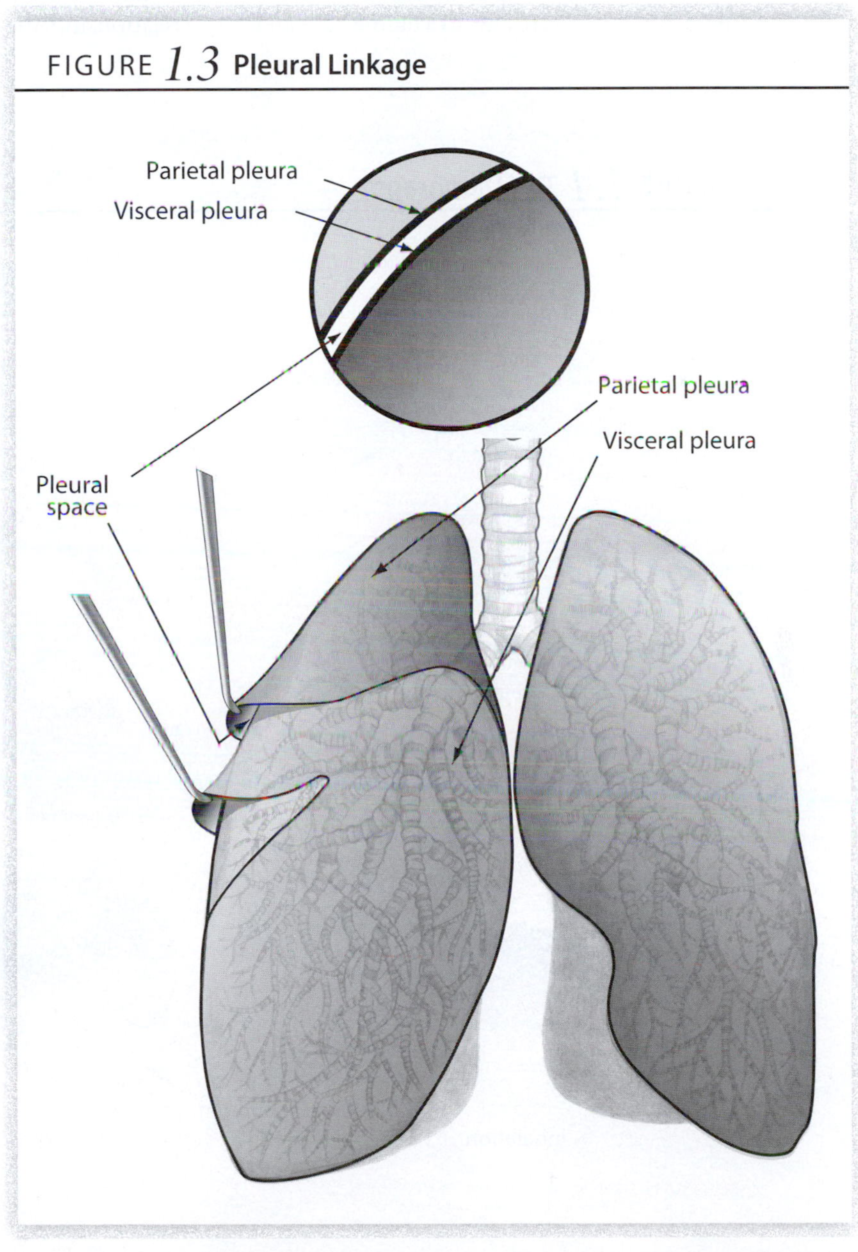

Inhalation and Exhalation. One cycle of respiration includes an inhalation and an exhalation phase. Inhalation depends on active muscle forces. In order to inhale, the thoracic cavity and lungs must expand. The expansion is achieved primarily via two muscles—the external intercostals and the diaphragm (Figure 1.4).

The 11 pairs of **external intercostal muscles** run between the ribs on either side (Figure 1.5). Their contraction pulls the rib cage in an upward and outward direction, expanding the thoracic cavity. The diaphragm attaches to the bottom six ribs on either side of the rib cage. At rest the muscle is shaped like an inverted bowl. Upon contraction the muscle flattens out, thus increasing the vertical dimension of the thoracic cavity. Contraction of the diaphragm and external intercostals increases the volume of the thoracic cavity and lungs. Because air pressure and air volume have an inverse relationship, the increased volume results

FIGURE 1.4 The Diaphragm

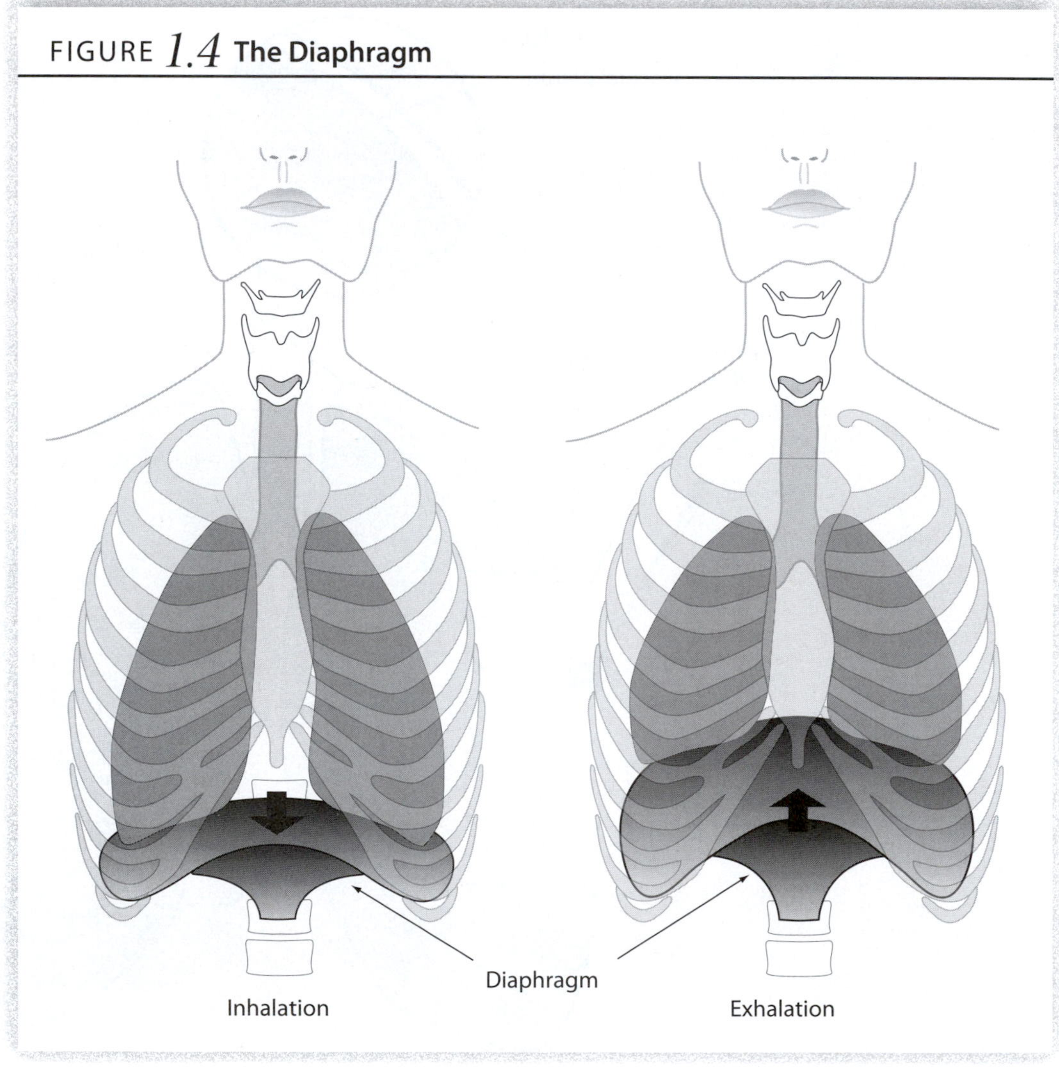

FIGURE 1.5 **Accessory Muscles of Respiration**

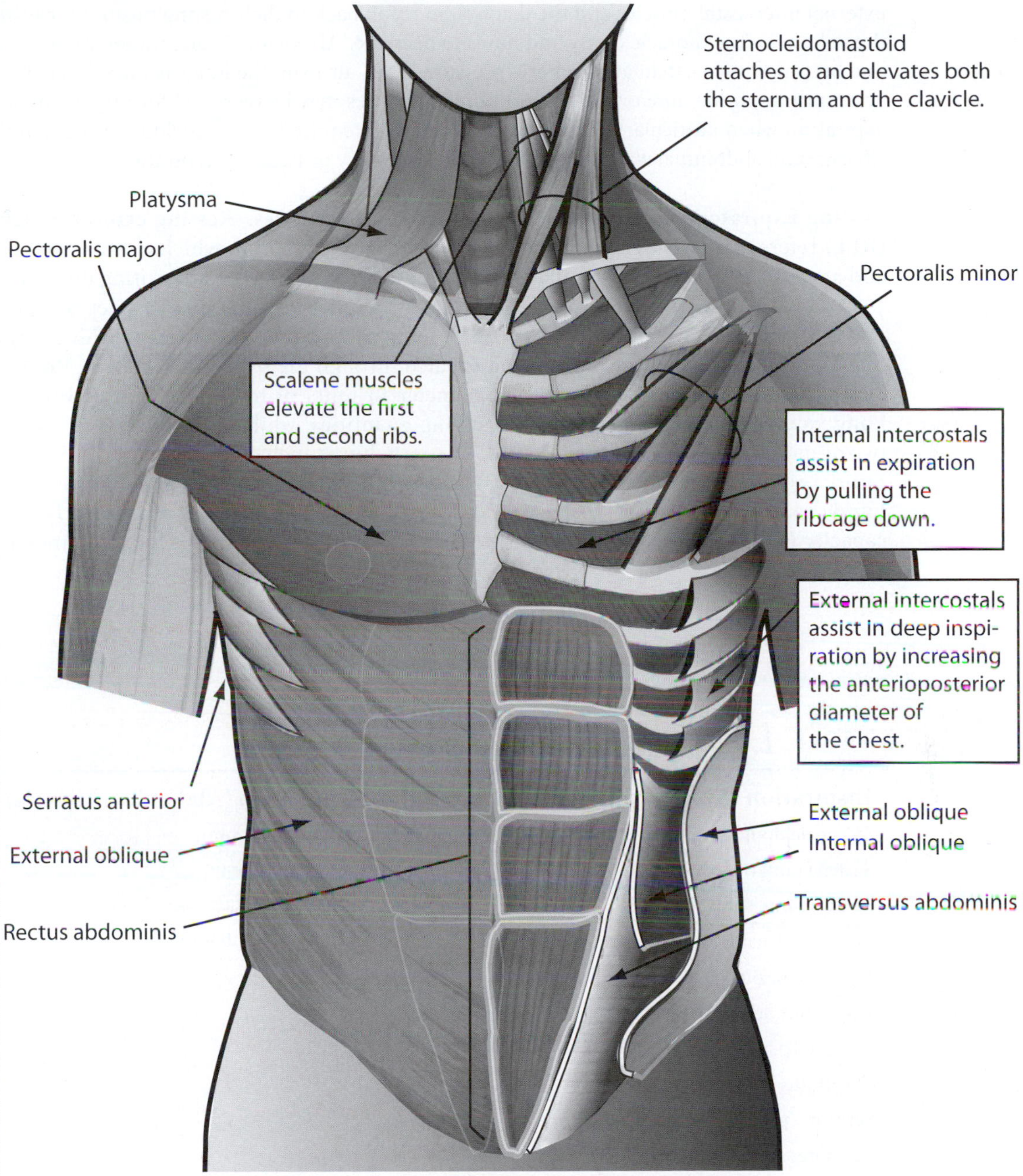

Sternocleidomastoid attaches to and elevates both the sternum and the clavicle.

Platysma

Pectoralis major

Pectoralis minor

Scalene muscles elevate the first and second ribs.

Internal intercostals assist in expiration by pulling the ribcage down.

External intercostals assist in deep inspiration by increasing the anterioposterior diameter of the chest.

Serratus anterior

External oblique

Rectus abdominis

External oblique

Internal oblique

Transversus abdominis

in a drop of pressure within the lungs (alveolar pressure). Air always flows from an area of higher pressure to an area of lower pressure. Consequently, air from the atmosphere is forced to flow into the respiratory system via the nose or mouth. The oxygen-rich air travels through the tracheobronchial tree to the alveoli, where gas exchange takes place. For exhalation the external intercostal muscles and the diaphragm recoil back to their resting positions, causing the volume of the thoracic cavity and lungs to decrease. Alveolar pressure therefore increases and becomes higher than atmospheric pressure. Thus air from the lungs is forced to exit the system through the nose or mouth. Additional muscles may be recruited for inspiration and expiration when particularly large volumes of air are required. These include muscles of the rib cage and abdominal wall. Table 1.1 lists the accessory muscles of respiration.

Resting Expiratory Level and Lung Volumes and Capacities. **Resting expiratory level (REL)** refers to a state of equilibrium in the respiratory system in which alveolar pressure and atmospheric pressure are equalized, and air is neither entering nor exiting the system. This occurs at the end of every inspiration and expiration. The endpoint of a quiet expiration is also called the **end-expiratory level (EEL).** Lung volumes and capacities provide a way of categorizing volumes of air inhaled and exhaled through the respiratory system. Volumes and capacities are measured with a spirometer in units of milliliters (ml) or liters (l). Lung volumes include single, nonoverlapping quantities, while lung capacities comprise two or more volumes (Wanger et al., 2005). Lung volumes include tidal volume (TV), inspiratory reserve volume (IRV), expiratory reserve volume (ERV), and residual volume (RV). Lung capacities include vital capacity (VC), inspiratory capacity (IC), functional residual capacity (FRC), and total lung capacity (TLC). Table 1.2 identifies the lung volumes and capacities.

TABLE 1.1 **Accessory Muscles of Respiration**

Inspiration (Muscles of the Rib-cage Wall)	Expiration (Abdominal Muscles)
Sternocleidomastoid	Rectus abdominis
Scalene (anterior, medial, posterior)	External oblique
Serratus anterior	Internal oblique
Pectoralis (major and minor)	Transverses abdominis
Upper trapezius	
Latissimus dorsi	
Iliocostalis lumborum	
Quadratus lumborum	
Serratus (posterior, superior, inferior)	
Levatores costarum	
Transverses thoracis	
Subclavius	

TABLE 1.2 **Lung Volumes and Capacities**

Lung Volumes	
Tidal volume (TV)	Volume of air inhaled and exhaled during a cycle of respiration; approximately 500 ml depending on age, gender, and level of physical exertion
Inspiratory reserve volume (IRV)	Volume of air that can be inhaled above TV
Expiratory reserve volume (ERV)	Volume of air that can be exhaled below TV
Residual volume (RV)	Volume of air remaining in the lungs after a maximum exhalation and that cannot be voluntarily expired
Lung Capacities	
Vital capacity (VC)	Volume of air that can be exhaled following a maximum inhalation (TV + IRV + ERV); approximately 5,000 ml depending on age and gender
Inspiratory capacity (IC)	Volume of air that can be inhaled from end-expiratory level (TV + IRV)
Functional residual capacity (FRC)	Volume of air remaining in the lungs and airways at the end-expiratory level (ERV + RV)
Total lung capacity (TLC)	Total amount of air that can be held in the lungs (TV + IRV + ERV + RV)

Source: Information from Wanger et al. (2005).

Volumes and capacities are often described in terms of the percentage of **vital capacity (VC)** expended. VC is the maximum amount of air one is able to voluntarily breathe in and out. REL occurs at around 35–40% of VC. At that point we can inhale 60–65% more air to fill the lungs to their maximum capacity and can continue to exhale below REL to 0% VC.

Life Breathing Versus Speech Breathing. While the same basic patterns of inspiration and expiration are involved in breathing for life (also called quiet or vegetative breathing) and breathing for speech, there are several crucial differences. In addition to fulfilling basic **ventilation** needs, breathing for speech requires integration of linguistic factors into the physiologic function. These include an adequate breath supply for the planned utterance, prosodic variations, changes in rate of speech and loudness levels, and inhaling at linguistically and conversationally appropriate junctures. Five major changes occur when switching from life to speech breathing, including location of air intake, ratio of time for inhalation versus exhalation, volume of air inspired, muscle activity for exhalation, and abdominal displacement (Table 1.3).

When a person is breathing for life, air is inhaled and exhaled via the nasal passageway, which effectively warms, moistens, and filters the air. Breathing for speech occurs via the oral passageway, allowing for a quicker inhalation and production of oral sounds on the exhalation.

TABLE 1.3 **Life Versus Speech Breathing**

	Life	Speech
1. Location of air intake	Nose	Mouth
2. Ratio of time for inhalation versus exhalation	Inhale: 40% Exhale: 60%	Inhale: 10% Exhale: 90%
3. Volume of air	500 ml 10% VC	Variable, depending on length and loudness of utterance; 20–25% VC
4. Muscle activity for exhalation	Passive; external intercostals and diaphragm relax	Active; thoracic and abdominal muscles contract to control recoil of rib cage and diaphragm
5. Abdominal position	Displaced outward relative to rib cage	Displaced inward relative to rib cage

The ratio of time for inhalation and exhalation in each respiratory cycle changes from nearly equal in life breathing (40% inhalation, 60% exhalation) to a considerably shorter and quicker inhalation and prolonged exhalation for speech (10% inhalation, 90% exhalation). This allows for a sufficient number of syllables per exhalation with quick replenishment of air that facilitates the uninterrupted flow of connected speech. The volume of air inhaled and exhaled also differs. During quiet breathing approximately 500 ml is inspired, depending on the age and gender of the individual. This amount is 10% of VC, which is approximately 5,000 ml. Inhalation for life breathing begins at REL (35–40% of VC) and goes up to a lung volume that is 50% of VC. The individual then exhales back down to REL. The volume inhaled for speech is variable, depending on the length and loudness of the upcoming utterance. Volumes for normal conversation typically occur in the mid-range of VC (35–60%) and are around twice as much as those involved in life breathing. At 60% of VC the corresponding alveolar pressure is approximately 10 cm H_2O, which is sufficient for most normal conversational utterances. This mid-volume range of VC is highly efficient because it requires very little respiratory muscle activity (Huber, 2008). For longer and louder utterances speakers inhale to higher lung volumes and continue the exhalation into lower volumes (Huber, 2008).

Switching from life to speech breathing changes the muscle activity required for exhalation. For both life and speech breathing, inhalation is an active process that requires muscular contraction to increase the volume of the thoracic cavity and lungs. Exhalation for life breathing occurs passively, as the respiratory tissues recoil back to their rest positions due to gravity, muscle relaxation, and elasticity of the lung tissue. For speech purposes the rate of recoil must be controlled in order to prolong the exhalation. For pressures above REL the muscles of inspiration continue to contract in order to provide a counteracting checking force that prevents the thoracic cavity and lungs from deflating too quickly. To access the expiratory reserve volume and continue speaking below REL, the abdominal muscles are recruited. Contraction of the abdominal muscles forces the abdominal wall to press inward on the abdominal contents (stomach, intestines, etc.). This, in turn, pushes the contents headward against the diaphragm, further decreasing the volume of the thorax and lungs so air continues to be exhaled. The internal intercostal muscles may also contract to depress the rib cage. Speaking at lung volumes below REL thus requires considerable muscular effort in order to continue decreasing the lung volume for exhalation and to prevent the rib cage from recoiling outward in an inspiratory direction. Finally, the shape of the chest wall differs for life and speech breathing. Recall that the chest wall includes the rib cage, diaphragm, abdominal wall, and abdominal contents. For speech breathing it has been reported that the abdomen is displaced further inward relative to the rib cage (Bailey & Hoit, 2002; Kalliakosta, Mandros, & Tzelepis, 2007). This positioning lifts the diaphragm (because of the upward pressure on the abdominal contents) and expands the lower rib cage. The muscle fibers of the diaphragm are thereby placed in an optimal position for generating quick strong contractions (Kalliakosta et al., 2007; Solomon & Charron, 1998). In addition, keeping the abdomen inward relative to the rib cage provides a platform against which the rib cage can move to control the varying lung volumes and air pressures necessary in connected speech (Bailey & Hoit, 2002). Movement of the rib cage is more efficient in changing lung volumes than movement of the abdomen because of the greater surface area of the lung (about three-quarters) that is adjacent to the rib cage (Connaghan, Moore, & Higashakawa, 2004; Kalliakosta et al., 2007). Therefore the rib-cage wall needs to move only one quarter of the distance that the abdominal wall does to achieve the same change in alveolar pressure (Kalliakosta et al., 2007).

NERVOUS SYSTEM CONTROL OF RESPIRATION

Respiration is controlled primarily by the medulla in the brainstem. The rate and depth of breathing is dependent on the levels of oxygen (O_2) and carbon dioxide (CO_2) in the bloodstream. O_2 and CO_2 receptors are located peripherally and in the central nervous system (CNS) (Zhang & Davenport, 2005). When O_2 levels decrease or when CO_2 levels increase, the receptors signal the CNS to increase respiratory drive with resulting increased inflow of O_2 (Zhang & Davenport, 2005). According to Zhang & Davenport (2005), other respiratory receptors that are involved in generating the respiratory rhythm produced in the brainstem (respiratory motor output) include **pulmonary stretch receptors (PSRs)** and **rapidly adapting receptors (RARs)** in the smooth muscles of the tracheobronchial tree. The PSRs sense the airway smooth muscle tone and project to the medullary respiratory neural network via the vagus nerve. The PSRs signal the transition from inspiration to expiration by inhibiting respiratory neuronal activity (Zhang & Davenport, 2005). RARs are sensitive to both mechanical and chemical changes and are stimulated by airway irritants.

While respiration is an autonomic process, higher brain centers can come into play, for example, in voluntary breath holding, or deliberately slowing down one's breathing rhythm. Control of breathing for vocalization and speech has been associated with the primary motor and sensory cortex, supplementary motor area, cerebellum, thalamus, and limbic system (Murphy et al., 1997; Wheeler & Sapienza, 2005). These structures are also involved in the conscious awareness of respiration, sensation of breathlessness, and subsequent enhanced breathing efforts (Wheeler & Sapienza, 2005). However, input from the medullary respiratory center can override the cognitive control. Thus, it is only possible for an individual to voluntarily hold his or her breath until CO_2 increases and O_2 decreases to a particular point, beyond which autonomic brainstem control takes over (Zhang & Davenport, 2005).

Phonatory System

FUNCTIONS OF THE LARYNX

The **larynx** is a complex structure formed by interlinked cartilages, membranes and ligaments, muscles, and soft tissues. While the larynx is the major structure involved in voice production, it also plays a crucial role in many biological functions. Because the larynx is continuous with both the trachea and the pharynx, it is involved in respiration, in swallowing, and in airway protection, as well as in phonation (Figure 1.6).

The larynx houses three pairs of folds that function as valves to open and close the airway. These include the aryepiglottic folds, false (ventricular) vocal folds, and true vocal folds. For respiration, the laryngeal valves are open, allowing air to flow freely into and out of the respiratory system. When greater amounts of air are needed, for example, during increased exertion, the glottis (space between the vocal folds) opens more widely to allow an increased flow of air through the system.

An important function of the larynx is airway protection during swallowing. For swallowing the entire larynx is raised by muscles in the neck and all three sets of folds close the larynx as the bolus of food enters the pharynx. The closure prevents food or liquid from entering the airway.

The larynx also protects the airway by means of coughing. Coughing is a reflex designed to expel any foreign objects from the airway and can be triggered by stimulation of the mucous

FIGURE 1.6 Location of the Larynx in Relation to the Pharynx and Trachea

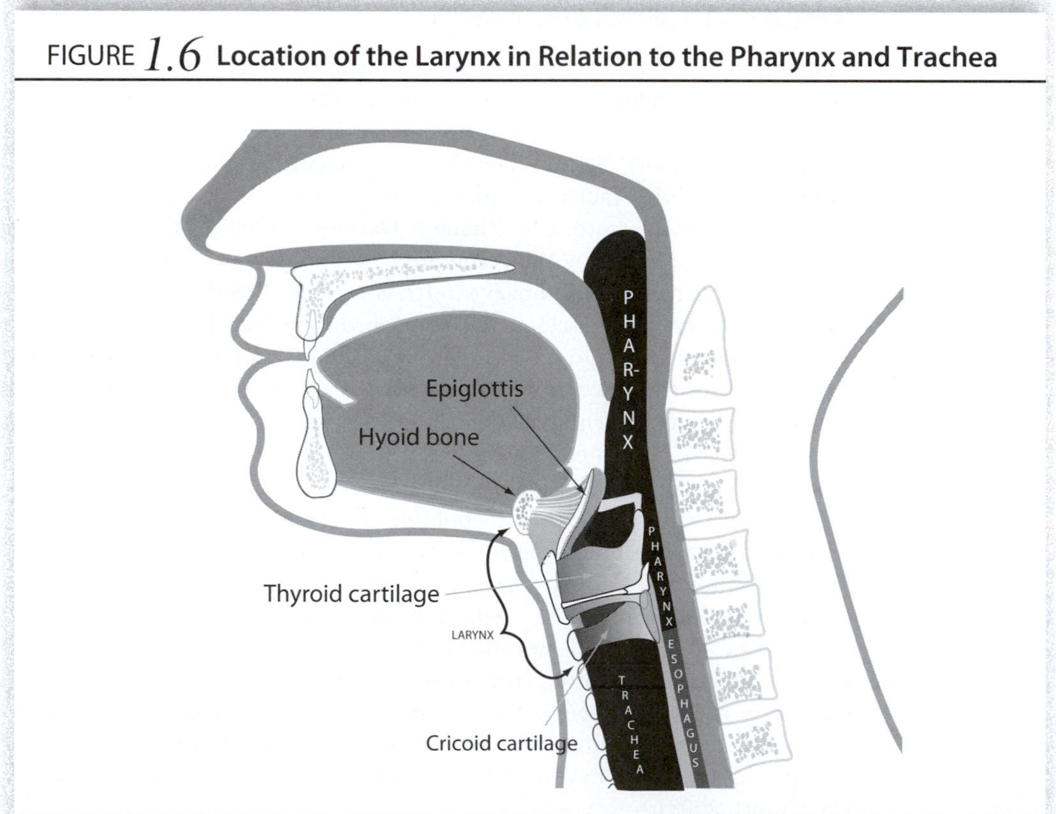

lining in the trachea, glottis, and supraglottic region (Ludlow, 2005). During a cough the vocal folds adduct with tremendous force in order to build up a strong stream of air beneath them. As the vocal folds abduct the air is released under high pressure, thereby expelling the foreign object.

Fixation of the chest is another laryngeal function. Bodily functions that require increased air pressure (e.g., excretion) are facilitated by tight closure of the glottis. This prevents air from escaping and raises the air pressure within the thoracic cavity.

The larynx is involved in emotional expression by means of reflexive vocalizations such as crying and laughing.

Finally, the larynx is involved in **phonation**, the process whereby exhaled air is converted into sound by means of vibration of the true vocal folds. The sound travels through the vocal tract where it is modified and resonated before exiting through the oral or nasal cavities. During speech the vocal folds constantly change their position and tension depending on which specific type of sound is being produced, that is, voiced or voiceless, high pitched or low pitched, louder or softer.

ANATOMY AND PHYSIOLOGY OF THE LARYNGEAL SYSTEM

A thorough understanding of the structure and function of the larynx is essential in order to determine how normal voice is produced, how breakdowns occur in voice production, and the effects of breakdowns on vocal function. This knowledge forms the foundation for planning and implementing appropriate diagnostic and therapeutic strategies for individuals with voice disorders.

The larynx is a small hollow tube-like structure situated between the 3rd–7th cervical vertebrae in the adult. It is held in place in the neck by a complex system of extrinsic muscles. It is made up of interconnecting cartilages, ligaments, membranes, and intrinsic muscles, and it houses three sets of soft tissue folds.

Framework of the Larynx. The supporting framework of the larynx is composed of one bone, nine cartilages, and two joints (Table 1.4).

TABLE *1.4* **Structures of the Laryngeal Framework**

Structures
Hyoid bone
Unpaired cartilages
Thyroid
Cricoid
Epiglottis
Paired cartilages
Arytenoids
Corniculates
Cuneiforms
Joints
Cricoarytenoid
Cricothyroid

The larynx is suspended from the **hyoid bone**, which is anatomically separate from the larynx, but functionally considered to be a part of the laryngeal system (Figure 1.7). The hyoid bone also forms the attachment for the root of the tongue. The bone consists of a body anteriorly and two pairs of horns (L. *cornua*) projecting from the body: the major horns, which form the sides of the bone, and the minor horns, which are small protrusions extending superiorly. The larynx is suspended from the hyoid bone by a sheet of membrane, the **thyrohyoid membrane**.

In addition to the hyoid bone, three unpaired and three paired sets of cartilages make up the supportive framework of the larynx (Figures 1.8 and 1.9). These cartilages are attached to each other by means of ligaments and membranes that allow them to change their relationships to each other. The three unpaired cartilages include the thyroid, cricoid, and epiglottis. The **thyroid** is the largest cartilage in the larynx. It is formed by two sheets (laminae) of hyaline cartilage, which are fused in the front and open in the back. The cartilage protrudes at an angle at the fusion, forming the "Adam's apple." This protrusion is typically more noticeable in men than in women, because the angle is more acute in men (90 degrees versus 120 degrees in women). Directly above the prominence is the V-shaped thyroid notch. Two sets of horns project from the posterolateral aspect of the thyroid cartilage. The superior horns project upward and connect the thyroid cartilage to the hyoid bone by means of the thyrohyoid ligament. This ligament is formed by the thickening of the lateral portions of the thyrohyoid membrane that connects the thyroid cartilage to the hyoid bone. The inferior horns project downward and form a joint with the cricoid cartilage. A slight ridge along the side of the thyroid lamina, called the oblique line, is where two of the extrinsic laryngeal muscles have their points of

FIGURE 1.7 **Hyoid Bone, Thyroid, and Cricoid Cartilages**

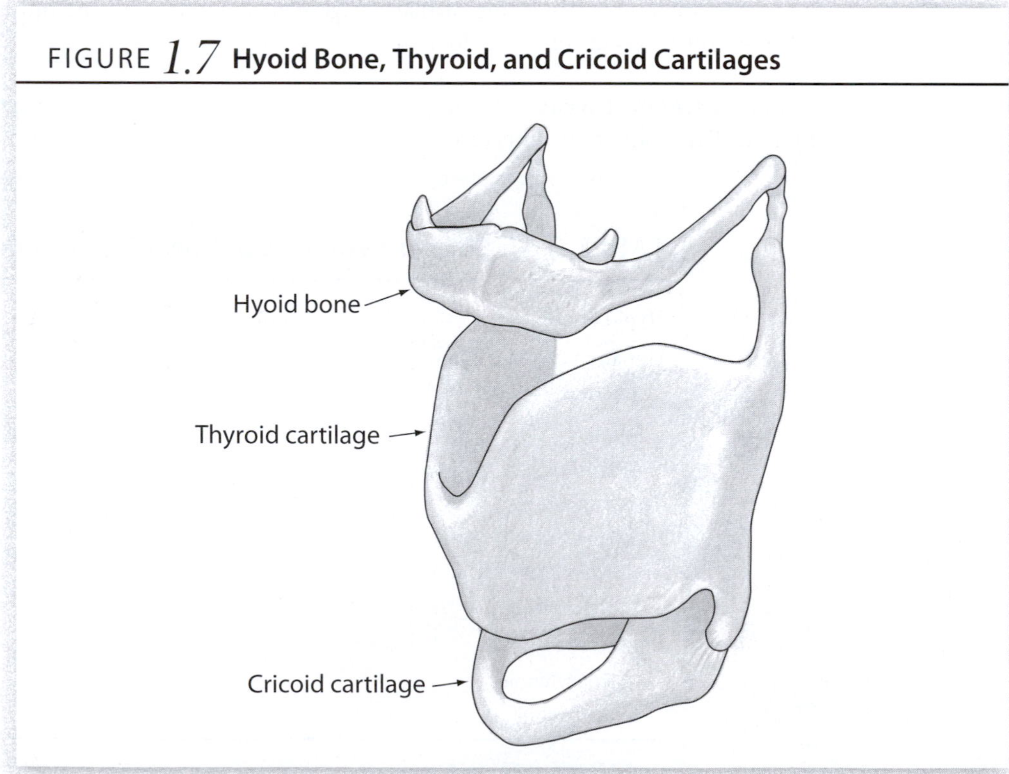

FIGURE 1.8 **Cartilages of the Larynx**

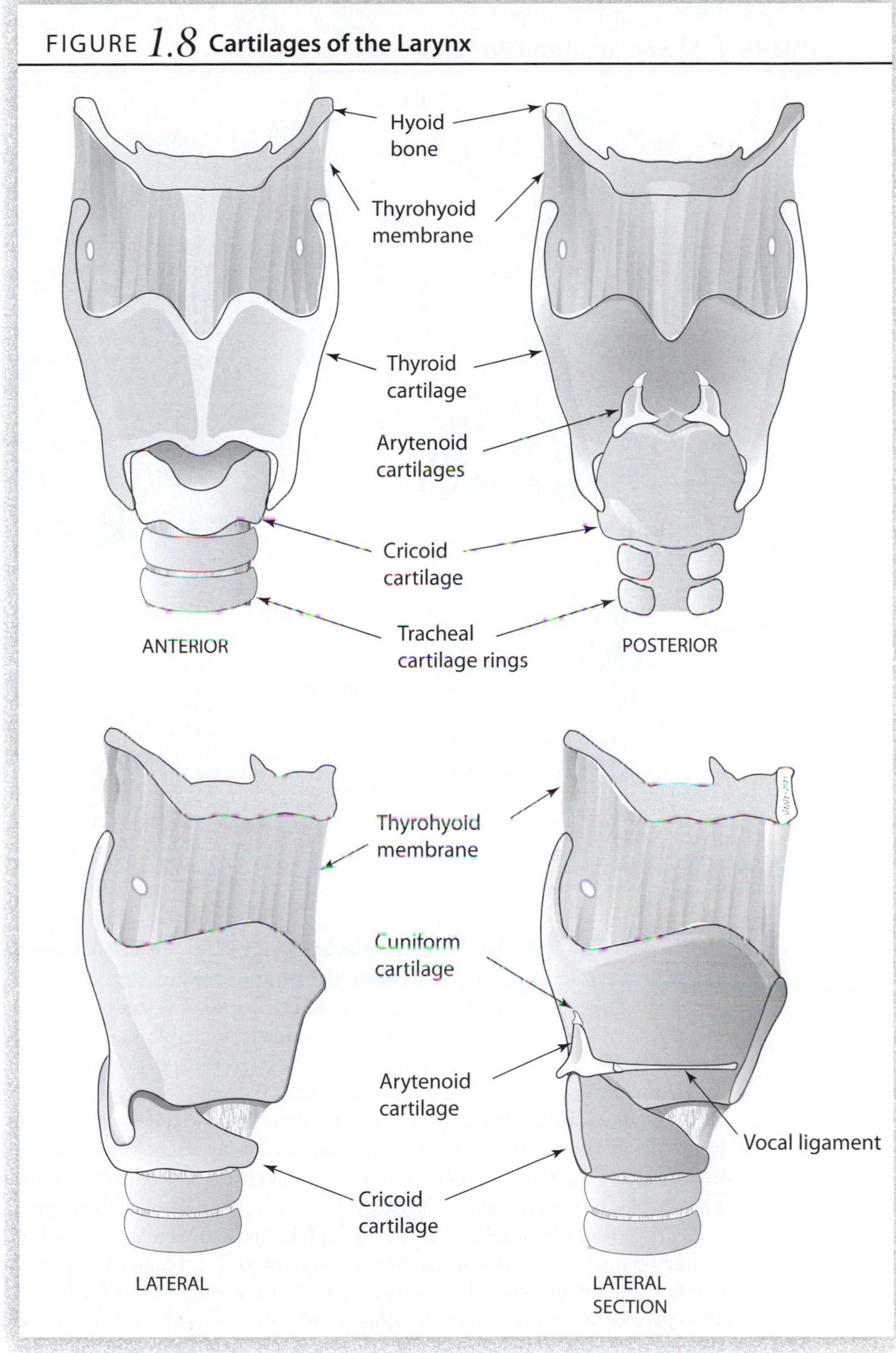

FIGURE *1.9* **Sectional and Posterior Views of the Larynx**

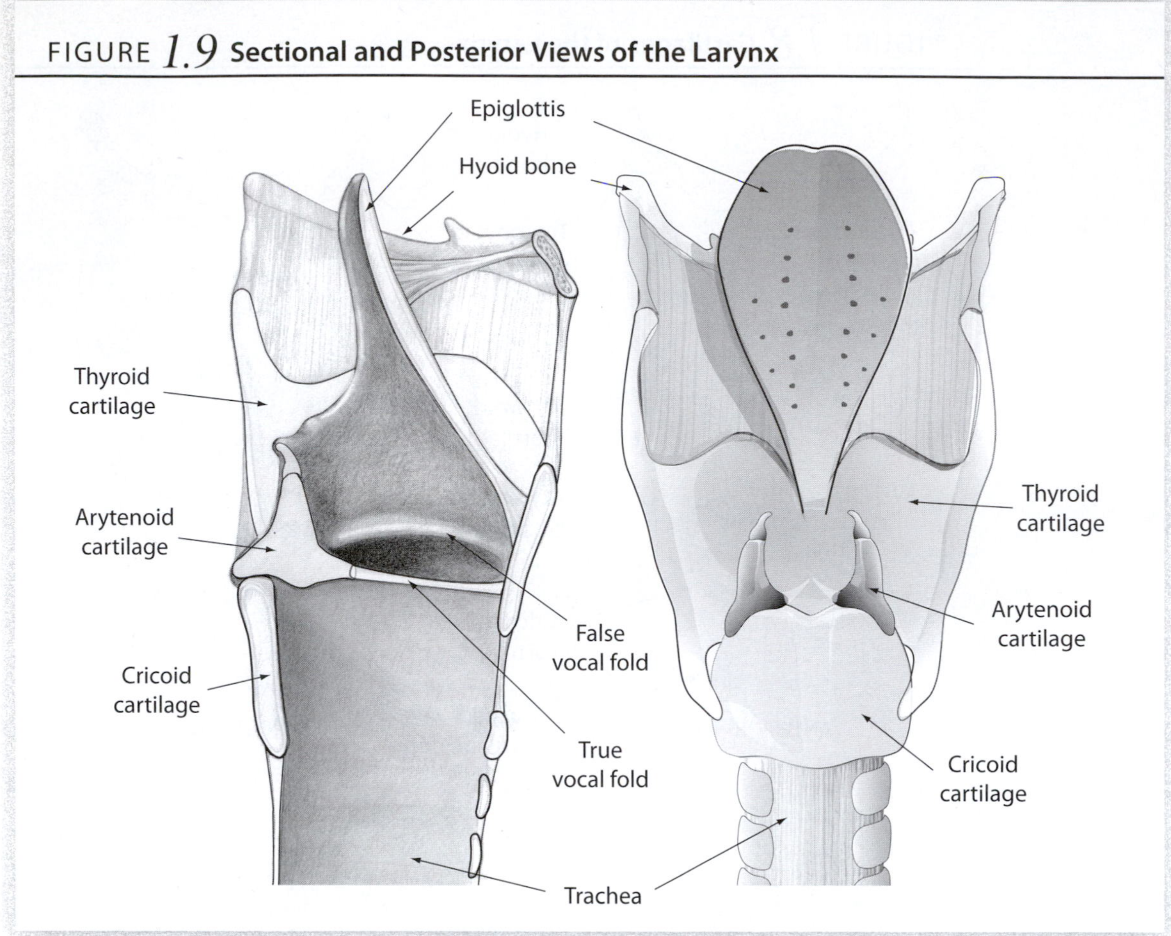

attachment. The true vocal folds are attached to the inner surface of the thyroid immediately below the thyroid notch at a point called the anterior commissure.

The **cricoid**, also composed of hyaline cartilage, is situated inferior to the thyroid. Unlike the thyroid this is a complete ring of cartilage, which is narrow in the front (the arch) and much broader and wider in the back. The posterior portion of the cricoid is called the **quadrate lamina** because of its squarish shape. The arch is only a few millimeters in height, while the quadrate lamina is approximately 30 mm high (Sataloff, 2005). The cricoid is located immediately superior to the trachea and connects to the trachea by means of the **cricotracheal membrane**. The **cricothyroid membrane** attaches the cricoid cartilage to the thyroid cartilage. The interior of the cricoid cartilage forms the narrowest point of the larynx.

The third unpaired cartilage is the **epiglottis**. This is a leaf-shaped, elastic cartilage attached by the thyroepiglottic ligaments to the thyroid cartilage and by the hyoepiglottic ligaments to the hyoid bone. The narrowest part of the epiglottis is the base, called the **petiole**. The space between the base of the tongue and the epiglottis forms the **vallecula**. This cartilage is more involved in swallowing than in phonation. During swallowing the epiglottis is pulled downward and backward. This movement closes the entrance to the larynx and prevents food or liquid from entering the airway.

The three paired cartilages include the arytenoids, corniculates, and cuneiforms. The **arytenoids** are located on the superior aspect of the quadrate lamina of the cricoid cartilage. They are small, cone-shaped cartilages, which are broad at their base and extend superiorly to a narrow tip or apex. The base of each arytenoid is complex in shape, with two processes projecting in different directions. The vocal process of each arytenoid projects anteriorly toward the thyroid cartilage; the muscular process projects posterolaterally. The vocal processes are composed of elastic cartilage, unlike the remaining portions of the arytenoids, which are formed of hyaline cartilage. The base of the arytenoid is concave, while the facet of the quadrate lamina is convex, forming an articulation between the cartilages. The arytenoids are extremely important for two reasons. First, the true vocal folds are attached to the vocal processes. The arytenoids are movable, so whenever they move, the vocal folds move as well. Second, the muscular processes form the point of attachment for muscles that adduct and abduct the vocal folds to open and close the glottis.

The corniculate and cuneiform cartilages are less important, and they may or may not be present in all individuals. The **corniculates** are small elastic cartilages located on the apex of each arytenoid cartilage. The **cuneiforms** are embedded within the aryepiglottic folds (described below). These may serve to give the aryepiglottic folds some degree of firmness that helps them to resist being pulled inward by negative pressure during inhalation.

Joints of the Larynx. There are two pairs of laryngeal joints, the cricoarytenoid joints and the cricothyroid joints, both of which play crucial roles in voice production (Figures 1.10 and 1.11).

The **cricoarytenoid joint** forms the connection between the concave base of each arytenoid cartilage and the convex superior surface of the quadrate lamina of the cricoid. This is a synovial diarthrodial joint, meaning that it has a relatively wide range of motion. It is lined with a synovial membrane that secretes synovial fluid. The joint allows the arytenoid cartilage to move in a back and forth rocking motion, as well as a medial/lateral gliding motion (Berry, Montequin, Chan, Titze, & Hoffman, 2003). These movements result in simultaneous bidirectional motion of the arytenoids (Letson & Tatchell, 2005). Thus, when the appropriate muscles contract, the arytenoid cartilages undergo a rotational movement. Depending on which muscle is contracted, the vocal processes either approximate medially and in a downward closing motion (toward one another), or laterally and in an upward opening motion (away from one another). Because the vocal folds are attached to the vocal processes, they follow the movement and are either brought toward or away from the midline. Thus it is the cricoarytenoid joints that control vocal fold adduction and abduction. Keep in mind, however, that it is not the joints themselves that cause the arytenoid cartilages to move. The joints merely permit the cartilages to be moved when the appropriate muscles are contracted.

The **cricothyroid joints** are located where the inferior horns of the thyroid cartilage connect to the articular facet at each side of the cricoid cartilage (Figure 1.12).

These are also synovial joints, allowing the thyroid cartilage to tilt superiorly and inferiorly and the cricoid cartilage to be tilted upward and backward. There is some question as to whether this joint permits the thyroid cartilage to glide anteriorly and posteriorly in addition to the tilting motion. Some researchers have argued for the existence of this type of movement (e.g., Maue & Dickson, 1971). Others have rejected the notion based on the orientation of the cricoid articular facets and the ligaments that limit movement of the cricothyroid joint (Hong, Kim, & Kim, 2001). Recently Hammer and colleagues (2010) concluded from their study on human cadavers that the joint allows horizontal and vertical gliding movements as well as rotation, but not in all individuals.

FIGURE 1.10 **Articular Facets of the Cricoid Cartilage**

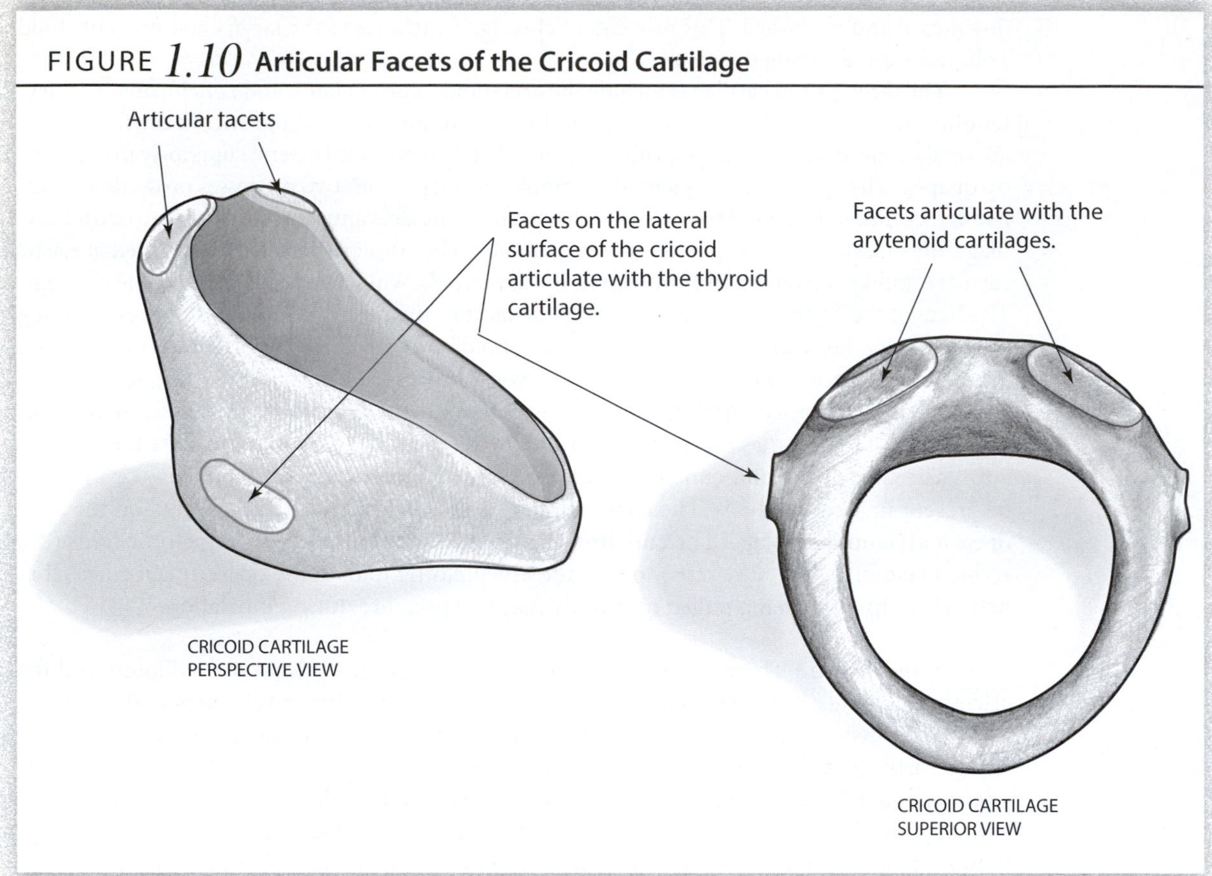

The effect of either the tilting downward of the thyroid cartilage toward the cricoid cartilage or the cricoid cartilage upward toward the thyroid cartilage is to increase the distance between the anterior commissure of the thyroid cartilage and the arytenoid cartilages (Figure 1.13).

As the vocal folds are attached at these two points, increasing the distance between them stretches and tenses the vocal folds. In turn, this increases their frequency (rate of vibration), resulting in a higher pitch. Decreasing the distance between the anterior commissure and the vocal processes shortens the vocal folds, decreasing frequency and pitch. The cricothyroid joints thus are involved in vocal pitch control. As with the cricoarytenoid joints, the joints themselves do not cause the movement of the cartilages, but they are the agents that allow movement to occur with muscle contraction.

Soft Tissues of the Larynx. The soft tissues of the larynx include extrinsic and intrinsic membranes, three sets of folds, and extrinsic and intrinsic muscles (Table 1.5).

Membranes. The extrinsic membranes link laryngeal structures to each other and to other structures on their external surfaces (Figure 1.14). They include the thyrohyoid membrane, cricotracheal membrane, and cricothyroid membrane.

FIGURE 1.11 Cricoarytenoid Joint

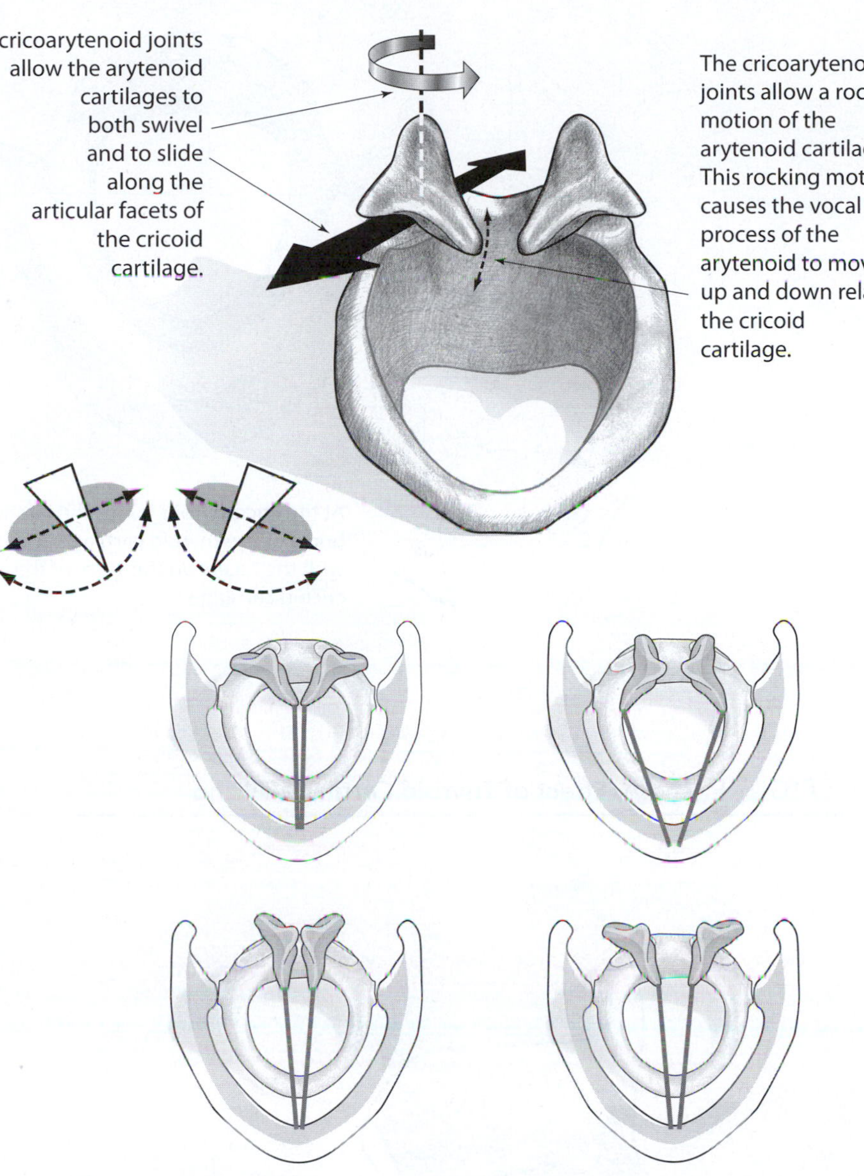

The thyrohyoid membrane connects the thyroid cartilage to the hyoid bone. This membrane is thickened in the central portion, called the **medial thyrohyoid ligament**. The lateral margins of the membrane are also thickened and form the **lateral thyrohyoid ligaments**. Small hyaline cartilages, the **triticeal cartilages**, may be found within the lateral thyrohyoid ligaments. The thyrohyoid membrane is pierced by blood vessels and nerves entering

FIGURE 1.12 **Cricothyroid Joint**

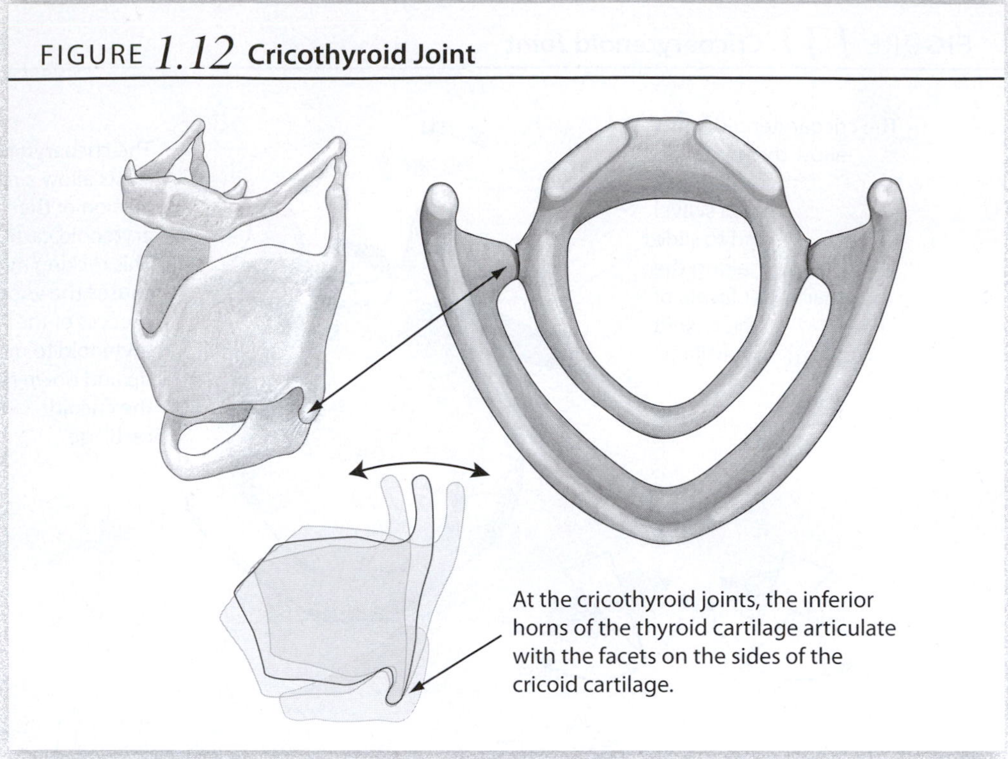

FIGURE 1.13 **Effect of Thyroid Cartilage Tilting**

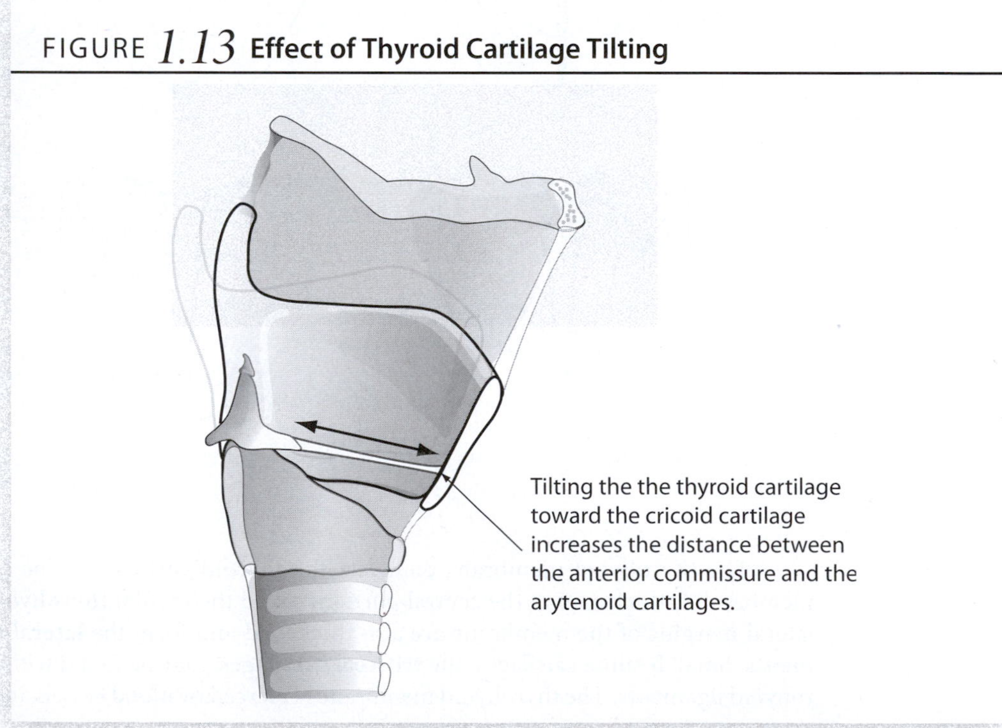

TABLE 1.5 Membranes and Folds of the Larynx

Membranes	
Extrinsic	**Intrinsic**
Thyrohyoid	Elastic membrane
Cricothyroid	Conus elasticus
Cricotracheal	Quadrangular membrane

Folds		
Aryepiglottic	**Ventricular (False)**	**True**
		Epithelium
		Lamina propria
		Thyroarytenoid muscle

the larynx. The cricotracheal membrane connects the cricoid cartilage to the first tracheal ring, and the cricothyroid membrane connects the external, anterior surfaces of the thyroid and cricoid cartilages.

The intrinsic membranes are located within the lumen of the larynx. An extensive membrane called the **elastic membrane** connects the entire inner framework. The inferior portion of this membrane is known as the **conus elasticus**, composed of the paired triangular membranes. The **triangular membranes** attach anteriorly to the thyroid and cricoid cartilages, inferiorly to the cricoid, and posteriorly to the vocal processes of the arytenoids (Sataloff, 2005). The superior margins of each of these membranes form the vocal ligament of the true vocal folds. The superior portion of the elastic membrane is called the **quadrangular membrane**, formed superiorly by the aryepiglottic folds and extending downward to become part of the false vocal folds.

Folds Within the Larynx. The larynx is a valve whose function is to open and close for vocalization, phonation, respiration, coughing, and swallowing. The valving is achieved by three different sets of tissue folds within the larynx. The three pairs of folds are located from superior to inferior and include the aryepiglottic folds, the false or ventricular folds, and the true vocal folds (Figure 1.15).

The **aryepiglottic folds** are bundles of connective tissue and muscle that run from the superior and lateral margins of the epiglottis to the apex of each arytenoid, forming a roughly oval-shaped sphincter. The elastic cuneiform cartilages are located within these tissues, providing a degree of firmness that enables the aryepiglottic folds to resist the negative pressures of inhalation. The aryepiglottic folds remain open during phonation and respiration, but close for swallowing. The muscle within these folds, the **aryepiglottic muscle**, is formed by fibers of the interarytenoid muscle (described later), which continue around the apex of the arytenoid and insert into the lateral border of the epiglottis. When the muscle contracts the epiglottis is pulled backward, thus covering the entrance to the larynx during swallowing.

FIGURE 1.14 **Extrinsic Membranes**

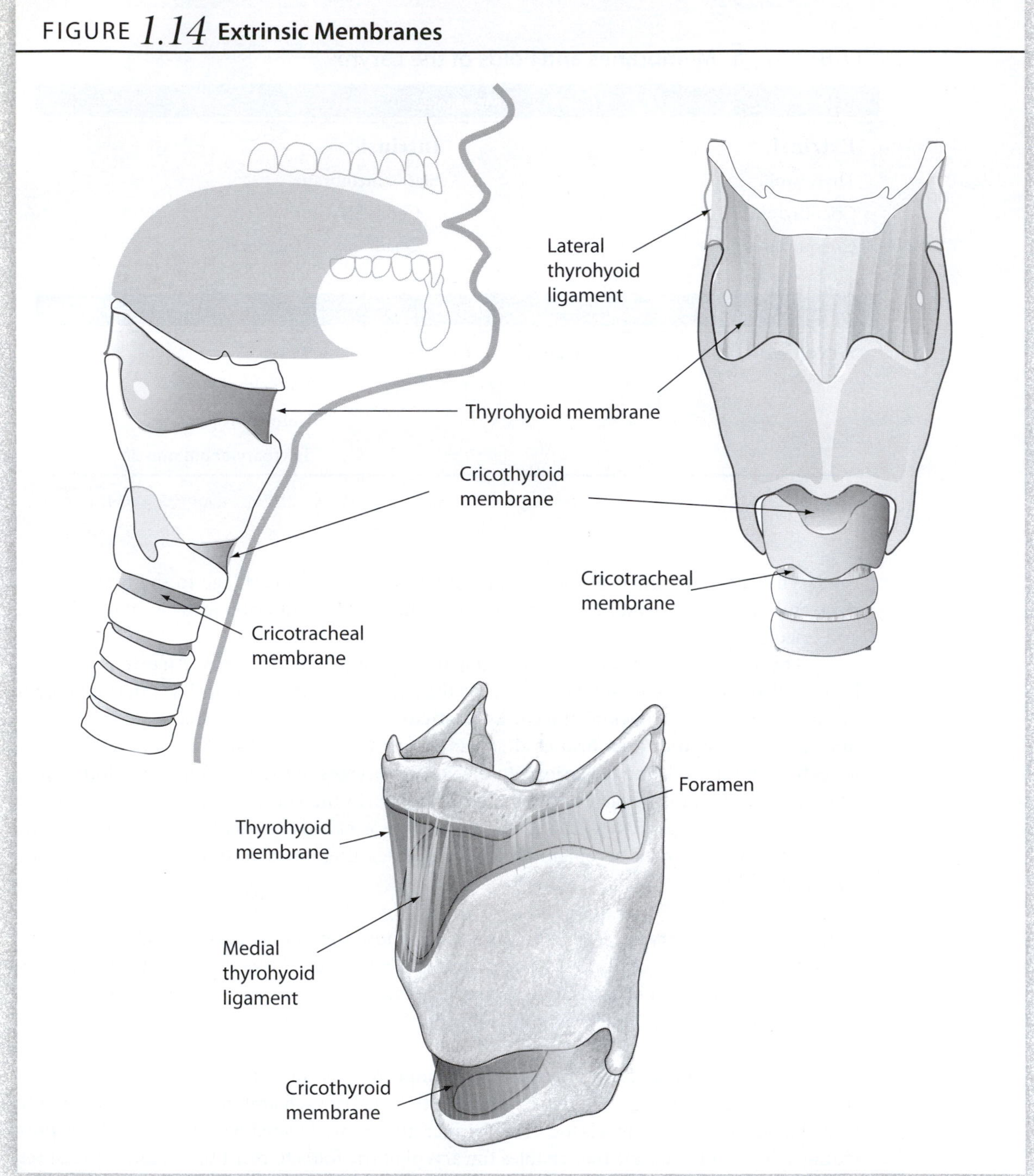

FIGURE 1.15 **Superior View of the Folds of the Larynx**

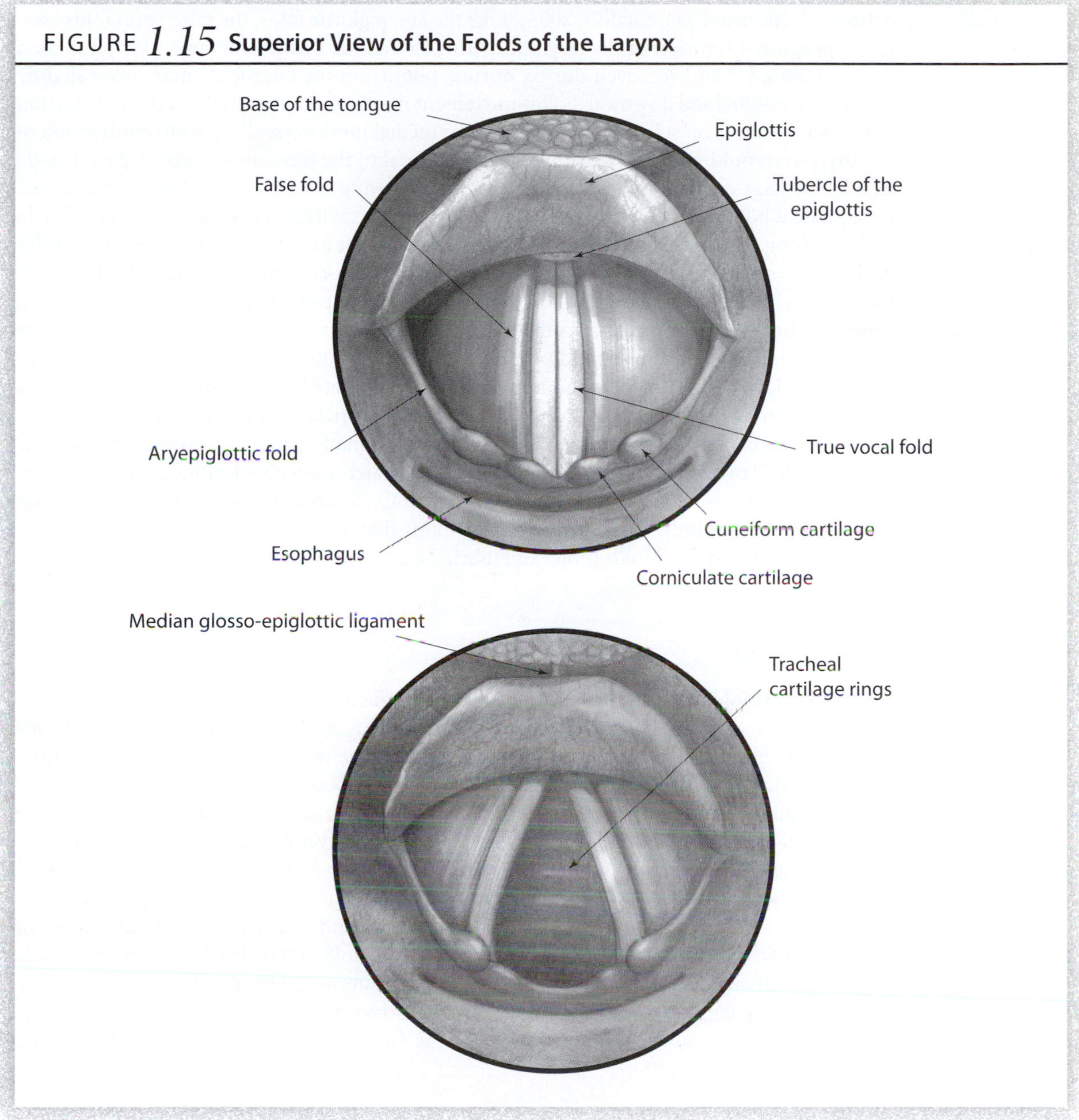

The **false** or **ventricular vocal folds** are located inferior to the aryepiglottic folds and superior to the true folds, and run parallel to the true folds. They do not extend toward the midline of the laryngeal lumen as far as do the true vocal folds. The false vocal folds are composed primarily of connective tissue and some muscle tissue (ventricularis muscle) and form the inferior borders of the quadrangular membrane. They contain numerous mucous glands and goblet cells that help to lubricate the true vocal folds beneath them (Agarwal,

Scherer, & Hollien, 2003; Sataloff, 2005). Like the aryepiglottic folds, the false vocal folds keep the **supraglottis** (portion of the larynx superior to the true vocal folds) open for phonation and respiration. However, even during normal phonation the false folds may move slightly toward the midline and downward. This movement may be due either to the active contraction of the ventricularis muscle, or to a more passive medial motion resulting from contraction of the **thyroarytenoid muscles**, which are located lateral to the false vocal folds (Agarwal et al., 2003). The false vocal folds close the larynx for swallowing as well as for other functions that necessitate a buildup of air pressure within the thoracic cavity, such as excretion, childbirth, and coughing. Because they contain very little muscle tissue and do not project medially as far as the true vocal folds, it takes a great deal of muscular effort to move the false folds toward the midline. There are occasions when the false folds do approximate during phonation, but generally these are not normal circumstances. Because the false vocal folds are more massive than the true vocal folds, the sound produced by their vibration tends to be very low pitched and strained. Occasionally, a person may voluntarily phonate by vibrating the false folds as a compensatory strategy when the true vocal folds are dysfunctional in some way.

Separating the false and true vocal folds is a small space, the **laryngeal ventricle** (Figure 1.16). Toward the front of the space there is a narrow opening leading to the **laryngeal saccule**. The saccule is a small area bounded by mucous membrane that contains the openings of 60–70 mucous glands (Sataloff, 2005). The fluids that are secreted by these glands help to keep the larynx and vocal folds moist and lubricated, which is crucial for laryngeal health and for normal phonation.

TRUE VOCAL FOLDS

The **true vocal folds** are extremely complex in their structure. They abduct to open the glottis for respiration and for the production of voiceless sounds, and adduct to close the glottis for swallowing and for the production of voiced sounds. The true vocal folds attach anteriorly at the anterior commissure of the thyroid cartilage and posteriorly to the vocal process of each arytenoid. The attachments are formed by the anterior and posterior macula flava. The **anterior macula flava** is an extension of the intermediate layer of the lamina propria and inserts into the anterior commissure tendon, called Broyle's ligament. The anterior commissure tendon connects to the midpoint of the thyroid cartilage. The posterior macula flava similarly arises from the intermediate layer of the lamina propria and attaches to the vocal process of each arytenoid cartilage via a transitional structure (Sataloff, 2005). This arrangement allows a systematic change in stiffness at both anterior and posterior attachments of the vocal folds, from the pliable vocal fold to the less pliable macula flava, to the relatively stiff cartilage. The change in stiffness may act as a protection for the vocal folds by cushioning them from the effects of vibration.

LAYERS OF THE VOCAL FOLDS

The true vocal folds are composed of five layers, each with a different cellular makeup and different biomechanical properties. From superficial to deep, the layers are the epithelium, superficial layer of the lamina propria (SLLP), intermediate layer of the lamina propria (ILLP), deep layer of the lamina propria (DLLP), and muscle.

Epithelium. The outermost layer of the vocal fold is composed of **epithelium** (Figure 1.17). Epithelial tissue covers all free surfaces and lines the cavities within our bodies, including the

FIGURE 1.16 True and False Vocal Folds and Laryngeal Ventricle

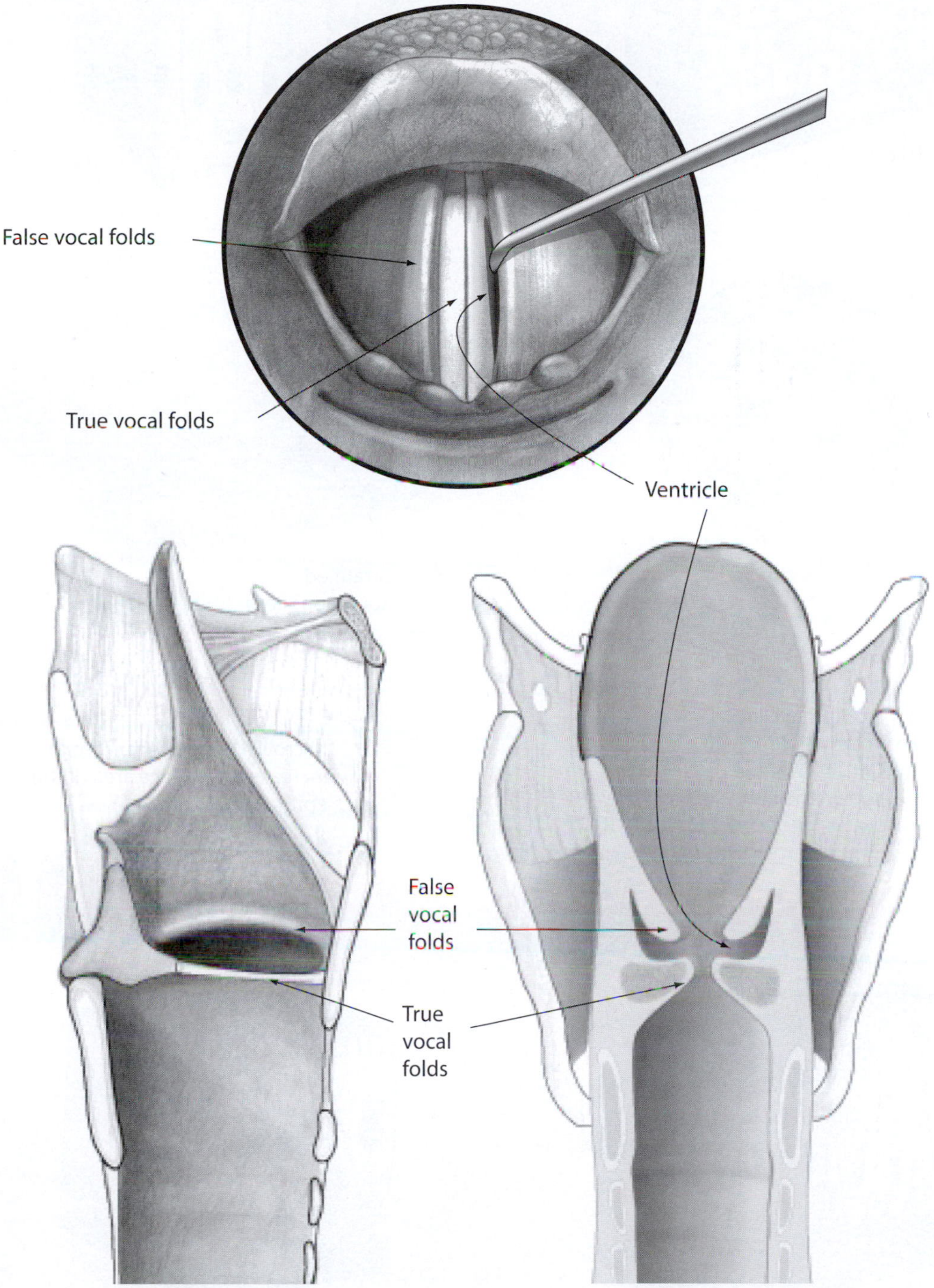

False vocal folds
True vocal folds
Ventricle
False vocal folds
True vocal folds

FIGURE 1.17 Epithelial Cells

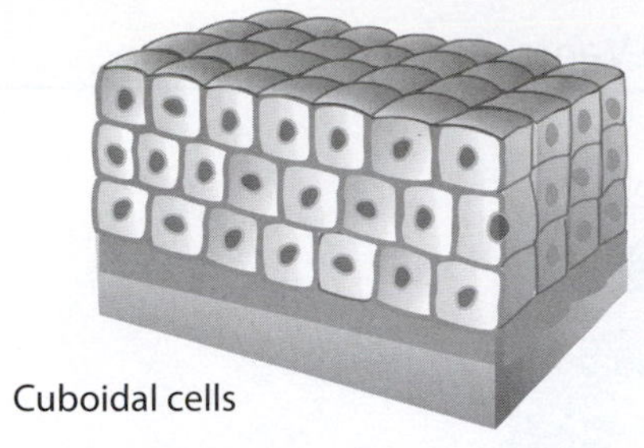

Cuboidal cells

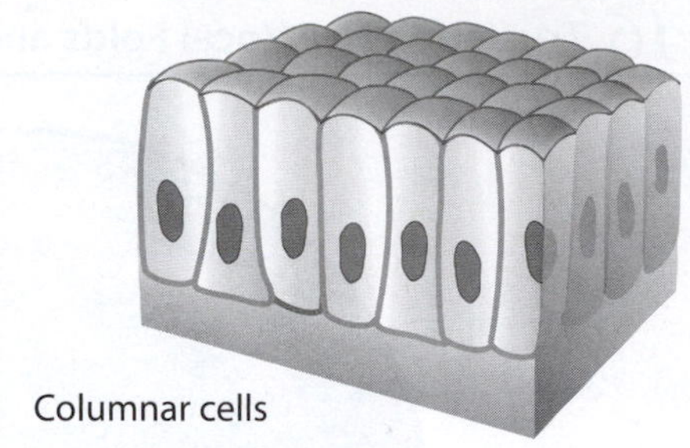

Columnar cells

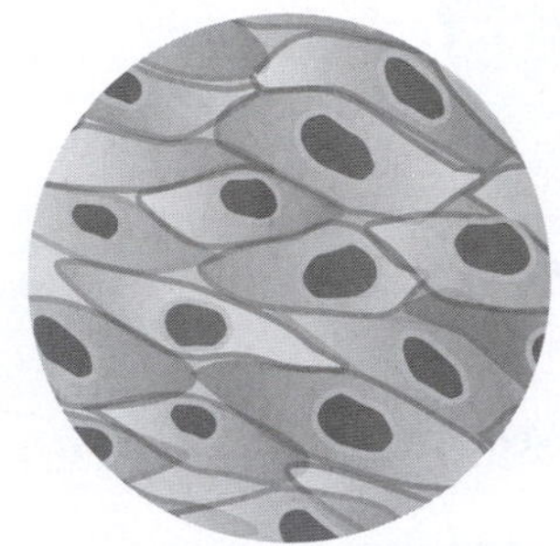

Squamous cells

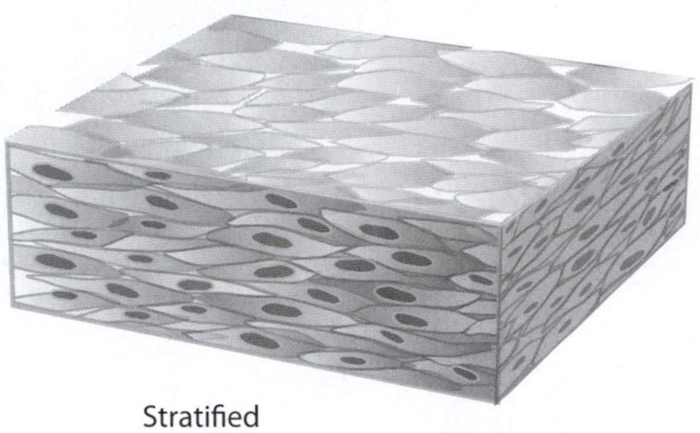

Stratified squamous cells

Cilia on the cells move in a wavelike motion and serve to move substances over the surface of the epithelium.

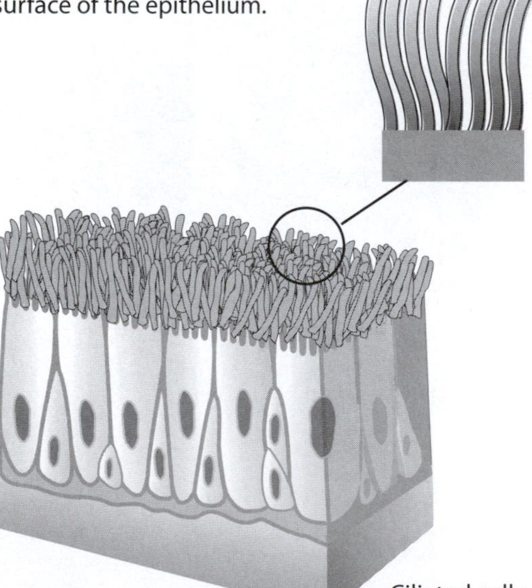

Ciliated cells

Microvilli on the cells serve to increase the surface area of the epithelium.

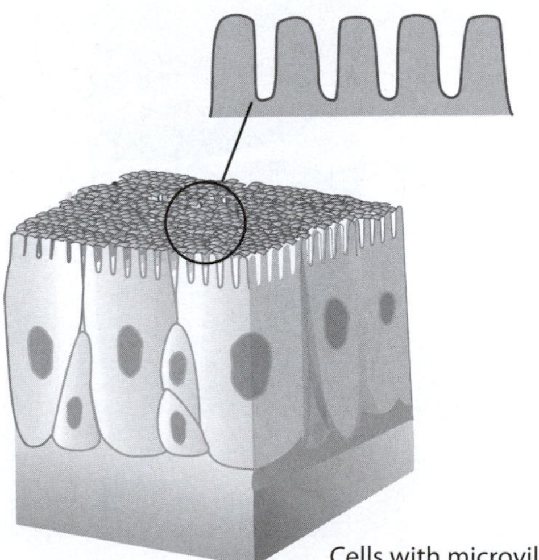

Cells with microvilli

oral and nasal cavities, pharynx, and respiratory passages. It also forms a covering for external surfaces, such as skin. There are many different types of epithelium, classified according to whether the epithelium is composed of a single layer of cells (simple epithelium) or more than one layer of cells (stratified). Pseudostratified epithelium looks stratified but contains only one layer of cells. Epithelium is also named according to the shape of the cells, which can be squarish (squamous), cube-shaped (cuboidal), or column-shaped (columnar). Epithelium can be ciliated or nonciliated. Different types of epithelium are specialized to perform different functions. For example, ciliated columnar epithelium, found within the trachea and bronchi, is involved in handling mucous secretions (Sataloff, 2005). Keratinized epithelium is found mainly in the skin and is highly waterproof due to the presence of keratin, a strengthening and waterproofing protein (Hickman, Roberts, & Larson, 2003). The epiglottis is lined with stratified columnar epithelium. The outermost surface of the true vocal folds is composed of nonkeratinizing stratified squamous cell epithelium. This type of epithelium is found mainly in wet cavities such as the oral and nasal cavities, and protects against abrasion and other forms of damage. The vocal fold epithelium thus helps to protect the vocal folds against the strong contact forces that occur during vibration. The vocal fold epithelium also plays an important role in maintaining vocal fold hydration. The tissue contains channels and microvilli. The channels allow fluid to move in and out of the vocal folds. Microvilli are tiny finger-shaped projections from the apical surface of the cells, which help to increase the surface area of the cell, thus facilitating absorption and secretion of fluids (Tillmann, Pietzsch-Rohrschneider, & Huenges, 1977).

The epithelium rests on a basement membrane, called the **basement membrane zone (BMZ).** The BMZ forms the attachment between the epithelium and the layer beneath it, the superficial lamina propria. The BMZ is made up of different types of collagen fibers in two layers, the **lamina lucida** and the **lamina densa.** These fibers anchor the layers to each other. The fibers are most numerous in the area of greatest vocal fold vibration.

Lamina Propria. Deep to the epithelium is a three-part layer of mucous membrane, the **lamina propria**, composed of different types of connective tissue.

Connective Tissue. Connective tissue consists of a small number of living cells called **fibroblasts** and a large amount of extracellular substance called matrix. The cells are embedded within the matrix. The **extracellular matrix (ECM)** is produced by the cells and gives the tissue its particular character (Figure 1.18). Matrix can be fluid (as in blood), flexible (as in cartilage), or rigid (as in bone). ECM is composed of networks of protein fibers embedded in a mixture of large **glycoproteins** (molecules that have short chains of carbohydrates attached to them) and **proteoglycans** (molecules that have more carbohydrate than protein) (Kimball, 2004). Different types of proteins with different characteristics are found in connective tissue. Two types of proteins are fibrous and interstitial (Table 1.6).

Fibrous proteins include collagen and elastin. **Collagens** are the primary proteins, which form the core of the connective tissue. Collagen is made up of fine, parallel fibrils of varying sizes that attach to each other and form bundles of fibers. Collagen possesses a great deal of **tensile strength** (force required to pull on a structure to its breaking point). **Elastin** fibers, on the other hand, are highly flexible, allowing for tissue recoil. Thus, collagen and elastin fibers provide structural support to the tissue, allow the tissue to maintain its shape and form, and give the tissue the ability to withstand stress (Ward, Thibeault, & Gray, 2002).

FIGURE 1.18 **Extracellular Matrix**

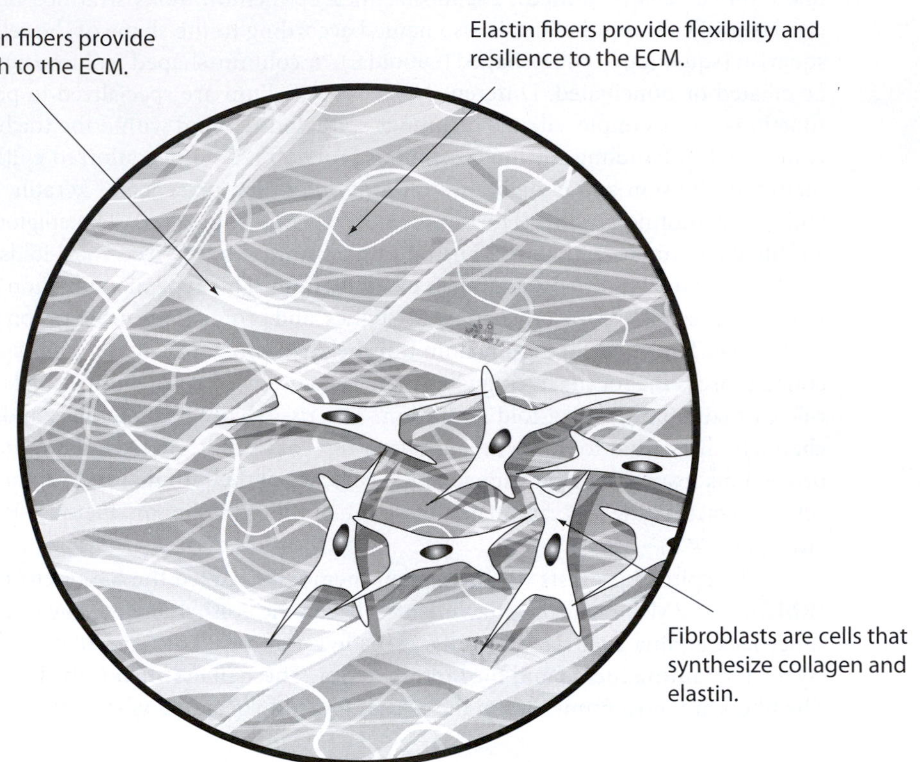

The extracellular matrix is the structure that surrounds and supports the cells of living tissue. The ECM is produced and maintained by the living cells within it. The structural proteins collagen and elastin are two of the most prominent components of the ECM.

TABLE 1.6 **Selected Components of Extracellular Matrix**

Fibrous proteins	
Collagen	Provides tensile strength to tissue
Elastin	Provides tissue flexibility and recoil
Interstitial proteins	
Hyaluronic acid	Tissue viscosity, wound healing
Fibronectin	Wound healing
Decorin	Regulates collagen thickness

Interstitial proteins provide connections between the collagen fibrils (Heinegard, Lidgren, & Saxne, 2003) and play a role in the vibratory characteristics of the vocal folds by influencing such factors as tissue viscosity, fluid content thickness, and the amount of collagen present in the tissue. Three interstitial proteins are **hyaluronic acid (HA),** or hyaluronan; fibronectin (FN); and decorin. HA is a large molecule that attracts water, resulting in the formation of a gel-like substance. Because of its fluid structure HA influences the degree of viscosity of a tissue. It also acts as a shock absorber by allowing the vocal fold tissue to resist being compressed. This helps to protect the vocal fold edges from the collision forces generated during vibration (Rousseau, Tateya, Lim, Munoz-del-Rio, & Bless, 2006; Ward et al., 2002). HA also plays a role in tissue osmosis and wound healing. Interestingly, it has been found that men have a higher concentration of HA in their vocal folds than women. This suggests that female vocal folds may be more prone to injury because of their less robust shock-absorbing and wound-healing capacity (Ward et al., 2002). Indeed, many studies have suggested that adult women do have a greater incidence of vocal nodules and other voice problems than do men. **Fibronectin (FN)** is another interstitial protein. It is particularly prevalent in tissues that have undergone some kind of trauma or injury and are in the process of healing (Hirschi, Gray, & Thibeault, 2002). A large amount of FN has been found in normal true vocal folds as well as in benign vocal fold tumors such as nodules and polyps. Hirschi et al. suggested that the presence of FN in normal vocal folds may be due to the constant low-grade trauma and resulting repair occurring from vocal fold vibration. The interstitial protein **decorin** is also found commonly in connective tissues. Decorin helps to regulate the thickness of collagen fibers by facilitating the combining of collagen fibrils to form bundles of fibers (Hedbom & Heinegard, 1993; Thibeault & Gray, 2005; Vogel, Paulsson, & Heingard, 1984).

Layers of the Lamina Propria. The lamina propria is composed of three layers: superficial, intermediate, and deep (Figure 1.19). The **superficial layer (SLLP),** also known as Reinke's space, is composed mostly of loosely organized elastin fibers. This layer is extremely compliant due to its ability to stretch and recoil, thus permitting easy movement during vocal fold vibration. In addition to the elastin fibers there is a high density of decorin in this layer (Branski, Verdolini, Sandulache, Rosen, & Hebda, 2006; Thibeault & Gray, 2005), as well as small amounts of collagen, hyaluronic acid (Hammond, Zhou, Hammond, Pawlak, & Gray, 1997), and fibronectin (Catten, Gray, Hammond, Zhou, & Hammond, 1998; Pawlak, Hammond, Hammond, & Gray, 1996). The **intermediate layer (ILLP)** contains elastin fibers, but the tissue is more densely organized than the superficial layer. The **deep layer of the lamina propria (DLLP)** contains mostly collagen. The intermediate and deep layers contain more fibrous and interstitial proteins than does the superficial layer. The amount of elastin and collagen increases from the superficial to the deep layers, but the highest density of elastin occurs in the intermediate layer (Thibeault & Gray, 2005). The ILLP also contains the highest concentration of HA.

Vocal Fold Muscle. The innermost layer of the vocal folds is composed of muscle tissue (the thyroarytenoid muscle), which is more dense and less flexible than the other layers. This muscle is described in more detail later in the chapter.

The vocal folds differ in their length among children, adult women, and adult men, and the ratio of the membranous to cartilaginous glottis also differs. The total length of the vocal folds in adult males ranges from around 17 to 21 mm while that of adult females ranges from 11 to 15 mm. Infant vocal folds are around 2.5–3 mm.

FIGURE 1.19 **Layers of the Vocal Folds**

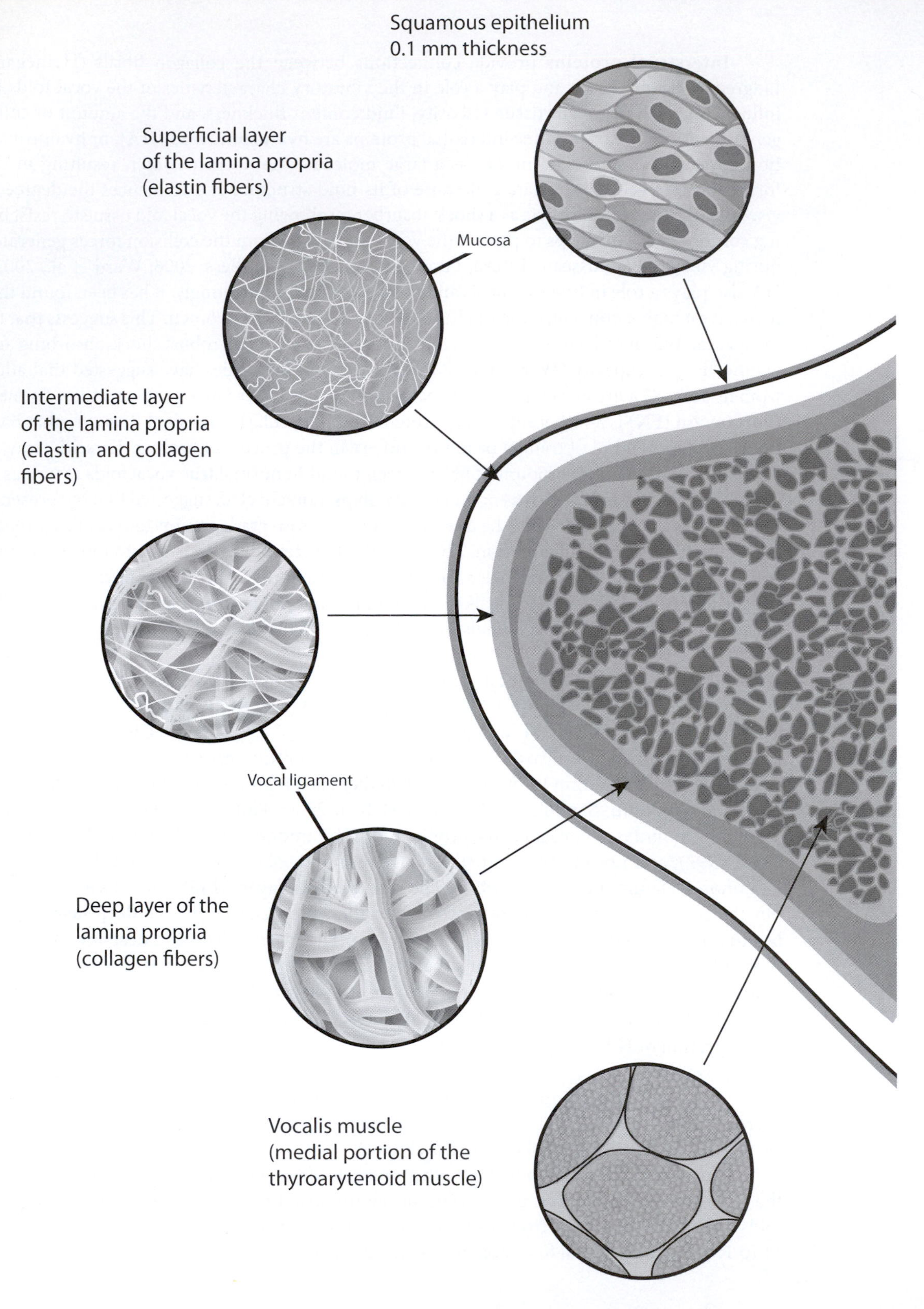

COVER-BODY MODEL OF THE VOCAL FOLDS

The **cover-body model** of the vocal folds (Figure 1.20) was first described by Hirano and his colleagues in the 1970s and 1980s (Hirano, 1974; Hirano, 1977; Hirano, Kurita, & Nakashima, 1981). The model is based on the stiffness characteristics of each layer of the vocal folds. Stiffness refers to how strongly a body resists being deformed or deflected by an applied force. The inverse of stiffness is compliance. The more compliant a body is, the less it resists being moved in some way. The cover-body model groups the five tissue layers into three distinct entities based on their biomechanical properties. The epithelium and SLLP are both compliant with similar movement characteristics and are together known as the cover. The ILLP and DLLP are stiffer than the epithelium and SLLP, and together form the transitional layer of the vocal ligament. The least compliant layer, the muscle, forms the body of the vocal folds. The differences between layers in stiffness and biomechanical characteristics result in the highly complex vibration of the vocal folds during phonation.

GLOTTIS

The true vocal folds run in an anteroposterior direction on either side of the lumen of the larynx. The space between the vocal folds is called the **glottis**, which is divided into the membranous and cartilaginous portions. The membranous portion comprises the anterior three-fifths

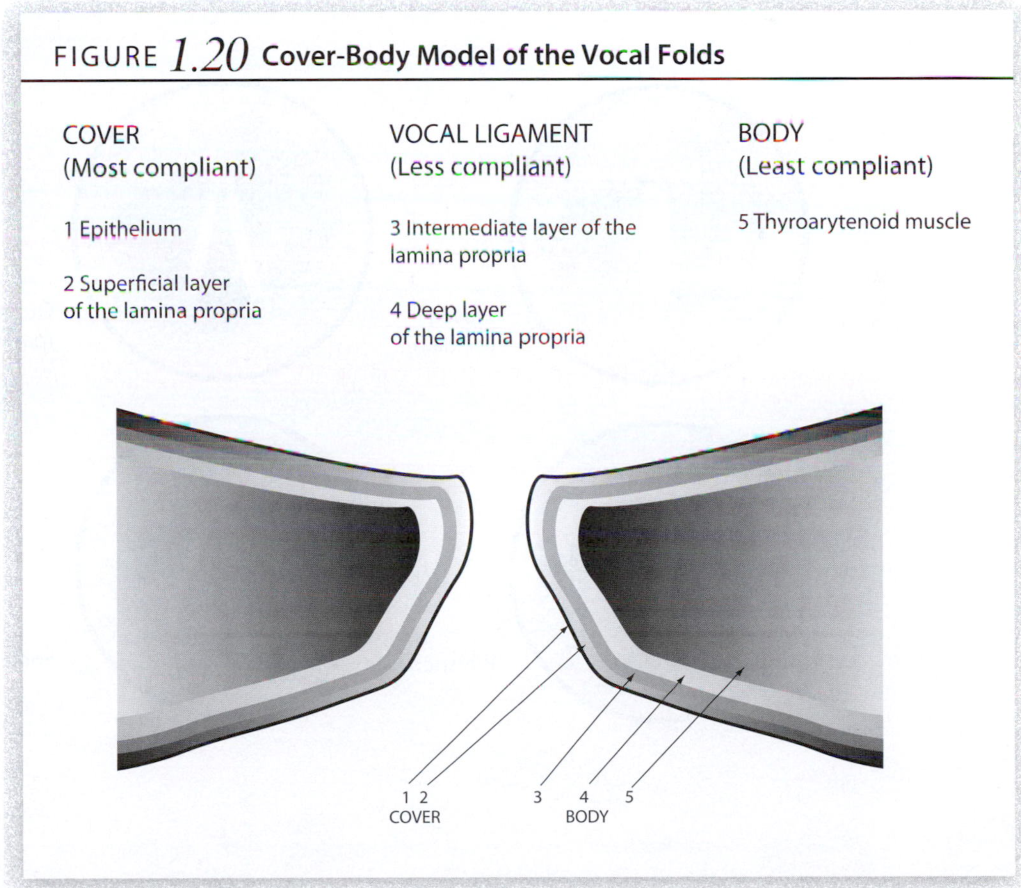

FIGURE *1.20* **Cover-Body Model of the Vocal Folds**

of the glottis in adults. This section of the glottic space is bounded on either side by soft tissue (that is, by the vocal folds). The greatest amplitude of vibration occurs at the midpoint of the **membranous glottis**, which is very elastic and therefore very flexible and responsive to the pressure changes that occur during vibration. The posterior two-fifths make up the **cartilaginous glottis**, so called because its boundaries are formed by the vocal folds where they attach to the vocal processes of the arytenoid cartilages. This portion of the structure does not usually participate as much in vibration except at extremely low pitches.

The glottis changes shape depending on the positioning of the vocal folds (Figure 1.21). For phonation of a voiced sound, the glottis is closed with the folds in a median position. Normal quiet breathing is associated with a somewhat open glottis, with the folds in a paramedian position. When large amounts of air are needed the glottis is very widely open with the folds in a position called forced abduction. Whispering is associated with a glottis that is closed along most of its length, but with a small posterior chink.

FIGURE 1.21 **Glottal Shapes**

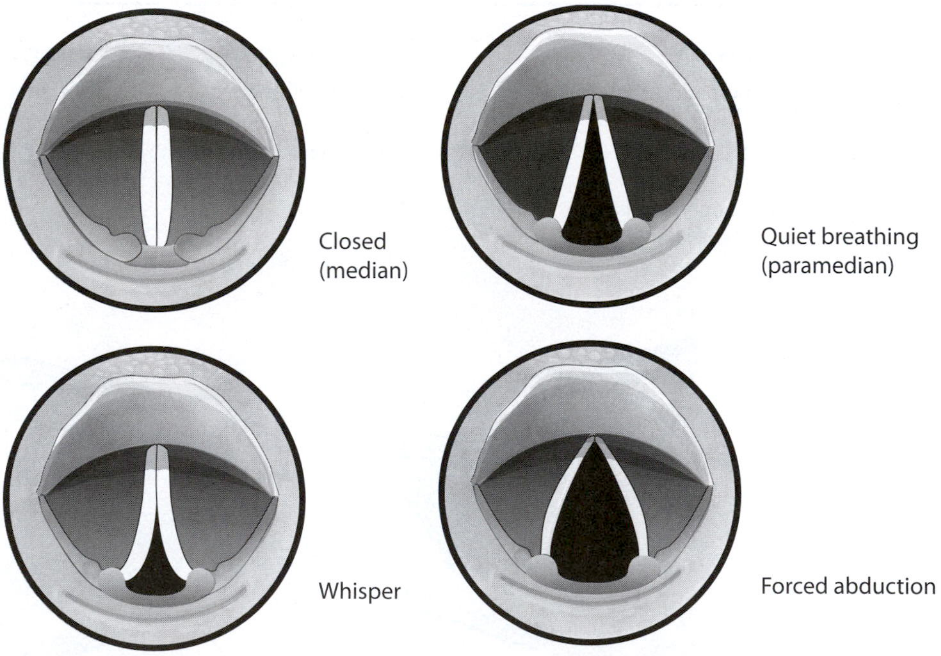

Closed (median)
Quiet breathing (paramedian)
Whisper
Forced abduction

MUSCLES OF THE LARYNX

Skeletal muscles, including those of the larynx, are made up of multiple individual muscle fibers (muscle cells), which are combined into bundles called fascicles (Figure 1.22). The basic elements of muscle fibers are contractile structures called **myofilaments.** These allow the muscle to shorten, thereby moving the structure(s) to which it is attached.

Muscles are composed of two major types of fibers, Type I and Type II (Table 1.7). Type II fibers are further subdivided into Types IIA, IIB, and IIX.

FIGURE 1.22 **Skeletal Muscle**

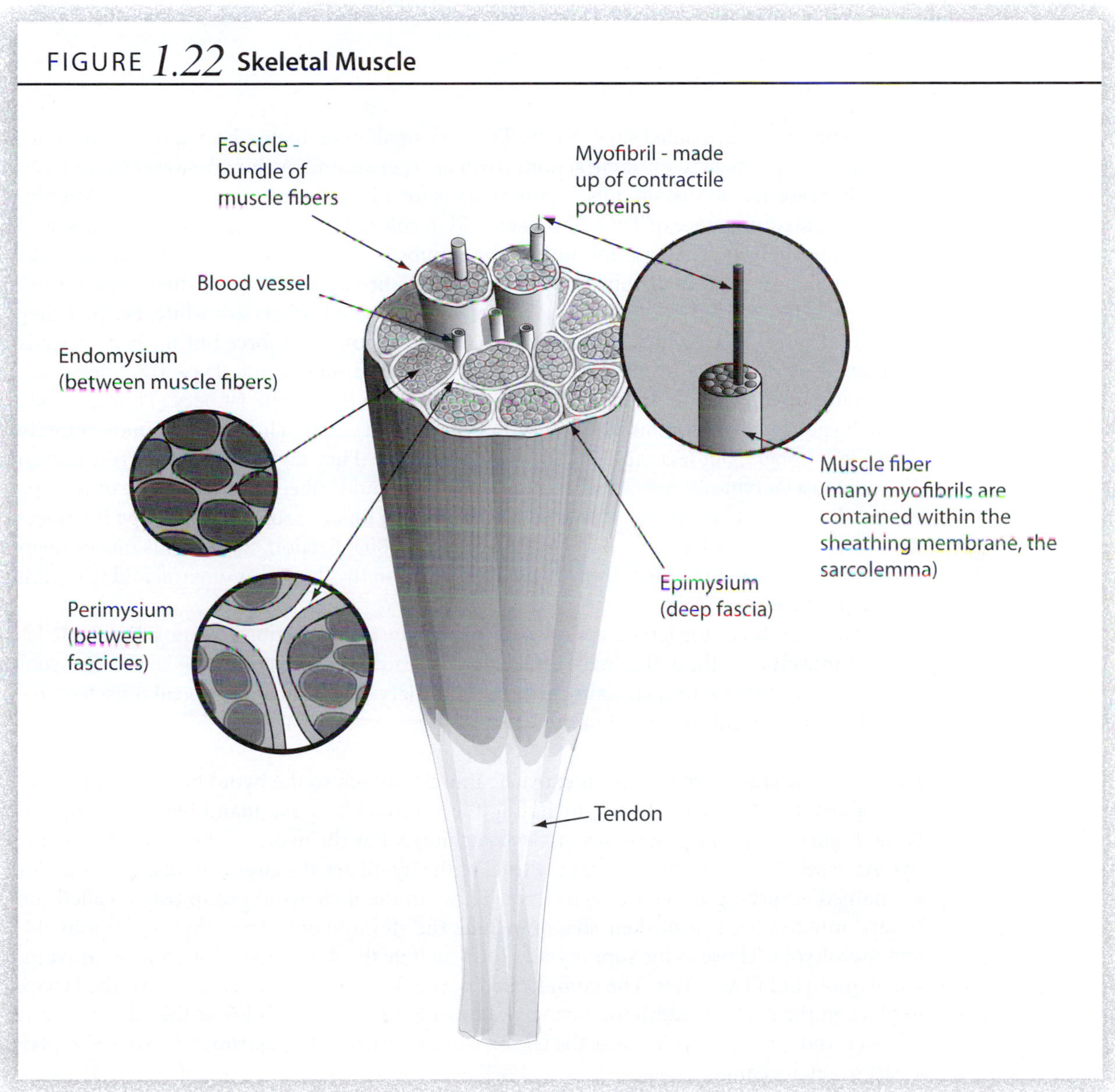

TABLE 1.7 **Type I and Type II Muscle Fibers**

Type I	Type II
Slow twitch	Fast twitch
Smaller diameter	Larger diameter
Slower contraction time	Faster contraction time
10–30 twitches per second	30–70 twitches per second
Fatigue resistant	Fatigue more quickly

Type I fibers are called slow twitch. They are small in diameter, have a slower contraction time, and produce 10–30 contractions (twitches) per second. Although slower to contract, these fibers are able to sustain muscle contractions for a long time without fatiguing. Muscles that have a predominance of Type I fibers are red in color, due to the many blood vessels used in their metabolism. They are found in large numbers in muscles that are associated with maintaining posture. Type II fibers, called fast twitch, fire at a higher rate than Type I fibers (30–70 twitches per second) but fatigue more quickly. Type II fibers are white, because they lack blood vessels. Fast twitch muscles generate large amounts of force but for brief periods of time. They dominate in muscles associated with rapid movement. Type IIX fibers have faster rates of contraction and lower levels of endurance than Type I fibers (Thomas et al., 2008). Type IIA fibers combine elements of Type I and Type II. They contract more rapidly than Type I fibers, but less rapidly than Type IIX fibers. They are also relatively resistant to fatigue. Muscles typically are comprised of both Type I and II fibers, but one or the other type will predominate. The intrinsic laryngeal muscles have a higher proportion of Type IIA fibers than most other muscles in the body (Brandon et al., 2003; Sataloff, 2005). This makes them particularly well suited to the extremely fast rates and lengthy durations of vocal fold vibration during phonation.

The muscles of the larynx are divided into extrinsic and intrinsic groups. **Extrinsic laryngeal muscles** are those that have one attachment to the cartilages of the larynx or hyoid bone, and the other to some structure external to the larynx. **Intrinsic laryngeal muscles** have both their attachments to or within the larynx.

Extrinsic Muscles. Two groups of extrinsic muscles attach to the hyoid bone and to structures above and below the hyoid, including the sternum, scapula, mandible, and temporal bone (Figure 1.23). The groups of muscles attaching below the hyoid are known as the **infrahyoids**, while those attaching above the level of the hyoid are the **suprahyoids**. The muscles are named according to their attachments. Those in the infrahyoid group (often called the "strap" muscles because of their shape) include the sternohyoid, sternothyroid, omohyoid, and thyrohyoid. Those in the suprahyoid group include the digastric, stylohyoid, mylohyoid, and geniohyoid (Table 1.8). The complicated network of extrinsic muscles keeps the larynx in place in the neck. In addition, during swallowing the infrahyoids lower the larynx within the neck and the suprahyoids raise the larynx within the neck. The extrinsic muscles also play a part in pitch change.

FIGURE 1.23 Extrinsic Muscles

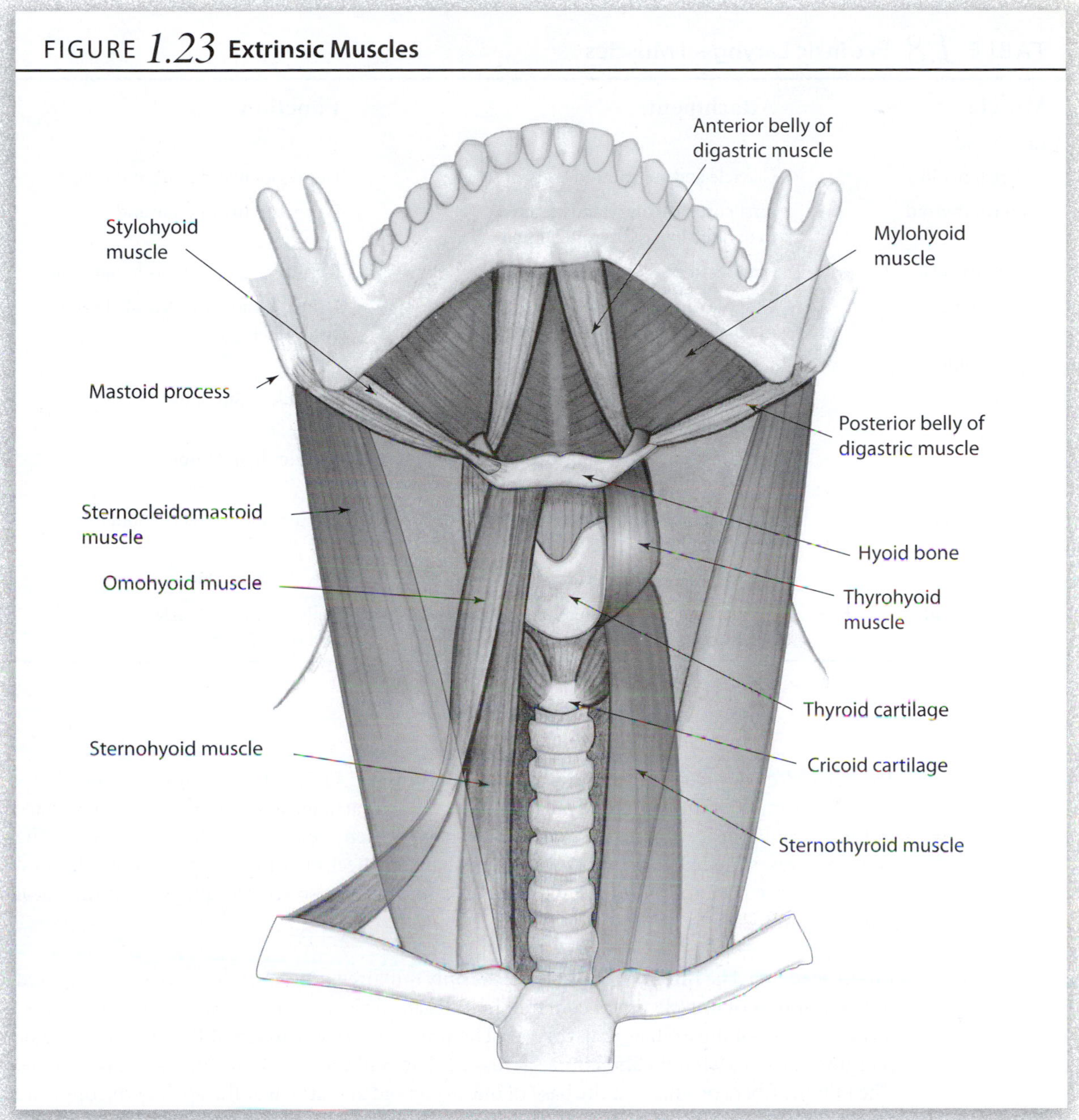

Intrinsic Muscles. There are five intrinsic muscles of the larynx, which perform the functions of adducting, abducting, tensing, and relaxing the vocal folds (Figure 1.24). One intrinsic muscle forms the body of the vocal folds. The intrinsic muscles are named according to their attachments. The muscles include the lateral cricoarytenoid, the interarytenoid, the posterior cricoarytenoid, the cricothyroid, and the thyroarytenoid (Table 1.9).

TABLE 1.8 **Extrinsic Laryngeal Muscles**

Muscle	Attachments	Function
Infrahyoids		
Sternohyoid	Clavicle and sternum to body of hyoid	Depresses hyoid bone and larynx
Sternothyroid	First costal cartilage and sternum to oblique line of thyroid lamina	Depresses hyoid bone and larynx
Omohyoid	Scapula to inferior border of hyoid	Depresses and retracts hyoid bone
Thyrohyoid	Oblique line of thyroid lamina to major horn of hyoid	Draws hyoid and thyroid closer to each other
Suprahyoids		
Digastric	Posterior belly: mastoid process of temporal bone to hyoid bone	Elevates hyoid bone
	Anterior belly: mandible to intermediate tendon of digastric muscle	Elevates hyoid bone
Stylohyoid	Styloid process of temporal bone to body of hyoid	Elevates and retracts hyoid bone
Mylohyoid	Body of mandible to hyoid	Elevates hyoid bone
Geniohyoid	Mental symphysis of mandible to body of hyoid bone	Pulls hyoid anteriorly and superiorly

Lateral Cricoarytenoid. The **lateral cricoarytenoid (LCA)** is a paired muscle with fibers coursing from the superior lateral portion of the cricoid cartilage to the anterior lateral surface of the muscular process of each arytenoid cartilage. When the muscle contracts it swings the vocal processes medially and downward. This has the effect of adducting the vocal folds and closing the membranous glottis (Figure 1.25). Contraction also stiffens all layers of the vocal folds (Sataloff, 2005).

Interarytenoid. The **interarytenoid (IA),** the only unpaired muscle of the larynx, is composed of two bundles of muscle fibers coursing in different directions across and between the posterior surfaces of the arytenoid cartilages. The transverse fibers attach at the lateral posterior margins of each arytenoid and course across the backs of the arytenoids in a sheet of muscle. The oblique fibers originate at the base of one arytenoid and attach at the apex of the opposite arytenoid. This results in a characteristic crossing pattern of the fibers. Contraction of this muscle pulls the arytenoid cartilages medially toward each other, adducting the vocal folds to close the cartilaginous glottis. Some of the oblique IA fibers continue laterally around the apex of the arytenoid and insert into the lateral margins of the epiglottis, forming the aryepiglottic muscle. When the aryepiglottic muscle contracts, the epiglottis is pulled downward and backward to cover the entrance to the larynx.

Posterior Cricoarytenoid. The paired **posterior cricoarytenoid (PCA)** muscle originates on the quadrate lamina of the cricoid cartilage. The fibers course upward and attach to the

FIGURE 1.24 Posterior View of Intrinsic Muscles

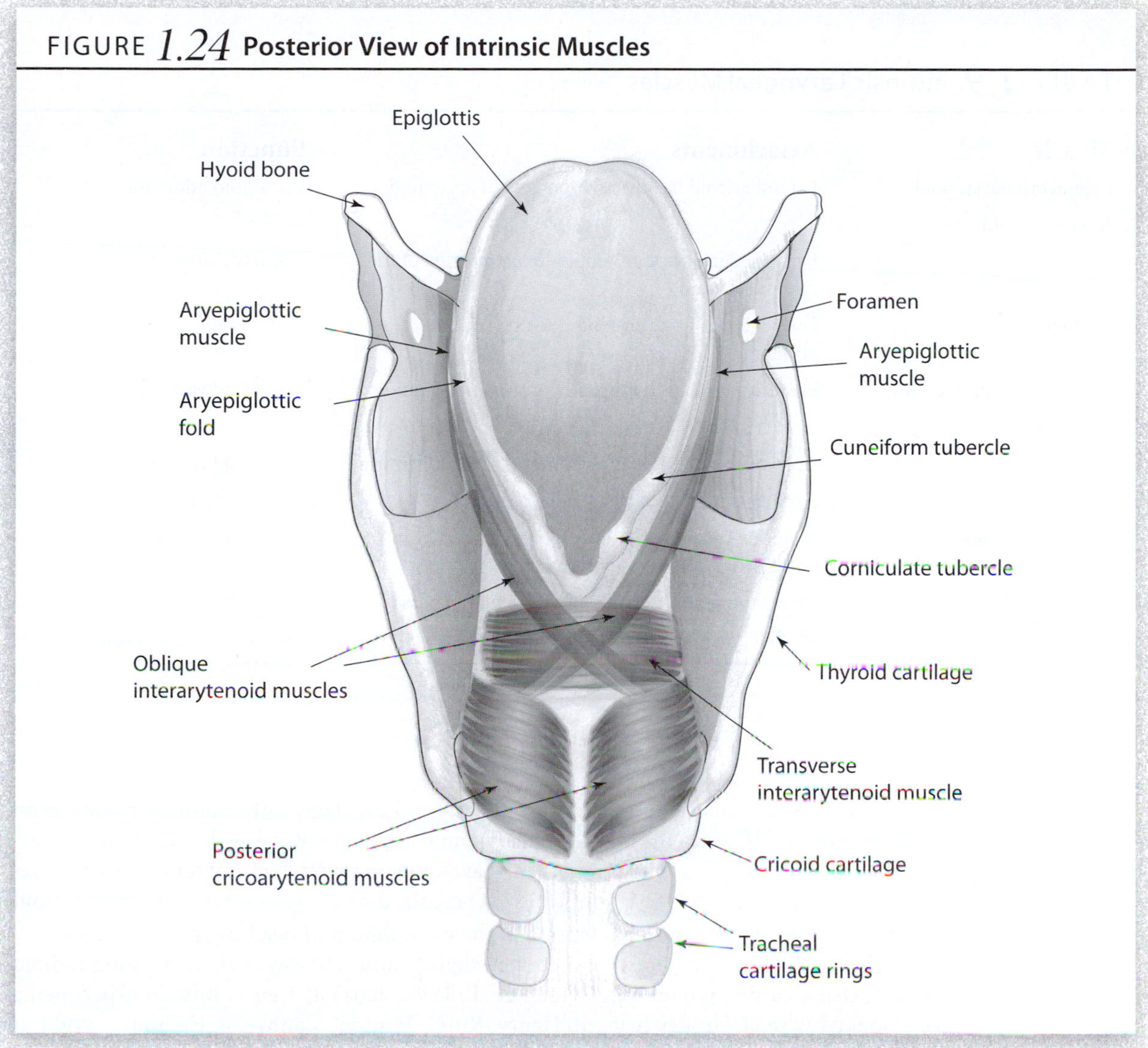

muscular process of each arytenoid, giving this large muscle a leaf-shaped appearance. Contraction rotates the vocal processes of the arytenoid cartilages laterally and upward, abducting the vocal folds and opening the glottis.

Cricothyroid Muscle. The **cricothyroid (CT) muscle** consists of two muscle bundles, the pars recta and the pars oblique (Figure 1.26). Both bundles of fibers originate at the lateral margins of the cricoid arch. The fibers of the pars recta course in a relatively vertical direction and attach to the inferior surface of the thyroid lamina. The oblique fibers course at a more oblique angle, inserting into the anterior surface of the inferior horn of the thyroid cartilage. This muscle, when contracted, tilts the thyroid cartilage downward toward the cricoid cartilage,

TABLE 1.9 **Intrinsic Laryngeal Muscles**

Muscle	Attachments	Function
Lateral cricoarytenoid	Lateral cricoid to muscular process of arytenoid	Vocal fold adductor
Interarytenoid		
Transverse	Lateral edge of one arytenoid to lateral edge of the other arytenoid	Vocal fold adductor
Oblique	Lateral base of one arytenoid to apex of other arytenoid	
Posterior cricoarytenoid	Posterior cricoid to muscular process of arytenoid	Vocal fold abductor
Cricothyroid		
Pars recta	Arch of cricoid to inferior border of thyroid lamina	Vocal fold tensor
Pars oblique	Arch of cricoid to inferior horn of thyroid	
Thyroarytenoid	Anterior commissure to base of arytenoid from vocal process to muscular process	Body of vocal fold
Thyromuscularis	Lateral portion inserting into muscular process	May shorten and slacken cover
Thyrovocalis	Medial portion inserting into vocal process	Exerts internal tension

or tilts the cricoid cartilage upward toward the thyroid cartilage. Either motion results in an increased distance between the thyroid and arytenoid cartilages. Because the vocal folds are attached anteriorly and posteriorly to these cartilages, they are stretched and tensed. This causes an increase in their rate of vibration, which is perceived as a higher pitch. The cricothyroid muscle thus regulates longitudinal tension of the vocal folds and resulting pitch changes.

The two bellies of the muscle function in slightly different ways to increase longitudinal tension. Using canine models (e.g., Hong et al., 1998, 2001) as well as human experiments with hooked wire electrodes (e.g., McHenry, Kuna, Minton, Vanoye, & Calhoun., 1997), it has been found that the pars recta is more effective in tensing the vocal folds than is the pars oblique. Hong et al. (2001) suggested that the pars recta is primarily involved in increasing longitudinal tension by rotating the thyroid cartilage down toward the cricoid in the vertical axis. They further proposed that the pars oblique moves the thyroid cartilage forward and the cricoid cartilage backward, with a corresponding increase of vocal fold length and tension. However, Ludlow (2005) noted that the action of the oblique portion is controversial. The contraction of the oblique was originally proposed to slide the thyroid cartilage forward over the cricoid cartilage, but this action has not been observed in humans. Further, such an action may not be physiologically possible because of the anatomical characteristics of the cricothyroid joint and the ligaments, which limit the extent of motion at the joint. Recently a third horizontal belly of the CT muscle has been identified (Mu & Sanders, 2009). Based on their investigation of human larynges, Mu and Sanders (2009) suggested that contraction of both the oblique and horizontal bellies has the effect of sliding the thyroid cartilage forward over the cricoid cartilage.

FIGURE *1.25* **Adductor and Abductor Muscles**

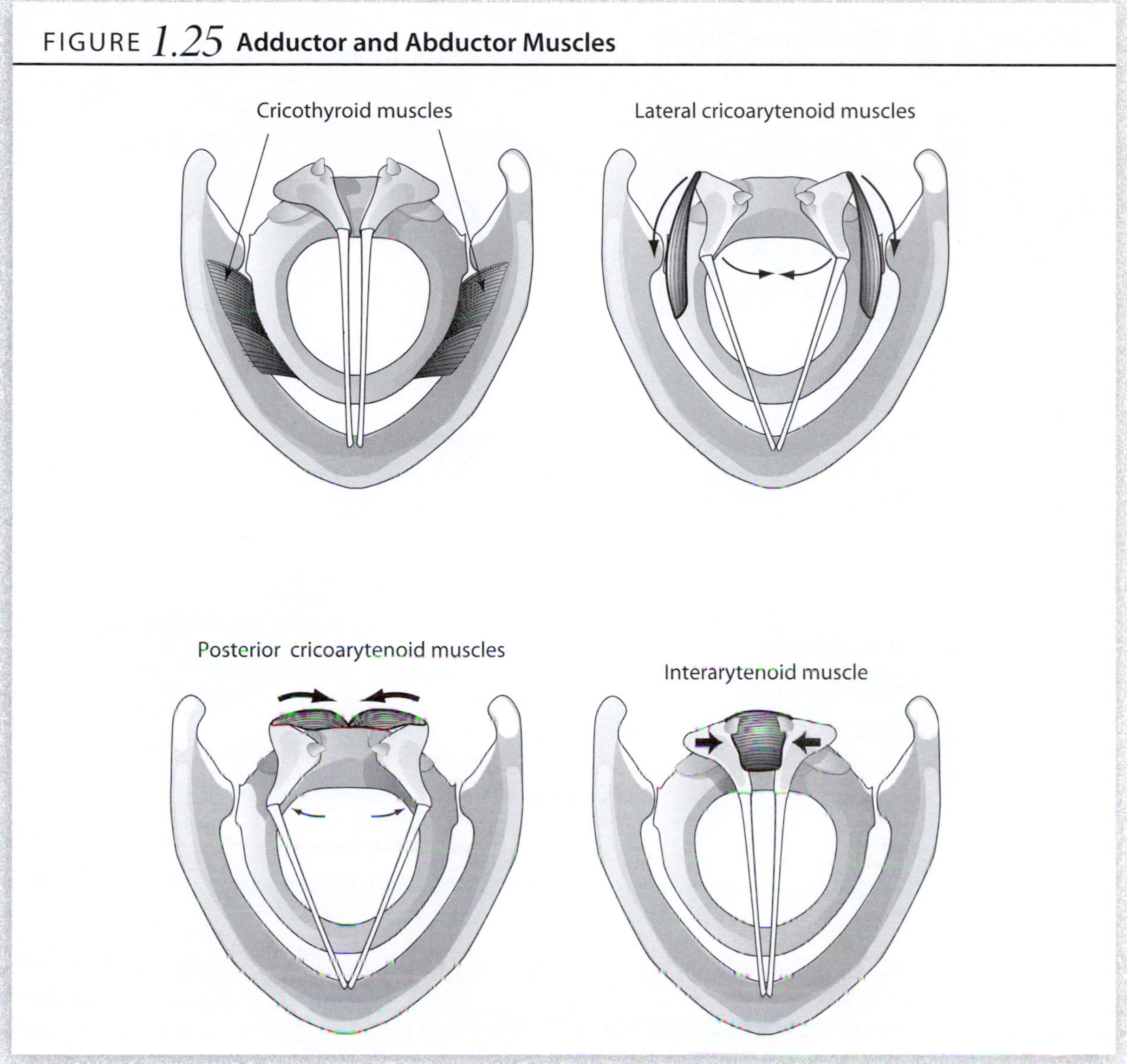

In addition to pitch regulation, the CT muscle plays an important part in respiration. It has been shown that CT activity increases greatly during respiration when increased air intake is required (Mu & Sanders, 2009). When the CT muscle contracts during deep breathing the anteroposterior dimensions of the glottis are increased, thus increasing the size of the airway and decreasing airway resistance (Hoh, 2005; Horiuchi & Sasaki, 1978).

Thyroarytenoid. The thyroarytenoid (TA) muscle has two sections: The more medial thyrovocalis fibers extend from the anterior commissure to the vocal processes of the arytenoid cartilages; the lateral thyromuscularis fibers extend from the anterior commissure to the muscular

FIGURE 1.26 Cricothyroid Muscle

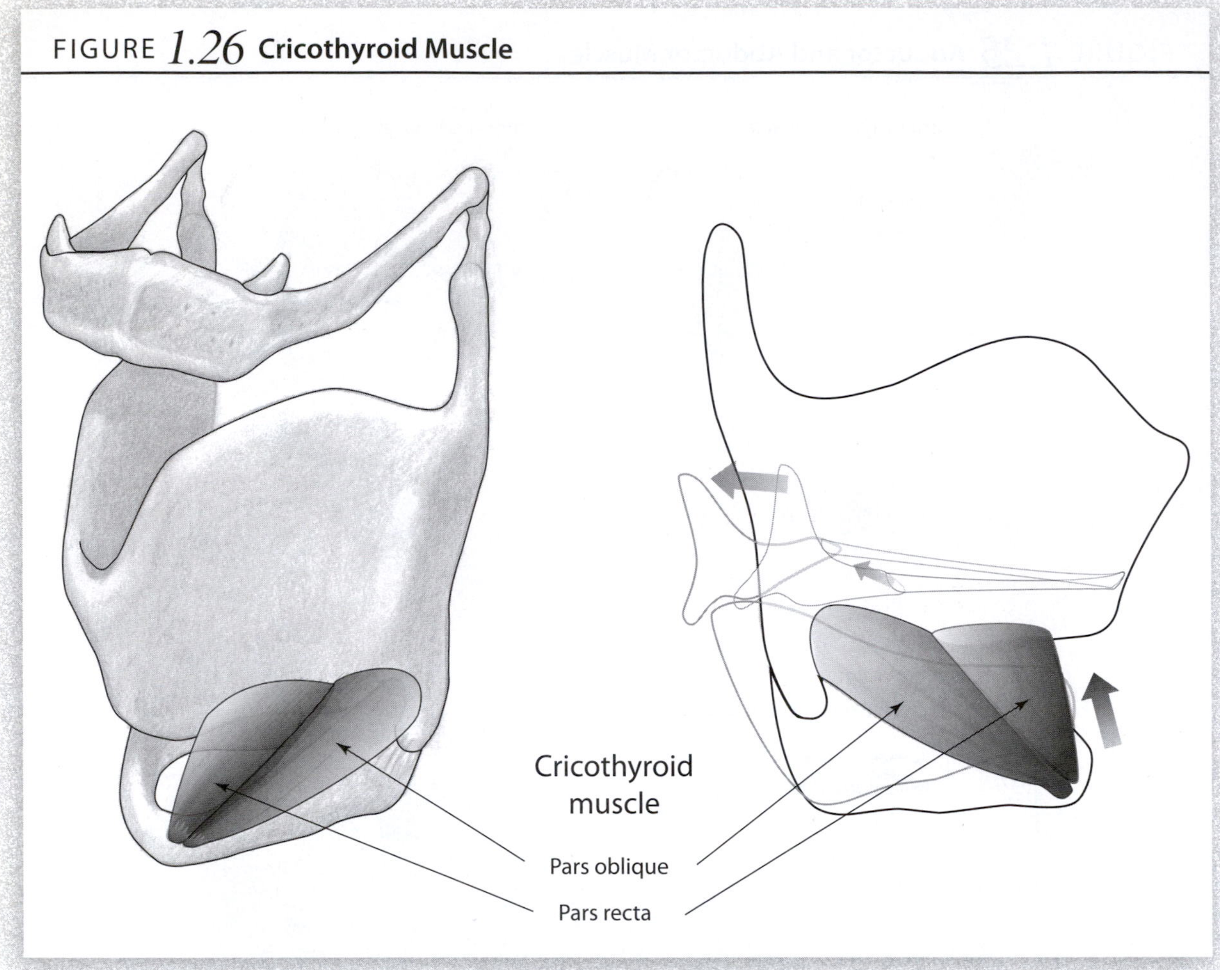

processes of the arytenoids (Figure 1.27). It has been proposed that the larger muscularis portion works to rapidly shorten the vocal folds, whereas the smaller vocalis fibers contribute to making finer tension adjustments along the vocal fold edge (Thomas, Harrison, & Stemple, 2008). The thyrovocalis muscle has been shown to be more active during vocal fold vibration than the thyromuscularis. In addition to active contraction, the TA forms the body of the vocal folds and is thereby acted upon indirectly by the functioning of the other intrinsic muscles.

While each intrinsic muscle has been described in terms of a specific function, it is important to keep in mind that all the intrinsic muscles work synergistically to regulate all aspects of laryngeal function in a highly complex and coordinated manner. Indeed, Poletto, Verdun, Strominger, and Ludlow (2004) found that the PCA was the only laryngeal muscle that was consistently associated with a specific function (glottal opening) in all their subjects in both speech and nonspeech activities. During speech tasks it has been reported that the CT and TA were associated with both vocal fold abduction and adduction (Ludlow, 2005). Nonspeech laryngeal activities such as sniffing and coughing tend to be more consistent in their muscular

FIGURE 1.27 Thyroarytenoid Muscle

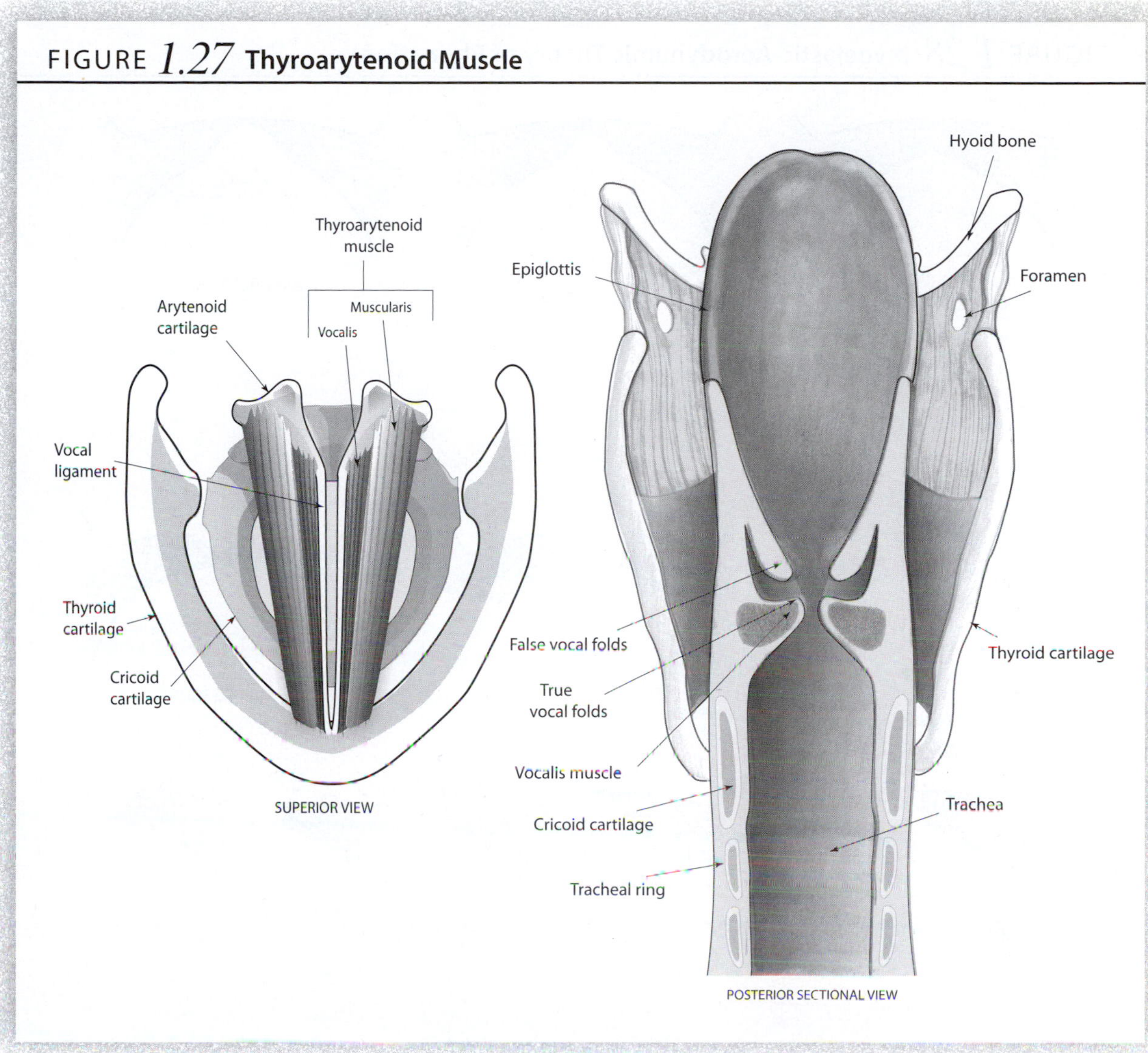

patterns. For example, the CT was correlated with vocal fold opening during a sniff, while the TA and LCA correlated with vocal fold closing when coughing (Poletto et al., 2004).

MYOELASTIC-AERODYNAMIC THEORY

The way that the vocal folds vibrate is described by the **myoelastic-aerodynamic theory** (Figure 1.28), based on seminal investigations of vocal fold function by Van Den Berg (1958). This theory describes one cycle of vocal fold vibration as an interaction of muscle forces, elastic recoil forces, and aerodynamic forces. The muscle force is the **medial compression** exerted by the LCA and IA muscles that adducts the vocal folds to close the glottis and initiate the vibratory cycle. The elastic recoil force is generated as the vocal folds are displaced

FIGURE 1.28 Myoelastic-Aerodynamic Theory of Phonation

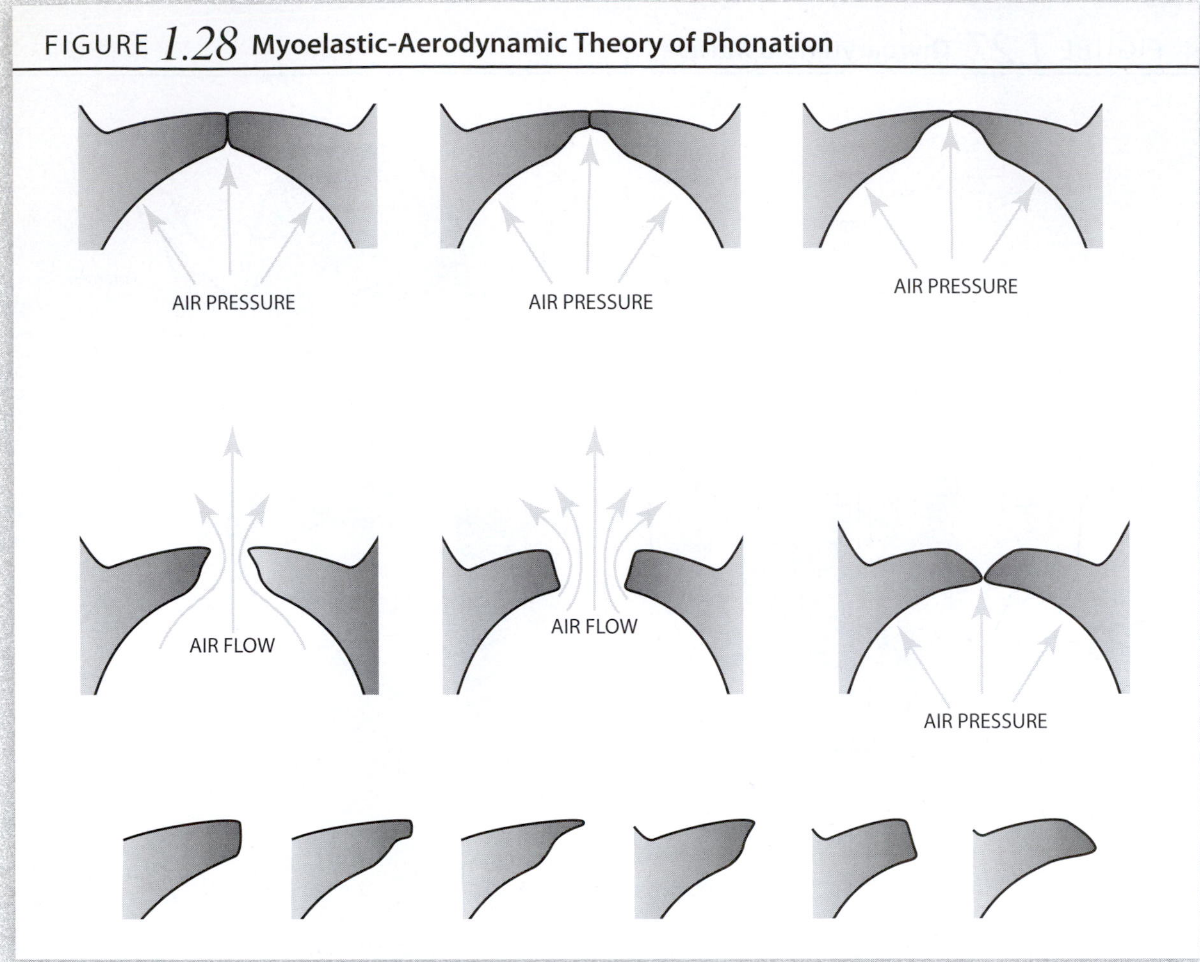

from their adducted position. Aerodynamic forces include positive and negative air pressures created during the vibratory cycle. Positive pressure acts to open the glottis; negative pressure acts to close it. Voice is produced on the exhalation of air, so when the vocal folds initially adduct, air is still flowing through the bronchi and trachea. This air is prevented from passing through the glottis by the adducted vocal folds. The air pressure underneath the vocal folds (**subglottal pressure**) therefore increases, until it reaches a point where it overcomes the medial compression. The positive subglottal pressure forces the glottis open, and a puff of air travels through the glottis and into the vocal tract. Once separated, the vocal folds close very quickly again due to the forces of elasticity and negative pressure. Elastic recoil of the vocal folds begins to return them to the midline, creating a negative pressure within the glottis. The negative pressure traveling through the glottis exerts a suction effect that draws the vocal folds together. The negative pressure is explained by an aerodynamic principle known as **Bernoulli's principle** and relates to the law of conservation of energy. Energy can be divided into two categories: kinetic and potential. Kinetic energy is associated with movement, whether it be the motion of waves, molecules, or objects. **Potential energy** is energy that is stored and may be released to become kinetic energy. The law of conservation of energy states that the overall amount of energy (that is, the sum of kinetic energy and potential energy) cannot change. If one form of energy increases, the other form must decrease in order for the total amount to remain constant. Bernoulli's principle states that as a fluid (gas or liquid) flows through a narrow channel or constriction, the speed of the flow (kinetic energy) increases, resulting in a decrease of pressure (potential energy). The narrowing glottis acts as the channel; thus the air passing through the glottis decreases in pressure, forcing the vocal folds back to the midline. The cycle then repeats itself. It is the interplay between positive and negative pressures that maintains the vocal fold vibration as long as medial compression continues to be exerted.

Scherer (2005) elaborated on the myoelastic-aerodynamic theory by taking into account the air pressures immediately above the vocal folds (supraglottal pressures), as well as glottal shape during vibration. As discussed above, the air flowing through the glottis decreases in pressure as the glottis closes. At the same time, the air that has already passed through the glottis travels up the vocal tract. The distance between the traveling body of air and the glottis increases, resulting in a negative pressure directly above the glottis. The supraglottal negative pressure reinforces the negative pressure within the glottis, which facilitates a greater closing force. Supraglottal pressure also affects the opening phase of the vibratory cycle. As the glottis opens due to positive pressure, the air flowing through the glottis meets the mass of air directly above it, creating compression of the air and increased positive air pressure. The positive supraglottal air pressure further raises the air pressure within the glottis, creating a stronger opening force.

Another factor that affects subglottal, glottal, and supraglottal pressures is the shape of the glottis during vibration (Scherer, 2005). When the vocal folds separate they are farther apart at their bottom margins and less so at the superior edges. This is known as a convergent shape. The convergent shape results in a positive pressure within the glottis, facilitating glottal opening. The opposite shape (divergent) occurs during glottal closure, where the glottis is narrower at the inferior margins and wider at the superior margins. As long as the glottal exit pressure is atmospheric or negative this shape lowers the pressure within the glottis, facilitating glottal closure (Figure 1.29).

One opening and one closing of the glottis constitutes one cycle of vibration (Figure 1.30). This process occurs hundreds of times per second depending on the individual's age and gender. The cycle of glottal opening and closing (called the **duty cycle**) repeats itself as long as medial compression continues to be exerted. The rate at which the vocal folds vibrate is measured in cycles per second, called **fundamental frequency (F0).** F0 is measured in **Hertz (Hz).** On average, adult men with longer and more massive vocal folds have an F0 ranging from 90–130 Hz; the average F0 of adult women with shorter and less massive vocal folds is around 180–230 Hz; and the F0 of young children is approximately 250–300 Hz.

Mucosal Wave. Vocal fold vibration is highly complex, due to the layered structure and different biomechanical characteristics of the cover, vocal ligament, and body. Rather than abducting and adducting in a rigid manner, the vocal folds approximate and separate in a rippling wavelike fashion called the **mucosal wave**. The rippling motion is related to the pliability of the cover in relation to the stiffer vocal ligament and body. The more pliable cover is able to slide easily over the inner layers of the vocal folds. As subglottal pressure builds up underneath the closed glottis, the head of the column of pressure forces the vocal folds to separate at their bottom edges, and the positive pressure continues to separate the folds in an upward direction. The air pressure immediately above the glottis is also positive, reinforcing the glottal opening.

FIGURE *1.29* **Convergent and Divergent Glottal Shapes**

When the vocal folds are shaped to produce a narrower opening at the top and wider opening at the bottom, air molecules passing through the vocal folds converge as they enter the supraglottal area.

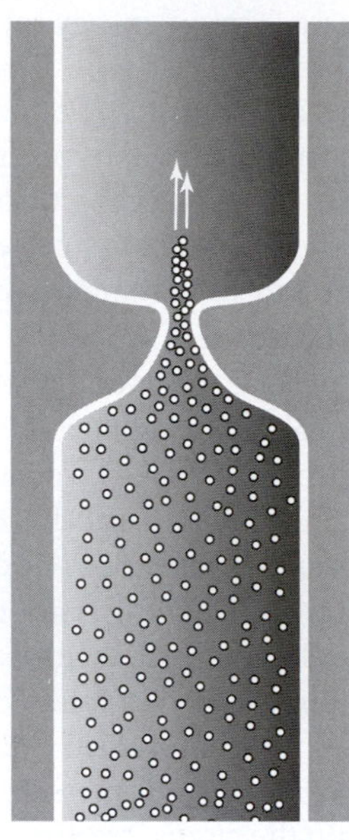

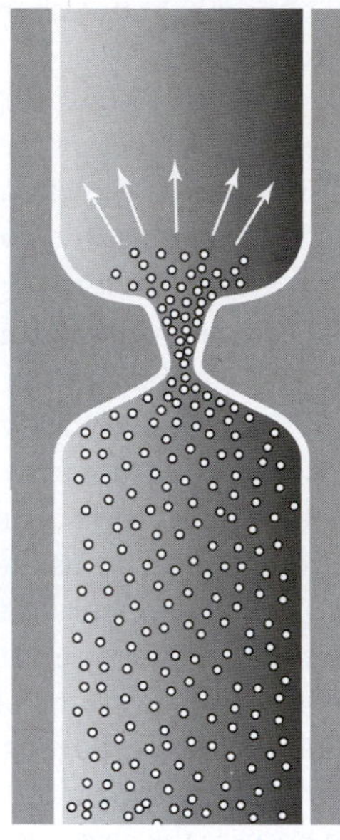

When the vocal folds are shaped to produce a narrower opening at the bottom and wider opening at the top, air molecules passing through the vocal folds diverge as they enter the supraglottal area.

FIGURE *1.30* **Cycle of Vocal Fold Vibration**

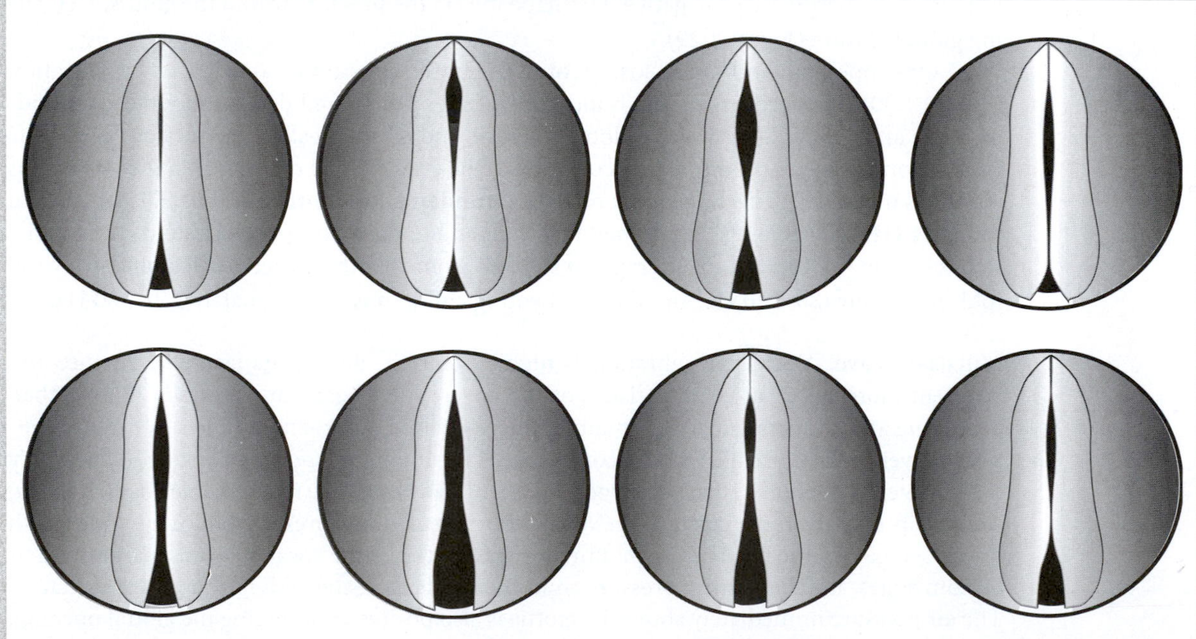

However, by the time the superior portion of the glottis is open, the inferior margins of the vocal folds are already moving toward the midline due to the negative pressure generated within the glottis. The glottal closing also proceeds from inferior to superior margins of the vocal folds. As the glottis is closing due to negative pressure, the supraglottic negative pressure further facilitates the closure. This slight time lag between the approximation and separation of the lower and upper edges of the vocal folds gives rise to a **vertical phase difference**. The vocal folds also open and close the glottis horizontally from anterior to posterior and posterior to anterior. In this case, in a motion rather like that of a zipper, the glottis opens first from the posterior portion at the vocal processes, and the opening travels toward the anterior commissure. Glottal closing occurs in the opposite direction, from anterior to posterior. This creates a slight time lag called the **longitudinal phase difference**. It is this complex vibration with the resulting mucosal wave that generates the rich, resonant sound of the human voice. Anything that interferes with the mucosal wave can result in **dysphonia**.

Phonation Threshold Pressure. Vocal fold vibration requires a buildup of subglottal pressure in order to be initiated. The minimum amount of subglottal pressure needed to set the vocal folds into vibration is known as the **phonation threshold pressure (PTP)** (Figure 1.31) and is measured in units of centimeters of water (cm H_2O).

The measure of cm H_2O is based on how much air pressure it would take to move a column of water a certain distance. To illustrate, if one blows into a U-tube containing a certain

FIGURE *1.31* **Phonation Threshold Pressure**

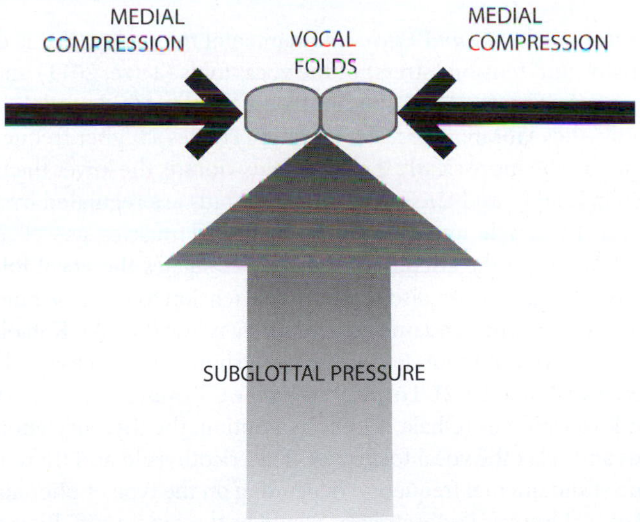

As medial compression increases, the subglottal pressure required to overcome it and set the vocal folds in vibration increases and the intensity of the resulting sound increases.

amount of water, the pressure of the air will displace the column of water a certain distance, depending on the amount of pressure exerted. The distance that the water is displaced is measured in cm H_2O. The minimum phonation threshold pressure needed to set the vocal folds into vibration is around 3 to 8 cm H_2O for normal conversational speech, but varies depending on pitch and loudness of the voice. Jiang et al. (1999) found average PTPs for normal speakers sustaining a vowel of 2.38 cm H_2O at 75 dB, 2.67 cm H_2O at 80 dB, and 2.98 cm H_2O at 85 dB. Rieves, Regner, and Jiang (2009) reported an average PTP of 3.68 cm H_2O for the normal speakers in their study. It has also been found that PTPs are higher for higher pitch levels, due to the fact that the increased longitudinal tension on the vocal folds during high pitches requires more subglottal pressure to initiate vibration. However, PTPs vary between and within individual speakers, depending on several factors. One of the most important factors is hydration of the vocal folds. Vocal folds that are well lubricated require less subglottal pressure to be set into vibration than those that are less well hydrated (Verdolini-Marston, Titze, & Druker, 1991). Another factor influencing PTP is fatigue. The more fatigued a speaker's voice, the higher the PTP required, and vice versa (Solomon & DiMattia, 2000). It has also been found that an individual speaking at his or her most comfortable pitch level requires a minimal amount of subglottal pressure to initiate vibration during phonation (Solomon, Ramanathan, & Makashay, 2007).

Changing Pitch and Loudness. As we speak, we constantly modify the pitch and loudness of our voice in order to express different emotions, as well as to signal different semantic and syntactic constructions. For example, with two identical sentences such as "Peter is eating," the only way to verbally distinguish between them as a statement or a question is to change the pitch at the end of the utterance. To signal the question "Peter is eating?" you would raise the pitch on "eating." To signal a statement, you would drop the pitch on "eating." Stress and emphasis also depend on subtle changes in pitch, loudness, and duration of vowels and/or syllables. To stress a syllable or word, these three elements are increased slightly relative to the adjacent syllables. Speakers also change loudness levels depending on the context in which they are communicating.

Fundamental Frequency and Pitch. Fundamental frequency (F0) is determined by the length, tissue density, and tension (stress) of the vocal folds (Titze, 2011) and corresponds to the perception of **pitch**. The more stretched and tense the vocal folds and the less the tissue density, the more rapidly they vibrate. The faster vibration creates a higher frequency and the perception of a higher pitch. The more slowly the vocal folds vibrate, the lower the frequency and the perception of pitch. Length and tension of the vocal folds are regulated by the cricothyroid muscles, the thyrovocalis muscle, and the extrinsic laryngeal muscles, as well as by subglottal pressure.

Contraction of the cricothyroid muscle elongates the vocal folds and stiffens the cover. The thyrovocalis muscle can also exert internal tension to increase rate of vibration when the CT muscles are relaxed and fundamental frequency is low (Owaki, Kataoka, & Shimizu, 2010). The posterior cricoarytenoid muscle has also been shown to be active at high pitches (Gay, Hirose, Strome, & Sawashima, 1972). To lower pitch, the CT muscle relaxes, as shown by decreased EMG activity at lower pitches (Ohala, 1972). In addition, the thyroarytenoid muscle can shorten the vocal folds and relax the vocal fold cover. The cricothyroid and thyroarytenoid muscles interact to influence fundamental frequency, depending on the type of phonation. According to Scherer (2005), if only the cover is vibrating, as would be the case in soft, high-pitch phonation, contraction of the thyroarytenoid should shorten and reduce the tension of the cover, with an associated decrease in F0. Conversely, during phonation that is loud and low-pitched, with the body of the vocal folds more fully participating in the vibration, contraction of the thyroarytenoid muscle will increase the effective tension of the entire vibrating structure, thus raising the F0.

Contraction of the extrinsic laryngeal muscles also affects F0 and pitch. The suprahyoid muscles pull the hyoid bone anteriorly, thus tilting the thyroid cartilage forward (Scherer, 2005). Forward tilt of the thyroid cartilage increases the distance between the anterior commissure and the arytenoid cartilages, thus stretching the vocal folds. F0, consequently, is raised. Conversely, contraction of the sternothyroid and sternohyoid muscles lowers the larynx, which has the effect of shortening the vocal folds and decreasing F0 (Honda et al., 1999; Ohala, 1972). F0 is also affected by subglottal pressure. It has been reported that increasing subglottal pressure by 1 cm H_2O increases F0 by 3–6 Hz (Baken, 2005; Scherer, 2005). This occurs because a greater subglottal pressure opens the vocal folds more widely, resulting in the vocal folds being more stretched. In turn this increases vocal fold tension, generating a higher F0.

By working together synergistically the CT and TA muscles, in combination with extrinsic laryngeal muscle contraction and subglottal pressure changes, allow a remarkable degree of fine and rapid control over vocal fold length and tension (Figure 1.32). This facilitates continuous, smoothly executed pitch changes during connected speech.

Intensity and Loudness. **Loudness** is the perceptual counterpart of vocal intensity or amplitude, measured in dB. Vocal intensity is controlled by degree of subglottal pressure and forcefulness of medial compression. In general, the greater degree of medial compression that is exerted, the higher is the subglottal pressure necessary to overcome the vocal fold resistance. When the folds are eventually forced apart, their amplitude of excursion is greater, and the force of closure is correspondingly greater as well. As a consequence, the sound wave is more intense. Finnegan, Luschei, and Hoffman (2000) reported that when subglottal air pressure is double the phonation threshold pressure, intensity increases to around 80 dB. Titze and Sundberg (1992) demonstrated that doubling subglottal pressure raises intensity by 6 dB. Intensity and F0 are strongly related, such that increases in intensity produce increases in F0 and

FIGURE 1.32 Contributors to Pitch

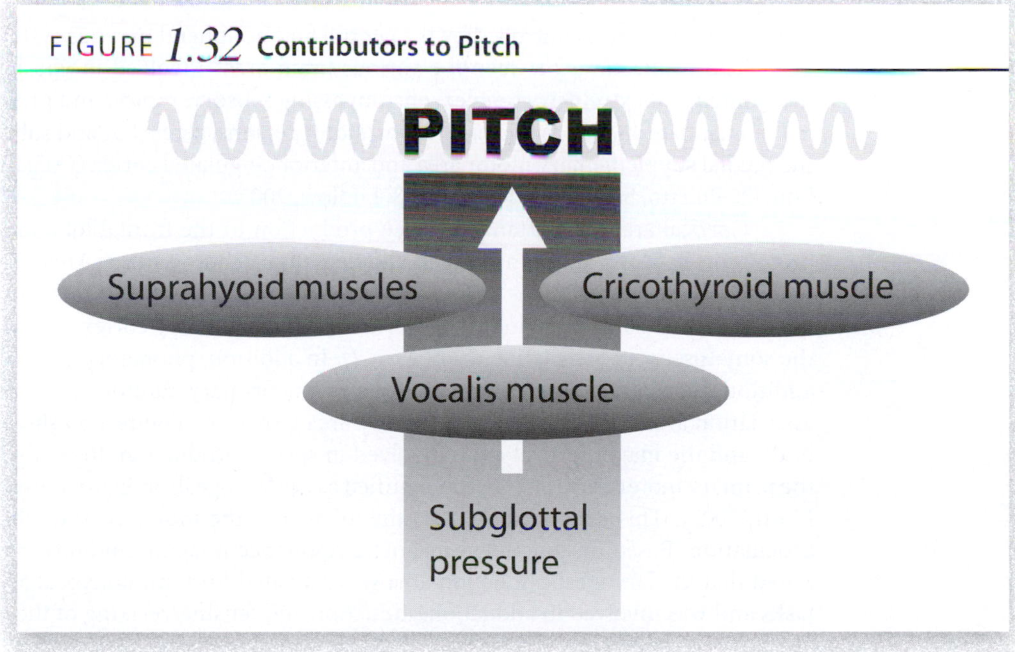

vice versa (e.g. Baker, Ramig, Sapir, Luschei, & Smith, 2001; Plant & Younger, 2000; Titze & Sundberg, 1992; Watson & Hughes, 2006). Intensity is regulated by the interaction between subglottal pressure generated by the respiratory system and glottal resistance generated by the laryngeal system. However, the specific patterns vary between speakers, with some individuals using primarily the respiratory system (i.e., increased subglottal pressure) to control loudness, some using primarily the laryngeal system (i.e., increased medial compression and/or vocal fold tension), and some using a combination of the two (Dromey, Stathopoulos, & Sapienza, 1992).

RESONANCE

The discussion thus far has focused on the role of the phonatory system in voice production. Vocal fold vibration generates the basic laryngeal tone. However, this is not the sound that is perceived by a listener. Once the sound is generated it is modified as it travels through the vocal tract. The vocal tract (pharynx, oral cavity, and nasal cavities) is an acoustic resonator that has multiple resonant frequencies called formants. The laryngeal sound is a complex periodic tone with a fundamental frequency and harmonics, which are whole number multiples of the fundamental frequency. As this sound travels through the vocal tract, those harmonics that fall close to a resonant frequency are amplified, while those that are farther from a resonant frequency are damped. This process of resonance modifies the acoustic quality of the sound. Different movements of the articulators change the vocal tract formants, resulting in different harmonics being amplified or damped. Resonant sounds such as vowels, diphthongs, glides, liquids, and nasals are characterized by specific relationships between the formants. Trained singers and speakers become adept at "tuning" the vocal tract formants by modifying their articulatory gestures in order to generate rich and resonant vocal qualities.

Nervous System Control of the Larynx

Laryngeal function is controlled by the central and peripheral nervous systems (Table 1.10).

The connections between the various brain areas involved in vocalization are widely distributed and extremely complex, encompassing sensory, motor, and premotor areas in the left hemisphere, as well as bilateral sensorimotor regions, cerebellar and subcortical areas, and the medial supplementary motor area and anterior cingulated cortex (Galgano & Froud, 2008; Loucks, Poletto, Simonyan, Reynolds, & Ludlow, 2007).

Cortical areas important for voice production in the frontal lobe include the primary motor cortex (Area 4), premotor and supplementary motor areas (Area 6), and Broca's area in the left hemisphere (Areas 44 and 45). Sensory areas within the parietal lobe also contribute to vocal motor control, including the primary somatosensory cortex (Areas 3, 1, and 2), and the somatosensory association area (Area 7). In addition, phonatory control is influenced by audition, represented in the temporal lobe by the primary auditory area (Area 41), auditory association area (Area 42), and Wernicke's area (Area 22). Figure 1.33 shows the lobes of the brain and the major cortical areas involved in speech production. Recently, a specific area in the primary motor cortex has been identified as the laryngeal/phonatory area (Brown, Ngan, & Liotti, 2007). This area is adjacent to the lip area in the motor cortex, which is involved in articulation. Based on functional magnetic resonance imaging findings, Brown et al. (2007) noted that the laryngeal/phonation area was activated for both nonvocal and vocal laryngeal tasks and was involved in adduction/adduction and tensing/relaxing of the vocal folds. Thus,

TABLE 1.10 **Nervous System Structures Involved in Phonation**

Structure	Function
Primary motor cortex	Initiates voluntary movement
Premotor area	Planning and selection of movement
Supplementary motor area	
Pyramidal system	
Corticospinal pathway	Fine control of voluntary movement mediated by spinal neurons
Corticobulbar pathway	Fine control of voluntary movement mediated by cranial neurons
Cerebellum	Regulates force, speed, range, timing, direction, and amount of displacement of movement; involved with posture and background muscle tone; coordinates muscle groups
Basal ganglia	Smoothes and refines intended movement by inhibiting excessive nerve impulses; substantia nigra produces inhibitory neurotransmitter dopamine
Thalamus	Integrates incoming sensory and outgoing motor information; influences level of consciousness and alertness; integrates emotional expression into motor activity
Periaqueductal grey	Coordinates respiratory and laryngeal motor patterns necessary for speech; involved in the expression of emotion
Vagus nerve	
Superior laryngeal	Innervates cricothyroid muscle
Recurrent laryngeal	Innervates lateral and posterior cricoarytenoid, thyroarytenoid, and interarytenoid muscles
Nucleus ambiguus	Houses motoneurons of the vagus nerve
Nucleus retroambiguus	Houses neurons that innervate muscles of the tongue, pharynx, soft palate, muscles of exhalation, and larynx
Laryngeal sensory receptors	Respond to touch, movement, vibration, changes in air pressure, chemical stimuli

this cortical area appears to be the major region for vocal control in humans. Brown et al. (2007) also posited the possible existence of an expiratory area in this region of motor cortex, which would facilitate the coordination of respiration and phonation for speech.

The primary motor cortex initiates motor impulses to be sent via nerve pathways to effect voluntary movement. Other areas such as the premotor cortex and the supplementary motor cortex are involved in planning and control mechanisms for voluntary movement (Murphy et al., 1997). These areas receive information from other brain areas including the basal ganglia and cerebellum that is used in the selection, planning, and refining of the movement prior to the actual initiation of the movement by the motor cortex.

PYRAMIDAL AND EXTRAPYRAMIDAL PATHWAYS

The neural pathways for voluntary vocalization arise in the sensory and motor cortex in both cerebral hemispheres. Nerve fibers that originate from the motor and sensory cortex in the frontal and parietal lobes of the brain project to other areas via two pathways: the **corticospinal**

FIGURE 1.33 **Cortical Areas Involved in Phonation**

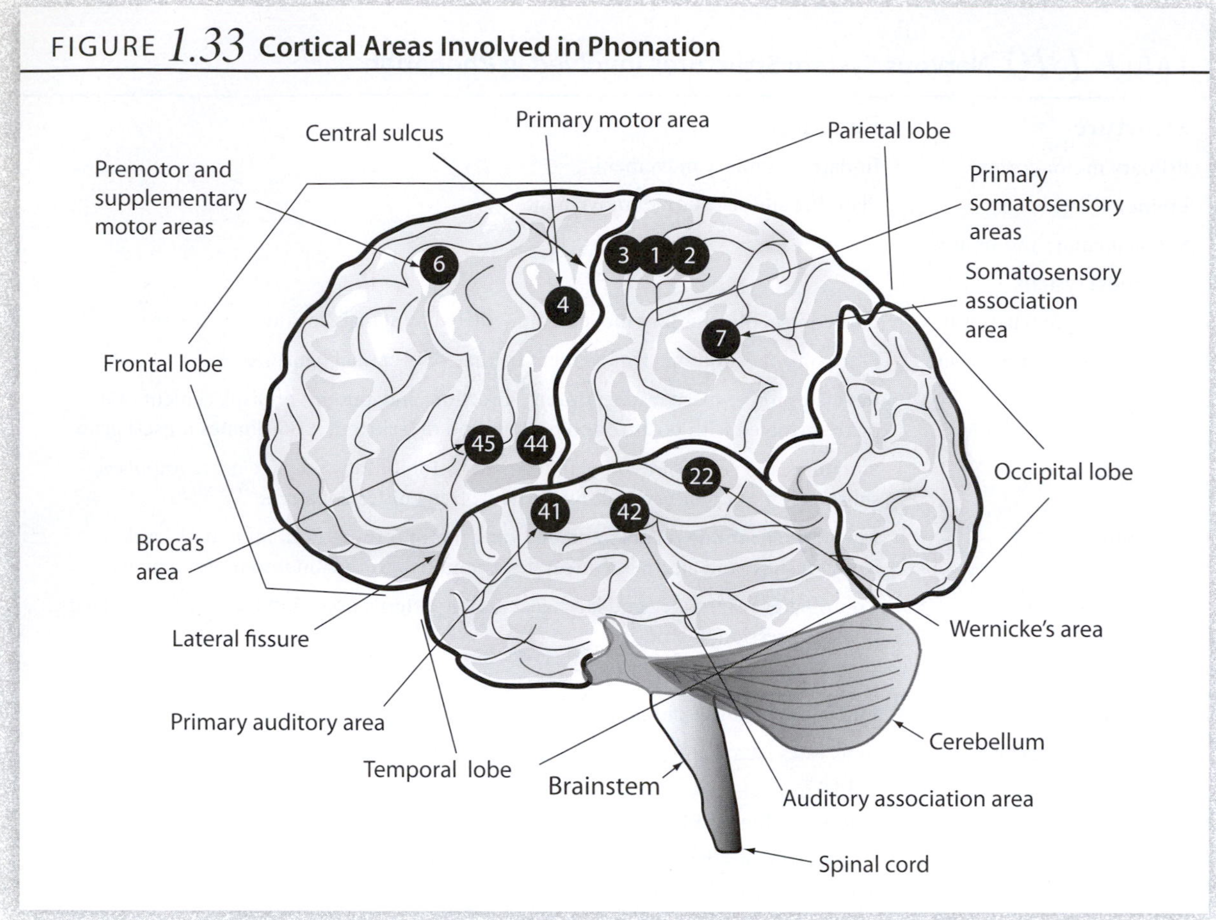

pathway and the **corticobulbar (corticonuclear) pathway**. These two pathways make up the so-called **pyramidal tract**, which is involved in fine control of all voluntary movement. The corticospinal tract arises from several cortical regions in the frontal lobe including the motor cortex, premotor area, and supplementary motor area, as well as the somatosensory cortex in the parietal lobe. Fibers in this pathway synapse directly with motor nerve cells in the spinal cord. At the medulla approximately 80% of the fibers on either side decussate and cross over to the contralateral (opposite) side, and continue to the spinal cord as the **lateral corticospinal tract**. The other 20% (**anterior corticospinal tract**) continue to descend on the ipsilateral (same) side of the body. This arrangement allows bilateral innervation of the structures involved in phonation.

The corticonuclear tract arises from the motor cortex in the frontal lobe and synapses with motor nuclei of cranial nerves V (trigeminal), VII (facial), X (vagus), and XII (hypoglossal). This is primarily an ipsilateral pathway, except for fibers of the facial nerve, which run both ipsilaterally and contralaterally. The motoneurons for the vagus nerve are located in the **nucleus ambiguus (NA)** within the medulla. Damage to the pyramidal pathways can result in weakness or spasticity of affected structures, including those involved in phonation.

The extrapyramidal tract is a more circuitous pathway that extends from the cortex to the brainstem or spinal cord through interconnections with the basal ganglia (also called the basal

FIGURE 1.34 **Cerebellum and Subcortical Areas Involved in Phonation**

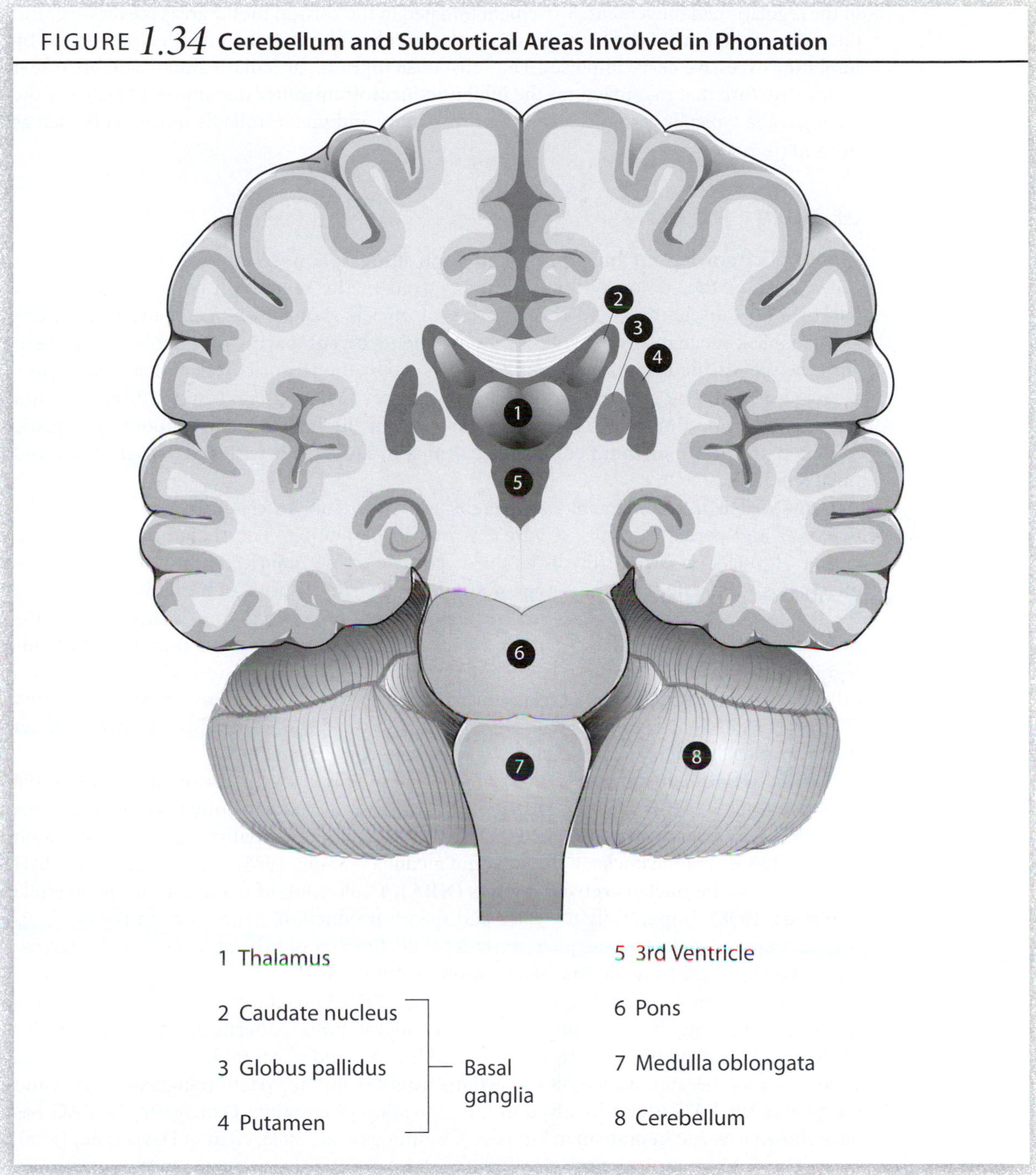

nuclei) and the cerebellum. The **basal ganglia** are subcortical clusters of nerve cells (nuclei) including the caudate nucleus, globus pallidus, putamen, and substantia nigra (Figure 1.34). These nuclei form part of multiple neural circuits that run between various areas of the cortex and subcortical regions including the thalamus. The basal ganglia play a critical inhibitory role in the regulation of movement. Movement initiated in the cortical motor areas is excessive, and one of the functions of the basal ganglia is to smooth and refine the intended movement by inhibiting excessive nerve impulses. The **substantia nigra** is particularly important, because it is this structure that manufactures the inhibitory neurotransmitter dopamine. Damage to the basal ganglia typically results in excessive involuntary and uncontrollable movements such as tics and tremors.

CEREBELLUM

The **cerebellum** has an integrating and controlling role over movements that arise in other parts of the motor system and is involved in the regulation of posture, balance, background muscle tone, and coordination of muscle groups. The cerebellum functions as a feedback mechanism for voluntary movements by comparing an ongoing movement with the specific neuromuscular commands issued by the motor cortex and correcting any detected errors. The cerebellum regulates the force, speed, range, timing, direction, and amount of displacement of movements throughout the body so that smooth synergistic muscle patterns are maintained. Damage results in movement patterns that are jerky and uncoordinated.

As well as the basal ganglia and cerebellum, other subcortical structures including the thalamus and periaqueductal grey are involved in phonation. The **thalamus** consists of a cluster of nuclei on either side of the third ventricle of the brain (Figure 1.34). Aside from olfaction, all nerve impulses traveling toward the brain from all areas of the body pass through the thalamus. The thalamus also receives motor nerve projections from many areas of the nervous system including basal ganglia, cerebellum, and cortex, making it an important integrating station for incoming sensory and outgoing motor information. The thalamus also influences an individual's level of consciousness and alertness, and it is involved in integrating emotional expression into motor activity. Damage to the thalamus has been shown to result in movement disorders such as dystonia (Lee & Marsden, 1994).

The **periaqueductal grey (PAG)** is an area made up of grey matter surrounding the cerebral aqueduct. It is a widely distributed area that adjoins with other subcortical areas including the thalamus (Sataloff, 2005). The PAG is connected anatomically to many brain areas, including cranial nuclei in the pons and medulla (Larson, 1985). Neurons from the PAG also project to the **nucleus retroambiguus (NRA),** a collection of nerve cells in the medulla (Holstege, 1998). Importantly for voice and speech production, neurons from the NRA innervate muscles of the tongue, pharynx, soft palate, muscles of exhalation (internal intercostals and abdominals), and larynx (Boers, Klop, Hulshoff, de Weerd, & Holstege, 2007; Davis, Zhang, & Bandler, 1996; Holstege, 1998; Sataloff, 2005). Thus the PAG seems to be important in coordinating the basic respiratory and laryngeal motor patterns that are necessary for speech, such as expiratory effort, vocal fold adduction, and vocal fold tension (Davis et al., 1996). Further, because it receives projections from the limbic system (cingulated gyrus and amygdala), the PAG is also involved in the expression of emotion. Damage to the PAG has been shown to result in mutism in humans (Cummings et al., 1983, cited in Davis et al., 1996).

Through the corticobulbar tract, humans have direct nerve pathways from the cortex to the nucleus ambiguus (NA) that houses the motoneurons of the vagus nerve (Larson, 1985; Simonyan and Jurgens, 2003). This direct connection is lacking in all other animals (Ludlow, 2005). Humans also have a motor pathway that encompasses nerve fiber projections between the limbic system, PAG, and NA. Thus human speakers appear to have two systems of control over vocalization. Cortical input to the laryngeal motoneurons is important for vocalization associated with purposeful speech, whereas the limbic system-PAG-NA pathway seems to be more involved in emotional vocalizations such as laughter, crying, screaming, and coughing (Davis et al., 1996; Larson, 1985; Ludlow, 2005).

CRANIAL NERVES

Motor output from the pyramidal and extrapyramidal systems and other subcortical and midbrain structures is transmitted to the cranial and spinal nerves that make up the peripheral nervous system. The larynx is innervated by cranial nerve X, the vagus (Figure 1.35), which also innervates the pharynx, palate, trachea, bronchi, lungs, heart, external ear, and parts of the gastrointestinal tract. There are two branches of the vagus that supply the intrinsic muscles of the larynx: the superior laryngeal nerve (SLN) and the recurrent laryngeal nerve (RLN).

The SLN has internal and external branches. The internal branch is sensory, and the external is motor, innervating the cricothyroid muscle. The other four intrinsic muscles are innervated by the RLN. This nerve is asymmetrical in its pathway. The right side extends into the chest where it loops underneath the subclavian artery of the heart and then courses upward alongside the trachea to enter the larynx. The left side extends even lower into the chest, winding underneath the aorta of the heart and then running upward to the larynx. The diameters of the nerve fibers in the right and left branches of the RLN also differ. Some authors have reported that the nerve fibers in the left RLN are larger in diameter than those on the right, possibly to compensate for the longer length, which could otherwise delay the arrival of the nerve impulse to the target muscle (Sataloff, 2005). Other researchers have found that the right RLN is larger in fiber area and perimeter than the left, and that any differences in conduction time between the right and left branches are insignificant in terms of vocal motor control (Jotz, de Campos, Rodrigues, & Xavier, 2011). The fact that the nerve runs so close to the heart means that it is also susceptible to damage from heart problems such as congestive heart failure and aortic aneurysms. Because the left side is longer than the right it is more susceptible to injury. In addition, the recurrent laryngeal nerve runs close to the thyroid gland and is prone to injury from thyroid surgery. Thus, trauma to the heart, lungs, and thyroid gland can affect vocal function. Damage to the superior and/or recurrent laryngeal nerves results in weakness or paralysis of laryngeal muscles.

REFLEXES

Laryngeal reflexes are important in laryngeal functions involved in airway protection. There are many different types of sensory nerve endings in the mucosal layers, joints, and muscles of the larynx. These nerve endings, called receptors, respond to different stimuli such as touch, movement, vibration, changes in air pressure, and chemicals. When stimulated, the receptors react by initiating a tight, reflexive closure of the laryngeal valves (the laryngeal adductor reflex) that protects the airway from foreign objects, or that forces the person to cough and expel the object (Aviv et al., 1999). In addition to airway protection, laryngeal reflexes may exert an influence on phonation. For example, within the laryngeal joints and muscles are proprioceptors that help to control laryngeal muscle tone (Ludlow, 2005). Sapir and colleagues (2000) proposed that the muscular and structural adjustments that occur during speech production may stimulate sensory receptors in the intrinsic and extrinsic laryngeal muscles, as well as in the mucosa, joints, and ligaments within and outside the larynx. These reflexes in turn influence vocal fold adduction, vocal fold length and tension, and subglottal air pressure levels. While laryngeal reflexes appear to play an important role in normal vocal

FIGURE 1.35 **Vagus Nerve**

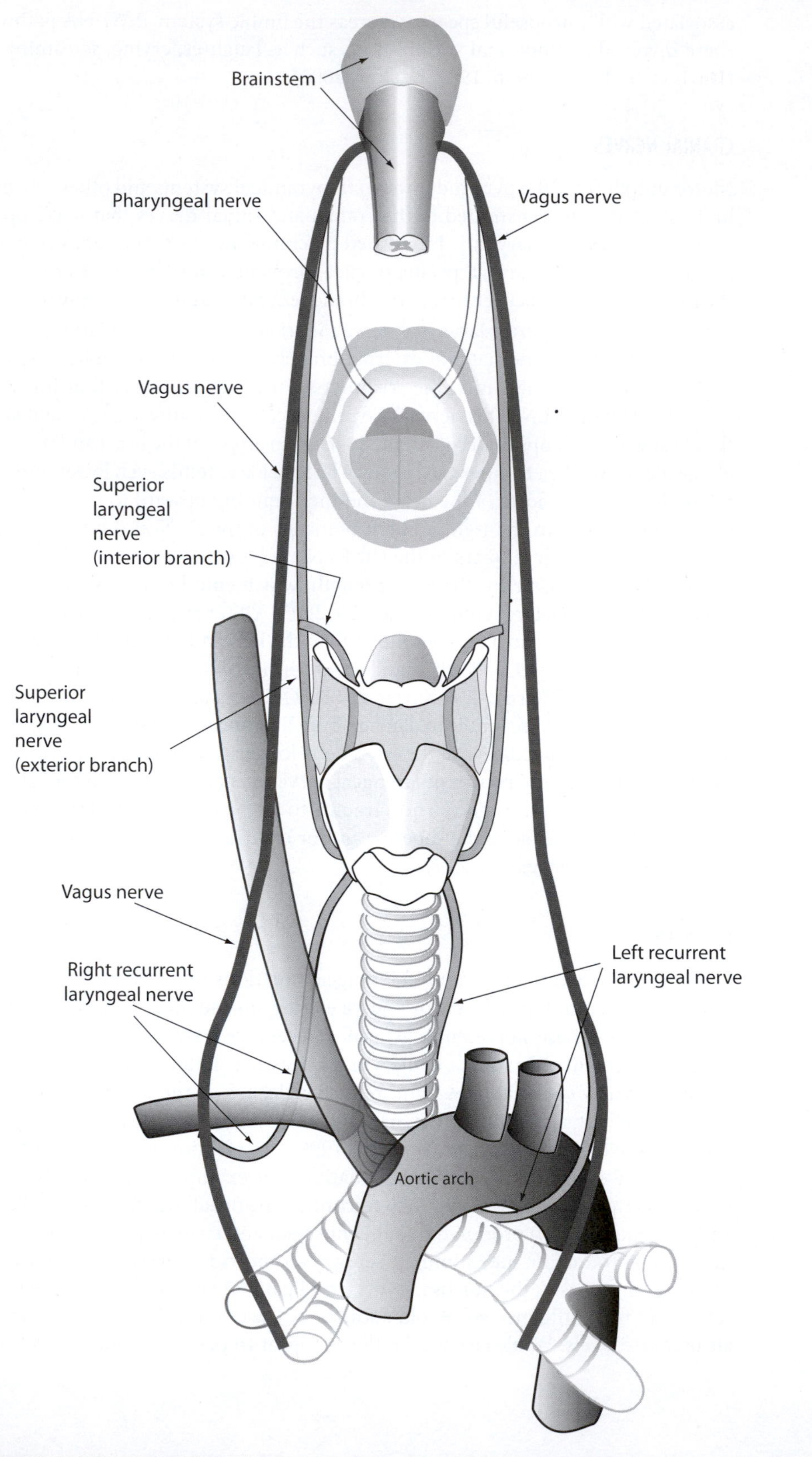

motor control, it has been suggested that lack of appropriate inhibition of these reflexes may be involved in disorders such as spasmodic dysphonia, hyperfunctional dysphonia, voice tremor, and stuttering. Dysfunctional muscle activity may occur because phonation produces vibration not only of the vocal folds themselves, but of all the adjacent tissues in the larynx. Because the sensory receptors in these tissues are stimulated by vibration, the reflexes must be inhibited during phonation so as not to interfere with voice production (Luschei, Ramig, Baker, & Smith, 1999).

Vocal Registers

The term **vocal register** is used widely in both singing and speech production contexts. In the singing context the term is used extremely loosely and can refer to a particular part of a singer's vocal range, a resonance area (e.g., head voice, chest voice), a particular vocal quality, or a region of the voice defined by vocal breaks (Echternach et al., 2010; McKinney, 1994). In the context of speech production, the term is more clearly defined in relation to voice physiology, acoustic and aerodynamic parameters of voice production, and perceptual characteristics. Much of the early research on registers in speech production was conducted by Hollien and his colleagues (e.g., Damste, Hollien, Moore, & Murry, 1968; Hollien, 1960, 1974; Hollien & Curtis, 1960; Hollien & Michel, 1968; Hollien & Moore, 1960; Hollien, Moore, Wendahl, & Michel, 1966; etc.). As used in speech contexts, a register refers to a particular range of vocal fundamental frequencies. Three registers are typically identified: pulse (also called glottal fry, vocal fry, or creak), modal, and loft (also called falsetto). Pulse is the lowest register, modal refers to the middle range of frequencies most often used in conversational speech, and loft is the highest register (Table 1.11). Each register has a distinctive perceptual quality associated with it, and each is produced by a different mode of vocal fold vibration. Some studies have found that there is little or no overlap between fundamental frequencies in different registers (e.g., Baken, 2005; Blomgren, Chen, Ng, & Gilbert, 1998; Hollien, 1974), while other researchers have reported that despite the differences in vocal quality, overlap can occur between fundamental frequencies across different registers (e.g., Riede & Zuberbuhle, 2003; Roubeau, Henrich, & Castellengo, 2009).

TABLE *1.11* **Registers**

	Modal	Pulse (Glottal Fry)	Loft (Falsetto)
Frequency	80–150 Hz (male)	30–80 Hz	> 300 Hz (m)
	180–230 Hz (female)		
	220–300 Hz (child)		> 500 Hz (f)
PTP	2–7.5 cm H_2O	2–5 cm H_2O	6–8 cm H_2O
Duty cycle	50/50	90/10	Never completely closed

Note: PTP: phonation threshold pressure.

MODAL REGISTER

Hollien and colleagues were the first to use the term **modal register** because it includes the range of frequencies typically used in speaking (i.e., the mode). This register is characterized by full participation of the cover and body during vibration. Individuals are able to generate the greatest range of intensities in this register. The duty cycle is characterized by relatively rapid onset, with a brief open phase followed by a longer closing phase and a short closed phase (Hollien, 1974). In this register PTP has been reported as around 2–7.5 cm H_2O (Blomgren et al., 1998; Jiang et al., 1999). The complete range of fundamental frequencies in modal register is around 75–450 Hz in men and around 130–520 Hz in women (Baken, 2005). Average speaking frequencies used in modal register have been reported as 211 Hz (range 175–266 Hz) for adult women and 117 Hz (range 86–170 Hz) for adult men (Blomgren et al., 1998).

PULSE REGISTER

Pulse register comprises the lowest range of fundamental frequencies an individual is able to produce. Males and females generate similar F0s averaging around 48 Hz (Blomgren et al., 1998). This is approximately one octave below the frequencies for the normal modal register for a male (Blomgren et al., 1998). To achieve this extremely low frequency the vocal folds are short and thick, and they vibrate extremely slowly. In addition, the false vocal folds appear to come into contact with the true folds, thus increasing the vibrating mass and decreasing the fundamental frequency (Blomgren et al., 1998; Hollien, 1974). The medial edges of the folds are loosely adducted, resulting in a decreased PTP, with reported values ranging from approximately 2 cm H_2O (Zemlin, 1998) to 5.5 cm H_2O (Blomgren et al., 1998). It has been proposed that the low F0 may be primarily determined by changes in subglottal air pressure, rather than by vocal fold length and tension (Blomgren et al., 1998; Riede & Zuberbuhle, 2003). In terms of the duty cycle the vocal folds are adducted for most (90%) of the cycle. Glottal opening and closing movements together only account for about 10% of the cycle. In addition, the vocal folds vibrate in a different manner than they do in modal. Instead of opening and closing the glottis once per cycle, they may approximate and separate partially once, twice, or three times (Blomgren et al., 1998) before completely adducting, a phenomenon known as multiphasic closure. This form of vibration results in the distinctive low-pitched, popping sound of pulse register.

LOFT REGISTER

Loft register comprises the highest range of fundamental frequencies and has been reported as 275–620 Hz in men and 490–1130 Hz in women (Baken, 2005). To achieve this very high frequency the cricothyroid muscle exerts a great deal of longitudinal tension. High-speed photography has shown that the folds appear very long and stiff, thin and sharp along the edges, with a tight and narrow glottis (Hollien, 1974; Van den Berg, 1958). The cover of the folds is lax, while the vocal ligament is tensed (Titze, 1994). The extreme tension on the vocal ligaments prevents the folds from adducting completely during vibration, resulting in reduced amplitude of vibration and a somewhat breathy quality. The extreme stiffness also results in a higher PTP of around 6–8 cm H_2O (Solomon & Di Mattia, 2000). In addition, because of the extreme tension on the vocal ligaments, the vocal ligament and body of the folds do not vibrate as fully as they do in modal and pulse registers, resulting in a less complex vibration and a thinner quality to the sound.

It is important to keep in mind that individuals make use of all three registers during speech and singing. Although modal is most commonly used for normal conversational speech, it is not unusual for individuals to drop their pitch into the pulse register at the ends of phrases and sentences, or to raise their pitch into the loft register when very excited. However, when either pulse or loft becomes the primary register used for conversational speech, this can create problems that may need to be remediated by a voice therapist.

chapter SUMMARY

THE RESPIRATORY SYSTEM provides the airstream that forms the basis of all voice and speech production. The respiratory system encompasses the oral and nasal cavities, pharynx, larynx, trachea, bronchi, bronchioles, alveolar sacs, and the lungs. The thorax and lungs act as an integrated unit due to pleural linkage. Thus, whenever the thoracic cavity is moved by active or passive forces, the lungs are moved as well. Inhalation and exhalation occur as alveolar pressure within the lungs increases and decreases, forcing air to either enter or exit the respiratory system. Lung volumes and capacities provide a way of categorizing volumes of air inhaled and exhaled through the respiratory system. Lung volumes include single, nonoverlapping quantities, while lung capacities comprise two or more volumes. Five major changes occur when switching from life to speech breathing, including location of air intake, ratio of time for inhalation versus exhalation, volume of air inspired, muscle activity for exhalation, and abdominal displacement.

The larynx is a small hollow, tubelike structure situated between the 3rd–7th cervical vertebrae in the adult. It is held in place in the neck by a complex system of extrinsic muscles. It is made up of interconnecting cartilages, ligaments, membranes, and intrinsic muscles, and houses three sets of soft tissue folds. Two pairs of synovial joints and five intrinsic laryngeal muscles allow the cartilages of the larynx to change positions relative to each other and thus to adduct, abduct, lengthen, and shorten the vocal folds. The vocal folds are complex layered structures composed of epithelium, connective tissue, and muscle. They abduct to open the glottis for respiration and for the production of voiceless sounds, and adduct to close the glottis for swallowing and for the production of voiced sounds. The myoelastic-aerodynamic theory describes one cycle of vocal fold vibration as an interaction of muscle forces, elastic recoil forces, and aerodynamic forces. Laryngeal function is controlled by the central and peripheral nervous systems. In addition to cortical areas, many subcortical and midbrain areas are involved in phonation, including the basal ganglia, cerebellum, periaqueductal grey, nucleus retroambiguus, and nucleus ambiguus. The final common pathway to the laryngeal and other muscles involved in phonation is made up of the cranial nerves, primarily the vagus nerve and its branches. Within the larynx itself, sensory receptors in the muscles, tissues, and joints are involved in reflexes that affect vocal fold closure and other functions.

Vocal registers refer to a particular range of vocal fundamental frequencies. Three registers are typically identified: pulse (also called glottal fry, vocal fry, or creak), modal, and loft (also called falsetto). Pulse is the lowest register, modal refers to the middle range of frequencies most often used in conversational speech, and loft is the highest register. Although modal is most commonly used for normal conversational speech, it is not unusual for individuals to drop their pitch into the pulse register at the ends of phrases and sentences, or to raise their pitch into the loft register when very excited. However, when either pulse or loft becomes the primary register used for conversational speech, this can create problems that may need to be remediated by a voice therapist.

review QUESTIONS

1. Explain how the lungs and thorax act as an integrated unit.
2. Describe the mechanics of inhalation and exhalation.
3. Define resting expiratory level and then identify the lung volumes and capacities.
4. List and explain the differences between breathing for life and breathing for speech.
5. Compare and contrast the aryepiglottic, false, and true vocal folds.
6. Describe the myoelastic-aerodynamic theory of vocal fold vibration and explain the occurrence of the mucosal wave.
7. Explain the mechanics of pitch and loudness regulation.
8. Identify and describe the cortical and subcortical structures important for phonation.
9. Describe the path of the vagus nerve and its role in phonation.
10. Compare the perceptual and acoustic characteristics of modal, pulse, and loft registers.

Chapter 2
Lifespan Changes in the Respiratory and Phonatory Systems

LEARNING OBJECTIVES

1. Identify similarities and differences between respiratory function in infants, children, and adults.
2. Describe structural differences between the infant and the mature larynx.
3. Identify changes in voice that occur during puberty.
4. Explain the influence of hormonal changes on voice.
5. Understand the structural and functional changes that occur within the larynx due to aging.

The voice changes dramatically over the lifespan, from the high-pitched crying of the infant to the thin, quavery voice often associated with the very old. These changes occur as the structures of the respiratory and laryngeal systems develop, mature, and decline, in conjunction with changes in neuromotor control of respiration and phonation. Other factors such as an individual's overall health, the type and amount of voice use, smoking, consumption of alcohol, presence of gastric reflux, and the individual's psychological state can also profoundly influence the voice over the course of time. This chapter focuses on changes in the structure and function of the respiratory and laryngeal systems, and the corresponding acoustic and perceptual characteristics of the changing voice over the lifespan.

Development and Maturation of Speech Breathing

Like other neuromotor skills, efficient speech breathing is a process that develops over time in conjunction with anatomical and physiological changes in the young child's respiratory system. Speech breathing has been conceptualized as progressing through periods of emergence, refinement, and adaptation (Boliek, Hixon, Watson, & Jones, 2009). The emergence period extends from birth to age 3 years. During this period infants and young children demonstrate some of the same breathing features for vocalization and speech as do older children, adolescents, and adults. These include initiating vocalizations in the midrange of predicted VC and at the beginning of the exhalation (Boliek, Hixon, Watson, & Morgan, 1996, 1997; Hoit, Hixon, Watson, & Morgan, 1990). Refinement is defined as the time during which speech in the young child has emerged but continues to progress toward the adult model (Boliek et al., 2009). Many changes occur during the emergence and refinement stages in terms of both structure and function of the respiratory system. These include increases in the size of the lungs with associated increases in lung volumes (Table 2.1); increases in the diameter and relative stiffness of

TABLE 2.1 Selected Respiratory Measurements Expressed in Liters at Different Ages (total lung capacity—TLC, vital capacity—VC, inspiratory capacity—IC, functional residual capacity—FRC, expiratory reserve volume—ERV, residual volume—RV, resting tidal volume—RTV)

Measure	Age	Male Mean	Female Mean
TLC	7	2.12	2.07
	10	3.14	2.98
	13	4.33	3.74
	16	6.20	4.98
	25	6.74	5.03
	50	7.05	5.31
	75	6.63	4.86
VC	7	1.67	1.58
	10	2.51	2.34
	13	3.55	2.99
	16	5.08	3.78
	25	5.35	3.93
	50	5.09	3.60
	75	4.47	2.94
IC	7	1.14	1.09
	10	1.74	1.55
	13	2.37	2.05
	16	3.26	2.43

TABLE 2.1 **(Continued)**

Measure	Age	Male Mean	Female Mean
	25	3.62	2.61
	50	3.59	2.38
	75	3.19	2.27
FRC	7	0.98	0.97
	10	1.40	1.43
	13	1.97	1.69
	16	2.94	2.56
	25	3.12	2.42
	50	3.46	2.93
	75	3.44	2.59
ERV	7	0.53	0.48
	10	0.77	0.78
	13	1.18	0.94
	16	1.81	1.35
	25	1.73	1.32
	50	1.50	1.22
	75	1.28	0.67
RV	7	0.45	0.49
	10	0.63	0.64
	13	0.79	0.76
	16	1.12	1.21
	25	1.39	1.10
	50	1.97	1.71
	75	2.16	1.92
RTV	7	0.20	0.19
	10	0.26	0.28
	13	0.39	0.35
	16	0.56	0.41
	25	0.56	0.46
	50	0.71	0.55
	75	0.53	0.54

Sources: Information from Hoit et al. (1989, 1990); Hoit & Hixon (1987).

the airways with an overall decrease in airway resistance; and ossification of the ribs, spinal column, and sternum resulting in increased chest wall stiffness and compliance of the respiratory system (Boliek et al., 2009). During the **adaptation period** the child's efficiency in breathing for speech continues to become increasingly adultlike as he or she continues to grow physically and, at the same time, becomes more linguistically adept.

While there are some similarities in speech breathing behaviors between younger and older children and adults, there are also many differences. Because of their smaller airways, young children generate higher pressures for speech than older children, and older children often use higher pressures than adults (Stathopoulos, 1986). In addition, young children tend to inhale more deeply and begin speaking at larger lung volumes than older children and adults (Solomon & Charron, 1998). This may be in order to take advantage of higher passive recoil forces at relatively high lung volumes. In addition to initiating speech at higher lung volumes, children sometimes end breath groups below REL (Boliek et al., 2009). The larger lung volumes are reflected in the percentages of VC children use for speech purposes compared to adults. Solomon and Charron (1998) found that infants use 25% and toddlers 13% of their predicted VC for a variety of vocalizations. Hoit et al. (1990) reported that 7-year-old children used approximately 18% VC for reading and conversational speech compared to older children who used 12–18% VC.

Children and adults use different amounts of rib-cage versus abdominal movement to change lung volumes for speech. Older children and adults use greater rib-cage than abdominal movement while infants use larger abdominal volumes (Solomon & Charron, 1998). As the child grows and the rib cage and abdomen become increasingly independent and less tightly coupled during speech breathing, the percentage of rib-cage contribution to volume change becomes systematically greater. Table 2.2 shows percentage of rib-cage contribution increasing from around 50% at age 4 years to 70–80% at age 16 years.

Changes in the respiratory system continue throughout the lifespan, including changes in lung volumes and capacities in young, middle-aged, and older adults (Table 2.1).

TABLE 2.2 Mean Percentage of Rib-Cage Contribution (% RC) to Volume Change in Resting Tidal Breathing at Different Ages

Age	Male	Female
4	52.85	52.85
5	61.35	61.35
6	51.07	51.07
7	69.36	60.50
10	64.64	59.51
13	75.51	63.39
16	71.23	80.44
25	80.95	69.71
50	80.59	79.38
75	85.02	89.39

Sources: Information from Boliek et al. (2009); Hoit & Hixon (1987); Hoit et al. (1989, 1990).

Other structural and physiological changes occur with aging, including a more convex thoracic shape, increased ossification and calcification of the costal cartilages, decreased strength of the respiratory muscles, loss of alveolar surface tension and pulmonary capillary blood volume, and decreased overall lung size (Huber & Spruill, 2008; Sperry & Klich, 1992). These changes result in decreased chest wall compliance, diminished elastic recoil pressures in the mid lung volume range, and reduced VC (e.g., Hoit & Hixon, 1987; Huber, 2008; Huber & Spruill, 2008; Sperry & Klich, 1992). To overcome this disadvantage, older adults have been shown to initiate speech at higher lung volumes (i.e., inhale more deeply) with correspondingly higher recoil pressures. In comparison to younger adults, older adults have been reported to demonstrate larger rib-cage and lung volume initiations and excursions, larger volumes of air expended per speech breath and per syllable, and fewer syllables per breath than younger adults (Hoit & Hixon, 1987; Hoit, Hixon, Altman, & Morgan, 1989; Huber & Spruill, 2008). One reason for initiating speech at higher lung volumes may be that inspiratory muscle force is better preserved than expiratory muscle function. Thus, it may be easier for older adults to achieve higher lung volumes to begin speech, rather than to use expiratory muscle effort to go to lower lung volumes (Huber & Spruill, 2008). Huber and Spruill (2008) noted that older adults also moved the abdomen for speech breathing more than younger adults, possibly as a compensation for the reduced elastic recoil. However, despite the changes in respiratory function with aging, healthy older adults are typically well able to generate and maintain adequate respiratory support for speech.

Structure and Function of the Larynx in Infancy and Childhood

Embryologically, the larynx is essentially developed by the end of the first trimester of pregnancy (Sataloff, Spiegel, & Caputo Rosen, 1998). However, there are many differences between the structure of the larynx at the time of birth and the more mature organ in terms of position of the larynx in the neck, shape and size of laryngeal cartilages, vocal fold length, and histological composition of the vocal folds (Table 2.3).

POSITION IN NECK

The position of the larynx in the neck, relative to the cervical vertebrae, is considerably higher in infants than in older children and adults. At birth and in early infancy the larynx is positioned at around the level of C3 to C4. The larynx gradually descends as the pharynx becomes longer and wider with maturation (Stemple, Glaze, & Klaben, et al., 2000) and continues to descend throughout life in both sexes. By puberty, the larynx is positioned at the level of C6 to C7.

CARTILAGES

At birth, the hyoid bone and cartilages are soft and flexible due to the small amount of calcium present in the structures. The hyoid bone in newborns overlaps the thyroid cartilage (Sapienza, Ruddy, & Baker, 2004), whereas in the mature larynx the two are separated by the fully developed thyrohyoid membrane. The immature hyoid is more pliable as it is not

TABLE 2.3 Characteristics of the Infant Larynx

Framework
Thyroid and hyoid attached
Bulky omega-shaped epiglottis
Position in neck
C3–C4
Vocal folds
1.25–3 mm
Undifferentiated lamina propria
F0
400–600 Hz

yet calcified and the horns of the hyoid have yet to develop. The thyroid cartilage is flatter in the immature larynx because the vertical prominence has not yet developed (Sapienza et al., 2004). The space between the thyroid and cricoid cartilages is small but will enlarge as the cricothyroid membrane grows. The arytenoid cartilages attain a larger size earlier than the other laryngeal cartilages and their relative size appears greater in the immature larynx than the mature larynx (Figure 2.1). In the infant the epiglottis is bulky and omega shaped, and only develops the adult shape by puberty. In addition, the infant epiglottis often touches the soft palate and is closer to the base of the tongue (Sapienza et al., 2004). Gradually the laryngeal skeleton separates and ossification of the hyoid bone and other cartilages begins.

VOCAL FOLDS

The vocal folds change over time in their overall length, in the relative proportions of the membranous and cartilaginous glottis, as well as in their histological composition (Figure 2.2). The newborn's vocal folds measure around 1.25 to 3 mm and the membranous and cartilaginous portions of the glottis are approximately equal (Sapienza et al., 2004; Stemple et al., 2000).

By adulthood, the female overall vocal fold length is 11–15 mm, and the male length is 17–21 mm. The cartilaginous portion in both males and females is around 2–3 mm, so the majority of growth in vocal fold length occurs in the membranous vocal folds. In addition, the downward tilt of the immature vocal folds becomes level in the mature larynx. In the infant, the mucosal cover of the vocal folds is very thick in relation to its length, and the intermediate and deep layers of the lamina propria are not differentiated into collagenous and elastic fibers (Colton, Casper, & Leonard, 2006; Mathieson, 2001; Sapienza et al., 2004). Tissue differentiation starts to develop between the ages of 1 to 4 years and is complete only by the end of puberty.

Infant and adult larynges also differ in terms of the narrowest portion of the larynx. In young children, the area below the vocal folds is the narrowest portion of the airway, with a diameter of approximately 4 mm (Sapienza et al., 2004). In adults the narrowest section of the

FIGURE 2.1 **Immature and Mature Larynx**

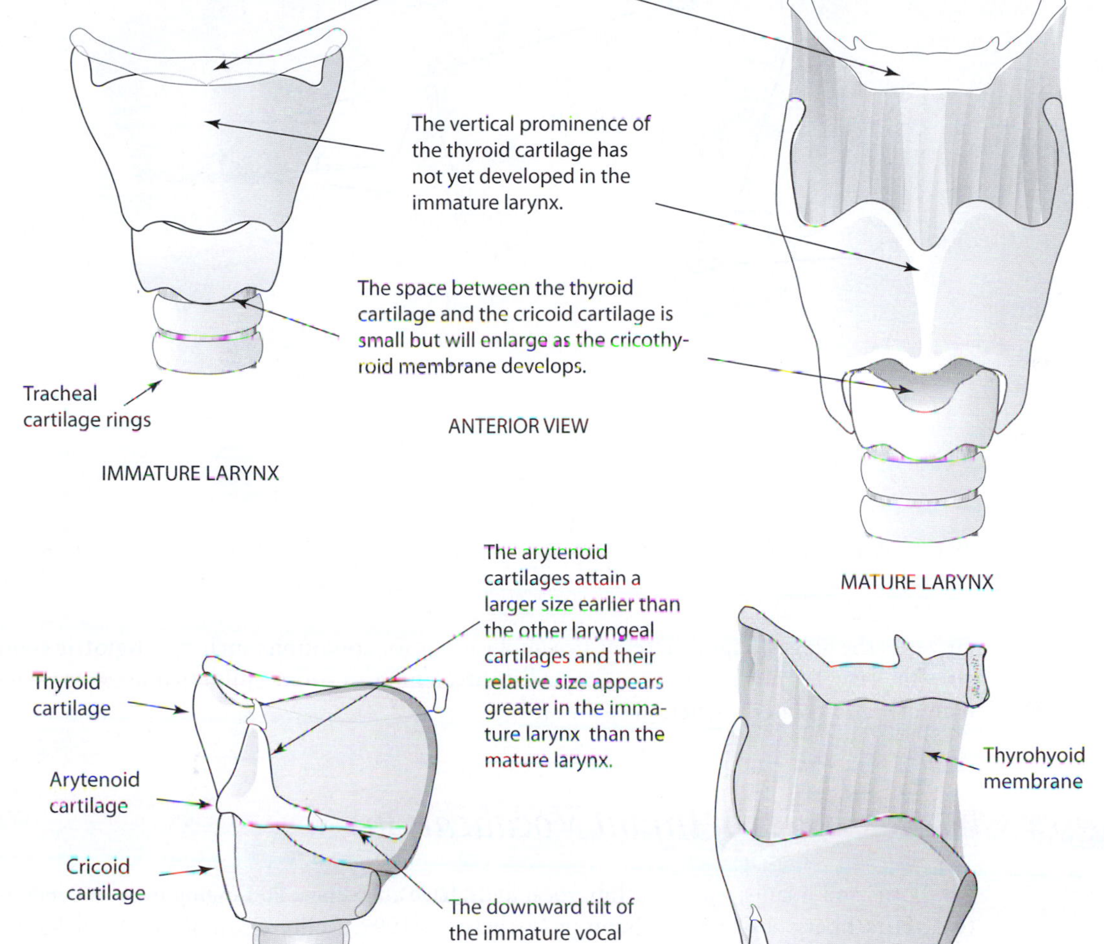

These illustrations highlight some of the major differences between the immature and the mature larynx. The relative increase in size would actually be greater than shown here. For the sake of clarity, the immature larynx has been depicted at a larger than true relative size.

FIGURE 2.2 **Infant Versus Adult Vocal Folds**

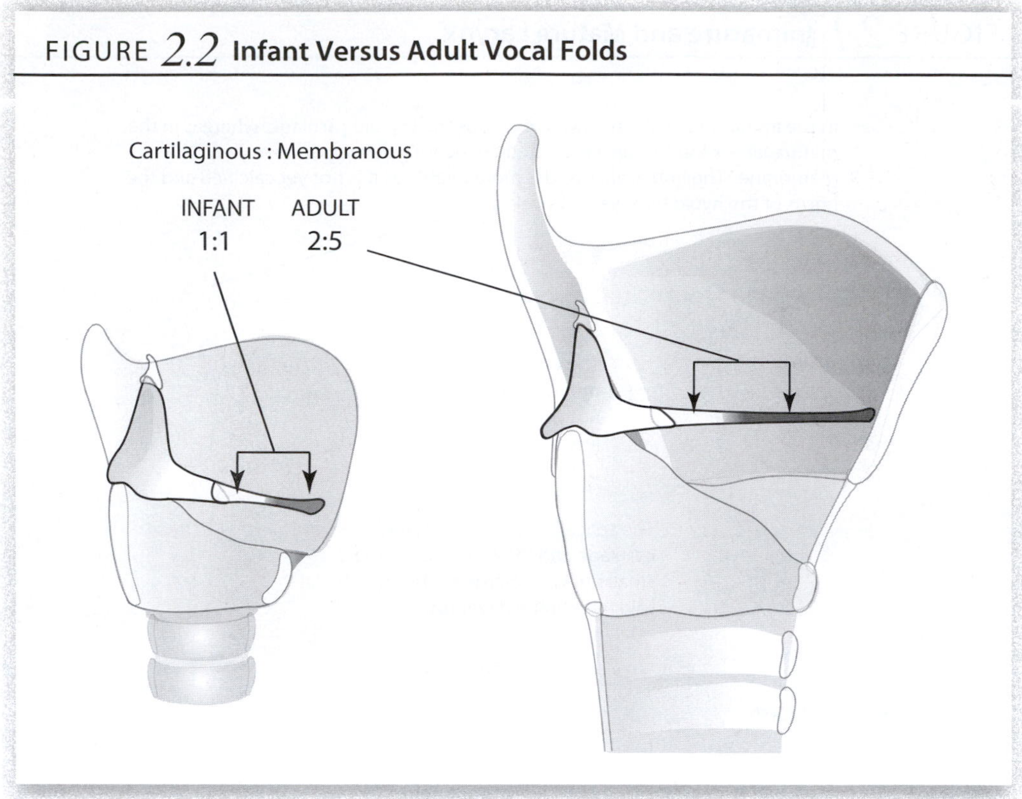

airway is the glottis. This difference has implications for conditions such as **subglottic stenosis**, which can be much more severe, even life threatening, in young children due to the smaller diameter and greater restriction of the airway.

Acoustic Characteristics of Infant Vocalizations

Newborns and infants, with their tiny vocal folds, have an average F0 ranging from 400–600 Hz (e.g., Hirschberg, 1999; Michelsson & Michelsson, 1999; Robb, Crowell, & Dunn-Rankin, 2007). A decrease in F0 with maturation is expected, given the increasing length and thickness of the developing vocal folds. However, F0 tends to be variable over the course of the child's first six months (Baeck & de Souza, 2006; Gilbert & Robb, 1996).

The F0 of infant cries and other vocalizations yields considerable information about the baby's neurological, physiological, and maturational status. Crying is a complex laryngeal motor activity occurring during exhalation, which requires the coordinated functioning of respiratory, laryngeal, and supralaryngeal muscles (Branco, Behlau, & Rehder, 2005). At birth and for the first weeks of life the vocalizations appear to be reflex indications of the infant's internal status, operating in an "on-off" manner with few changes in intensity and duration (Gilbert & Robb, 1996; Michelsson & Michelsson, 1999). At this early stage of life the baby does not have much neuromuscular control over laryngeal function, and most of the sounds he or she produces are cries, coughs, and burps. As the child gains more control, he or she is able to produce a more varied repertoire of sounds, as well as a wider range of pitch and loudness levels. Some different types of vocalizations that have been identified as the baby matures include cry, short cry, coo, wail, moan, squeal, laugh, croak, and raspberry (Scheiner, Hammerschmidt, Jurgens, & Zwimer, 2002). With continued development the baby cries in a more purposeful and goal-directed manner in response to hunger, pain, discomfort, fright, and distress.

One reason for the interest in the infant cry is the information cries provide regarding nervous system status and physiological function. Maturation of the nervous system allows the infant a greater degree of laryngeal muscle control as well as greater control over subglottal air pressure (Scheiner et al., 2002). Researchers have reported that F0 is increased in premature infants, and the more immature the baby, the higher the F0. Two reasons have been proposed to explain this phenomenon. First, the higher F0 in premature infants may be related to the smaller vocal folds resulting from size differences at birth (Goberman & Robb, 1999). Second, preterm infants may display a more stressful response to pain stimuli (Goberman & Robb, 1999). Pain crying is characterized by an increase of tension in the laryngeal, pharyngeal, supraglottic, and facial muscles (Branco, Fekete, Rugolo, & Rehder, 2007). The increased tension has the effect of raising F0. F0 is also higher in babies with diseases affecting the central nervous system (Lind & Wermke, 2002; Michelsson & Michelsson, 1999) and in malnourished infants who presumably sustained nervous system damage resulting from the malnutrition (Donzelli et al., 1994). In some conditions such as **apnea of infancy (AOI)**, the baby's F0 may be lower than expected. AOI is defined as an unexplained cessation of breathing for 20 s or longer, or a shorter respiratory pause in breathing accompanied by **bradycardia** (slowness of the heartbeat), **cyanosis** (purplish coloration of the skin and mucous membrane due to deficient oxygenation of the blood), pallor, and/or marked hypotonia (Robb et al., 2007). Robb et al. (2007) compared pain-induced crying episodes of healthy infants to those with AOI. They reported an average F0 of 463 Hz for the healthy babies compared to 435 Hz for the unhealthy babies and ascribed the lower F0 to a decrease in laryngeal muscle tone. They also found that infants with AOI took a longer time to respond to the stimulus than the healthy infants, reflecting a longer time for the nervous system to interpret the pain stimulus.

Infant crying is important not only for survival but also as the beginning of human vocal communication (Michelsson & Michelsson, 1999). Researchers have related early vocalizations to the beginning of speechlike behaviors. Scheiner et al. (2002) proposed five preverbal stages in the infant's vocal development. In stage 1 (0–1 month) there is no systematic differentiation between opening and closing of the vocal tract. In stage 2 (2–3 months) different types of vocalizations start to occur, including the first appearance of laughing. In stage 3 (4–6 months) the baby starts to engage in vocal play, exploring sounds such as squealing, growling, and producing noises by blowing air, food, or saliva through the pharynx and oral cavities. Babbling starts to occur in stage 4 (7–10 months), and stage 5 (11 months) sees an expansion of babbling with alternating syllables and different consonantal and vocalic elements. Buder et al. (2008) noted the existence of at least three recognizable categories of phonation types occurring in most infants: a mid-pitch category (vowel-like sounds, full vowels, or quasivowels); a high-pitch category (squeals or squeaks); and a category that can be either low or mid pitch with a very harsh vocal quality (growls). The authors speculated that these vocalization types may represent the first contrastive vocal categories that are created by the infant, and thus reflect an early ability to form the phonemes of language.

Childhood

In the childhood years the larynx starts to increase in size and to descend in the neck. The vocal folds lengthen, and differentiation of the layers of the lamina propria begins. The primary acoustic manifestation of these changes is a drop in F0 from the infant level to around 230–250 Hz by the preteen years. Table 2.4 displays the average F0 of boys and girls at various ages reported in the literature. Table 2.5 shows the decrease in F0s of boys and girls measured in a longitudinal study initially at ages 6, 8, and 10 years, and again 42 months later. The data in Table 2.4

TABLE 2.4 F0 (in Hz) for Boys and Girls Reported in the Literature for Different Age Groups

Author(s)	Age	Boys/Girls/Combined	F0
Weinrich et al. (2005)	6.0–6.11	C	248.3
	7.0–7.11	C	271.5
	8.0–8.11	C	294.4
	9.0–9.11	C	278.4
	10.0–10.11	C	266.9
Nicollas et al. (2007)	6	B	268.90
	6	G	260.92
	7	B	252.70
	7	G	255.98
	8	B	259.42
	8	G	282.83
	9	B	233.04
	9	G	264.28
	10	B	255.23
	10	G	251.73
	11	B	228.70
	11	G	244.84
	12	B	234.42
	12	G	239.43
Whiteside et al. (2002)	6	B	264.6
	6	G	239.6
	8	B	250.6
	8	G	251.8
	10	B	222.4
	10	G	231.3

TABLE 2.4 (Continued)

Author(s)	Age	Boys/Girls/Combined		F0
Whiteside & Hodgson	6	B		248.80
(2000)	6	G		242.43
	8	B		255.43
	8	G		234.40
	10	B		223.95
	10	G		226.98
Ferrand & Bloom (1996)	3–4	B		256.91
	3–4	G		249.43
	5–6	B		256.09
	5–6	G		243.07
	7–8	B		234.36
	7–8	G		252.75
	9–10	B		240.50
	9–10	G		253.81
Chen et al. (2009)	4	C	/a/	334.00
			/i/	358.00
			conv	297.00
			story	307.00
			play	418.00

TABLE 2.5 Changes in F0 (in Hz) over a 42-Month Period, from First Measurement (M1) to Second Measurement (M2)

	Age at M1	F0 at M1	Age at M2	F0 at M2	Change
Boys	6	264.6	10	211.7	52.9
Girls	6	239.6	10	205.8	33.8
Boys	8	250.6	12	194.7	55.9
Girls	8	251.8	12	193.1	58.7
Boys	10	222.4	14	163.9	58.5
Girls	10	231.3	14	204.1	27.2

Source: Information from Whiteside et al. (2002).

demonstrate a range of F0s for children ages 4–12 years, ranging from a low of 222 Hz to a high of 418 Hz. Inspection of Table 2.5 indicates a consistent decrease in F0 from ages 6 to 14 years for both boys and girls. At age 6 the F0 is around 265 Hz for boys and 240 Hz for girls. By age 14 the F0 has decreased in boys by over 100 Hz to approximately 164 Hz; F0 in girls has decreased by around 36 Hz to 204 Hz.

Other acoustic parameters of children's voices that have been examined include **harmonics-to-noise ratios (HNR)** and vocal dynamic capabilities. Children have been reported to obtain significantly lower harmonics-to-noise ratios than adults (e.g., Ferrand, 2000; Glaze, Bless, Milenkovic, & Susser, 1988). Young children also have been shown to have restricted dynamic vocal capabilities compared to adults (McAllister, Sederholm, Sundberg, & Gramming, 1994). These differences likely result from the anatomically immature structure of children's vocal folds, including the less differentiated lamina propria, the different ratios of the length of the membranous and cartilaginous glottis, as well as the high F0s, which result in fewer glottal source harmonics (Ferrand, 2000).

Puberty

Puberty is a time of enormous growth and change affecting many bodily systems including the larynx. Growth is regulated by the male and female sex hormones, which can be classified as **androgens** (male) or **estrogens** (female). These classes of hormones are present in both males and females, although in different proportions. Greater levels of androgens (testosterone) are found in males, and greater levels of estrogen are present in females. While laryngeal growth occurs in both sexes, it is particularly pronounced in males due to the release of androgens (Gugatschka et al., 2010; Puts, Hodges, Cardenas, & Gaulin, 2007; Raj, Gupta, Chowdhury, & Chadha, 2010). Growth of the laryngeal cartilages contributes to the overall enlargement of the larynx, with male larynges increasing two to three times more than their female counterparts in both anteroposterior dimensions and weight (Kahane, 1982). The vocal folds also grow in length with a reported average increase of 11.57 mm in males and 4.16 mm in females (Kahane, 1982). This translates into an increase of 63% for males and 34% in females (Kahane, 1982). The angle of the thyroid cartilage also changes differentially. In the male larynx the angle decreases to a more acute 90 degrees, while the female remains at 120 degrees. This change in angle contributes to the more noticeable "Adam's apple" in males. In both sexes the shape of the epiglottis changes, becoming both larger and flatter.

During this time of growth and change the vocal ligament continues the process of differentiating into separate layers with different cellular compositions. In addition, the larynx descends to the level of C6 or C7, resulting in a longer vocal tract, which changes the resonating characteristics as well as the pitch of the voice.

These changes typically occur over a long period of time and are usually more noticeable in males. Boys going through the voice change tend to experience pitch breaks, during which the voice pitch abruptly shifts upward or downward. The boy may also go through periods of hoarse voice. These pitch breaks and vocal quality changes can be embarrassing for some boys, although most go through this time without any problems. In general, the male's F0 decreases steadily throughout this period. For males, the decrease in F0 corresponds to a pitch drop of around one octave, while the F0 decrease for females corresponds to a pitch drop of around 2.5 semitones.

Longitudinal studies of boys undergoing voice change have shown that the age of onset of puberty, duration, and ending time are extremely variable. Hollien, Green, and Massey,

TABLE 2.6 Stages of Voice Changes in Boys from Childhood through Puberty Based on Range of F0 (in Hz) and Average Range of Speaking F0 (SF0, in Hz)

Stage	Range of F0	Average Range SF0
1	220–698	220–260
2	208–523	220–247
3	175–440	196–233
4	147–370	175–185
5	123–311	131–165
6	98–294	110–139

Source: Information from Cooksey (2000).

(1994) reported that the majority of males in their investigation demonstrated the onset of adolescent voice change between the ages of 12.5 and 14.5 years. However, there were some who began the process as early as age 10.5 years and others whose onset did not begin until 16.5 years. The authors also noted that approximately 25% of the subjects had not completed the voice change process within the 5-year period of the study. Based on this finding Hollien et al. (1994) suggested that the completion of adolescent voice change may continue until age 18 for boys in the United States. In addition, the duration of the process was also highly variable. While the average duration of the change was 18 months, the shortest duration was 8 months, and one subject took over 4 years to complete the process.

There is some evidence that voice change in boys occurs in specific stages. Fuchs et al. (2007) proposed that prepubertal voice change can be divided into three time periods: the premutation, the mutation, and the postmutation. Typical signs of mutation include a restriction of the pitch range and an increased perception of roughness in the voice. Fuchs et al. (2007) examined 21 boys in a longitudinal study using acoustic analysis of jitter, shimmer, and other acoustic parameters reflecting noise in the voice signal. The average age at the first examination was 11.2 years, and the beginning of the mutation period occurred at an average age of 14.2 years. Fuchs et al. found that all acoustic parameters changed significantly 6 months before the actual voice changes were perceptible and suggested that this represented the premutation stage. Cooksey (2000) identified six stages that occurred in the same sequence for all boys but at variable times and rates for individuals. Each stage is characterized by its range of F0s and average speaking F0 (Table 2.6).

The Adult Voice

After puberty the voice and F0 stabilize. The larynx is fully mature at this point, with its adult size, shape, and structure, including differentiated vocal ligaments. The adult female voice is often characterized by a slight degree of **breathiness** resulting from a posterior glottal gap during vocal production (e.g., D'haeseleer, Depypere, Claeys, Wuyts, Baudonck, & Van Lierde 2011; Linville, 1992; Schneider & Bigenzahn, 2003; Sodersten & Lindestad, 1990; Sodersten, Hertegard, & Hammarberg, 1995). After puberty the female voice is subject to fluctuations resulting from cyclical hormonal changes related to menstruation. Voice is a secondary sexual characteristic influenced by fluctuating levels of estrogens, progesterone, and androgens (Abitbol, Abitbol, & Abitbol, 1999). Estrogen and progesterone act together to cause cyclical menstrual changes in women during the childbearing years. These two hormones have different effects on the larynx. Estrogen causes increased secretion of the glandular cells above and below the vocal fold edges, which reduces mucosal viscosity (Abitbol et al., 1999; D'haeseleer, Depypere, Claeys, Van Borsel, & Van Lierde, 2009; Morris, Gorham-Rowan, & Harmon, 2011). Progesterone causes reduction in secretions of the glandular epithelium and dehydration of the mucosa, as well as tissue congestion, increased mucosal viscosity, and thinning of the vocal fold mucosa (Abitbol et al., 1999; D'haeseleer et al., 2009; Morris et al., 2011). Androgens also cause a reduction in glandular secretions and loss of hydration, as well as atrophy of the laryngeal mucosa. Androgens have an irreversible masculinizing effect in women (Abitbol et al., 1999; D'haeseleer et al., 2009). The F0 in women taking testosterone for medical purposes has been reported to decrease from 228.47 Hz to 112.74 Hz (Damrose, 2008).

Postpubertal girls and women may be affected vocally by the fluctuating hormone levels during the menstrual cycle (Hamdan, Mahfoud, Sibai, & Seoud, 2009). A premenstrual vocal syndrome has been identified, characterized by vocal fatigue, decreased range with a loss of high tones, loss of vocal power, and loss of certain high harmonics (Abitbol et al., 1999). The symptoms occur in about one-third of women and usually begin approximately 4–5 days before menstruation (Raj et al., 2010). The effects may be particularly evident in singers, who have reported experiencing difficulty reaching high notes and reduced vocal flexibility during the premenstrual phase of the cycle (Morris et al., 2011; Ryan & Kenny, 2009). Not all women, however, experience vocal effects. Some of the female singers in Ryan and Kenny's study reported no significant adverse effects of their cycle, while others reported a range of problems and reductions in their vocal quality, particularly during the first seven days of the cycle. Visual evaluation of vocal fold structure and function at the time of ovulation and at the premenstrual phase has demonstrated edema of the mucosa, thickened and diminished glandular secretions, reduced amplitude of vibration, and vascular disturbances of the vocal folds (Abitbol et al., 1999). Oral contraceptive pills reduce the fluctuation of hormones across the menstrual cycle (Morris et al., 2011) and have been reported to be helpful in improving vocal quality and in reducing vocal symptoms during the menstrual cycle (e.g., Amir, Biron-Shental, Tzenker, & Barer, 2005; Ryan & Kenny, 2009). Hormonal influences during pregnancy also affect vocal production in some women. Hamdan et al. (2009) reported that during pregnancy 8–12% of the women in their study demonstrated symptoms of dysphonia including **vocal fatigue** and **hoarseness**.

The Aging Voice

The topic of the aging voice has become an important focus for researchers and clinicians over the past several decades, as the number of people over age 65 continues to increase in the United States. One question in particular is extremely important, and that is, what are the normal effects of aging on the voice, and how can they be distinguished from pathological voice changes? This question has implications for clinical diagnosis and management. Vocal aging is a complex process with many parameters that influence the rate and extent of the aging, as well

TABLE 2.7 Parameters of Vocal Aging

Structural and physiological laryngeal changes
Acoustic characteristics
Listener perception
Gender
Overall health status
Related/unrelated vocal disorders

as many consequences resulting from the vocal aging itself. Any model of vocal aging must therefore take into account many factors, including the structural and physiological changes that occur in the larynx, the individual's overall state of health, which plays an important role in the rate and extent of these changes, the acoustic characteristics that are a consequence of the structural and physiological changes, the way in which the voice is perceived by listeners, the influence of gender, and related or unrelated vocal disorders (Table 2.7).

Before discussing the structural and functional changes that occur with aging, we need to keep in mind three points. First, age-related changes do not occur suddenly. Kahane (1990) studied cellular and tissue changes in normal male and female larynges. The age of the specimens ranged from the third through the eighth decades. Age-related changes began in the thirties in males and the forties in females. As the age of the specimen increased, so did the extent of the changes. Thus, the changes tend to be very gradual and to become more pronounced with advancing age. Second, laryngeal changes are extremely variable between individuals. Individuals age at different rates and even within the same individual the rate and extent of aging varies between different bodily systems. Third, gender differentially affects the laryngeal aging process. It has been well established that males' laryngeal systems begin the decline process sooner than females,' and the amount of degeneration is greater in males than in females (Case, 2002; Linville, 2001). Women are also affected by menopause at the end of the childbearing years resulting from changes in the ratios of the sex hormones. During menopause estrogen and progesterone levels decrease and the influence of androgens becomes more pronounced (D'haeseleer et al., 2009; Lindholm, Vilkman, Raudaskoski, Suvanto-Luukkonen, & Kauppila, 1997). The increased effects of androgen result in reduced glandular secretions and loss of hydration of the vocal folds (Abitbol et al., 1999). Laryngeal symptoms that have been reported during and after menopause include vocal fatigue, decreased **vocal intensity**, decreased range, loss of timbre, muscular atrophy, thinning of the vocal fold mucosa, reduced amplitude during phonation, asymmetry of vibration between the right and left vocal folds, microvarices, reduced motion of CA joints; mild swelling of the vocal folds either of the free edges or in Reinke's space; huskiness, hoarseness, changes in vocal quality, reduced flexibility; dryness of the throat, frequent throat clearing, and lower frequency levels (Abitbol et al., 1999; Biever & Bless, 1989; D'haeseleer et al., 2009 Raj, Gupta, Chowdhury & Chadha, 2010). In addition, menopause has been associated with a higher prevalence of **gastroesophageal reflux disease (GERD)**, which affects laryngeal function (D'haeseleer et al., 2009).

STRUCTURAL CHANGES

All aspects of laryngeal structure start to show evidence of changes by the third or fourth decade of life. These structural changes can result in changes in the function of the vocal mechanism, leading to noticeable acoustic and perceptual effects. We will discuss changes that occur to the laryngeal cartilages, joints, muscles, epithelium, and lamina propria.

Cartilage. Aside from the apex and vocal processes of the arytenoid cartilages and the epiglottis, the laryngeal cartilages are composed of hyaline. This type of cartilage ossifies with age. The movements of the cartilages therefore become less flexible, potentially affecting vocal fold vibration. Ossification begins as early as the third decade and increases with advancing age (Casiano, Ruiz, & Goldstein, 2010; Fatterpekar, Mukherji, Rajgopalan, Lin, & Castillo, 2004; Mupparapu & Vuppalapati, 2005). Other researchers have found that the ossification process begins much earlier than the third decade. For example, Strauss (2000) reported finding calcification/ossification of the cricoid cartilage in the majority of the healthy children and adolescents aged 6–16 years in the study. Some researchers have reported that the thyroid cartilage is more frequently ossified than the cricoid, and that ossification is more prevalent and more extensive in men than in women (e.g., Mupparapu & Vuppalapati, 2005; Yeager, Lawson, & Archer, 1982).

Joints. Like other joints in the body, the cricoarytenoid and cricothyroid joints are subject to degenerative changes such as surface erosion, thinning of the articular surfaces, breakdown/disorganization of the collagen fibers in the cartilage matrix, changes in the synovial membrane, and surface irregularities (Hodge, Colton, & Kelley,2001; Kahn & Kahane, 1986; Linville, 2001; von Leden & Alessi, 1994). Changes of the surrounding structures such as muscular atrophy and fibrosis also affect joint function (Casiano et al., 2010). Because these changes are particularly evident in the cricoarytenoid joint, the range of motion of the arytenoid cartilages may be limited, reducing the degree and extent of vocal fold adduction and **abduction**. In addition, vocal fold movement patterns may become less smooth and less well coordinated, resulting in breathiness and/or weakness in the voice (Kahn & Kahane, 1986; Linville, 2001; Paulsen, Bernhard, & Tillmann, 1998).

Muscles. As muscles age, the muscle fibers become replaced by loose connective tissue and fat (Thomas et al., 2008; von Leden & Alessi, 1994). In particular, the thyroarytenoid muscle tends to atrophy, resulting in decreases in fiber diameter and degeneration of muscle tissue (Kersing & Jennekens, 2004). The number and size of fast twitch muscles decreases, and the remaining muscle tissue must in essence work harder to achieve the same function (Thomas et al., 2008). The speed, force, strength, and endurance of muscle contractions are lessened resulting in incomplete approximation of the vocal folds during phonation. These muscle changes probably contribute to the weak and breathy quality in some elderly speakers (Baker, Ramig, Luschei, & Smith, 1998). Changes also occur in nervous system innervation of laryngeal muscles, including a decrease in the number of motor neurons innervating the fast Type II muscle fibers; a decline in the number of myelinated and unmyelinated fibers within peripheral nerves; and changes in the thickness and regularity of the myelin sheath (Thomas et al., 2008; Tiago, Pontes, & Campones do Brasil, 2007). These changes have the effect of decreasing the speed of nerve conduction to the muscles, and thus reducing muscle efficiency.

Epithelium and Lamina Propria. There are numerous degenerative changes to the epithelium and layers of the lamina propria that contribute to vocal changes. Some of the changes are more prevalent in males; others occur more often in females. The epithelium has been reported to thicken in females (von Leden & Alessi, 1994). The epithelium may also become dehydrated, due to atrophy of the mucous glands, infiltration of fats into the glands, and fibrotic changes. Laryngeal glandular secretions are crucial in the protection and lubrication of the vocal folds (Gracco & Kahane, 1989). With aging, these secretions decrease in quantity and quality. The dry epithelium interferes with normal vocal fold vibration by increasing the stiffness of the cover (Gracco & Kahane, 1989). This can affect the regularity and symmetry of vocal fold vibration, resulting in increased vocal effort, vocal fatigue, and poorer voice quality (Linville, 2001).

The lamina propria also undergoes degenerative changes. As discussed in Chapter 1, elastin and collagen fibers are important components of the lamina propria. Collagen fibers help to maintain structural integrity, and elastic fibers give resilience and stiffness to the tissue (Linville, 2001). With aging, changes occur in the structure of these fibers as well as their relative proportions. Rather than running parallel to the edge of the vocal fold, collagen fibers separate and become irregularly arranged. Elastic fibers become fragmented and less dense, particularly in males (Linville, 2001; von Leden & Alessi, 1994). The deep layer becomes thicker, with an increase in collagen fibers (Hirano, Kurita, & Sakaguchi, 1989; von Leden & Alessi, 1994). These changes in the lamina propria may alter the viscoelastic properties of the vocal folds (Pontes, Brasolotto, & Behlau, 2005) and contribute to bowing and irregularities along the medial edge. As a result, vocal fold vibration becomes less efficient with accompanying acoustic and perceptual changes such as breathiness and weakness (Sato & Hirano, 1997).

The consequence of the loss of muscle mass and tonicity, connective tissue changes, cartilage ossification, decreased lubrication of the folds, and diminished respiratory power is a loss of fine vocal motor control. The vocal folds lose their ability to modulate precisely their rate and amplitude of vibration. This loss of control is manifested in various ways in the acoustic signal that is generated, and the perceptual results of the acoustic changes.

ACOUSTIC EFFECTS

One of the most robust findings in the literature on vocal aging is that fundamental frequency (F0) changes as the vocal mechanism ages (Table 2.8).

Some researchers have reported an increase in F0 in elderly men (Harnsberger et al., 2010; Linville, 2001; Xue & Deliyski, 2001), while other researchers have found no significant changes in young versus older males (e.g., Ma & Love, 2010). In male speakers whose F0 does change, the increase is probably due to the thinning and stiffening of the vocal fold tissue that results from muscle atrophy and connective tissue changes. F0 changes in males have been linked to hormonal factors. Gugatschka et al. (2010) reported that F0 in older males was related to levels of androgens (testosterone) and estrogens in the blood. Specifically, F0 was significantly higher in males who had lower levels of estrogens. In addition, the speakers with reduced estrogen levels demonstrated a shift of the voice range, with increased highest and lowest frequencies. Conversely, higher testosterone levels have been linked to a lower F0 (Evans, Neave, Wakelin, & Hamilton, 2008).

Female F0 tends to decrease with age by around 10–35 Hz (Brown, Morris, & Michel, 1989; Ferrand, 2002; Higgins & Saxman, 1991; Linville & Fisher, 1985; Teles-Magalhaes, Pegoraro-Krook, & Pegoraro, 2000). Inspection of Table 2.8 indicates a range of F0s in older women ranging from approximately 160–186 Hz, compared to the range in young women of approximately 191–224 Hz. The lowering may be accounted for, in part, by postmenopausal edema, which increases vocal fold mass and decreases the rate of vibration (e.g., Pontes et al., 2005). The edema may not only increase the mass of the vocal folds, but may also change the

TABLE 2.8 Selected F0 Values (in Hz) for Young, Middle-Aged, and Older Adults Reported in the Literature

Ma & Love (2010)			
	Young men	**Middle-aged men**	**Older men**
/a/	120.95		123.50
Phrase	108.03		110.00
Reading	114.26		114.63
	Young women	**Middle-aged women**	**Older women**
/a/	224.05		186.05
Phrase	191.41		160.15
Reading	196.97		171.39
D'haeseleer et al. (2011)			
	Young women	**Middle-aged women**	**Older women**
/a/	202.00	190.00	
Speech	200.00	184.00	
Schneider & Bigenzahn (2003)			
	Young women	**Middle-aged women**	**Older women**
Speech	217.00		
Ferrand (2002)			
	Young women	**Middle-aged women**	**Older women**
/a/	209.68	204.49	175.23
Xue & Deliyski (2001)			
	Young women	**Middle-aged women**	**Older women**
/a/	243.97		187.70
	Young men	**Middle-aged men**	**Older men**
	145.22		127.62

contour and shape of the vocal folds (Biever & Bless, 1989). Another reported postmenopausal change that may affect vocal fold vibratory patterns is drying of the laryngeal mucosa (Gorham-Rowan & Laures-Gore, 2006).

Another reported acoustic result of laryngeal aging is an increase in F0 variability. That is, during prolongation of isolated vowels the vocal folds are less able to maintain the consistent muscle force and tension necessary for stable vibration. The decrease in phonatory stability manifests as a higher standard deviation of the fundamental frequency (F0sd) and decreased periodicity of vocal fold vibration (e.g., Biever & Bless, 1989; Ferrand, 2002; Gorham-Rowan & Laures-Gore, 2006; Vipperla, Renals, & Frankel, 2010).

Intensity levels in elderly speakers have also been studied. While younger and older speakers use the same laryngeal and respiratory mechanisms to control vocal intensity (Baker et al., 2001; Hodge, Colton, & Kelley, 2001), many older speakers have been shown to have reduced intensity ranges and levels (de Menezes & Vicente, 2007; Kozlakowski, 2003). Both Baker et al. (2001) and Hodge et al. (2001) found that the young and older speakers in their studies controlled vocal intensity in comparable ways and generated comparable levels of subglottal pressure, but the older individuals obtained lower intensities across soft, comfortable, and loud conditions. The decreased intensity may result from the laryngeal changes associated with aging, as well as from respiratory factors such as reduced strength of the respiratory muscles, decreased elastic recoil of the lungs, lower lung pressures, and smaller vital capacities.

Another common finding in elderly speakers is increased breathiness characterized by unusually high airflows during speech, larger lung volumes per breath, and more breath expended per syllable (Melcon, Hoit, & Hixon,1989). This is likely due to the loss of fine laryngeal muscle control, which results in bowing of the folds and lack of complete approximation during vibration. Greater breathiness also probably contributes to the decreased intensity evident in many older individuals. Laryngoscopic studies have shown that elderly women often demonstrate a more anterior glottal gap during phonation, probably resulting from atrophy and degeneration of laryngeal tissue (Gorham-Rowan & Laures-Gore, 2006). Breathiness has been found to differentiate older females from both middle-aged and young females (Harnsberger et al., 2010).

PERCEPTUAL FINDINGS

Laryngeal function carries considerable information about speaker identity. Listeners use variations in acoustic cues to make judgments regarding individuals' ages, personality characteristics, social status, physical traits, and emotional states (Imhof, 2010; Teshigawara, Amir, Amir, Wlosko, & Avivi, 2007). Listeners have been shown to be quite accurate in judging speaker age from purely auditory cues. For example, Harnsberger, Shrivastav, Brown, Rothman and Hollien (2008) examined the responses of college students to male and female young, middle-aged, and older talkers. The perceived age of the talkers corresponded very closely to their chronological ages. Reubold, Harrington, and Kleber (2010) examined F0 from archived broadcasts of the Queen of England and other noted actors and speakers (males and females) in the speakers' earlier ages (34–43) and later years (64–73). They reported that the F0 values were lower for all speakers in the later broadcasts. They presented samples of these earlier and later broadcasts to listeners, who correctly judged the perceived ages in the 2 conditions based on the changes in F0. Debruyne and Decoster (1999) conducted a study in which listeners rated male and female voices as young or old. The women's voices that were perceived as older were characterized by a lower speaking F0 and a decreased HNR, indicating an increased level of noise in the voice. Listeners judged men's voices as sounding older based on a higher speaking F0 as well as decreased HNR.

While F0 appears to be the most salient cue to speaker age, other vocal aspects also affect listener judgments, such as increased hoarseness, breathiness, reduced intensity, less pitch variability, and **vocal tremor**. Rate of speech has also been found to influence listener perception of speaker age. Speakers who are perceived as old have significantly slower speaking rates compared to those perceived as young (e.g., Harnsberger et al., 2010). Gender has been found to play a role in the interpretation of vocal cues. Reportedly, a female with a breathy voice is perceived as more feminine, prettier, petite, and vivacious, whereas a male with the same voice characteristics is perceived as relatively young and more artistic (Imhof, 2010).

Perceptions and judgments of the elderly voice seem to be indicative of attitudes toward elderly people in general, at least in the United States. The stereotypical "old" voice has been referred to as the voice of senescence, or as a senile voice. Both of these terms have a negative connotation. This seemingly negative attitude toward the elderly voice, and by extension, toward elderly individuals, has been explored in various studies. Deal and Oyer (1991) had speakers ranging in age from 41 to 83 years rated on a 7-point "pleasantness" scale by groups of listeners ranging from college age to 80. The youngest speakers were rated the most pleasant, and all other age groups were rated progressively less pleasant. Young listeners consistently made judgments nearer the unpleasant end of the scale than did older listeners. Newsom and Robbins (2010) reported that older listeners were not as sensitive to voice age as younger groups and did not perceive older voices as necessarily older sounding, whereas younger listeners perceived older voices more negatively. Interestingly, this stereotyping is even more negative for elderly women than it is for elderly men. Ryan and Capadano (1978) reported that female speakers perceived as elderly were viewed negatively as "reserved, passive, out of it, and inflexible." Older-sounding male voices were rated as "inflexible," but this was considered to be a sign of authority, and as such was not seen as particularly negative. More recent research confirms that listeners associate older-sounding voices with fewer positive stereotypes, and the older the voice is perceived, the more negatively it is judged (Lee, Mazloff, & Henry, 1999).

HEALTH STATUS AND AGE-RELATED VOCAL DISEASES

There is a strong relationship between vocal capacity and general health. Ringel and Chodzko-Zajko (1987) found that younger unhealthy patients exhibited vocal characteristics similar to those of much older people. Conversely, better physiological health was associated with increased laryngeal control. Orlikoff (1990) reported significant differences between healthy young adult men and healthy elderly men on F0 and amplitude standard deviations as well as on levels of noise in the voice. These differences were even larger when the younger speakers were compared with elderly men with cardiovascular conditions such as atherosclerosis. In a study by Xue and Mueller (1997), physically active elderly speakers were judged as chronologically younger than those who were more sedentary. The active participants also exhibited a smaller standard deviation of F0 and lower levels of jitter than the less active group.

Not only does overall physiological condition influence vocal function, but there are many age-related disorders that directly impact the laryngeal mechanism, such as pulmonary diseases like emphysema and chronic obstructive pulmonary disorder. Pulmonary diseases can disrupt airflow and influence loudness and pitch control. Coronary artery disease impairs respiratory function as well as laryngeal and pulmonary blood supply, and changes in voice quality may be an important diagnostic sign in some cases of hypertension. Central nervous system diseases affect laryngeal control, and many are associated with the aging process. For instance, **amyotrophic lateral sclerosis** generally develops in the fifth and sixth decades and is marked by progressive dysphonia and eventual **aphonia**. Pseudobulbar palsy secondary to multiple strokes is also commonly associated with aging and results in excessively tense vocal fold **adduction**, with a characteristic strain-strangled voice quality. **Parkinson's disease** is one of the most common neurological diseases in elderly individuals, with an incidence of 1% of the population over age 50. This disorder often results in a reduction in laryngeal muscle mobility, leading to reduced loudness and restricted pitch range.

PRESBYPHONIA

Based on the age-related changes described above, some authors have used the term **presbyphonia** to describe the aging of the laryngeal mechanism. Thomas and Stemple (2007) characterized presbyphonia in terms of auditory-perceptual changes, visual perceptual changes, and acoustic changes. Auditory-perceptual changes include altered pitch, hoarseness, breathiness, strain, and slowed rate. Visual perceptual changes include bowing of the vocal fold edge, vocal fold atrophy, a spindle-shaped gap during phonation, and edema (in females). Acoustic changes include increased F0 in males, decreased F0 in females, decreased intensity, and increased noise-to-harmonics ratio. Presbyphonic changes have been found to be relatively common in groups of healthy elderly individuals and can adversely impact quality of life (e.g., Golub, Chen, Otto, Hapner, & Johns, 2006; Turley & Cohen, 2009).

CLINICAL IMPLICATIONS

Because of all these age-related physiological, acoustic, and perceptual changes, it is crucial to account for the variable of age when assessing vocal function. Otherwise, the effects of normal aging on laryngeal performance could be mistaken for those of laryngeal pathology. Both normal aging and disease can result in voice tremor, laryngeal tension, air loss and breathiness, and hoarseness. It is therefore crucial to try to tease out which characteristics may be indicative of normal aging, and which may be related to underlying structural or physiological pathology. With this knowledge, clinicians will be better prepared to successfully treat elderly individuals with voice problems.

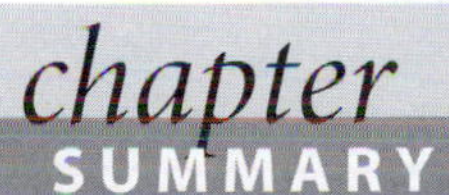

chapter SUMMARY

EFFICIENT SPEECH BREATHING is a process that develops over time in conjunction with anatomical and physiological changes in the young child's respiratory system. Changes in the respiratory system continue throughout the lifespan, including changes in lung volumes and capacities in young, middle-aged, and older adults.

There are many differences between the structure of the larynx at the time of birth and the more mature organ in terms of position of the larynx in the neck, shape and size of laryngeal cartilages, vocal fold length, and histological composition of the vocal folds. Newborns and infants, with their tiny vocal folds, have an average F0 ranging from 400–600 Hz. Infant cries provide information regarding nervous system status and physiological function. Maturation of the nervous system allows the infant a greater degree of laryngeal muscle control as well as greater control over subglottal air pressure. Infant crying is important not only for survival but also as the beginning of human vocal communication. During puberty laryngeal growth occurs in both sexes, but it is particularly pronounced in males due to the release of androgens. During this time of growth and change the vocal ligament continues the process of differentiating into separate layers with different cellular compositions. In addition, the larynx descends to the level of C6 or C7 resulting in a longer vocal tract, which changes the resonating characteristics as well as the pitch of the voice.

After puberty the voice and F0 stabilize. The larynx attains its adult size, shape, and structure, including differentiated vocal ligaments. The adult female voice is often characterized by a slight degree of breathiness resulting from a posterior glottal gap during vocal production. Postpubertal girls and women may be affected vocally by fluctuating hormone levels during the menstrual cycle. Vocal aging is influenced by many factors, including the structural and physiological changes that occur in the larynx, the individual's overall state of health, the acoustic characteristics that are a consequence of the structural and physiological changes, the way in which the voice is perceived by listeners, the influence of gender (i.e., menopause in women), and related or unrelated vocal disorders. The term *presbyphonia* has been coined to characterize the aging of the laryngeal mechanism. The variable of age must be taken into consideration when assessing vocal function. Otherwise, the effects of normal aging on laryngeal performance could be mistaken for those of laryngeal pathology.

review QUESTIONS

1. Explain the terms *emergence*, *refinement*, and *adaptation* in relation to speech breathing in children.
2. Describe changes in lung volumes and capacities that occur from infancy to adulthood.
3. Compare and contrast the framework of the larynx in infants and adults.
4. Discuss the importance of the infant cry.
5. Explain the influence of hormonal changes on voice in puberty and adulthood.
6. Identify the structural and functional changes that occur within the larynx due to aging, and explain how these contribute to changes in vocal output in older men and women.
7. Explain what is meant by the term *presbyphonia*. Do you think this is an appropriate description of the aging voice? Why or why not?
8. Explain the clinical significance of differentiating between normal laryngeal changes due to the aging process and disease states of the larynx.

Chapter 3

Considerations in Voice Treatment

LEARNING OBJECTIVES

1. Understand what is meant by the term *normal voice.*
2. Become familiar with the terminology used to describe perceptual and acoustic aspects of voice disorders.
3. Appreciate the value of the team approach in the clinical management of voice disorders.
4. Identify levels of prevention and application to voice disorders.
5. Gain familiarity with the World Health Organization's International Classification of Functioning, Disability, and Health.
6. Understand the effects of different classes of medications on vocal function.
7. Appreciate the role of multicultural factors in the provision of clinical services for individuals with voice disorders.
8. Identify principles of evidence-based practice and treatment efficacy and their application to voice disorders.

Before turning our attention to the evaluation and treatment of voice problems, it is important to consider factors that provide a framework for and can affect the provision of clinical services for individuals with voice disorders. It is also necessary to become familiar with the terminology used to describe normal voice as well as perceptual and acoustic aspects of voice disorders. This chapter begins with a discussion of what constitutes normal voice, followed by a definition of abnormal voice. Descriptions of commonly used perceptual and acoustic terms related to vocal output are presented. The discussion then turns to the interrelatedness of causes of voice disorders, the importance of the team approach to diagnosis and treatment, and the role of prevention in voice disorders. The World Health Organization's International Classification of Functioning, Disability, and Health is described and the relevance of this classification system to voice is emphasized. This is followed by information regarding the effects of drugs on the voice, including a description of many commonly used medications. The influence of cultural factors that may affect voice treatment is explored, and selected examples are presented of cultural attitudes toward disability. Finally, the increasing importance of evidence-based practice and treatment efficacy in voice disorders is discussed.

Normal Voice

For any voice disorder, perhaps the most important question to be asked is "How does this person's voice differ from normal, and what are its characteristics?" To answer this question one must understand what is meant by normal voice. This is not as easy as it seems, because it is very difficult to pin down exactly what constitutes a normal voice. Normal voices differ depending on a wide array of variables, including the speaker's sex, age, build, culture, region, personality, and health status (Table 3.1). Normal voice is also very much a function of the listener's perception. A trained voice therapist, for example, might consider a young woman's voice that is slightly low-pitched and husky to be deviant and in need of remediation, whereas the same voice might be considered attractive by the individual herself and by her family and friends. The production of voice also is a physical phenomenon, and physical sensations may be perceived by the speaker during phonation. Even if the voice sounds clear and pleasant to listeners, if the speaker feels strain or discomfort or fatigue in producing the voice, it cannot be considered normal (Karnell et al., 2007). Another factor that complicates the definition of normal voice is the individual's level and degree of voice usage. A voice that might feel and sound perfectly normal and acceptable for a person who does not depend on the voice for his or her livelihood may be unacceptable in quality or effort to a professional voice user such as a singer, actor, or teacher. Thus, it is clear that normal voice is a multidimensional entity that encompasses many different physical, perceptual, and lifestyle aspects.

A comprehensive definition of normal voice includes factors relating to the vocal output such as pitch, loudness, and quality; physical aspects of voice production such as effort, pain, discomfort, strain, and fatigue; and lifestyle considerations such as degree and purpose of daily voice use. Thus, the voice can be defined as normal when the quality is clear; pitch and loudness are appropriate for age, sex, and situation; the voice is produced without undue effort, pain, strain, or fatigue; and the voice is satisfactory to the speaker in terms of fulfilling his or her occupational, social, and emotional vocal needs (Table 3.2). When any of these aspects of voice production is compromised, a voice disorder may result.

TABLE 3.1 Aspects of Normal Voice

Speaker	Sex, age, build, culture, personality, health status
Listener perception	Expectations, experience, training, culture
Physical sensations	None, strain, effort, fatigue
Voice usage	Professional or nonprofessional voice user

TABLE 3.2 Vocal Dimensions of Normal Voice

Clear quality
Pitch and loudness appropriate for age, sex, and situation
No effort, pain, strain, fatigue
Fufills occupational, social, and emotional vocal needs

Terminology

It is important for professionals who provide services to people with voice disorders to use consistent terminology that promotes clarity of communication within and among different disciplines. In the field of voice disorders, auditory-perceptual and acoustic terms are commonly used to describe a speaker's vocal output. Perceptual terms are those that involve a subjective judgment of voice on the part of a speaker or listener. Perceptual judgments are influenced by an individual's experience, his or her expectations of what a normal voice should sound like, cultural factors, geographic location, age and gender of the listener, and age and gender of the speaker. Perceptual impressions can relate to vocal fold vibratory patterns, resonance characteristics of the voice, and/or respiratory factors.

PERCEPTUAL TERMS

The term used to describe any vocal dysfunction is *dysphonia*. Dysphonia is defined as an impairment of the speaking or singing voice (ASHA, 2005b). A voice can be dysphonic in terms of pitch, loudness, and/or quality (Table 3.3).

The terms used to describe pitch and loudness problems are relatively straightforward. Pitch can be too low, too high, monotone, or unstable. Pitch breaks occur when the voice abruptly changes to either a higher or lower pitch. Pitch can also fluctuate in a rhythmic manner resulting in a tremor. **Diplophonia** refers to the perception of two different pitches being produced simultaneously. Pitch range can be reduced, resulting in a voice that sounds monotonous or monopitch. Loudness level can be inadequate, excessive, monoloud (inadequate variation), or uncontrolled. Perceptual terms related to vocal fold vibratory patterns include breathy, harsh/rough, hoarse, strained, and strained/strangled. A breathy voice is characterized by air loss through loosely or hypoadducted vocal folds. Breathiness is often accompanied by low intensity. Hoarseness sometimes is used interchangeably with the more generic descriptor dysphonia. Hoarseness results from excessive noise in the vocal signal giving the voice a rough, raspy quality. Sometimes the hoarseness has a wet, gurgly sound to it, caused by an accumulation of mucus on the vocal folds. **Harshness** results from irregular vocal fold vibration creating noise in the lower frequencies accompanied by breathiness. The terms *strained* and *strained/strangled* denote excessive laryngeal muscular effort during voice production. **Voice arrests** refer to complete cessation of voicing for a brief period of time; aphonia is the complete lack of voicing. Perceptual terms related to resonance characteristics

TABLE 3.3 Perceptual Terms Describing Types of Dysphonia

Pitch	Loudness	Quality
Too low	Inadequate	Hoarse
Too high	Excessive	Harsh
Monotone	Monoloud	Tense
Unstable	Unstable	Strained
Tremor	Tremor	Breathy
Diplophonia		Rough
		Weak
		Hypernasal
		Hyponasal
		Nasal emission
		Cul-de-sac resonance

of the voice include hyper- and hyponasality. **Hypernasality** refers to a voice that sounds overly nasalized, usually due to problems with velopharyngeal function. Hyponasality indicates a lack of nasal resonance, particularly on nasal sounds and vowels, and may result in a muffled **voice quality**. **Nasal emission** refers to the audible release of air through the nose and ranges from barely audible to extremely loud and distracting. Nasal emission usually occurs in the case of cleft palate or velopharyngeal inadequacy. Typically the nasal emission occurs on stops and fricatives, which require a buildup of oral pressure for their production. **Cul de sac resonance** is the term used to describe a voice that sounds muffled and low in volume. This quality results when the vocal signal is blocked from exiting through the oral or nasal cavities by some type of obstruction such as large tonsils or a deviated septum (Kummer, 2007). Respiratory terms that are associated with voice problems include stridor and dyspnea. **Stridor** refers to noisy inhalation and/or exhalation that indicate airway obstruction. **Dyspnea** refers to a subjective feeling of difficulty breathing. It is important to keep in mind that pitch, loudness, and quality problems can occur either alone or, more commonly, in various combinations. A person whose voice is hoarse may also have a very low pitch and reduced loudness. Another person may sound both hypernasal and have an excessively high pitch. A third person may exhibit stridor and a harsh voice, and so on.

ACOUSTIC TERMS

Acoustic terms are descriptors derived from acoustic analysis of the voice signal, which are assumed to be more objective than perceptual judgments. The most commonly used acoustic measures include fundamental frequency, frequency variability, maximum phonational frequency range, intensity/amplitude, intensity/amplitude variability, and dynamic range.

TABLE 3.4 **Commonly Used Acoustic Terms, Descriptions, and Units of Measure**

Term	Description	Measure
Fundamental frequency (F0)	Rate of vocal fold vibration	Hz
Frequency variability	Changes in F0 during isolated vowels or conversational speech	Standard deviation of F0 (F0SD); pitch sigma
Maximum phonational frequency range	Complete range of possible F0s a person can generate	Hz; octaves
Intensity/amplitude	Degree of vocal fold excursion	Decibels (dB)
Intensity/amplitude variability	Changes in intensity/amplitude during isolated vowels or conversational speech	Standard deviation of dB (dBSD)
Dynamic level	Complete range of intensities/amplitudes a person can generate	dB
Jitter	Cycle-to-cycle frequency variability	%; msec
Shimmer	Cycle-to-cycle amplitude variability	%; dB
Harmonics-to-noise ratio Noise-to-harmonics ratio Signal-to-noise ratio	Ratio between periodic and aperiodic components in the voice	dB

Measures of the degree of noise in a voice are also common in clinical practice and include jitter, shimmer, and various ratios of harmonic to inharmonic components in the voice (Table 3.4).

Fundamental frequency (F0) is the acoustic correlate of the vocal pitch. It reflects the rate at which the vocal folds vibrate and is measured in Hertz (Hz). F0 can be measured in an isolated vowel or in connected speech. F0 in connected speech is often referred to as **speaking fundamental frequency (SFF)**. **Frequency variability** refers to changes in F0 indicated by the standard deviation of F0 (F0SD). It is obtained either in connected speech or in an isolated vowel. F0 variability is typically greater in connected speech because of the large F0 variations associated with intonational patterns, and less in an isolated vowel, which requires a constant level of vocal fold length and tension to maintain a relatively constant F0. Sometimes the standard deviation is converted to semitones and measured in a unit called *pitch sigma*. **Maximum phonational frequency range (MPFR)** refers to the complete range of F0s a person is able to generate from the lowest to highest excluding pulse but including falsetto, measured in Hz or in octaves. It indicates the physiological limits of an individual's frequency-regulating mechanism.

Intensity and amplitude both correspond perceptually to the loudness of a person's voice. Intensity is measured in dB (**decibel**) IL (intensity level) and **amplitude** is measured in dB SLP (sound pressure level). Very often these terms are used interchangeably. **Average intensity** is the intensity measured over an utterance, either connected speech or an isolated vowel. **Intensity variability** refers to the changes in intensity occurring within an utterance and can be measured by the standard deviation. **Dynamic range** refers to the complete range of intensities a person is capable of generating from the softest phonation produced without whispering to the loudest. Intensity depends to a certain extent on fundamental frequency. Individuals are able to produce more intense utterances in the middle of their frequency range, with a narrower dynamic range at higher and lower frequencies.

Because of the neurological and biomechanical characteristics of vocal motor function, normal voice is not perfectly periodic and always contains a slight degree of noise. The level of aperiodicity can be quantified by calculating the minute fluctuations in frequency and amplitude that occur between individual cycles of vibration. Cycle-to-cycle frequency variations are known as **jitter**, which is measured as a percentage or in milliseconds. Cycle-to-cycle variation in amplitude is referred to as **shimmer**, measured in dB or as a percentage. Other measures of spectral noise include harmonics-to-noise ratio (HNR), noise-to-harmonics ratio (NHR), and **signal-to-noise ratio (SNR)**. These measures quantify the ratio between the harmonic (periodic) and inharmonic (aperiodic) components of the voice and are measured in dB.

Causes of Voice Disorders

Causes of voice disorders tend to be multifactorial. Dysphonia may result from structural problems within or outside of the larynx, neurological problems, lifestyle habits and choices, medications, psychological problems, systemic diseases of the body, physical injury to the larynx, digestive disorders, respiratory disorders, and unknown causes (Table 3.5).

Keep in mind that while we will discuss laryngeal disorders separately for the sake of convenience, in reality it is more common to find multiple causes of voice disorders. For example, a person with a neurological disorder that affects the voice may also have related or unrelated **stress** issues, a vocally demanding lifestyle, and a poor diet. The individual may, in addition, use compensatory vocal strategies that may obscure or worsen the underlying problem. Another fairly common situation is for a psychological stressor to initiate or exacerbate a neurological problem. Often, too, individuals may have problems of the digestive system such as gastroesophageal reflux disease (GERD), which can cause, exacerbate, or coexist with voice problems. Because many, if not most, voice disorders are multifactorial, it is often very difficult to tease out the causes and effects of the dysphonia. Therefore, when evaluating and treating an individual with a voice disorder, it is critical that the clinician take into account not only the patient's dysphonia, but his or her lifestyle, medical history, social and vocational factors, and cultural attitudes and beliefs. Without a complete picture of the individual within his or her everyday environment, it is possible that important information relating to the disorder will not be detected.

Team Approach to Diagnosis and Treatment of Voice Disorders

Over the past few decades it has become widely recognized that no one professional is able to offer a patient all the care that he or she needs. This has resulted in a multidisciplinary approach, in which a team of professionals contribute their expertise to the diagnosis, evaluation, and

TABLE 3.5 **Causes of Voice Disorders**

Structural/Organic Problems
Congenital
Acquired
Physical Injury
Mechanical
Thermal
Chemical
Neurological Problems
Congenital
Acquired
Lifestyle
Degree and style of voice usage
Occupational vocal requirements
Diet
Tobacco consumption
Alcohol consumption
Exercise habits
Psychological Problems
Emotional or mental disorders
Everyday stresses/conflicts
Systemic Diseases
HIV/AIDS
Arthritis
Medications
Prescription
Over-the-counter
Respiratory Problems
Asthma
Allergies
Idiopathic

clinical management of individuals with voice disorders. Many multidisciplinary voice centers have been established, and patients may be referred to the center by a general or specialist physician, by a speech-language pathologist, or by a classroom teacher or singing teacher. The core clinical unit in such centers typically comprises the **otolaryngologist**, the speech-language pathologist, and the patient and/or parents/caregivers. An otolaryngologist is a physician who specializes in the diagnosis and treatment of patients with ear, nose, and throat disorders (ENT). This is the professional who makes a medical diagnosis of the patient's condition and prescribes any appropriate medications, surgical procedures, and/or voice therapy. The speech-language pathologist assesses the patient's voice using **auditory-perceptual evaluation** as well as acoustic and aerodynamic instrumentation. The speech-language pathologist also provides behavioral voice treatment, keeps ongoing data regarding the individual's vocal progress, and assesses the patient's voice at appropriate intervals. The patient or patient's parents/caregivers contribute valuable input regarding the patient's progress, impact of treatment, lifestyle changes, and sociocultural information.

In addition to the core team, a collateral team may be established to contribute additional professional expertise depending on the patient's situation and problem (Table 3.6).

The team is coordinated by a case manager, typically the otolaryngologist or the speech-language pathologist. Teams may meet on a regular basis or as needed to discuss aspects of the patient's clinical management and to ensure that the patient is receiving ongoing quality care that is individually tailored to meet his or her specific needs. This type of multidisciplinary team approach ensures that patients receive the best possible care for their voice problems.

TABLE 3.6 Core and Collateral Teams for Voice Disorders

Core Team
Otolaryngologist
Speech-language pathologist
Patient/parents/caregivers
Collateral Team
Audiologist
Classroom teacher
Neurologist
Endocrinologist
Nurse
Social worker
Respiratory therapist
Allergist
Gastroenterologist
Psychotherapist
Vocal coach
Physical therapist
Occupational therapist

However, even if not a member of a team, it is important that speech-language pathologists make referrals to appropriate professionals as the need dictates for their clients. For example, a clinician working with an individual who complains of extreme stress at work and occurrences of acid reflux may refer the individual to a psychotherapist and a physician in order to deal most effectively with all issues that may be contributing to the voice problem.

Prevention of Voice Disorders

The concept of prevention of disorders has been around for many years and has become an important focus for speech-language-hearing professionals. The American Speech-Language-Hearing Association (ASHA) recognized the critical role of prevention in the field of communication disorders with its adoption in 1988 of a Position Statement titled "The Prevention of Communication Disorders" (available from www.asha.org/docs/html/PS1988-00228.html). The ASHA bylaws also emphasize that one of the purposes of the association is to promote investigation and prevention of disorders of human communication (Article II.4; available from www.asha.org/docs/html/BY2008-00284.html#sec1.1.2). The concept of prevention does not negate the need for traditional speech-language services of identifying and treating communication disorders, but rather expands the focus and broadens the scope of practice. Prevention is categorized as primary, secondary, or tertiary. Table 3.7 lists definitions of terms commonly used in relation to prevention.

PRIMARY PREVENTION

Primary prevention aims to entirely eliminate or prevent the onset of a disorder by reducing a person's susceptibility to the disorder, or by reducing exposure of a susceptible individual to that disorder (ASHA, 1991; Marge, 1984). Immunization is an example of primary prevention that has been extremely successful in reducing the spread of diseases such as poliomyelitis and smallpox. In terms of voice disorders, education is a powerful tool in primary prevention. Many disorders that result from undesirable practices are amenable to prevention, such as **phonotraumatic** behaviors, smoking, substance abuse, and poor diet. Awareness of the harmful effects of these behaviors can motivate an individual to reduce their frequency and thereby prevent a voice problem from developing. For example, an important primary prevention strategy to reduce the incidence of laryngeal cancer is public education regarding the effects of smoking. Another example is a primary prevention program designed to teach principles of good vocal technique to individuals who use their voices professionally. Such programs can be very effective. For example, Bovo, Galceran, Petrucelli, and Hatzopoulos (2007) implemented a vocal care course for teachers. The course comprised lectures focusing on symptoms of vocal fatigue, reduction in the amount of voice usage, and strategies for non–vocally damaging techniques of classroom management. On a questionnaire administered three months after completion of the course, 85% of the teachers reported that they practiced good vocal habits, and 90% had adopted strategies for reducing vocal demand in the classroom.

Children also benefit from primary prevention. Most childhood dysphonia is a consequence of vocally traumatic behaviors (Flynn, 1983), so it makes sense to reduce the incidence of vocal problems through prevention programs (Kahane & Mayo, 1989). School screenings to detect vocally damaging behaviors and other conditions that can affect voice (e.g., hearing loss) can be a quick and cost-effective means of preventing the occurrence of future vocal problems

TABLE 3.7 **Terminology Relating to Prevention**

Term	Description
Primary prevention	Elimination or inhibition of the onset and development of a communication disorder by altering susceptibility or reducing exposure for susceptible persons
Secondary prevention	Early detection and treatment of communication disorders; early detection and treatment may lead to the elimination of the disorder or the retardation of the disorder's progress, thereby preventing further complications
Tertiary prevention	Reduction of a disability by attempting to restore effective functioning; major approach is rehabilitation of the individual
At risk	Potential to develop a disorder based on specific biological, environmental, or behavioral factors; term may apply to an asymptomatic population
Incidence	Rate of new occurrences of a condition in a population free of the disorder within a specified time period
Prevalence	Total rate or proportion of cases in a population at or during a specified period of time
Epidemiology	Observational science that investigates distribution and determinants of diseases and disorders in populations
Wellness	Development and maintenance of an optimal level of competence appropriate to any given stage of the life cycle

Source: Reprinted with permission from *Prevention of Communication Disorders* [Position Statement]. Available from www.asha.org/policy.

(Holland & DeJarnette, 2002; Kahane & Mayo, 1989). Nilson and Schneiderman (1983) described a prevention program for second- and third-grade students and their teachers. The program included a basic overview of the vocal mechanism and voice production, descriptions of adequate and inadequate voice qualities, and identification of damaging vocal behaviors. Students and teachers demonstrated significant improvement in their knowledge of vocal health care. Importantly, participants retained this information 5 months after the end of the program, and no new cases of deviant voice quality were found during rescreening of the children who participated in the program.

Flynn (1983) proposed three specific types of primary prevention activities for speech-language pathologists practicing in a school setting. These include providing information to parents and teachers regarding the effects of vocally traumatic behaviors as well as other conditions that can affect voice (e.g., allergies); helping parents and teachers to focus children's attention on sounds in their environment including people's voices; and explaining the structure and function of the larynx to groups of teachers and children. ASHA (1991) identified primary prevention activities including those targeted at teachers,

TABLE 3.8 **Examples of Prevention Activities for Speech-Language Pathologists Targeted at Various Groups**

Teachers	Collaborate with classroom teachers to identify children at risk for voice problems
	Provide classes for teachers to educate them about normal and disordered vocal function
	Provide lectures and discussions on healthy vocal usage in life choices and biology classes in junior and senior high schools
	Expand school prevention programs to day care providers
Administrators	Inform school administrators about prevention efforts and activities
Parents	Inform parents of their role in identification and prevention
Clients	Refer clients who smoke to cessation programs as part of their treatment for voice disorders
	Refer clients who abuse alcohol to alcohol treatment centers
	Inform clients how to eliminate vocally damaging behaviors and how to avoid or limit use of the voice in unhealthy situations
	Encourage clients to develop new ways to deal with daily tension and environmental stress
	Encourage clients to avoid use of nonmedicinal drugs and prescription drugs if at all possible
	Refer individuals with early warning signs of laryngeal cancer to an otolaryngologist
General public	Develop and distribute information on the vocal symptoms that are early warning signs of laryngeal cancer and on the importance of medical assessment when symptoms appear

Source: Reprinted with permission from *Prevention of Communication Disorders Tutorial* [Relevant Paper]. Available from www.asha.org/policy.

at school administrators, at parents, at clients, and at the general public. These activities can be adapted by the speech-language professional for voice usage (Table 3.8).

SECONDARY PREVENTION

Secondary prevention focuses on the early detection and treatment of communication disorders. This can help to eliminate or slow the progress of the disorder. For example, diagnosing and treating laryngeal cancer in the early stages can help to prevent the spread of the disease and the necessity of having a total laryngectomy. Similarly, treating **polyps** in the earliest stages of their development can eliminate the need for surgery. Secondary prevention of phonotraumatic behaviors in children can help to avoid long-term patterns of maladaptive vocal use and habituated hyperfunctional vocal production.

TERTIARY PREVENTION

Tertiary prevention refers to the reduction of a disability by using various clinical management techniques to restore normal functioning to the extent possible. Most of the treatment strategies employed in the clinical management of voice disorders fall into the tertiary category of prevention.

INTERNATIONAL CLASSIFICATION OF FUNCTIONING, DISABILITY, AND HEALTH (ICF)

A voice disorder can impact an individual's ability to function effectively in different areas of life. Quality of life describes a person's well-being in physical, economic, social, communicative, and psychological domains (Ma & Yiu, 2001; Smith et al., 1996). People with voice disorders may experience many negative effects that can adversely impact their quality of life, including job loss or change, social isolation, depression, and difficulty being understood (Smith et al., 1996).

In order to fully describe the effect of any disorder on an individual's life, the World Health Organization (WHO) in 1980 proposed a model (the International Classification of Impairment, Disabilities, and Handicap) that takes into account the individual's physical (or mental) impairment, the level of disability resulting from the impairment, and the handicapping effect of the disability. The model also takes into account the individual's environment, cultural values and beliefs, goals, expectations, standards, and concerns (Gasparini & Behlau, 2007; Konnai, Jayaram, & Scherer, 2008; Krischke et al., 2005).

In this model impairment refers to the bodily problem and its effect on the functioning of the structure. A voice-related example would be unilateral **vocal fold paralysis** that results in a dysphonic voice. Disability is defined as the impact on performance due to the impairment. A person with a dysphonic voice may experience difficulty in any or all aspects of communication. Handicap can result from the impact of the disability on the individual's social, environmental, or economic functioning. Because of different personalities and ways of dealing with life events, differences in support networks and resources, and differences in vocal needs and usage, two people who have similar types and degrees of dysphonia may have vastly different levels of handicap. Factors such as duration of the disorder, the conditions surrounding its onset, the age and social setting of the patient, employment status, profession, the individual's personality, rate of disease progression, past experiences with vocal function, and the person's general health may have a positive or negative on a patient's quality of life and degree of handicap (Murry, Medrado, Hogikiyan, & Aviv, 2004; Wheeler, Collins, & Sapienza, 2006). For example, an opera singer who depends on her voice for her career may be considerably more handicapped by a mild dysphonia than a nonprofessional voice user with a more severe dysphonia.

Since the WHO first proposed the model, it has been updated and was endorsed in 2001 by all 191 member states as the international standard to describe and measure health and disability (WHO, 2001). Now called the **International Classification of Functioning, Disability, and Health (ICF),** the second edition reflects more current thinking and terminology. The term "limitation of activities" is used in preference to "disability level," and "handicap" is replaced by "restriction in participation." These changes recognize that physical/mental health, limitation of activity, and restriction in participation are interdependent, and that this relationship in turn is impacted by environmental, social, and personal factors. The ICF sets forth a framework for describing the health status of a person from both an individual and a societal perspective. The latest version of the ICF (2001) emphasizes health and wellness rather than disease and disability, and it places health and functioning in the context of biological, psychological, and environmental factors. A major advantage of the ICF is that it facilitates a standard terminology that can be used worldwide to promote communication among health care professionals and others involved in health care delivery. Table 3.9 identifies and defines major components of the ICF.

There are two basic categories in the ICF: body functions and structures and activities and participation. Body functions include all anatomical, physiological and psychological

Xerostomia is the most common side effect in the vocal tract and has been associated with more than 500 medications to date (Porter, Scully, & Hegarty, 2004). The dryness can also affect the mucosa of the vocal folds. The viscosity of secretions is directly related to available body water, so any agent that affects the body's water content can affect the level of laryngeal moisture. Lubrication can also be impaired by changes in the normal balance and consistency of laryngeal secretions. Proper lubrication of the vocal folds is critical for their unrestricted movement and generation of a normal mucosal wave. Dry vocal folds require greater phonation threshold pressure (PTP) to be set into vibration, which is more effortful and can result in vocal fatigue (e.g., Sivasankar & Fisher, 2002). Roh, Kim, and Kim (2008) tested vocal function in healthy young men after participants took drugs to dry the mouth, and reported that phonatory effort scores, frequency and intensity values, and PTPs were significantly affected in the xerostomia group.

Medications can affect laryngeal function by side effects other than dehydration and changes in mucosal secretions. For example, painkillers (analgesics) such as aspirin and nonsteroidal anti-inflammatories such as ibuprofen can increase the risk of hemorrhage because they interfere with the ability of the blood to form clots (Murry, McRoy, & Parhizkar, 2007). People who use their voices excessively are particularly prone to **vocal fold hemorrhage** when taking aspirin. Psychoactive medications include antidepressants, mood stabilizers, antianxiety drugs, and antipsychotic drugs. These can affect vocal function by affecting the central nervous system and resulting in temporary or permanent side effects such as dyskinesia, tremor, ataxia, or **dysarthria** (Thompson, 1995). These medications may also cause or worsen reflux, or contribute to vocal fold dehydration. Other potential side effects of various pharmacologic agents include agitation, anxiety, confusion, delirium, depression, hallucinations, mania, paranoia, nervousness, and sleep disturbances (Abaza et al., 2007).

Commonly used medications include antihistamines, expectorants, cough suppressants, blood pressure medications, antireflux medications, painkillers, steroids, hormones, neurologic medications, and psychotropic medications. Table 3.10 provides a listing of selected drug classes and their potential effects on vocal production.

Antihistamines. Antihistamines are used to alleviate the symptoms of allergies. These medications affect the salivary glands and mucus-secreting membranes of the respiratory tract and have the effect of reducing and thickening upper respiratory tract secretions (Abaza et al., 2007; Sataloff et al., 1998; Thompson, 1995). In turn this can produce a dry cough, further interfering with phonation. Additional side effects reportedly can include hoarseness, sore throat, voice changes, laryngitis, and increased phonatory effort (Murry et al., 2007). The newer antihistamines such as Claritin often have less of a drying effect.

Mucolytics. Mucolytics (expectorants) increase the quantity of and help to thin mucosal secretions, which may counteract the effects of antihistamines. These medications are relatively harmless and may be helpful for people who complain of thick secretions, frequent throat clearing, or postnasal drip.

Antitussives. Antitussives (cough suppressants), particularly those that contain codeine, often include agents that dry vocal tract secretions (Thompson, 1995). In addition, antitussives may include antihistamines as one of the ingredients, which worsen the dehydration of the tissues.

Antihypertensives. Antihypertensives (blood pressure medications) dry the mucous membranes of the upper respiratory tract. In addition, they are often used in combination

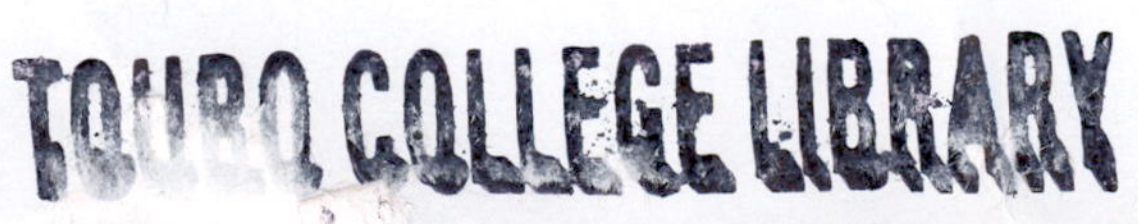

TABLE 3.10 **Selected Classes and Brands of Drugs and Potential Side Effects on Vocal Function**

Drug Class	Name	Potential Effects on Voice
Antianxiety	Valium	Dysarthria, tremor
	Xanax	Mucosal drying
	Librium	Ataxia
Anticholinergic	Parsidol	Mucosal drying
Anticonvulsant	Neurontin	Ataxia
	Tegretol	Ataxia
	Dilantin	Ataxia; dysarthria
Antidepressant (Tricyclic)	Elavil	Mucosal drying
Antihistamine	Allegra	Mucosal drying
	Benadryl	Mucosal drying
	Claritin	Mucosal drying
	Dimetapp	Mucosal drying
	Zyrtec	Mucosal drying
Antihypertensive	Acebutolol	Dry cough
	Toprol	Bronchial spasms
	Accupril	Dry cough; sore throat
	Lasix	Dehydration
	Calan	
Antipsychotic	Clozaril	Tremor, hypokinesia, ataxia, dysarthria
	Haldol	Mucosal drying; **tardive dyskinesia**
	Orap	Mucosal drying; tardive dyskinesia; ataxia
	Thorazine	Tardive dyskinesia
Antispasmodic	Baclofen	
	Botox	Breathiness; weakness
Antispasticity	Zaniflex	Mucosal drying
Bronchodilator	Albuterol	
	Isuprel	Mucosal drying; pharyngeal irritation
	Serevent	
COMT inhibitor	Tasmar	Dyskinesia
Corticosteroid	Prednisone	Susceptibility to infections
Dopamine agonist	Parlodel	Mucosal drying; dyskinesia

TABLE 3.10 (Continued)

Drug Class	Name	Potential Effects on Voice
Dopamine agonist	Parlodel	Mucosal drying; dyskinesia
Dopaminergic	Symmetrel	Mucosal drying
Dopamine replacement	L-Dopa	Mucosal drying
	Sinemet	
Monoamine oxidase inhibitor	Nardil	Mucosal drying; edema
MAO-B inhibitor	Selegiline	Mucosal drying; dyskinesia
Mood stabilizer	Lithium	Hypothyroidism
Penicillin	Amoxil	Glossitis; mucosal drying
Psychostimulant	Ritalin	Mucosal drying; tremor
Sedative hypnotic	Prosom	Hypokinesia
	Ambien	Mucosal drying
Selective serotonin reuptake inhibitor	Prozac	
	Paxil	Mucosal drying
	Zoloft	Mucosal drying; tremor

with diuretic medications that decrease the total amount of body water and contribute to the dehydration (Thompson, 1995). Antihypertensives may also aggravate gastric reflux due to their action on the smooth muscle of the lower esophagus (Rammage, Morrison, & Nichol, 2001).

Antisecretory Drugs. Reflux medications are used to treat gastroesophageal reflux disease (GERD) by neutralizing gastric acid with antacids, inhibiting acid secretions by way of **H2 blockers**, or completely blocking the stomach's production of acids with **proton pump inhibitors**. Some of these medications may have a drying effect on vocal tract secretions (Lawrence, 1987). Other serious potential side effects of such antisecretory agents are confusion, delirium, depression, hallucinations, nervousness, and mania (Abaza et al., 2007).

Corticosteroids. Steroids are prescribed for many conditions including infections, trauma, and immune system disorders. Inhaled steroids used to treat asthma or chronic bronchitis may irritate the laryngeal tissues or generate a laryngeal yeast infection (Rammage et al., 2001). Side effects of inhaled steroids may include wasting of the thyrovocalis muscle and bowing of the vocal folds, inflammation, and fungal growth on the vocal folds (Sataloff, Hawkshaw, & Anticaglia, 2005).

Hormones. Hormones can change the fluid content or the structure of the vocal folds. For example, androgens may be used to treat disorders such as endometriosis, or may be included as part of chemotherapy regimens for some breast cancers (Thompson, 1995). They may also be used to treat postmenopausal sexual dysfunction. However, they may produce permanent lowering of F0 in females and coarsening of the voice (Abaza et al., 2007; Murry et al., 2007; Sataloff et al., 1998). Some birth control pills have a relatively high level of progesterone, and these are most likely to produce androgen-like changes in the voice. Currently most oral contraceptives marketed in the United States are appropriately balanced in terms of estrogen-progesterone content. Some hormones, rather than creating voice problems, help to alleviate potential problems. For example, hormone replacement therapy with estrogen can prevent the edema and lowering of F0 that often accompany the menopausal and postmenopausal periods in a woman's life (Abaza et al., 2007; Murry et al., 2007).

Neuroleptics. Neuroleptics (neurologic medications) are used to treat conditions such as Parkinson's disease, **multiple sclerosis**, **myasthenia gravis**, amyotrophic lateral sclerosis, and others. These types of medications target the central and/or peripheral nervous systems and can have nervous system side effects including tremors, ataxia, and dysarthria.

The National Institutes of Health provides a detailed and complete list of medications and side effects on their website at www.nlm.nih.gov/medlineplus/druginfo/drug_Aa.html.

MULTICULTURAL FACTORS IN CLINICAL MANAGEMENT OF VOICE DISORDERS

Multicultural considerations have become an integral part of the research and clinical foundation in the area of voice disorders. Over the past decade, the influence of social and cultural factors on the perception of acceptable voice quality and on the perception of voice disability has become widely recognized. Cultural, dialectical, and language-based expectations influence what is considered normal vocal quality (Thibeault, 2006) and acceptable vocal patterns and usage. In the United States, standards of speech and voice are based on white, middle to professional class, educated monolingual speakers of General American English (Grosjean, 1989; Kohnert, Kennedy, Glaze, Kan, & Carney, 2003). However, this norm does not apply to a large segment of the United States population. According to the 2010 census (U.S. Bureau of the Census, 2010), 72.4% of the population is White, an increase of 5.7% since the 2000 census, and 12.6% is African American, representing an increase of 12.3% since 2000. American Indian and Alaska Natives make up 0.9% of the population, an increase of 18.4% over 2000 numbers. The percentage of Asians is 4.8, an increase of 43.3%. Hispanic and Latino individuals comprise 16.3%, increasing by 43% since 2000. Native Hawaiian and Other Pacific Islander groups represent 0.2% of the U.S. population, up by 35.4%. Other groups not specifically identified make up 6.2%, an increase of 24.4%, and individuals who reported belonging to two or more groups increased by 32% to 2.9% of the population. Over the past decade every state has increased in population, primarily from immigration from Asia, Mexico, Central America, Africa, South America, Europe, and the Middle East (Kohnert et al., 2003). This makes it imperative for speech-language pathologists to understand and appreciate the traditions, values, and beliefs of cultures other than their own. In particular, clinicians must be aware that perceptions of disability, including communicative disability, can vary between cultures in terms of perception of severity, impact on life, beliefs regarding etiology, and preferences for treatment (Salas-Provance, Erickson, & Reed, 2002). Values, attitudes, and beliefs regarding health and disability may be influenced by the degree of individualism versus collectivism in a specific culture. Individualist societies such as the United States tend to place more emphasis on individuals' personal goals; collectivist societies such as those in Asia and South America place more emphasis on group goals (Yiu, Ho, Ma, Abbott, & Branski, 2009).

Appreciating the critical importance of the role of multicultural factors in the provision of services for individuals with communication disorders, the American Speech-Language-Hearing Association (ASHA) published a Knowledge and Skills Statement in 2004 titled "Knowledge and Skills Needed by Speech-Language Pathologists and Audiologists to Provide Culturally and Linguistically Appropriate Services" (available from www.asha.org/docs/html/KS2004-00215 .html). This document notes:

> Cultural diversity can result from many factors and influences including ethnicity, religious beliefs, sexual orientation, socioeconomic levels, regionalisms, age based peer groups, educational background, and mental/physical disability. In the US, racial and ethnic projections for 2000–2015 indicate that the percentage of racial/ethnic minorities will increase to over 30% of the total population. By 2010 children of immigrants will represent 22% of the school age population. Every clinician has a culture, just as every client/patient has a culture. Only about 7% of the total ASHA membership is from a racial/ethnic minority background. Regardless of our personal culture, practice setting, or caseload demographics, we must strive for culturally and linguistically appropriate service delivery. For example, we must consider how communication disorders or differences might be manifested, identified, or described in our clients'/patients' cultural and linguistic community. This will inform all aspects of our practice including our assessment procedures, diagnostic criteria, treatment plan, and treatment discharge decisions. The ASHA Principles of Ethics state "Individuals shall not discriminate in the delivery of professional services" (ASHA, Principles of Ethics I, Rule C). This mandates that clinicians continue in lifelong learning to develop those knowledge and skills required to provide culturally and linguistically appropriate services.

The 2004 ASHA Statement provides specific guidelines for providing appropriate services to individuals from diverse cultures (Table 3.11).

Applying these principles to voice disorders, ASHA (2004) mandated that knowledge and skills must be related to (a) current research on preferred practice patterns in the identification/assessment and treatment/management of resonance and voice disorders; (b) community standards of typical resonance and voice patterns; and (c) application of the standards of the clients' speech/communication community for dismissal/discharge criteria.

Becoming culturally competent to provide services has been described by Camphina-Bacote (1993) as a four-stage process. The first stage involves becoming aware of differences in other cultures. The second stage involves obtaining information from various resources to facilitate clinical management strategies appropriate to individuals from different cultures. It is vital to gather information from different cultural and linguistic groups in order to fully understand the impact of a communication disorder on a person's life. This knowledge is essential in determining clinical goals and educating patients and their families about the clinical process (Altenberg & Ferrand, 2006). The third stage is devoted to the development of professional skills to assess the client's cultural values, beliefs, and practices including the client's perception of disability. In the fourth stage professionals should feel comfortable interacting with clients from diverse backgrounds.

Mahendra, Battle, and Payne (2006) proposed several steps when first meeting with a patient from a different culture. These include calling to introduce oneself and explaining what will happen at the first meeting; asking specific questions to determine the need for an interpreter; obtaining some background knowledge about the client's ethnic community; and obtaining information about length of time in the United States, educational experiences, languages spoken and/or understood, socialization patterns, and religious affiliations. Armed with this knowledge, the practitioner is in a strong position to incorporate the individual's values and wishes into an integrated treatment plan.

TABLE 3.11 **ASHA Knowledge and Skills for Cultural and Linguistic Competence**

a. Understand the influence of one's own beliefs and biases in providing effective services
b. Maintain respect for an individual's race, ethnic background, lifestyle, physical/mental ability, religious beliefs/practices, and heritage
c. Appreciate the influence of the clients/patient's traditions, customs, values, and beliefs related to providing effective services
d. Identify the impact of assimilation and/or acculturation processes on the identification, assessment, treatment, and management of communication disorders/differences
e. Recognize the clinician's own limitations in education/training in providing services to a client/patient from a particular cultural and/or linguistic community
f. Implement appropriate intervention and assessment strategies and materials, such as food, objects, and/or activities that do not violate the patient's/client's values and/or that may form a constructive bridge between the client's home culture and community or communication environment
g. Maintain appropriate communications with clients, caregivers, and significant others, so that the values imparted in the counseling are consistent with those of the client
h. Appreciate the need to refer to/consult with other service providers with appropriate cultural and linguistic proficiency, including a cultural informant/broker
i. Understand the ethical responsibilities of the clinician concerning the provision of culturally and linguistically appropriate services

Source: Reprinted with permission from *Knowledge and Skills Needed by Speech-Language Pathologists and Audiologists to Provide Culturally and Linguistically Appropriate Services.* Available from www.asha.org/policy. Copyright 2004 American Speech-Language-Hearing Association. All rights reserved.

Cultural Views on Disability. The views of various cultures toward disability have been well described in the disability literature. Three brief examples are provided as an illustration.

Hispanic. Hispanic cultures have a collectivist orientation in which the well-being of the group is more important than that of the individual. Thus an individual's disability is "owned" by all family members (Salas-Provance et al., 2002). Salas-Provance et al. reported that members of the Hispanic culture often distinguish between the disability and "the normal child within." In this view, as long as the affected individual has no physical illness or disease and is able to attend to daily living at his or her present level of functioning, he or she is considered to be healthy. At the same time, however, traditional views of "machismo" may contribute to the denial of a disability (Salas-Provance et al., 2002). Some men may refuse to participate in a rehabilitation program, seeing participation as a sign of weakness. Women, on the other hand, may deny the impact of a disability in order to meet cultural expectations of endurance of the hardship of the disability.

Korean. The Korean view of the universe is holistic and spiritual, and health is considered to depend on the interactions between environmental, social, and physiological domains (Erickson, Devlieger, & Moon Sung, 1999). Illness results from disturbances in physical, psychological, or spiritual factors, or a combination of any of these. The traditional Korean medicine called *hanbang* incorporates the factors of health, wholeness, and balance (Erickson et al., 1999). Individuals in the Korean culture may be comfortable using a combination of traditional and Western medicine. This was apparent in a survey of 30 Korean-American women carried out by Erickson et al. (1999). Almost three quarters of the respondents suggested prayer as a cure or preventive method for hearing problems. The strong influence of religion in this culture should be taken into account in clinical management, together with the common use of herbal medicines and acupuncture. At the same time, however, many Korean Americans also believe strongly in the Western view of the causes and treatment of disabilities, and they see no difficulties in combining both types of treatment.

Chinese. The Chinese culture rewards conformity, obedience, and passivity, as opposed to the North American culture, which rewards creativity and independence (Fung & Roseberry-McKibbin, 1999). American children are expected to participate in class, ask questions, and demonstrate independent thinking. Chinese children are taught to be polite and respectful of their teachers, and they do not make direct eye contact, which is considered rude and disrespectful. Cantonese speakers are also taught to not show emotions in public, particularly negative emotions. Clinicians should realize that when a Cantonese speaker nods, he or she is not necessarily indicating agreement, but just that he or she understands what is being conveyed (Fung & Roseberry-McKibbin, 1999). Fung and Roseberry-McKibbin noted that a Cantonese-speaking client may be quite angry with the clinician or frustrated with treatment and the clinician may never know about it. Thus when the client does not attend scheduled treatment sessions or answer phone calls, the clinician may be bewildered because everything seemed to be going so smoothly. Americans prize frankness, but speech-language pathologists need to be very sensitive to the fact that parents may not want to discuss their child's problem. It may be difficult for some Cantonese-speaking parents in the United States to accept that their child has special education needs or a speech disorder. Speech-language professionals also should be aware of linguistically based voice differences. Cantonese speakers in the United States may be perceived as speaking too quickly and loudly, and they may need to learn to monitor their rate and volume (Fung & Roseberry-McKibbin, 1999). In addition, because Cantonese is a tonal language that uses pitch phonemically to distinguish words, a speaker with a Cantonese accent may sound monotonous to listeners used to the wider range of pitch inflections used in English.

Perception of Voice Disorders. Altenberg and Ferrand (2006) investigated how different groups (monolingual English, English/Russian bilingual speakers; English/Cantonese bilingual speakers) perceived individuals with voice disorders. Results indicated that listeners' perceptions became increasingly negative as the severity of the disorder increased. Even mild disorders elicited more negative attitudes than normal voices. While this pattern was the same for each of the three groups, the Cantonese-English bilinguals rated individuals with severely disordered voices more negatively than did English monolinguals. This may be interpreted as a lesser degree of acceptance of individuals with voice disorders. Thus the degree of negativity toward individuals with voice disorders, particularly severe disorders, can vary depending on linguistic and cultural background.

Yiu et al. (2009) evaluated groups of Chinese (Hong Kong) and North American (Pittsburgh) dysphonic speakers' self-perceptions of their voice disorder in terms of activity limitations and participation restrictions. The two groups demonstrated similar levels of voice impairment. However, the Hong Kong group perceived their daily activities and social functions to be more severely restricted than the Pittsburgh group. The Chinese speakers also felt more emotional distress regarding the voice problem. Yiu et al. (2009) emphasized that management of voice problems should extend beyond the impairment level to include social and cultural factors.

Cultural Factors and Vocal Health. Differences in the perception of voice and vocal health occur not only between cultures, but within cultures as well. Individuals within a culture have different ethnicities, varying socioeconomic and educational levels, different religious beliefs, and different family backgrounds (Erickson et al., 1999). These factors can influence an individual's perspective on health and disability. For example, Verdolini and Ramig (2001) assessed self-perceived voice problems in African American and Caucasian choral singers. Questions targeted health, medications, hygiene, voice use and training history, perceived voice problems, and treatment-seeking patterns around voice problems. Fifty percent of the African American singers reported current perceived hoarseness compared to 35% of Caucasian singers. The Caucasian singers with hoarseness were more likely to have sought treatment or to intend to seek treatment for their voice problems than the African American singers. In addition, the Caucasian subjects appeared to be more influenced by their own perceptions of the problem, while the African American subjects appeared to be more influenced by the opinions of others regarding treatment for the voice problem. Thus, intervention models may need to be different across different sectors of the population (Verdolini & Ramig, 2001).

Cultural phenomena such as dietary habits and occupational trends can also influence laryngeal health. Holland and DeJarnette (2002) suggested that culturally rooted dietary habits, often reinforced by conditions of poverty or low socioeconomic potential, can contribute to or exacerbate GERD and/or laryngopharyngeal reflux (LPR) and put minority groups at higher risk for cancer. It is well established that fatty and fried foods, spicy foods, tomato-based foods, alcohol, and caffeine can cause or worsen acid reflux (e.g., Sataloff et al., 2006). In addition, certain foods such as fats and those with high levels of curing agents are known to increase the risk of some cancers (Holland & De Jarnette, 2002). Hargreaves, Baquet, and Gamshadzahi (1989) reported that foods eaten by African Americans tended to be high in protein, fat, and carbohydrates, and low in the healthier nutrients, fiber, thiamine, riboflavin, vitamins A and C, and iron. These dietary factors may contribute to the higher incidence of laryngeal cancers in African American men and women reported by the American Cancer Society (2009). Changes in lifestyle and foods that are often prescribed for GERD and LPR may be particularly challenging for persons from cultural groups such as African Americans and Latinos who prefer foods that tend to aggravate LPR (Holland & De Jarnette, 2002). The preference for spicy foods may be particularly difficult to resist during cultural celebrations and holidays.

Occupational trends among minority populations can increase the risk of laryngeal diseases including cancer. Minority groups in the United States have historically been overrepresented in low-paying, high-risk jobs (Smart & Smart, 1997), and have thus been exposed to toxic and carcinogenic agents used in manufacturing and processing jobs. Different ethnic groups may also be genetically predisposed to various conditions that influence voice production. For example, a variety of respiratory difficulties have been noted in the Chinese population including chronic cough, postnasal drip, chronic bronchitis, bronchial asthma, and pulmonary tuberculosis (TB; Holland & DeJarnette, 2002). According to the Centers for Disease Control and Prevention, the incidence figures for 1990 showed that minorities account for the greatest incidence of TB. It has been noted that some races have less resistance to TB, which suggests a genetic predisposition to the disease (Holland & DeJarnette, 2002).

Anatomic and Acoustic Factors Related to Ethnic and Linguistic Background. Researchers have investigated respiratory, laryngeal, and supralaryngeal differences between certain races and ethnic groups. In a very early study, Boshoff (1945) reported differences in laryngeal size between black and white South African cadavers. Williams (1975) found differences in pulmonary function (total lung capacity, vital capacity, and residual volume) between black and white individuals in the United States. More recently, Xue and Hao (2006) measured the lengths and volumes of the oral cavity, pharyngeal cavity, and vocal tract in male and female White American, African American, and Chinese individuals. They reported differences between groups for oral volume and total vocal tract volume. Specifically, Chinese male speakers had significantly larger oral volume and total vocal tract volume than both white and black American male speakers. White American female speakers had significantly larger pharyngeal volume than both African American and Chinese female speakers. The authors suggested that these differences may indicate that speakers from different races have different vocal tract configurations that contribute to differences in voice quality. Listeners are able to detect voice differences between ethnic groups of speakers in connected speech as well as in isolated vowels. Walton and Orlikoff (1994) contended that these differences appear to be associated with vocal differences rather than dialectical or linguistic differences. However, Holland and DeJarnette (2002) argued that acoustic differences between African American and Caucasian voice qualities are related to oral traditions of African American speech. They noted that according to the acoustic evidence, African American speakers appear to have low F0s and tend to use the higher end of the range more than the lower end. The authors described the intonation characteristics used by African American speakers as including the use of a wide range of pitches that frequently shift to falsetto register to emphasize particular points; frequent use of level and rising final pitch contours on all sentence types; and use of falling pitch contours to express yes and no questions (which in Standard American English requires a rising intonation). Altenberg and Ferrand (2006) suggested that acoustic patterns may be related to specific language use. They examined F0 as an indication of code switching in young adult English/Russian female bilingual speakers and English/Cantonese female bilingual speakers. Mean F0s were compared in each language and in English with those of a monolingual English-speaking group. The English/Russian bilinguals consistently demonstrated a higher mean F0 in Russian than they did in English. Mean F0 did not change with language switch for the English/Cantonese speakers. There were no significant differences between the groups in their English productions. Andrianopoulos, Darrow, and Chen (2001a) also found that male and female speakers of Mandarin had a considerably higher F0 than African American, white, and Indian speakers of Hindi. Table 3.12 lists some reported values for fundamental frequency for various racial, cultural, and linguistic groups of various ages.

While it is not clear whether the reported acoustic and quality differences are related to anatomical, physiological, and/or sociocultural factors, it seems likely that a combination of these factors results in perceptible differences in vocal output between various cultural and linguistic groups. It is essential that these differences be taken into account when providing professional services to speakers from different cultural, racial, and ethnic groups. Further, it is important to keep in mind that listeners' reactions to voices are influenced by cultural values and social attitudes (Altenberg & Ferrand, 2006).

EVIDENCE-BASED PRACTICE

The notion of **evidence-based practice (EBP)** originated in the medical and allied health professions and has become extremely important in the fields of speech-language pathology and audiology. EBP is a three-pronged approach to clinical management that involves providing

TABLE 3.12 **Selected Reported Fundamental Frequencies (F0, in Hz) for Children (C) and Adults (A) for Different Racial, Cultural, and/or Linguistic Groups**

Author(s)	Groups	C/A	F0 (Hz)
Altenberg & Ferrand (2006)	English monolingual females	A	185
	English/Russian bilingual females	A	190 (Eng) 208 (Rus)
	English/Cantonese bilingual females	A A	182 (Eng) 174 (Cant)
Andrianopoulos et al. (2001)	African American males	A	127
	African American females	A	227
	Indian (Hindi) males	A	137
	Indian (Hindi) females	A	251
	Chinese (Mandarin) males	A	154
	Chinese (Mandarin) females	A	266
	White males	A	128
	White females	A	233
Awan & Mueller (1996)	African American males	C	241
	African American females	C	231
	Hispanic males	C	248
	Hispanic females	C	248
	White males	C	240
	White females	C	243
Hudson et al. (1981)	African American males	A	110
	African American females	A	193
	White males	A	116
	White females	A	217

TABLE 3.12 (Continued)

Author(s)	Groups	C/A	F0 (Hz)
Walton & Orlikoff (1994)	African American males	A	108
	White males	A	107
Wheat & Hudson (1988)	African American males	C	219
	African American females	C	211

patients with the best possible services based on combining evidence from the research literature with clinical expertise and the individual's specific needs, wishes, and values. Thus, EBP fits into a multicultural framework as such practice cannot be separated from the patient's family and cultural background, belief system, and attitudes about disability.

Recognizing the importance of EBP, ASHA published a Position Statement on Evidence-Based Practice in Communication Disorders (2005, available from www.asha.org/docs/html/PS2005-00221.html). This document emphasizes the obligation of all speech, language, and hearing professionals to incorporate the principles of EBP into their clinical practice. ASHA's position is as follows:

> It is the position of the American Speech-Language-Hearing Association that audiologists and speech-language pathologists incorporate the principles of evidence-based practice in clinical decision making to provide high-quality clinical care. The term evidence-based practice refers to an approach in which current, high-quality research evidence is integrated with practitioner expertise and client preferences and values into the process of making clinical decisions. In making clinical practice evidence-based, audiologists and speech-language pathologists—Recognize the needs, abilities, values, preferences, and interests of individuals and families to whom they provide clinical services, and integrate those factors along with best current research evidence and their clinical expertise in making clinical decisions; Acquire and maintain the knowledge and skills that are necessary to provide high quality professional services, including knowledge and skills related to evidence-based practice; Evaluate prevention, screening, and diagnostic procedures, protocols, and measures to identify maximally informative and cost-effective diagnostic and screening tools, using recognized appraisal criteria described in the evidence-based literature; Evaluate the efficacy, effectiveness, and efficiency of clinical protocols for prevention, treatment, and enhancement using criteria recognized in the evidence-based practice literature; Evaluate the quality of evidence appearing in any source or format, including journal articles, textbooks, continuing education offerings, newsletters, advertising, and Web-based products, prior to incorporating such evidence into clinical decision making; Monitor and incorporate new and high-quality research evidence having implications for clinical practice.

In order to facilitate the use of EBP, ASHA has established a National Center for Evidence-Based Practice in Communication Disorders. The center maintains a list of clinical practice guidelines, publishes systematic reviews of relevant literature, and carries out its own systematic literature reviews of various topics (Kent, 2006).

Benefits of EBP. There are many benefits to both patients and professionals in applying the principles of EBP to clinical management of patients with voice disorders. By evaluating new information, clinicians are more likely to understand how a treatment works to effect desired changes in communication (Meline & Paradiso, 2003). This allows therapeutic strategies to be adjusted in response to individual patient needs (Bernstein Ratner, 2006). Thus, patients receive services that are specifically tailored to their unique individual and sociocultural circumstances. Using research evidence in conjunction with clinical expertise to guide evaluation and treatment maximizes the probability of a successful patient outcome. For speech-language pathologists, EBP can help in selecting the most appropriate treatment approach for the patient, making an informed prognosis, and determining the likely cost-effectiveness of the intervention (Worrall & Bennett, 2001). Thus, EBP is a means of increasing clinician accountability, including accountability to government agencies and third-party payers who require evidence of the effectiveness of clinical services for payment purposes (Justice & Fey, 2004; Mullen, 2007). A further benefit of EBP is that it sets a standard for what is considered an acceptable procedure (Plante, 2004). For example, the **Lee Silverman Voice Treatment** has been shown in numerous studies to increase loudness in patients with Parkinson's disease and is well established as an effective treatment protocol. The chewing technique, used to decrease hyperfunctional voice use, has not been systematically investigated, and by this standard, it could not be considered an effective treatment strategy.

Speech-language pathologists are becoming aware of the importance of evidence-based practice in the best interests of their clients. Survey studies have found that the vast majority of speech-language professionals surveyed demonstrated generally positive attitudes toward research and EBP, were confident in their ability to read and understand research literature, and recognized the importance of keeping up-to-date with research (e.g., Meline & Paradiso, 2003; Zipoli & Kennedy, 2005).

Drawbacks of EBP. EBP provides a systematic and reasoned approach to clinical management of patients with communication disorders. However, there are some drawbacks to the wholehearted application of experimental research to clinical practice. The gold standard of research is considered to be randomized controlled studies, in which subjects are assigned randomly to experimental and control groups. The groups are compared on a target variable, with other variables being held constant. However, human communication is a highly variable behavior, and randomized controlled studies are specifically designed to eliminate or reduce variability. Yorkston et al. (2001) argued that the variability inherent in patients with voice disorders, as well as the variability of the treatment approaches tailored to fit each client's individual profile of strengths and weaknesses, means that speech-language professionals need experimental research designs that will reflect this heterogeneity rather than mask it. Individual patients seen by speech-language pathologists may differ in important respects from the group data obtained in large randomized studies, so the treatment under consideration may or may not be relevant to the individual. Further, speech-language professionals often see patients with chronic impairment and associated disability in which cognitive, communication, and behavioral impairments interact with each other in complex ways in an ever-changing environment

(Ylvisaker et al., 2002). Another factor to be taken into account is that treatment regimes may be too complex, too intense, or too long in duration, and may not be appropriate for individual clients even if the treatment is shown to be effective (Worrall & Bennett, 2001). Thus, the evidence obtained from large studies is not always relevant to particular patients. Despite these drawbacks, the adoption of evidence-based practices in voice therapy is a necessary goal, and continued rigorous research demonstrating cause-effect relationships between specific treatment techniques and the desired voice outcome is a crucial basis to achieving this goal.

TREATMENT EFFICACY

Treatment efficacy is a broad term that includes treatment effectiveness, treatment efficiency, and treatment effects. Treatment effectiveness relates to whether the target treatment works, and if so, for which patients. Treatment efficiency refers to the ability of the treatment to achieve the objectives and goals with the minimum expenditure of time and cost. Efficiency also relates to whether one treatment works better than another (Ramig & Verdolini, 1998). Treatment effects refer to ways in which the treatment modifies the target behavior(s). Behavioral voice treatment has been shown overall to be efficacious. Voice treatment can resolve a voice disorder when medical intervention is not warranted, and/or may reduce the need for surgery or other medical intervention (ASHA, Treatment Efficacy Summary). In 2005, a Consensus Statement regarding voice therapy in the treatment of dysphonia was developed by the American Academy of Otolaryngology—Head and Neck Surgery Committee on Speech, Voice, and Swallowing, in conjunction with Special Interest Division 3 of the American Speech-Language-Hearing Association, (Voice and Voice Disorders). The statement is summarized as follows: "It is the consensus of these committees that voice therapy by a licensed speech language pathologist is important for effective medical and surgical treatment of the patient with dysphonia. Voice therapy should be an integral part of the treatment plan of the patient until optimal patient response is achieved." Studies have demonstrated the efficacy of behavioral voice treatments in improving voice function and reducing the recurrence of laryngeal pathology (Ramig & Verdolini, n.d.). For example, Carding, Horsley, and Docherty (1998) conducted a prospective controlled group study of effectiveness of direct, indirect, and no therapy on patients with nonorganic dysphonia. Patients were randomly assigned to one of three groups. Outcomes were measured by means of a patient questionnaire of vocal performance, auditory-perceptual voice quality ratings, and acoustic analysis. The authors reported that 14 of 15 patients in the direct therapy group showed the greatest improvement, with a voice quality within normal limits. These individuals reported a return to normal voice use and function. Seven patients in the indirect group showed considerable voice improvement, 5 showed minimal or no change, and 3 showed deterioration. Thirteen of the control patients showed either no improvement or further deterioration of vocal function. In a more broadly based study John, Enderby, and Hughes (2005) used a benchmark tool (Therapy Outcome Measure) comparing voice therapy services in seven voice centers in the United Kingdom. The measure evaluated impairment (degree of severity of the voice disorder), disability/activity (degree of limitation in use of voice to communicate), handicap/participation (amount of disadvantage to social participation), and well-being (effect on emotion/level of distress). The authors reported that the majority of patients made a positive change on each of the four dimensions. Patients completing their full treatment had the best outcomes.

chapter SUMMARY

NORMAL VOICE is a multidimensional entity that encompasses many different physical, perceptual, and lifestyle aspects. Voice is defined as normal when the quality is clear; pitch and loudness are appropriate for age, sex, and situation; the voice is produced without undue effort, pain, strain, or fatigue; and the voice is satisfactory to the speaker in terms of fulfilling his or her occupational, social, and emotional vocal needs. Auditory-perceptual and acoustic terms are commonly used to describe a speaker's vocal output. Perceptual terms are those that involve a subjective judgment of voice on the part of a speaker or listener. Acoustic terms are descriptors derived from acoustic analysis of the voice signal and are assumed to be more objective than perceptual judgments.

Dysphonia may result from structural problems within or outside of the larynx, neurological problems, lifestyle habits and choices, medications, psychological problems, systemic diseases of the body, physical injury to the larynx, digestive disorders, respiratory disorders, and unknown causes. The ideal approach to treatment is multidisciplinary in which a team of professionals contribute their expertise to the diagnosis, evaluation, and clinical management of individuals with voice disorders. Prevention of voice disorders is an important aspect of treatment. Prevention is categorized as primary, secondary, or tertiary. A focus on prevention expands the focus and broadens the scope of practice in the field of voice.

The International Classification of Functioning, Disability, and Health (ICF) sets forth a framework for describing the health status of a person from both an individual and a societal perspective and places health and functioning in the context of biological, psychological, and environmental factors. This classification system emphasizes health and wellness rather than disease and disability.

Medications help to alleviate many acute and chronic disorders and have contributed enormously to improved quality of life for millions of people. However, most medications have side effects, and many have the potential for affecting vocal function.

Over the past decade, the influence of social and cultural factors on the perception of acceptable voice quality and on the perception of voice disability has become widely recognized. Cultural, dialectical, and language-based expectations influence what is considered normal vocal quality and acceptable vocal patterns and usage. Cultural factors have also been implicated in vocal health.

Evidence-based practice is a three-pronged approach to clinical management that involves providing patients with the best possible services based on combining evidence from the research literature with clinical expertise and the individual's specific needs, wishes, and values. Behavioral voice treatment has been shown overall to be efficacious. Treatment efficacy is a broad term that includes treatment effectiveness, treatment efficiency, and treatment effects. Treatment effectiveness relates to whether the target treatment works, and if so, for which patients. Treatment efficiency refers to the ability of the treatment to achieve the objectives and goals with the minimum expenditure of time and cost. Treatment effects refer to ways in which the treatment modifies the target behavior(s).

review QUESTIONS

1. What factors need to be taken into account when trying to define normal voice and when dealing with an individual with a voice problem?
2. Identify and define perceptual and acoustic terms used in the diagnosis and treatment of voice disorders.
3. Describe the core and collateral members on a voice team and the responsibilities of each member.
4. Identify the three levels of prevention and provide examples of each.
5. Compare and contrast the 1980 and 2001 versions of the World Health Organization classification of disability and functioning.
6. Discuss the importance of xerostomia as a side effect of many classes of medications.
7. Develop a detailed protocol for dealing with a client from a different cultural background in preparation for an upcoming voice assessment. Provide a rationale for each step of the protocol.
8. Identify the benefits and drawbacks of evidence-based practice and apply these to a hypothetical clinical situation for a patient from a minority background.

Chapter 4

Diagnosis and Evaluation of Voice Disorders

LEARNING OBJECTIVES

1. Identify major areas to be addressed in the case history.
2. Appreciate the importance of quality of life measures in the evaluation process.
3. Understand the informal and formal procedures involved in the perceptual evaluation of the patient's voice.
4. Describe commonly used instrumental measures of vocal function including endoscopy and videostroboscopy.
5. Identify and define acoustic measures used to assess vocal output.
6. Describe electroglottography and how it may be used in the evaluation process.
7. Identify aerodynamic measures used in vocal function assessment.
8. Describe advantages and disadvantages of laryngeal electromyography in distinguishing between causes of vocal fold immobility.

The voice is the end result of the complex integration and coordination of many structural and physiological systems. It reflects the internal and external status of the individual, such as short-term and long-term physical status, emotional status, and psychological status. The voice is an important tool for social communication and is also strongly related to one's professional/vocational and/or educational status. The voice is influenced by cultural context and societal expectations. Because of the multitude of variables associated with voice, the diagnosis and evaluation of voice disorders is necessarily a complex and multidimensional undertaking.

The chapter begins with a brief summary of the roles of the otolaryngologist and speech-language pathologist in the diagnostic process. A detailed discussion of the components of a comprehensive voice evaluation is then presented. Attention is focused on the case history including quality of life issues, auditory-perceptual evaluation of voice, and instrumental measures of vocal function. Commonly used acoustic, electroglottographic, and aerodynamic measures are described, and the role of laryngeal electromyography is noted. The chapter concludes with an example of a diagnostic report that illustrates many of the described measures.

The primary aims of the voice evaluation are to determine the existence of a problem; discover the cause of the problem; describe the symptoms of the problem; assess the severity of the problem; investigate the effects of the problem on the patient's life; and determine the most effective ways to treat the problem. The many diverse aspects that may contribute to the disorder—respiratory, laryngeal, digestive, social, emotional, and so on—are best assessed and treated in a holistic manner, with members of the team contributing their expertise in their respective areas. Open communication and coordination among all professionals involved in the evaluation maximizes the probability for successful treatment outcomes. The specific members on the team depend on the individual's vocal problems and needs. As discussed in Chapter 3 the core team includes the otolaryngologist, speech-language pathologist, and patient/parents/caregivers. The collateral team may include a singing teacher, voice coach, neurologist, pulmonologist, endocrinologist, gastroenterologist, allergist, counselor, social worker, and classroom teacher.

The otolaryngologist is the medical specialist who examines the patient's larynx using direct or endoscopic laryngoscopy to detect any structural pathology or functional problems. The otolaryngologist usually makes the decision about whether to treat the voice problem using surgical, pharmacological, and/or behavioral methods. The speech-language pathologist may also carry out endoscopic laryngeal examination of the patient. The speech professional uses auditory-perceptual, acoustic, and/or aerodynamic means to evaluate the quality, pitch, and loudness characteristics of the patient's voice and to determine the overall severity of the dysphonia. The speech-language pathologist investigates the individual's vocal usage in different situations, vocal habits, and vocal technique. He or she takes an extensive case history of the patient. This includes medical information to determine if the individual has any coexisting disorders, what medications he or she is taking, previous conditions, and onset and course of the disorder. Information regarding the person's emotional status is also important to determine whether the patient is currently undergoing or has undergone conflict, stress, or anxiety that could be contributing to the voice problem. Finally, it is the speech-language pathologist's responsibility to design and implement a therapeutic regimen based on the information obtained from the evaluation. All diagnostic and assessment procedures should be carried out in accordance with ASHA's (2004) preferred practice patterns for the assessment of voice disorders (see Appendix 1).

Components of the Evaluation Process

The voice evaluation is typically divided into several components. These include the patient interview and case history, laryngeal examination, perceptual and instrumental assessment of voice, interpretation of test results, prognosis, and recommendations for treatment (Table 4.1). If possible, team members should discuss their findings after each phase of the evaluation and contribute their ideas to the clinical picture (Gartner-Schmidt & Rosen, 2009). After the evaluation process is complete the team members formulate a treatment plan based on all findings.

CASE HISTORY

The first step in the evaluation process is the case history interview. During this interview the speech-language pathologist gathers information from the patient and/or other people in the patient's life about the history and current features of the problem. Because the voice is a

TABLE 4.1 Components of a Comprehensive Voice Evaluation

Case history	Medical
	Psychosocial
	Professional/vocational/educational
	Interpersonal
	Lifestyle/diet/tobacco/alcohol/caffeine
Quality of life	Voice Handicap Index
	Voice Activity and Participation Profile
	Voice-Related Quality of Life
	Glottal Function Index
	Parent proxy questionnaires
Auditory-perceptual	CAPE-V
	GRBAS
	Counting (endurance, fatigue)
	Hard glottal attacks
	Cough
Laryngeal examination	Indirect (mirror) laryngoscopy
	Rigid/flexible endoscopy
	Videostroboscopy
	Laryngeal electromyography
Acoustic analysis	Mean fundamental frequency (sustained vowel, connected speech)
	Maximum phonational frequency range
	Frequency variability
	Mean intensity (sustained vowel, connected speech)
	Dynamic range
	Voice range profile
	Jitter/shimmer
	Harmonics-to-noise ratio/noise-to-harmonics ratio/normalized noise energy
	Electroglottography
Aerodynamic analysis	Air volume
	Glottal airflow
	Subglottal pressure
Phonatory/respiratory efficiency	Maximum phonation time
	s/z ratio

multidimensional entity, it is important that the case history be broadly based in order to elicit information regarding all aspects of the individual's life that may affect vocal function. The case history allows the evaluator to obtain a detailed understanding of the person's disorder, including the onset of the problem, how the problem has (or has not) changed over time, and the current status of the problem. Tables 4.2 and 4.3 provide samples of case history forms for adults and children, respectively.

TABLE 4.2 Sample Case History Form for an Adult

Name:	DOB	Age	M	F
Address:				
Occupation:				
Marital status:				
Children (names and ages):				
Phone: Home	Work		Cell	
Email:				
Referred by:				

Voice History

What is the problem that brings you here today?

When did you first start to notice this problem?

Have you ever experienced any previous voice changes or difficulties? If yes, explain.

How would you describe the severity of your voice problem?

Has the problem changed since you first noticed it? If yes, explain.

Prior to today, did you consult a health professional about this problem? If yes, who?

Have you ever been treated by an ear, nose, and throat doctor (ENT) in the past? If yes, explain.

Have you ever been seen by a speech-language pathologist in the past? If yes, explain.

Has anyone in your family ever had a voice problem? If yes, explain.

Voice Symptoms

How would you describe your voice symptoms (e.g., hoarse, breathy, tight, strained, weak, monotonous)?

Does your voice change during the day? If yes, explain.

On a 5-point scale where 1 = very mild and 5 = very severe, how would you rate your vocal symptoms?

On a scale of 0–5, where 0 = never and 5 = always, how often do you do the following?

Shout or scream

Talk loudly

Talk a lot

Talk over noise

Use the phone

Sing

TABLE 4.2 (Continued)

Physical Symptoms

Do you have any burning, soreness, tickling, or irritation in your throat?
Do you sometimes have the sensation of a "lump" in the throat?
Do you have any aching or tightness in your throat?
Do you ever feel tension in your neck area?
Does your voice get tired easily?
Do you feel as if you have to strain to produce voice?
Do you feel as if you need to cough or clear your throat a lot?
Do you ever lose your voice completely? If yes, explain.
Do you ever have difficulty swallowing? If yes, explain.
Do you often get sore throats?
Do you have difficulty projecting your voice?

Medical History

Have you had any major surgeries or illnesses? If yes, describe.
Have you ever been intubated (breathing tube)? If yes, describe.
Do you have any neurological conditions? If yes, describe.
Do you have any respiratory problems (e.g., asthma, allergies, postnasal drip)? If yes, describe.
Do you have acid reflux or heartburn? If yes, describe.
Do you have any hormonal problems (e.g., hypo- or hyperthyroidism)? If yes, describe.
If you are a female, do you take oral contraceptives or other hormonal medications? If yes, describe.
List all medications you take, including prescription, over-the-counter, vitamins, and supplements.
Check if you have ever had any of the following:

AIDS	Arthritis	Cancer
Chronic fatigue	Depression	Diabetes
Dizziness	Ear infections	Ear pain/tinnitus
Eating disorder	Headaches	Hearing loss
Heart disease	Hiatal hernia	Nasal blockage
Neck injury	Psychiatric disorder	Seizures
Sinus problems	Sleep problems	Stroke
Temporomandibular joint problems	Weight loss	Tremor
Ulcer		

Occupational Voice Demands

Are you a professional voice user (e.g., teacher, salesperson, customer service representative, etc.)? If yes, explain.
Are you a professional or amateur singer? If yes, explain.
On a scale of 1–5 where 1 = very little and 5 = excessive, how would you characterize your daily average voice use?
Is there a high level of noise in your workplace? If yes, explain.
Are you exposed to fumes, pollutants, and other irritants in your workplace (e.g., ammonia, chemicals, dust, etc.)? If yes, explain.

(continued)

TABLE 4.2 Sample Case History Form for an Adult (Continued)

Lifestyle Considerations

How many people live in your house?
How many children live with you?
Do you have an active social life? Explain.
Does anyone in your family or your social circle have a hearing loss?
What are your hobbies?
Do you participate in activities such as debate, cheerleading, singing, etc.? If yes, explain.
Do you smoke? If yes, how many cigarettes/cigars per day?
If not, did you smoke previously? When?
Do you drink alcohol? If yes, how much per week?
Do you drink caffeinated beverages (e.g., tea, coffee, soda)? If yes, how many per day?
How much water do you drink per day?
Do you exercise on a regular basis? If yes, how often per week?
Do you have a healthy diet? Explain.

TABLE 4.3 Sample Case History Form for a Child

Child's name:	DOB	Age	M	F
Mother's name:				
Occupation:		Phone:		
Father's name:				
Occupation:		Phone:		
Home phone:				
Parent cell phone:				
Home address:				
Other children (names and ages):				
School:		Grade:	Teacher:	
Referred by:				

Voice History

What is the problem with your child's voice that brings you here today?
When did you first start to notice this problem?
Has your child ever experienced any previous voice changes or difficulties? If yes, explain.

TABLE 4.3 (Continued)

How would you describe the severity of your child's voice problem?
Has the problem changed since you first noticed it? If yes, explain.
Prior to today, did you consult a health professional about this problem? If yes, who?
Has your child ever been treated by an ear, nose, and throat doctor (ENT) in the past? If yes, explain.
Has your child ever been seen by a speech-language pathologist in the past? If yes, explain.
Has anyone in your family ever had a voice problem? If yes, explain.

Voice Symptoms

How would you describe your child's voice symptoms (e.g., hoarse, breathy, tight, strained, weak, monotonous)?
Does your child's voice change during the day? If yes, explain.
On a 5-point scale where 1 = very mild and 5 = very severe, how would you rate your child's vocal symptoms?
Does your child frequently cough or clear his or her throat?
Does your child have any difficulty breathing or swallowing?
Does your child often complain of a sore throat?
Does your child's voice sound worse at different times of day?
On a scale of 0–5, where 0 = never, and 5 = always, how often does your child do the following?
Shout or scream
Talk loudly
Talk a lot
Cry
Make car/animal noises
Talk over noise
Use the phone
Sing
Cough and/or clear his or her throat
Participate in sports activities or cheerleading activities that require extremely loud volumes

Developmental History

Did you have any problems during your pregnancy with this child or any of your other children?
Did your child meet developmental milestones (sitting, walking, talking, etc.) within the normal time range?
Does your child have normal hearing?
How does your child perform academically?

Medical History

Does your child often complain of a sore throat?
Does your child lose his or her voice every time he or she has a cold?
Has your child had any major surgeries or illnesses? If yes, describe.
Has your child ever been intubated (breathing tube)? If yes, describe.
Does your child have any neurological conditions? If yes, describe.
Does your child have any respiratory problems (e.g., asthma, allergies, postnasal drip)? If yes, describe.
Does your child have acid reflux or heartburn? If yes, describe.

(continued)

TABLE 4.3 Sample Case History Form for a Child (Continued)

Does your child have any hormonal problems (e.g., hypo- or hyperthyroidism)? If yes, describe.
List all medications your child takes, including prescription, over-the-counter, vitamins, and supplements.
Does your child have a hearing loss or frequent ear infections?
Was your child intubated at birth or later? If yes, describe.

Social Development

How would you describe your child's social skills (e.g., outgoing, shy, independent, neat, withdrawn, interested)?
Does your child participate in activities such as sports, debate, cheerleading, drama, singing?
Does your child attend social events such as parties, concerts, sports events?
Does your child express his or her feelings as appropriate?

The interview begins by questioning the patient or parent/caregiver regarding his or her perceptions of the voice problem and history of this or previous problems. The medical history is important to determine if, and to what extent, medically related factors may have contributed to the development of the voice disorder. The individual (or parent/caregiver) is questioned about past surgeries, particularly laryngeal, head and neck, chest, or heart surgeries. If the patient has been hospitalized, it is important to learn if he or she was intubated, and for how long. Questions are asked about the existence of chronic disorders such as arthritis, and whether the individual uses over-the-counter or prescribed medications. If the patient is a female, it is necessary to find out if she uses oral contraceptives or is undergoing hormone replacement therapy. The presence of any neurological problems, respiratory problems, gastrointestinal tract problems, allergy-related problems, psychiatric problems, congenital anomalies, or hearing loss is noted. Complaints of physical symptoms related to the voice may be assessed on a scale such as the Vocal Tract Discomfort Scale (Mathieson et al., 2009) (Table 4.4).

When questioning the patient or the patient's caregiver(s) about his or her social and professional/vocational/educational lives, the objective is to probe the amount and type of voice use in different situations, as well as to determine if the individual is subjected to stress, anxiety, and tension that may contribute to the voice problem. Questions focus on the patient's home life, family relationships, social network, hobbies, and work- or school-related issues. Lifestyle questions elicit information regarding the individual's tobacco, caffeine, and alcohol usage; eating habits; and occupational or educational demands.

The interview process provides an excellent opportunity for the clinician to informally evaluate the patient's voice in a conversational setting. Aspects to be noted include the overall level of severity of dysphonia and the presence of specific voice qualities such as hoarseness, roughness, breathiness, strain, tension, and weakness. The clinician notes whether the individual's voice quality fluctuates or is consistent. Pitch and loudness levels are considered, and the clinician notes any pitch breaks, diplophonia, voice arrests, stridor, hyper- or hyponasality, hard glottal attacks, and excessive coughing or throat clearing. The examiner can also observe if there is any visible tension around the patient's laryngeal area. The speech-language pathologist takes note of the individual's sitting and standing posture, as well as breathing patterns such as shallow, exaggerated, abdominal, thoracic, or clavicular breathing (Gilman & Hapner, 2006).

TABLE 4.4 **Vocal Tract Discomfort Scale**

The following are symptoms or sensations that you may feel in your throat, which may occur as part of your voice problem. Please indicate the frequency with which they occur and the severity of the symptom or sensation, by circling a number in the appropriate column.

Patient identifier ____________________

Date ______________________________

	Frequency of sensation/symptom							**Severity of sensation/symptom**						
	0	1	2	3	4	5	6	0	1	2	3	4	5	6
	never	*sometimes*		*often*		*always*		*none*	*mild*		*moderate*		*extreme*	
Burning	0	1	2	3	4	5	6	0	1	2	3	4	5	6
Tight	0	1	2	3	4	5	6	0	1	2	3	4	5	6
Dry	0	1	2	3	4	5	6	0	1	2	3	4	5	6
Aching	0	1	2	3	4	5	6	0	1	2	3	4	5	6
Tickling	0	1	2	3	4	5	6	0	1	2	3	4	5	6
Sore	0	1	2	3	4	5	6	0	1	2	3	4	5	6
Irritable	0	1	2	3	4	5	6	0	1	2	3	4	5	6
Lump in throat	0	1	2	3	4	5	6	0	1	2	3	4	5	6

Source: From "Laryngeal Manual Therapy: A Preliminary Study to Examine Its Treatment Effects in the Management of Muscle Tension Dysphonia," by L. Mathieson, S. P. Hirani, R. Epstein, R. J. Baken, G. Wood, and J. S. Rubin, 2009, *Journal of Voice, 23,* pp. 358–359. Copyright 2009 by The Voice Foundation. Reprinted with permission.

Also important is to judge the patient's vocal endurance or fatigue, and to note if the voice deteriorates or improves with use during the interview.

Quality of Life. A critical element of the evaluation process is to obtain the individual's perception of the impact of the voice disorder on his or her life using an appropriate quality of life (QOL) measure. This information helps the clinician to obtain a comprehensive view of the patient's functioning in all aspects of his or her life including any limitations of activity and restriction in participation. QOL information helps to provide the best possible treatment for the patient, as well as serving as an important outcomes measure.

Measures that assess the impact of health issues on quality of life have been around for some decades and are widely used in many health fields. Only since the mid-1990s, however, have tools been developed to apply these concepts to voice. Several such tools have been developed over the past few years (Table 4.5).

The Voice Handicap Index (VHI) developed by Jacobson et al. (1997) is a 30-item questionnaire, with questions divided into physical, functional, and emotional categories (Table 4.6).

The patient rates each statement on a 5-point scale (0 = never had the experience, 1 = almost never, 2 = sometimes, 3 = almost always, 4 = always). The functional scale includes statements that describe the impact of the patient's voice disorder on daily activities. The physical scale contains statements representing the patient's perceptions of any

TABLE 4.5 Adult and Pediatric Voice-Related Quality of Life Instruments

Instrument	Developer(s)	Categories
Adult		
Voice Handicap Index (VHI)	Jacobson et al. (1997)	Physical, Functional, Emotional
Voice Activity and Participation Profile (VAPP)	Ma & Yiu (2001)	Job, Daily Communication, Social, Emotional
Voice-Related Quality of Life (V-RQOL)	Hogikyan et al. (2000)	Physical, Social-Emotional
Voice Outcome Survey (VOS) (Unilateral vocal fold paralysis)	Gliklich et al. (1999)	Functional, Social, Work
Voice Symptom Scale (Voiss)	Dreary et al. (2003)	Communication, Physical, Emotional
Vocal Disability Coping Questionnaire (VDCQ)	Epstein et al. (2009)	Information seeking, Problem solving, Avoidance, Social withdrawal
Pediatric		
Pediatric VHI (pVHI)	Zur et al. (2007)	Same as adult
Pediatric VOS (PVOS)	Hartnick et al. (2003)	Physical, Social, School
Pediatric V-RQOL (PVRQOL)	Boseley et al. (2006)	Same as adult

TABLE 4.6 Voice Handicap Index

F1	My voice makes it difficult for people to hear me
P2	I run out of air when I talk
F3	People have difficulty understanding me in a noisy room
P4	The sound of my voice varies throughout the day
F5	My family has difficulty hearing me when I call them throughout the house
F6	I use the phone less often than I would like
E7	I'm tense when talking with others because of my voice
F8	I tend to avoid groups of people because of my voice
E9	People seem irritated with my voice
P10	People ask 'What's wrong with your voice?'
F11	I speak with friends, neighbors or relatives less often because of my voice
F12	People ask me to repeat myself when speaking face to face
P13	My voice sounds creaky and dry

TABLE 4.6 **(Continued)**

P14	I feel as though I have to strain to produce voice
E15	I find other people don't understand my voice problem
F16	My voice difficulties restrict my personal and social life
P17	The clarity of my voice is unpredictable
P18	I try to change my voice to sound different
F19	I feel left out of conversations because of my voice
P20	I use a great deal of effort to speak
P21	My voice is worse in the evening
F22	My voice problem causes me to lose income
E23	My voice problem upsets me
E24	I am less outgoing because of my voice problem
E25	My voice makes me feel handicapped
P26	My voice "gives out" on me in the middle of speaking
E27	I feel annoyed when people ask me to repeat
E28	I feel embarrassed when people ask me to repeat
E29	My voice makes me feel incompetent
E30	I'm ashamed of my voice problem

Source: From "The Voice Handicap Index (VHI): Development and Validation," by B. J. Jacobson, A. Johnson, C. Grywalski, A. Silbergleit, G. Jacobson, M. S. Benninger, and C. W. Newman, 1997, *American Journal of Speech-Language Pathology, 6*, p. 68. Copyright 1997 by the American Speech-Language-Hearing Association. Reprinted with permission.

physical pain or discomfort in and around the larynx as well as his or her voice quality. On the emotional scale the patient provides information regarding his or her feelings about the voice disorder. The higher the score, the greater the patient's perception of disability created by the voice problem. The scale is scored out of a total possible number of points of 120. A score of 0–30 indicates a low perception of voice-related handicap; a score between 31 and 60 points indicates a moderate level of handicap; and a score greater than 60 points indicates a severe level of handicap (Jacobson et al., 1997). The VHI is the most commonly used quality of life instrument for voice disorders and has been translated into many languages including Greek (Helidoni et al., 2008), Hebrew (Amir et al., 2006), Chinese (Lam et al., 2006), and Portuguese (Gasparini & Behlau, 2007; Guimaraes & Abberton, 2004). It has been validated in occupations including teaching, professional speaking, and singing (Franic, Bramlett, & Bothe, 2005), and it has been modified for use for partners of individuals with voice problems (Zraick et al., 2007).

The Voice-Related Quality of Life (V-RQOL) measure developed by Hogikyan, Wodchis, Terrell, Bradford, and Esclamado (2000) assesses the impact of the voice problem in the social-emotional and physical domains, as well as the patient's perception of his or her voice quality during the two-week period preceding the assessment. There are 10 questions, which are rated in terms of severity on a 5-point scale (Table 4.7).

TABLE 4.7 Voice-Related Quality of Life

I have trouble speaking loudly or being heard in noisy situations.
I run out of air and need to take frequent breaths when talking.
I sometimes do not know what will come out when I begin speaking.
I am sometimes anxious or frustrated (because of my voice).
I sometimes get depressed (because of my voice).
I have trouble using the telephone (because of my voice).
I have trouble doing my job or practicing my profession (because of my voice).
I avoid going out socially (because of my voice)
I have to repeat myself to be understood.
I have become less outgoing (because of my voice).
The overall quality of my voice during the last two weeks has been (please circle)
Poor Fair Good Very good Excellent

Source: From "Voice-Related Quality of Life (V-RQOL) Following Type I Thyroplasty for Unilateral Vocal Fold Paralysis," by N. D. Hogikyan, W. P. Wodchis, J. E. Terrell, C. R. Bradford, and R. M. Esclamado, 2000, *Journal of Voice, 14*, p. 381.

The Voice Disability and Coping Questionnaire (VDCQ), developed by Epstein, Hirani, Stygall, and Newman (2009), is a 15-item instrument that uses a 6-point scale to assess how the individual copes with the effects of a voice disorder (Table 4.8).

Coping refers to the individual's cognitive and behavioral efforts to manage the stress of illness and is directly related to physical and functional outcomes of illness (Zraick & Jacobson, 2008). Coping can be problem-focused or emotion-focused. A problem-focused approach is one in which the individual tries to solve the problem by changing the environment to reduce the impact of the stress; in an emotion-focused approach the individual attempts to control or discharge the emotions generated by the stressful situation (Epstein et al., 2009). The VDCQ identifies four coping strategies: social support, information seeking, passive coping, and avoidance. The authors noted that the questionnaire can be used to identify adaptive and maladaptive coping strategies used by the patient, and thus help to guide intervention.

Several of the QOL instruments, including the VHI, have been modified for use as parent proxy questionnaires for children with voice disorders (see Table 4.5). The VHI has been modified for pediatric use as the Pediatric VHI (Zur et al., 2007), and the V-RQOL has been modified for pediatric use as the Pediatric V-RQOL (Blumin, Keppel, Braun, Kerschner, & Merati, 2008). Table 4.9 displays the Pediatric VHI.

The focus on children is a recent acknowledgment that quality of life issues are as important for children as they are for adults. Parent proxy questionnaires are thought to be a valid means of obtaining information about the child's QOL. Young children may not be able to fully understand their disorder or its effect on their present and future functioning (Boseley, Cunningham, Volk, & Hartnick, 2006; Hartnick 2002). The child's parents may have a clearer understanding of how the voice problem affects his or her academic, social, and interpersonal functioning (Hartnick, Volk, & Cunningham, 2003). However, recent qualitative studies have

TABLE 4.8 Vocal Disability Coping Questionnaire

Frequency of usage: 0 = never; 1 = almost never; 2 = sometimes; 3 = quite often; 4 = very often; 5 = always

1. It helps me to cope with my voice problem if other people are sympathetic.
2. I try to avoid situations where my voice problem would become evident.
3. I find myself wishing that I never had a voice problem.
4. I try to find as much information as possible about my voice problem.
5. I find it easier to cope with my voice problem by expressing my feelings outwardly.
6. I find it easier to cope with my voice problem by telling myself not to think about it.
7. I find talking with friends and family about my voice problem helpful.
8. I find it easier to cope with my voice problem by finding out as much about it as I can.
9. I keep any worries I may have about my voice problem to myself.
10. I take the view that there is little I can do about my voice problem.
11. I find it easier to live with my voice problem if I do not use my voice.
12. Having a voice problem has helped me find some important truth about my life.
13. I find it easier to cope with my voice problem if I ask the doctor questions about it.
14. I find it easier to cope with my voice problem by avoiding being with people in general.
15. I find it easier to cope with my voice problem by wishing that it would go away or somehow be over with.

Source: From "How Do Individuals Cope with Voice Disorders? Introducing the Voice Disability Coping Questionnaire," by R. Epstein, S. P. Hirani, J. Stygall, and S. P. Newman, 2009, *Journal of Voice, 23*, p. 213, Copyright 2009 by The Voice Foundation. Reprinted with permission.

TABLE 4.9 Pediatric Voice Handicap Index

Subject Number: ________________ Date: ___________

I would rate my/my child's talkativeness as the following:

1	2	3	4	5	6	7
Quiet Listener			Average Talker			Extremely Talkative

Instructions: These are statements that many people have used to describe their voices and the effects of their voices on their lives. Circle the response that indicates how frequently you have the same experience:

0 = never 1 = almost never 2 = sometimes 3 = almost always 4 = always

Part I-F

1. My child's voice makes it difficult for people to hear him/her.	0 1 2 3 4
2. People have difficulty understanding my child in a noisy room.	0 1 2 3 4

(continued)

TABLE 4.9 **Pediatric Voice Handicap Index (Continued)**

3. At home we have difficulty hearing my child when he/she calls through the house.	0 1 2 3 4
4. My child tends to avoid communicating because of his/her voice.	0 1 2 3 4
5. My child speaks with friends, neighbors, or relatives less often because of his/her voice.	0 1 2 3 4
6. People ask my child to repeat him/herself when speaking face-to-face.	0 1 2 3 4
7. My child's voice difficulties restrict personal, educational and social activities.	0 1 2 3 4
Part II-P	
1. My child runs out of air when talking.	0 1 2 3 4
2. The sound of my child's voice changes throughout the day.	0 1 2 3 4
3. People ask "What's wrong with your child's voice?"	0 1 2 3 4
4. My child's voice sounds dry, raspy, and/or hoarse.	0 1 2 3 4
5. The quality of my child's voice is unpredictable.	0 1 2 3 4
6. My child uses a great deal of effort to speak (e.g., straining).	0 1 2 3 4
7. My child's voice is worse in the evening.	0 1 2 3 4
8. My child's voice "gives out" when speaking.	0 1 2 3 4
9. My child has to yell in order for others to hear him/her.	0 1 2 3 4
Part III-E	
1. My child appears tense when talking to others because of his or her voice.	0 1 2 3 4
2. People seem irritated with my child's voice.	0 1 2 3 4
3. I find other people don't understand my child's voice problem.	0 1 2 3 4
4. My child is frustrated with his/her voice problem.	0 1 2 3 4
5. My child is less outgoing because of his/her voice problem.	0 1 2 3 4
6. My child is annoyed when people ask him/her to repeat.	0 1 2 3 4
7. My child is embarrassed when people ask him/her to repeat.	0 1 2 3 4

Overall Severity Rating of Voice

(Please place "X" mark anywhere along this line to indicate the severity of your child's voice; the verbal descriptions serve as a guide)

Normal	Severe

Source: From "Pediatric Voice Handicap Index (pVHI): A New Tool for Evaluating Pediatric Dysphonia," by K. B. Zur, S. Cotton, L. Kelchner, S. Baker, B. Weinrich, and L. Lee, 2007, *International Journal of Pediatric Otorhinolaryngology, 71*, p. 79. Copyright 2007 by Elsevier. Reprinted with permission.

revealed that children with voice problems as young as age 2 years are aware of and often concerned about their voices. Concerns expressed by children and adolescents include physical issues such as running out of air, effort in initiating vocalization, sore throat when vocalizing; functional issues such as being asked to speak up, difficulty talking on the phone, and being teased; and emotional issues such as voice-related feelings of anger, sadness, irritation, and frustration (Connor et al., 2008; Verduyckt, Remacle, Jamart, Benderitter, & Morsomme, 2010). Thus, it is important that a quality of life instrument be developed specifically to assess children's own perceptions of the impact of the voice disorder on their everyday lives.

Despite some concerns regarding the development and validation of these voice-related quality of life measures, their use provides clinicians a way to track and measure treatment effectiveness. These measures also help speech-language pathologists to gain insight into the patient's expectations of the rehabilitation process and treatment outcomes (Branski et al., 2009).

AUDITORY-PERCEPTUAL EVALUATION

Following the case history interview including administration of appropriate quality of life measures, the patient undergoes a series of assessments aimed at determining the nature and severity of his or her voice problem. The evaluation typically includes auditory-perceptual and instrumental measures. Auditory-perceptual measures require the clinician to make a subjective judgment of aspects of the person's voice, such as the overall level of severity, the appropriateness of the pitch and loudness levels, and the quality of the voice. In addition, auditory-perceptual evaluation allows the clinician to obtain a comprehensive overview of the speaker's voice, to describe specific aspects of the voice, to identify and define the extent of the vocal problem, and to plan, monitor, and measure the outcome of therapeutic intervention (Carding, Carlson, Epstein, Mathieson, & Shewell, 2000).

Auditory-perceptual evaluation is often considered a "gold standard" that provides a real-life basis of comparison between the patient's voice and a reference group of normal voices (e.g., Solomon, Helou, & Stojadinovic, 2009). Perceived voice quality by self and others is the means by which an individual's vocal and communicative effectiveness is judged. Thus the patient's perception of the initial severity of the disorder forms an important basis for later decisions regarding the success of treatment and patient satisfaction (Eadie et al., 2009; Kelchner et al., 2008).

During the auditory-perceptual evaluation the clinician asks the patient to perform various vocal activities designed to assess aspects of vocal production such as respiratory-phonatory efficiency, vocal endurance, reflexive laryngeal function, and presence of musculoskeletal tension (Table 4.10).

Simple and noninvasive measures such as maximum phonation time (MPT) and the s/z ratio provide information regarding the individual's respiratory support for speech and glottal efficiency in converting the exhaled air into voiced sound. To obtain MPT the patient is asked to take as deep a breath as possible and sustain the vowel /a/ for as long as possible. This is often done at three pitch levels: comfortable pitch, high pitch, and low pitch. Adults should be able to sustain voicing for least 20 seconds, and children for 10–15 seconds. MPT is often reduced in individuals with dysphonia (e.g., Speyer et al., 2008). It is very commonly used as an outcomes measure that reflects changes in glottal efficiency, particularly in patients who have undergone treatment for conditions that impair glottal efficiency such as unilateral vocal fold paralysis. The s/z ratio compares the individual's ability to sustain the voiceless and voiced fricatives. The patient is asked to take the deepest breath possible and sustain /s/ for as long as possible; then he or she is asked to do the same for /z/. The time recorded for /s/ is divided by the time for /z/. The normal ratio is around 1.0–1.4, indicating that the individual is able to sustain respiration without voicing (/s/) and with voicing (/z/) for approximately equal amounts of time. Ratios greater than 1.4 demonstrate that the patient is not able to sustain the voiced sound for as long as the voiceless sound, and this may indicate impaired glottal efficiency. However, recent research has demonstrated that there is considerable variability in the s/z ratios of healthy speakers with no voice problems, and there is substantial overlap in the ratios of those with and without laryngeal pathology (Gelfer & Pazera, 2006).

TABLE 4.10 **Vocal Activities in an Auditory-Perceptual Evaluation**

Phonatory-respiratory efficiency
Maximum phonation time
s/z ratio
Vocal range
Pitch range
Loudness range
Physical
Endurance testing
Musculoskeletal tension test
Laryngeal function
Hard glottal attack
Cough
Laugh
Clear throat

The patient's maximum ranges of pitch and loudness are assessed. In terms of pitch, he or she is asked to sing a scale reaching the highest and lowest notes possible, excluding pulse register but including falsetto. The normal pitch range is around two and one half to three octaves for adults, and around two octaves for children. To determine loudness range, the patient is asked to count starting from the softest voice possible and then gradually increasing to the loudest possible. To test vocal endurance the individual is asked to count vigorously to at least 100. The presence of musculoskeletal tension is determined by palpating the external laryngeal musculature with the patient identifying any points of pain or tenderness. A pattern of hard glottal attacks is evaluated as the patient counts from 80 to 90, stopping between each number. Reflexive laryngeal valving is assessed by asking him or her to cough forcefully, to say "uh-huh," laugh, and clear the throat. This is important information for disorders such as **spasmodic dysphonia**, in which the patient may have normal reflexive vocal function, but impaired function for phonation. A weak cough often accompanies vocal fold paralysis or **paresis**.

In addition to these vocal activities, the patient's voice is rated on some kind of scale. Auditory-perceptual rating instruments include equal-appearing interval scales, semantic differential scales, and visual analogue scales. Equal-appearing interval scales comprise a series of numbers that represent levels of severity of a particular aspect of voice. For example, quality may be rated from 0 to 5, with 0 representing normal quality and 5 representing severely deviant quality. The same type of scale could be used for pitch and loudness, or other vocal features. Semantic differential scales present a series of polar opposites related to voice, for example, normal–abnormal; pleasant–unpleasant; weak–strong; high pitch–low pitch; and so on. The evaluator determines where the patient's voice falls on a 5- or 7-point scale between the polar opposites. Visual analogue scales allow the examiner a more finely graded continuum for rating the voice. These scales typically present a 100 mm horizontal line for specific vocal

TABLE 4.11 GRBAS Voice Rating Scale

0 = normal
1 = slight
2 = moderate
3 = extreme

Grade (degree of hoarseness or voice abnormality):
Roughness (auditory/acoustic impression of irregularity of vibration)
Breathiness (auditory/acoustic impression of degree of air leakage)
Asthenic (weakness or lack of power)
Strain (auditory/acoustic impression of hyperfunction

Check for presence of the following:
Tremor
Pitch variation
Loudness variation
Voice interruption
Other

features such as hoarseness, breathiness, harshness, and strain. Normal values are toward the left side of the line, and abnormal values toward the right side of the line. The evaluator marks the point on the line that corresponds to his or her perception of the voice abnormality.

An equal-appearing interval scale that is used commonly in Europe and is becoming more widely recognized in the United States is the GRBAS scale (Table 4.11).

This scale was developed by the Committee of Phonatory Function Tests of the Japan Society of Logopedics and Phoniatrics (Hirano, 1981). The five items on the scale are grade (G), rough (R), breathy (B), asthenic (A), and strained (S). Each of these features is rated on a 4-point scale on which 0 represents normal and 3 indicates an extreme problem. This scale has been shown to be a reliable measure and is recommended for clinical and research purposes by the European Research Group on the Larynx (Mathieson, 2001).

Recently, a group of clinicians and researchers in ASHA's Special Interest Division on Voice and Voice Disorders developed a visual analogue scale to evaluate voice (Kempster, Gerratt, Verdolini, Barkmeier-Kraemer, & Hillman, 2009). Called the Consensus Auditory-Perceptual Evaluation of Voice (CAPE-V), it is designed to facilitate a standardized approach to evaluating and documenting vocal function and voice quality (Table 4.12).

The authors incorporated several principles into the development of this instrument. First, the selected vocal dimensions should reflect a minimal set of clinically meaningful perceptual voice parameters. Second, procedures and results should be easy and efficient to obtain. Third, procedures and results should be applicable to a broad range of vocal pathologies and clinical settings; and fourth, ratings should be reliable within and across clinicians. The protocol examines vocal features in different contexts including vowel prolongations, sentence repetition, and connected speech. Vocal features that are evaluated include overall

TABLE 4.12 **Consensus Auditory-Perceptual Evaluation of Voice (CAPE-V)**

Tasks

Sustained vowels /a/ and/i/ for 3–5 seconds duration each sentence production:

a. The blue spot is on the key again.
b. How hard did he hit him?
c. We were away a year ago.
d. We eat eggs every Easter.
e. My mama makes lemon muffins.
f. Peter will keep at the peak.

Spontaneous speech in response to "Tell me about your voice problem" or "Tell me how your voice is functioning."

Legend C = Consistent I = Intermittent

MI = Mildly Deviant, MO = Moderately Deviant, SE = Severely Deviant

				Score
Overall Severity	______	______	______	/100
	MI	MO	SE	
Roughness	______	______	______	/100
	MI	MO	SE	
Breathiness	______	______	______	/100
	MI	MO	SE	
Strain	______	______	______	/100
	MI	MO	SE	
Pitch	______	______	______	/100
	MI	MO	SE	
Loudness	______	______	______	/100
	MI	MO	SE	

Resonance

Other (diplophonia, glottal fry, falsetto, asthenia, aphonia, pitch instability, tremor, wet/gurgly, strained/strangled)

Normal ____________________ Other (Provide description): ____________________

Source: From "Consensus Auditory-Perceptual Evaluation of Voice: Development of a Standardized Clinical Protocol," by G. B. Kempster, B. R. Gerratt, K. Verdolini Abbott, J. Barkmeier-Kraemer, and R. E. Hillman, 2009, *American Journal of Speech-Language Pathology, 18*, p. 128. Copyright 2009 by the American Speech-Language-Hearing Association. Reprinted with permission.

severity (the clinician's global integrated impression of voice deviance), roughness (perceived irregularity in the voicing source), breathiness (audible air escape), strain (perception of excessive vocal effort/hyperfunction), pitch (perceptual correlate of F0), and loudness (perceptual correlate of intensity). The form also provides space for the clinician to rate other perceptual aspects of the individual's voice such as spasm, tremor, diplophonia, falsetto, glottal fry, and so on. Features are rated on a 100 mm horizontal line, where the left of the line indicates a more normal voice feature, and the right end of the line indicates a more severe level. For every feature the mark on the line is converted to a quantitative score by measuring the distance from the mark to the left point of the line. Thus a mark measured to be 75 mm from the left point is given a score of 75/100. The higher the score, the more severe the rated feature. Features are also noted to be consistent or intermittent. This instrument is becoming widely used in the United States and has been reported to demonstrate empirical validity (Zraick et al., 2010). Additional information regarding the CAPE-V is available from www.southalabama.edu/alliedhealth/speechandhearing/jestis/SLP%20551/551%20CAPEV.pdf.

Patient self-perception scales are also becoming more popular. Bach, Belafsky, Wasylik, Postma, and Koufman (2005) developed the Glottal Function Index (GFI), which has been used at the Center for Voice Disorders of Wake Forest University for many years. This is a 5-point equal-appearing interval scale that assesses the patient's perception of glottal dysfunction. A GFI score greater than 4 is considered to reflect problems in vocal function (Table 4.13).

Auditory-perceptual measurement of voice is the most often used clinical evaluation method (Oates, 2004). While auditory-perceptual assessment is considered the "gold standard," there are several disadvantages associated with these measures. First, definitions of commonly used terms (hoarseness, breathiness, roughness, strain, tense) are not standardized, making the judgments very subjective. Consequently it is difficult or impossible for clinicians from different settings to communicate accurately about a patient with a voice problem. Second, voice quality is multidimensional and is influenced by factors such as pitch, loudness, articulatory precision, rate of speech, and resonance characteristics. Traditional perceptual labels such as "roughness" or "breathiness" are one-dimensional and do not take the interdependence of factors into account (Schaeffer & Sidavi, 2009). Third, while the clinician can form a good idea about the sound of a patient's voice, it is not possible to analyze the actual vocal fold behavior that produced this quality. The fourth disadvantage is the commonly reported lack of reliability of perceptual ratings between and within raters, regardless of their degree of sophistication and expertise (e.g., Kreiman & Gerratt, 2010). Also unknown is how individual differences in perception influence clinician judgment (Kelchner et al., 2008). Despite these drawbacks, there is evidence that different types of scales for perceptual ratings are reasonably reliable, and commonly used terms to describe voice quality features have reasonable validity in terms of their relationship with underlying vocal tract physiology and acoustic features (Oates, 2004).

TABLE 4.13 Glottal Function Index

On a scale of 0 (no problem) to 5 (severe problem) within the last month, how did the following problems affect you?

1. Speaking took extra effort
2. Throat discomfort or pain after using your voice
3. Vocal fatigue (voice weakened as you talked)
4. Voice cracks or sounds different

Source: Information from Bach et al. (2005).

In sum, auditory-perceptual evaluation is considered an indispensable tool for patient and clinician judgment of voice functioning (Kempster et al., 2009).

INSTRUMENTAL MEASURES

Instrumental measures include those that measure vocal fold structure and function directly or indirectly, as well as measures of acoustic and aerodynamic aspects of vocal function. Over the past several decades the wide availability of computerized instrumentation has vastly expanded the scope of voice assessment and evaluation. Visual-perceptual, acoustic, and aerodynamic measures are used to determine the existence of a voice problem, assess the severity or stage of progression of the voice problem, and identify the source of the problem. Such measures also enable quantitative documentation of vocal function and assessment of treatment efficacy (Mehta & Hillman, 2007). Perceptual judgments alone may not allow for precise tracking of the patient's progress, because the ear may not be sensitive enough to detect small but significant changes in voice characteristics indicating that a treatment procedure is working (Awan, 2001). It is important, however, that the professional using the instrument is knowledgeable about the equipment and skilled in interpreting the information obtained. It is also vital that the device be properly calibrated and maintained in order to yield meaningful data. Instrumental measures include indirect and direct laryngoscopy, endoscopy, videostroboscopy, and acoustic and aerodynamic measures.

Indirect Laryngoscopy. Indirect (mirror) laryngoscopy has been used since the mid 19th century as a means of determining the physical structure and function of the vocal folds. In this procedure the patient is seated upright. The patient protrudes his or her tongue, and the laryngologist gently pulls on the tongue using a piece of gauze. The examiner then inserts a laryngeal mirror (much like a dental mirror) into the oropharynx region over the tongue. The back of the mirror may actually touch and raise the velum. The examiner wears a headband that has a light attached to it. The light is focused on the mirror, providing a mirror image of the vocal folds. As in all mirror images the reflection is reversed in terms of left and right. Once the laryngeal reflection is obtained, the patient is asked to prolong the /i/ vowel, which helps to raise the epiglottis and expose the vocal folds. Indirect laryngoscopy allows the examiner to detect gross tissue changes (e.g., **nodules** and polyps), vocal fold paralysis or weakness, and infections of the larynx (Case, 2002). Normal phonation, however, cannot be visualized.

Direct Laryngoscopy. Direct laryngoscopy involves anesthetizing the patient so the laryngoscope can be placed directly into the throat via the oral cavity. With this method, the larynx can be visualized in detail, allowing detection of tiny changes in tissue structure. In addition, surgery can be performed with special microlaryngeal instruments that are inserted through the laryngoscope. Typically, the laryngoscope is also attached to a video camera and the image is displayed on a monitor. This method is more invasive than indirect laryngoscopy, but it allows a more thorough scrutiny of the laryngeal structures.

Endoscopy. Endoscopic procedures use either a flexible or rigid endoscope that is inserted into the patient's pharynx to illuminate the larynx. The procedure may be done either via the patient's nose or mouth. When done via the nose, a very thin, flexible tube is inserted through the nostril into the pharynx. When done via the oral cavity, a rigid scope is used. Either way, the image is typically projected onto a video monitor, using a magnifying scope and video camera. Laryngeal endoscopy has many advantages. First, the patient is awake so the risks inherent in general anesthesia are avoided. Second, the procedure allows detailed examination of the structure and function of the larynx. Use of the rigid scope does not permit examination of phonatory function during connected speech as the patient is restricted to phonation of the /i/ vowel. However, the procedure yields a high-quality image of the larynx. Vocal fold changes at different pitch levels are also well visualized.

With **nasoendoscopy** the patient is able to phonate relatively normally, so that vocal fold vibratory patterns during phonation can be evaluated. This is particularly important for movement disorders such as spasmodic dysphonia and **paradoxical vocal fold dysfunction**, in which the structures appear normal but abnormalities in function can be detected. As the flexible endoscope is inserted the examiner evaluates the individual's nasal cavity and nasopharynx. This can provide information about nasal contributions to the voice disorder, such as nasal septal deviation, adenoid hypertrophy, or allergic or infectious sinonasal disease that may cause thick secretions and frequent throat clearing (Nunez & Rosen, 2005; Roehm & Rosen, 2004). As the larynx comes into view it is first examined at rest, while the individual breathes quietly. The normal position of the vocal folds at rest is predominantly abducted, adducting slightly with expiration and abducting during inspiration (Heman-Ackah & Barr, 2006). The examiner notes any evidence of inappropriate vocal fold adduction during inspiration or expiration (Nunez & Rosen, 2005). The resting position and muscle activity of the vocal folds can provide helpful information about possible causes of the voice problem. For example, a median position of one or both folds usually implies vocal fold fixation either from paralysis, **scar**, or joint immobility, while a paramedian position is usually associated with paresis, scarring, or CA joint dysfunction; spontaneous activity at rest is usually caused by tremor or spasms (Heman-Ackah & Barr, 2006).

Following the assessment at rest, the individual's phonatory behavior is examined. During phonation the supraglottic and pharyngeal muscles should be relaxed, with most movement occurring in the true vocal folds (Heman-Ackah & Barr, 2006). Table 4.14 lists typical phonatory activities performed during endoscopy, with associated laryngeal findings and possible etiologies.

The patient is asked to prolong the /i/ vowel at a comfortable pitch, and then at higher and lower pitches. The examiner notes the presence of any lesions or masses on the vocal folds, any vocal fold atrophy, and the degree of vocal fold mobility (Nunez & Rosen, 2005; Roehm & Rosen, 2004). The patient is then asked to say /hi/ /hi/ /hi/ or /he/ /he/ /he/ with a breath or a sniff in between each syllable, which causes the vocal folds to alternately adduct and abduct. This procedure tests the agility and fatigability of the vocal folds and allows for the detection of slowed or reduced vocal fold movement (Heman-Ackah & Barr, 2006; Nunez & Rosen, 2005; Roehm & Rosen, 2004). The patient's ability to change pitch is evaluated by having him or her phonate the /i/ vowel continuously from lowest to highest and highest to lowest (Heman-Ackah & Barr, 2006). During this maneuver the individual's vocal folds should lengthen symmetrically. Lack of lengthening indicates possible involvement of the superior laryngeal nerve or fixation of one or both cricothyroid joints.

Other tasks may be done to test for specific disorders. For example, when spasmodic dysphonia is suspected, the individual is asked to count. Counting tasks are useful to assess for abductor spasms during the voiceless sounds and for adductor spasms during voiced sounds (Heman-Ackah & Barr, 2006). Coughing, whistling, singing, and talking at a higher than normal pitch may also be helpful in detecting cases of spasmodic dysphonia. Excessive tightening of the true vocal folds and contraction of the supraglottic, pharyngeal, and strap muscles during phonation may indicate muscle tension dysphonia (Heman-Ackah & Barr, 2006). **Muscle tension dysphonia** is typically characterized by anterior-to-posterior or lateral-to-medial squeezing of

TABLE 4.14 Phonatory Tasks Used in Endoscopy, Associated Vocal Findings, and Possible Etiologies

Task	Finding	Etiology
Normal respiration	Paradoxical vocal fold motion	PVFD or **dystonia**; reflux laryngitis
	Tremor	**Essential tremor**, neuromuscular disorder
	Erythema and edema of posterior larynx and/or arytenoids	Extra esophageal reflux
/i/	Vocal fold immobility	Vocal fold paresis, paralysis, arytenoid dislocation, posterior glottic web
	Vocal fold atrophy	Presbylaryngis
/he/ /he/ /he/	Vocal fold immobility	Vocal fold paralysis, arytenoid dislocation, glottic web
	Relative unilateral slowing of vocal fold mobility, decreased vocal fold adduction	Vocal fold paresis
Glissando /i/	Inability to lengthen vocal folds	Superior laryngeal nerve paralysis, cricothyroid joint dysfunction
Whistle, laugh, cough	Normal glottic opening despite restriction during respiration	PVFD
	Decreased vocal fold range of motion	Vocal fold paresis, recovering vocal fold paralysis
"We see three green trees"; "You should use new blue shoes"	Anterior-posterior supraglottic shortening, false vocal fold hyperadduction	Muscle tension dysphonia, functional dysphonia
Observation of connected speech	Tremor	Essential tremor, neuromuscular disorder
"Buy Bob a baseball"; "Pay Paul a penny"	Periodic breathy breaks	Abductor spasmodic dysphonia

Source: Information from Roehm & Rosen (2004).

the false vocal folds and pharyngeal muscles. Typically this behavior is present consistently throughout an entire sample of running speech. In cases of suspected muscle tension dysphonia, the patient may be asked to engage in spontaneous speech, which may reveal hyperfunctional laryngeal behaviors. This exercise can also be used as a starting point for behavioral therapy as the patient visualizes precisely what he or she is doing during speech (Nunez & Rosen, 2005; Roehm & Rosen, 2004).

It is important to ensure the patient's comfort during endoscopic examination. Rigid endoscopy via the oral cavity can cause gagging if the endoscope comes into contact with the posterior oral or pharyngeal structures. Discomfort during nasoendoscopy may occur from resistance of the nasal passageway to the instrument or from stimulation of the pharynx and larynx from contact with the endoscope. Particularly in children, discomfort may interfere with the individual's ability to perform the phonatory activities (Hay, Oates, Giannini, Berkowitz, & Totenberg, 2007). A topical anesthetic may be used in the nasal cavity to facilitate the passage of the endoscope. With either type of scope, patients and parents/caregivers should be familiarized with the procedure before the actual insertion of the scope to maximize comfort and minimize apprehension.

Videostroboscopy. Endoscopy may be used in conjunction with **videostroboscopy**. Stroboscopy works by shining a light source onto a moving object and periodically interrupting the light source. The observer views only the phase of movement exposed by the light, and any movement that occurs between the flashes of light is not seen (Case, 2002). This generates what is essentially an optical illusion, allowing an observer to view moving objects as though they are stationary or in slow motion. In laryngeal stroboscopy the light source is directed through the endoscope to illuminate the larynx. The instrument has two modes based on the timing of the interruptions to the light source. In walking mode (also called running or traveling mode) the rate of strobe light illumination is timed to be approximately 2 Hz different from the patient's F0 (Poburka, 1999). The vocal folds are therefore illuminated at consecutive points over many vibratory cycles (Figure 4.1). The resulting apparent "slow motion" view of the vocal folds is made up of "snapshots" of a sequence of cycles, with each snapshot having been taken at a different stage in each cycle (Mathieson, 2001). Viewers perceive an integrated image rather than a series of disjointed movements because the human eye can only perceive a maximum of five images per second (Stemple, 2000). Stimuli that are presented faster appear as a single ongoing image. This is similar to what happens when we set a fan into motion. As the fan begins to spin, we see the blades rotating individually. However, as the fan speeds up, we are no longer able to perceive the blades separately, but perceive instead what looks like one blade spinning extremely rapidly. Similarly, when the strobe light illuminates the larynx at a much faster

FIGURE 4.1 **Different Points of Vocal Fold Vibration Illuminated by Stroboscopy**

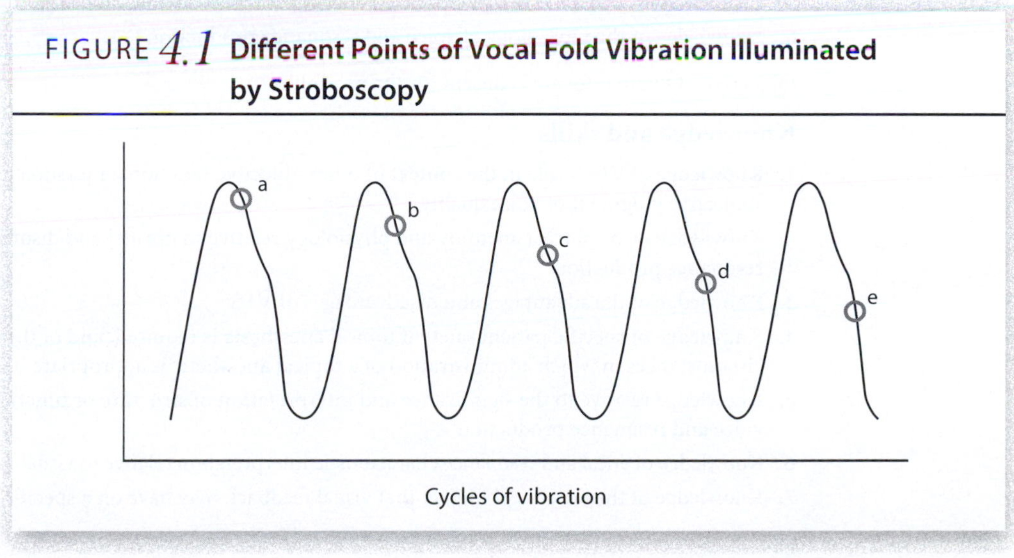

rate than five images per second, we perceive what seems to be continuous motion of vocal fold vibration. In stopped or locked mode the light is exactly timed to the patient's F0 so flashes occur at the same point in each successive cycle. In this mode the vocal folds appear to be stationary as long as the vibration is regular and periodic (Deliyski, 2007; Hapner & Johns, 2007; Poburka, 1999; Walker & Messing, 2006).

Videostroboscopy is performed either by an otolaryngologist and/or speech-language pathologist. ASHA has recognized endoscopic imaging techniques as being within the scope of practice for speech-language pathologists for the purpose of diagnosing and treating patients with voice or resonance/aeromechanical disorders (ASHA, 2004). Table 4.15 identifies the objectives for vocal tract visualization and imaging and the knowledge and skills needed by speech-language pathologists to achieve the objectives.

Endoscopic imaging has become the gold standard of evaluation of laryngeal structure and function. Aspects that are assessed include pliability or stiffness of the vocal fold cover, vocal fold vibratory patterns, involvement of supraglottic structures, and the adequacy of the mucosal wave (Walker & Messing, 2006). Table 4.16 lists the following specific aspects of vocal fold structure and function that are commonly evaluated via videostroboscopy.

TABLE 4.15 Knowledge and Skills Required for Vocal Tract Visualization and Imaging

Objective: Qualify the patient for the procedure

Knowledge and skills

1. Understanding of photographic principles of VES and its use as a diagnostic tool
2. Knowledge of how to assess patient physiology
3. Knowledge of particular patient physiology
4. Skills in the performance of VES and clinical interpretation
5. Understanding the patient's physical and emotional receptivity to the procedure
6. Knowledge of the physiology of voice and resonance production

Objective: Obtain informed consent for the procedure

Knowledge and skills

1. Knowledge of VES's role in the context of other objective functional measures of the voice and subjective judgment of voice quality
2. Knowledge of vocal tract anatomy and physiology relative to normal and disordered voice and resonance production
3. Knowledge of the advantages and disadvantages of VES
4. Knowledge of specific patient safety if topical anesthesia is required, and of the setting and/or circumstances in which administration of a topical anesthetic is appropriate
5. Knowledge relative to the significance and interpretation of structure or function deviation to voice and resonance production
6. Knowledge of vocal and resonance characteristic interpretation relative to visualization of pathology
7. Knowledge of the emotional impact that visual feedback may have on a specific patient

TABLE 4.15 (Continued)

Objective: To perform the procedure alone or with others

Knowledge and skills

1. Knowledge of laryngeal and velopharyngeal anatomy and physiology
2. Skill in the technique of rigid fiberoptic oral endoscopy, flexible fiberoptic videonasoendoscopy, or stroboscopic light used to image the vocal tract in a manner that yields maximum quality recordings
3. Skill in the techniques of obtaining a videotape of the viewed image
4. Knowledge of potential risks to the patient
5. Knowledge of various approaches to becoming trained to perform VES
6. Knowledge/skill of administration of topical anesthetic to accomplish VES with maximal safety and minimal discomfort to the patient
7. Knowledge of universal precaution procedures that protect both clinician and patient from accidental exposure to disease
8. Knowledge of the clinical significance of obtained image to make appropriate referrals when necessary. This requires additional understanding of the visual image dependence on
   a. elicited tasks
   b. examiner and patient response to the obtained image
9. Knowledge of the ability to organize, store, retrieve VES data for quality assurance and treatment efficacy purposes, and medical-legal documentation

Objective: To interpret the effects of vocal behavior on the laryngeal anatomy as well as the laryngeal anatomy effects on laryngeal physiology in conjunction with medical colleagues, and concisely describe VES findings and interpretations for professional communication purposes

Knowledge and skills

1. Knowledge of laryngeal physiology
2. Knowledge of pathology of the larynx
3. Knowledge of the relative effectiveness of therapy, surgery, or medication in the management of specific disorders or diseases of the larynx
4. Knowledge of professional communication skills in describing/interpreting VES findings
5. Reporting effectively and clearly

Objective: To interpret the effects of velopharyngeal behavior on resonance as well as the velopharyngeal function effects on voice physiology in conjunction with medical colleagues, and concisely describe VES findings and interpretations for professional communication purposes

Knowledge and skills

1. Knowledge of velopharyngeal physiology
2. Knowledge of the impaired function of the velopharynx
3. Knowledge of the relative effectiveness of therapy, surgery, or medication in the management of specific disorders involving the velopharynx
4. Knowledge of professional communication skills in describing/interpreting VES findings
5. Reporting effectively and clearly

(continued)

TABLE 4.15 Knowledge and Skills Required for Vocal Tract Visualization and Imaging (Continued)

Objective: To design and implement appropriate treatment or response to diagnostic procedure

Knowledge and skills

1. Skill in the technique of laryngeal and velopharyngeal imaging that provides guided real-time patient visual feedback
2. Skill necessary to obtain laryngeal and velopharyngeal images during conversational speech
3. Knowledge in interpretation of obtained images and application to management techniques
4. Knowledge of vocal tract compensatory adjustments
5. Knowledge of biofeedback reinforcement strategies
6. Knowledge of appropriate medical/behavioral management techniques to observed behaviors and laryngeal and velopharyngeal status

Source: ASHA (2004). Reprinted with permission from *Knowledge and Skills Required for Vocal Tract Visualization and Imaging*. Available from www.asha.org/policy.

TABLE 4.16 Aspects of Vocal Fold Structure and Function Typically Evaluated via Videolaryngostroboscopy

Aspect Evaluated	Description
Vocal fold edge	Smoothness of medial margins of the vocal folds
Glottic closure	Degree and pattern of closing during a cycle of vibration
Extent of opening	Degree of vocal fold opening when maximally abducted
Phase closure	Open and closed phases should be roughly equal
Mucosal wave	Should travel from inferior to superior margins of the folds and spread laterally
Presence/extent of nonvibrating portion	Any portion of the vocal fold(s) that does not participate in vibration (a dynamic segment)
Amplitude of vibration	Extent of lateral excursion of the vocal folds
Phase symmetry	Degree to which both folds reach midline and maximum abduction at the same time
Periodicity/regularity	Degree of similarity of successive cycles of vibration
Supraglottic activity	Degree of medial compression or anterior-posterior compression of the false vocal folds
Vertical approximation	Degree to which both folds are on the same vertical plane

Vocal fold edge: Normally the free margins or edges of the vocal folds are straight and smooth. If the edge looks uneven or rough, this may indicate some kind of structural problem, such as edema or a nodule.

Glottic closure: This feature is evaluated in terms of both degree and pattern of closure during a cycle of vibration, at the point when the vocal folds are maximally adducted. The closure may be complete (fully closed along the entire glottis), inconsistent (some opening in some portion of the glottis), or incomplete (never fully closed). Different patterns of glottic closure have also been described. A posterior chink indicates that the membranous glottis is closed but the cartilaginous glottis is open. This pattern is often seen in women with no laryngeal pathology and appears to be a normal aspect of phonation. However, a large chink can be associated with muscle tension. An anterior chink indicates that some portion of the anterior glottis is not closing properly. An hourglass pattern results when there are both anterior and posterior chinks with only the middle portion of the glottis achieving closure. This is often associated with bilateral nodules. The chink may be irregular along the edges as a result of scarring or other lesions. A bowed or spindle-shaped glottis is open in the midportion but closed at the anterior and posterior margins. It can result from many different conditions, including aging. Closure can also be variable, showing any combination of the above patterns.

Extent of opening: This term refers to the amount of opening when the vocal folds are in their most abducted position during phonation. This parameter is rated from very slight to extreme opening.

Phase closure: A cycle of vibration is typically divided into three phases: the opening part of the open phase, the closing part of the open phase, and the closed phase (Poburka, 1999). The open/closing and closed phases of the vocal folds in modal register should be approximately equal in each cycle. An excessively long closed phase indicates that the vocal folds are hyperadducting, whereas an excessively long open phase reflects hypoadduction. An increased open phase is often seen in cases of vocal fold paralysis, presbylaryngis, or glottal lesions, whereas an increased closed phase is most often due to hyperfunction (Walker & Messing, 2006).

Presence/extent of mucosal wave: Normally, the mucosal wave travels from the bottom to the top surface of the vocal folds and also spreads laterally across their superior surface. The wave should be seen to travel at least half the width and length of the visible fold during normal pitch and loudness conditions (Walker & Messing, 2006). A lesion on the folds will hamper or prevent the wave at that point, which is seen as a nonvibrating or adynamic segment.

Amplitude of vibration: Refers to the extent of lateral excursion of the folds. In normal vibration the fold should travel approximately half of the visible width of the fold (Walker & Messing, 2006). Amplitude tends to decrease when the vocal folds are stiffer and when the wave comes into contact with lesions. The symmetry of amplitude is also noted, that is, whether each fold opens to the same point on either side of the glottis.

Phase symmetry: Indicates the degree to which both folds reach the midline and point of maximum opening at the same time, demonstrating that both are vibrating at the same frequency. Asymmetry can indicate differences in the position of the vocal folds, as well as differences in mass, tension, and elasticity between the folds resulting from lesions, scar, paralysis, or other problems (Walker & Messing, 2006).

Periodicity/regularity: This refers to a sequence of cycles that may be regular, irregular, or inconsistent. Periodicity can be demonstrated when the strobe image is set to its locked phase. In this setting periodic vibration results in the image appearing to be very still; an unstable image suggests that the vibration is aperiodic.

Supraglottic activity: Refers to false vocal fold activity during phonation. The false folds are sometimes seen to constrict in an anterior-posterior and/or lateral-medial direction in cases of hyperfunctional phonation, muscle tension dysphonia, and **adductor spasmodic** dysphonia.

Vertical level of vocal fold approximation: The vocal folds are normally on the same vertical plane. Planes may be different in cases of dislocation of an arytenoid or unilateral paralysis.

Videostroboscopic features are typically rated on a 6- or 7-point scale, such as the commonly used Stroboscopic Assessment of Voice (Table 4.17).

TABLE 4.17 **Stroboscopy Rating Form**

Glottic Closure

On plane

Off plane

Hourglass | Complete | Incomplete | Irregular | Posterior gap | Anterior gap | Spindle gap

Supraglottic Activity

0	1	2	3	4	5
Slight compression				Ventricular phonation	

Vertical Level

0	1	2	3	4	5
Glottic plane				Off plane	

TABLE 4.17 (Continued)

Vocal Fold Edge

Left

0	1	2	3	4	5

Right

0	1	2	3	4	5
Straight/smooth					Rough/irregular

Amplitude

Left

0	1	2	3	4	5

Right

0	1	2	3	4	5
Normal					Barely perceptible/no visible movement

Mucosal Wave

Left

0	1	2	3	4	5

Right

0	1	2	3	4	5
Normal					Absent

Nonvibrating Portion

Left

0	1	2	3	4	5

Right

0	1	2	3	4	5
None	20%	40%	60%	80%	100%

Phase Closure

−5	−4	−3	−2	−1	0	1	2	3	4	5
Open phase predominates				Normal			Closed phase predominates			

Phase Symmetry

0	1	2	3	4	5
Symmetrical					Always asymmetrical

Regularity

0	1	2	3	4	5
Regular					Always irregular

Source: From "A New Stroboscopy Rating Form," by B. J. Poburka, 1999, *Journal of Voice, 13*, pp. 403–413. Copyright 1999 by The Voice Foundation. Reprinted with permission.

Advantages and Disadvantages of Endoscopy and Stroboscopy. Endoscopy (with or without stroboscopy) has many benefits and some limitations (Table 4.18).

Advantages include the detailed examination and documentation of laryngeal structure and function; forward, reverse, and frame-by-frame playback, which can be used for patient education; and the ability to annotate single and multiple frame hard copy color photographs (Leonard et al., 2002). Stroboscopy is very useful for assessing alteration or interruption of the mucosal wave, differentiating nodules from submucosal cysts, assessing vocal fold mobility and tone following paralysis, and assessing superior laryngeal nerve paralysis. It is also useful for identifying early or small lesions such as nodules, **papilloma**, and carcinoma.

Despite the clear advantages, there are several limitations of endoscopy and stroboscopy that should be kept in mind. A major limitation arises from the nature of the technology itself. Because the stroboscopic illumination is triggered by and linked to the patient's F0, the vibratory patterns of individuals with moderately or severely dysphonic voices, voice breaks, or diplophonia cannot be validly interpreted (Hapner & Johns, 2007; Mortensen & Woo, 2008; Patel, Dailey, & Bless, 2008; Walker & Messing, 2006). This is due to the fact that the aperiodic vocal fold vibration causes the light to become asynchronized with the actual phase of vocal fold movements (Deliyski, 2007). Another limitation is that the optic devices that are used can result in distortions of the image. Further, the vocal folds can only be viewed from above, so the degree of glottal closure during vibration can only be inferred (Hapner & Johns, 2007). An additional disadvantage is that the patient's phonation during the procedure is not truly representative of his or her normal conversational speech, even

TABLE 4.18 Advantages and Disadvantages of Laryngeal Endoscopy and Stroboscopy

Advantages
Detailed assessment and documentation of laryngeal structure and function
Forward/reverse function
Frame-by-frame playback
Ability to generate color photographs
Disadvantages
Stroboscopy is not valid for moderately to severely dysphonic voices
Image distortion
Vocal folds can only be viewed from above
Phonation is not completely representative of normal connected speech
Rigid scope requires substantial patient cooperation
Interpretation is subjective
Rating forms are not standardized

Sources: Information from Deliyski (2007); Hapner & Johns (2007); Hartnick & Zeitels (2005); Kelchner et al. (2007); Leonard et al. (2002); Mortensen & Woo (2008); Patel et al. (2008); Stemple et al. (2000); Walker & Messing (2006).

with the use of flexible nasoendoscopy. With a rigid endoscope the utterance is even less representative, because it is limited to the /i/ vowel. Use of a rigid endoscope also requires substantial patient cooperation (Hapner & Johns, 2007; Hartnick & Zeitels, 2005). Use of a rigid scope in children may be particularly difficult due to the shape of the juvenile epiglottis, the possibility of enlarged tonsils that reduces the size of the posterior oral cavity, and the child's relatively small oropharynx (Kelchner et al., 2007).

Interpretation of the obtained image poses a potential problem because it is subjective and relies on visual perception. This leads to poor reliability between and within raters (Hapner & Johns, 2007; Walker & Messing, 2006). In addition, there is a large amount of variability in structure and function of the human larynx, and normal variation may be mistaken for an abnormality (Stemple et al., 2000). Finally, rating forms are not standardized, and the level of training and experience of examiners varies (Hapner & Johns, 2007; Walker & Messing, 2005).

High-Speed Digital Imaging. Recently, high-speed digital imaging (HSDI) has become a viable option for visualizing the structure and function of the larynx. High-speed equipment can record with sampling rates of 2,000–4,000 frames per second (fps), allowing each individual cycle of vibration to be recorded and analyzed (Mortensen & Woo, 2008). This overcomes the problem of videostroboscopy, which has a maximum recording rate of 30 fps and cannot capture individual cycles of vibration (Patel et al., 2008). Because HSDI is independent of the individual's F0, it allows for detailed evaluation of vocal fold vibratory patterns in patients who demonstrate voice breaks, diplophonia, and severe dysphonia (Mortensen & Woo, 2008; Patel et al., 2008). However, HSDI is not widely available, and even when it is, this technology should be viewed as a supplement to stroboscopy, and not as a replacement (Patel et al., 2008).

ACOUSTIC ANALYSIS

Acoustic analysis of the patient's vocal output is a popular way of assessing vocal function. From the acoustic analysis, inferences can be made about vocal fold vibration. Acoustic analyses are widely used because the instrumentation is easily available and relatively inexpensive. The equipment does not require extensive training to use effectively, and it is safe and noninvasive. Acoustic analysis provides visual and quantifiable information that can be used as a baseline measure, as a form of **biofeedback** in treatment, for documentation of the patient's progress in therapy, and as an outcome measure.

Many computerized acoustic devices are available commercially, including the Visi-Pitch and Computerized Speech Lab (CSL) by KayPentax, Dr. Speech Science for Windows by Tiger Electronics, and the C-Speech system by Milenkovic. The Multidimensional Voice Program (MDVP) that is available on the CSL is widely used internationally. These programs perform similar types of analyses, including variables related to fundamental frequency (F0), intensity, quality, and periodicity.

Measurement of acoustic output obtained during selected phonatory activities yields useful information about the patient's vocal mechanism. For example, average values of F0 and intensity contribute information regarding the individual's typical or habitual voice use. Maximum performance ranges provide data on the anatomical integrity and/or physiological capability of the laryngeal structure (Koschkee & Rammage, 1997). Measures of periodicity reflect the regularity and stability of vocal fold vibration and the degree of noise in the individual's vocal output.

Frequency Measures. Commonly measured attributes related to F0 include average F0, maximum phonational frequency range, and frequency variability.

Average Fundamental Frequency. Fundamental frequency (F0) refers to the rate of vibration of the vocal folds and corresponds (although not linearly) to the perceptual impression of pitch. Average F0 is measured in isolated vowels and in reading or speaking tasks. Average F0 in connected speech is often called speaking fundamental frequency (SFF). Average F0 is helpful in comparing the patient's F0 to norms that have been established for men, women, and children. See Table 4.19.

TABLE 4.19 Average F0 (in Hz) for Different Age Groups Reported in the Literature

Author(s)	Age Group	M	F	Race
Robb & Saxman (1985)	11–25 (mos)	357	357	
McGlone & Shipp (1971)	13–23 (mos)	443	443	
Eguchi & Hirsch (1969)	3	298	298	
	4	285	285	
	5	289	289	
Awan & Mueller (1996)	5–6	240	243	W
	5–6	241	231	AA
	5–6	249	248	H
Weinberg & Bennett (1971)	5	252	248	
	6	247	247	
Wheat & Hudson (1988)	6	219	211	AA
Ferrand & Bloom (1996)	3–6	256	246	
	7–10	237	253	
Sorenson (1989)	6	251	296	
	7	288	258	
	8	229	251	
	9	221	266	
	10	220	229	
Pederson et al. (1990)	8.6–12.9		256	
	13–15.9		248	
	16–19.8		241	
Bennett (1983)	8.2	234	235	
	9.2	226	222	
	10.2	224	228	
	11.2	216	221	

TABLE *4.19* **(Continued)**

Author(s)	Age Group	M	F	Race
Fitch (1990)	21-26	109	210	
Kent (1994)	20.3	120		
	47.9	123		
	73.3	119		
	85	136		
Hollien & Shipp (1972)	20–29	120		
	30–39	112		
	40–49	107		
	50–59	118		
	60–69	112		
	70–79	132		
	80–89	146		
dePinto & Hollien (1982)	18–25	229		
Morgan & Rastatter (1986)	20–24	228		
Pegoraro Krook (1988)	20–29	195		
	30–39	195		
	40–49	191		
	50–59	182		
	60–69	181		
	70–79	188		
	80–89	188		
Russell et al. (1995)	65–68	181		
Brown et al. (1996)	21–33	136		
	20–22	189		
	40–54	128		
	42–50	186		
	69–87	134		
	65–89	175		
Honjo & Isshiki (1980)	69–85	162	177	

Values for postlingual children and adults are for conversational speech or oral reading. Some studies included race as a factor: White (W), African American (AA), Hispanic (H). Unless otherwise stated, ages are in years.

Note: Some values have been rounded to the nearest whole number.

Table 4.19 clearly demonstrates the link between age and F0. Infants have the highest F0, which decreases by around age 3 years. Thereafter F0 remains in the range of approximately 220–250 Hz for both boys and girls until puberty. The male F0 drops by around 100 Hz and reaches the adult level between 110–130 Hz. F0 values for elderly males are somewhat higher than those for younger adults, ranging from approximately 130 Hz to 160 Hz. This increase reflects the vocal fold atrophy that tends to occur in males with advancing age. F0 values for females drop slightly after puberty, to around 180–230 Hz. This level decreases in elderly women to around 175 Hz. The drop is usually attributed to postmenopausal effects such as greater fluid retention in the tissues and changes in the contour of the vocal folds.

Maximum Phonational Frequency Range. Maximum phonational frequency range (MPFR) refers to the extent of F0s the speaker can produce from lowest (excluding pulse register) to highest, including falsetto. This is a useful measure of the physiological limits of laryngeal function in terms of vocal frequency. Frequencies are typically obtained beginning at the person's most comfortable (habitual) level and then phonating downward and upward to the most extreme levels possible (e.g., Zraick et al., 2002). MPFR is expressed in Hz, octaves, or semitones. Most normal speakers have a range of around 2.5 octaves or 30 semitones (ST). The lowest frequency adult males are able to produce is around 80 Hz, and the highest is in the 700 Hz range; adult females produce a low F0 of approximately 135 Hz and a high level that can reach over 1,000 Hz (Colton, Casper, & Leonard, 2006). Clinically, it has been found that physical condition affects MPFR more than either age or sex. Older speakers in good health tend to have a larger range than younger speakers in poor health. Neurological diseases such as amyotrophic lateral sclerosis and Parkinson's disease have been shown to reduce MPFR (e.g., Gamboa et al., 1997; Silbergleit, Johnson, & Jacobson, 1997). Robinson, Mandel, and Sataloff (2005) reported that mean MPFR in men with superior laryngeal nerve paresis was 15 ST compared with 36 ST in healthy speakers and 21 ST in women with SLN paresis compared with 35 ST in healthy females.

Frequency Variability. Frequency variability reflects the variations in F0 during an isolated vowel or connected speech. It is measured either as the standard deviation of F0 in Hz (SDF0), or in semitones (pitch sigma). Frequency variability can be used as an index of vocal fold vibration stability or as a measure of intonational appropriateness. When a speaker sustains an isolated vowel, the standard deviation of F0 should be small (less than 10 Hz), indicating normal laryngeal motor control. During connected speech the standard deviation of F0 should be larger, reflecting the increases and decreases in F0 that are characteristic of the linguistic and intonational patterns of a language. People constantly change their F0 levels as they speak to reflect different emotions, different types of accenting and syllable stress, and different grammatical constructions. These F0 changes contribute to the overall melody, or prosody, of speech. A certain amount of frequency variability is desirable in a speaker's voice, depending on the individual's age, sex, social situation, mood, dialect, and culture. This variability is something that speakers of a particular language in a particular culture intuitively recognize. Too much or too little frequency variability sounds wrong and can indicate a functional, organic, or neurogenic voice problem. Standard deviation of F0 in normal conversational speech is around 20–35 Hz (Ferrand, 2007). In terms of pitch sigma, the value should be around 2–4 semitones (Colton et al., 2006). Research has indicated that F0 variability can be a sensitive indicator of disease. For example, Harel, Cannizzaro, and Snyder (2004) showed that changes in frequency variability were detected in a patient with Parkinson's disease five years prior to the diagnosis and to the onset of clinically noticeable symptoms.

Intensity Measures. Intensity corresponds perceptually to vocal loudness. Intensity can be measured in terms of average intensity of an isolated vowel or connected speech, intensity variability, and intensity range (dynamic range). Intensity can be measured with commercially available acoustic instruments and can also be measured by means of a sound level meter, easily available from electronics stores. While norms for frequency variables are plentiful, those for intensity are not.

Average Intensity. Intensity level depends to a large degree on situational factors. Someone whispering in a church would probably want to use a lower intensity level than when he or she is yelling for their favorite team in a football game. Average dB values reported for single words were around 65–77 dB for females and 70–80 dB for males; values for reading were 68 dB for females and 70 dB for males (Colton & Casper, 1996).

Dynamic Range. To obtain the dynamic range, the person is asked to phonate a vowel as softly and as loudly as possible at a comfortable frequency level. In terms of dynamic range, a value of approximately 30 dB indicates normal voice function for adults (Rammage et al., 2001). Maximum intensity levels have been reported to be around 100–110 dB SPL, and minimum levels not involving whispering are around 40 dB (Colton & Casper, 1996; Kent, 1994).

The Voice Range Profile. A handy way of integrating vocal frequency and intensity information is through the voice range profile (VRP), also called the phonetogram. This is a graph that plots F0 along the horizontal axis and intensity along the vertical axis. The graph yields a visualization of phonational frequency range in comparison to dynamic range. The individual is asked to phonate a vowel at different frequencies at his or her softest and loudest levels. This results in an upper and a lower contour. The upper contour represents the speaker's maximum intensity at different frequencies, and the lower one represents his or her minimum intensity at those frequencies. The VRP thus provides an indication of the person's maximum physiological vocal function. VRPs have a characteristic shape, reflecting the physiological features of the human voice production system. The shape is roughly similar to an oval, with narrower endpoints and a more expanded midportion. This shape results from the typical relationship between the range of frequencies and amplitudes that can be generated by the laryngeal system (Figure 4.2). Humans have a far greater dynamic range in the middle of the frequency range, whereas the dynamic range shrinks considerably at very high or very low frequencies. In the middle of the frequency range an individual can generally vary the intensity by 20–30 dB, whereas at the ends of the frequency range he or she may only be able to vary the intensity by a few decibels (Titze, 1994).

The graph gives very useful information for several reasons. First, the VRP can help to determine the physiological limits of an individual's voice, because the dynamic and phonational frequency ranges are directly related to the person's ability to control the vocal folds (DeLeo LeBorgne & Weinrich, 2002; Sulter, Schutte, & Miller, 1995). Because the graph provides information regarding the interaction between frequency and intensity, it can identify a speaker's physiological and vocal limitations (DeLeo LeBorgne, 2007; Wuyts, Heylen, Mertens, De Bodt, & Van de Heyning, 2002). A person who has difficulty in achieving normal frequency and amplitude ranges will demonstrate a restricted or compressed VRP, with the upper and lower contours closer together than normal (e.g., Ma et al., 2007). Second, the VRP can show the impact of behavioral or surgical intervention on an individual's voice by displaying and quantifying changes in the patient's frequency and intensity ranges and the

FIGURE 4.2 Voice Range Profile

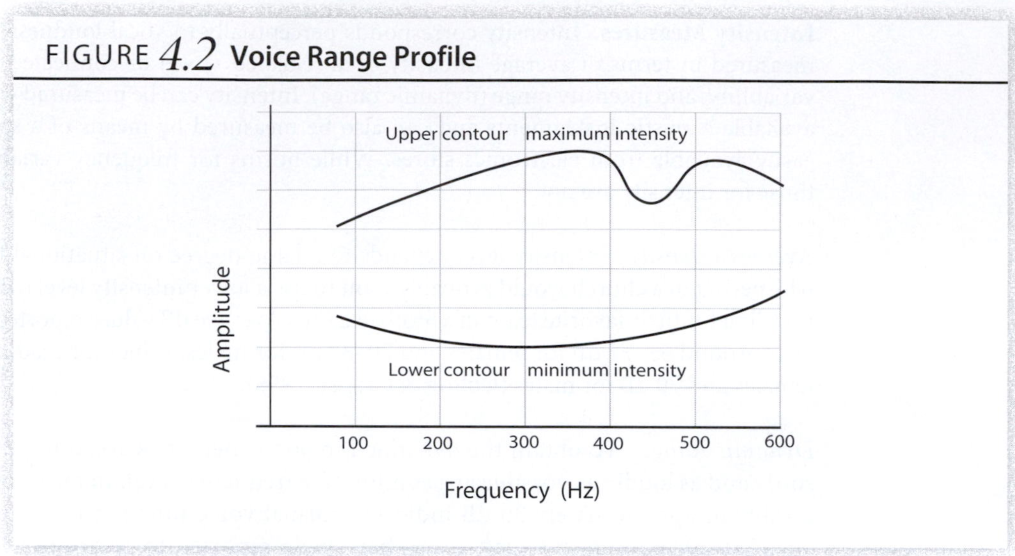

interaction between them. An expanded VRP after treatment would show graphically that the patient's phonational and/or dynamic range has increased. For example, Speyer, Wieneke, van Wijck-Warnaar, and Dejonckere (2003) evaluated VRPs before and after a program of voice therapy in patients with dysphonia related to a diverse range of etiologies. The authors reported that the graph in many patients did not conform visually to the smooth oval contour seen in vocally healthy speakers. Some subjects had separated voice areas, jagged boundaries of the lower or upper contour, or restricted phonation in the higher registers. After therapy patients demonstrated a larger VRP, reflecting an expansion of MPFR and dynamic range. VRPs are also helpful for singers and professional voice users to monitor changes in vocal range (DeLeo LeBorgne & Weinrich, 2002; Stemple et al., 2000).

Vocal Perturbation and Noise Measures. Measures of voice quality and periodicity include jitter, shimmer, and harmonics-to-noise ratio/noise-to-harmonics ratio/signal-to-noise ratio.

Jitter and Shimmer. Perturbation measures quantify the degree of periodicity and stability of vocal fold vibration. Perturbation refers to frequency and amplitude variations in successive cycles of vocal fold vibration. Frequency perturbation is called jitter and is measured either as a percentage of the average F0 or in milliseconds; amplitude perturbation is referred to as shimmer and is measured either as a percentage of average amplitude or in dB. A certain amount of variability is inherent in vocal fold vibration, which is therefore never completely periodic. The expected level of jitter in the normal human voice is around 0.2 to 1.0%, and that of shimmer is less than 5% or 0.5 dB.

Harmonics-to-Noise Ratio. Because there is always a slight degree of aperiodicity in vocal fold vibration, the sound produced has both harmonic (periodic) and inharmonic (aperiodic) components. There are several measures that quantify the ratio of periodic to aperiodic components in the voice, including harmonics-to-noise ratio (HNR), noise-to-harmonics ratio (NHR), and signal-to-noise ratio (SNR), all measured in dB. In a normal voice the harmonic components should predominate, yielding either a high harmonics-to-noise or signal-to-noise ratio, or a low noise-to-harmonics ratio.

Jitter, shimmer, and noise measures are the most frequently described in the voice literature (Yan, Damrose, & Bless, 2007). These measures have been utilized as a basis of comparison between vocally healthy speakers and those with various voice disorders. In addition, comparisons have been made of vocally disordered individuals before and after voice treatment. Disorders that have been described include partial **laryngectomy** (e.g., Bertino, Bellomo, Ferrero, & Ferlito, 2001; Pfuetzenreiter, Dedivitis, Queija, Bohn, & Barros, 2010), dysarthria following stroke (e.g., Wang, Kent, Kent, Duffy, & Thomas et al., 2009), **Huntington's disease** (Garcia, Cobeta, Martin, Alonso-Navarro, & Jimenez-Jimenez, 2009), superior laryngeal nerve paresis (Robinson et al., 2005), vocal fold microsurgery (Finck, Harmegnies, Remacle, & Lefebvre, 2009), effects of asthma medications (e.g., Balter, Adams, & Chapman, 2001), vocal fold nodules in children (e.g., Niedzielska, 2001), effects of microsurgery to remove vocal fold polyps (Petrovic-Lazic, Babac, Vukovic, Kosanovic, & Ivankovic, 2009), unilateral vocal fold paralysis (Sridhara, Ashok, Raghunathen, & Mann, 2003), and cochlear implant users (e.g., Evans & Deliyski, 2007).

Advantages and Disadvantages of Acoustic Analysis. There are numerous advantages and some disadvantages of acoustic measurement (Table 4.20).

Acoustic measures are noninvasive, provide quantitative data that indirectly reflect vocal fold vibration, and are easily obtainable through a variety of user-friendly computerized systems (Eadie & Doyle, 2005; Leonard et al., 2002). Such measures are useful in detecting subtle aspects of laryngeal function that may not be auditorily perceptible but that indicate some kind of problem in vocal fold vibration. Acoustic measures are also used widely as a baseline before treatment and to document changes in the patient's vocal output following behavioral, medical, and surgical interventions. Acoustic measures can be useful in validating and/or supplementing information obtained through auditory-perceptual evaluation. Acoustic analysis of the vocal signal is useful as feedback for patients and can provide evidence for the success of therapeutic interventions (Rodriguez-Parra, Adrian, & Casado, 2007; Smits, Ceuppens, & De Bodt, 2005). The numerical output provided by acoustic analysis can indicate the degree of dysphonia severity, and it provides a means to communicate this information to all stakeholders such as voice clinicians, patients, third-party payers, and physicians (Maryn, Corthals, Van Cauwenberge, Roy, & De Bodt, 2009).

However, while acoustic measures are widely used and can provide much useful information regarding an individual's vocal function, there are some drawbacks. One of the most important limits of acoustic analysis is the problem in analyzing voices that are severely aperiodic. Acoustic analysis is based on identifying individual cycles of vocal fold vibration. A voice that is highly aperiodic contains unidentifiable glottal cycles, and the resulting numerical data is likely to be invalid (Eadie & Doyle, 2005). Another disadvantage is that these measurements are highly sensitive to external noise, and their validity is dependent on the environment in which they are obtained (Deliyski, Evans, & Shaw, 2005). In addition, the quality of the hardware and software (microphone, computer soundcard, etc.) used to obtain acoustic measures influences the resulting data. Interpretation of the obtained numerical data may sometimes be difficult because the relationship between the acoustic values and vocal fold function is not direct. Clinicians may collect a variety of acoustic measurements without having a clear idea of what the numbers mean or how to best use the information for diagnostic and treatment purposes (Leonard et al., 2002). Other sources of potential error include the method of signal acquisition, the effects of microphone type and placement during signal acquisition, and the

TABLE 4.20 **Advantages and Disadvantages of Acoustic Analysis**

Advantages
Noninvasive and safe
Easily obtainable
Quantitative data
Can detect subtle aspects of laryngeal function
Can be used as a baseline measure
Can document changes in vocal output
Can validate/supplement auditory-perceptual information
Can be useful for patient feedback and motivation
Can be used as outcomes measures
Can be used as a communication tool
Disadvantages
Not valid for moderate/severe dysphonia
Instrumentation is sensitive to external noise
Validity of analysis depends on the quality of the hardware and software
Indirect relationship between acoustic values and vocal fold function
Interpretation of numerical data may be difficult
Quality of the input depends on microphone placement
Difficult to compare values across settings because of differences in the computer programs used to calculate acoustic values
Lack of correspondence between acoustic measure and auditory-perceptual judgments

Sources: Information from Bhuta et al. (2004); Deliyski et al. (2005); Eadie & Doyle (2005); Kent et al. (2003); Leonard et al. (2002); Maryn et al. (2009); Rodriguez-Parra et al. (2007); Smits et al. (2005).

temporal duration of the signal under analysis (Kent, Vorperian, Kent, & Duffy, 2003). Further, measurements of the same signal made with different software systems may not yield comparable values, largely because of differences in the computer programs used to calculate the values (Kent et al., 2003). This makes it difficult or impossible to compare information across speakers and settings.

Another issue in acoustic measurement is the lack of correspondence between acoustic measures, auditory-perceptual features of the voice, and quality of life issues (e.g., Bhuta, Patrick, & Garnett, 2004; Eadie & Doyle, 2005). For example, Wheeler et al. (2006) acoustically analyzed the voices of patients with mild dysphonia, and patients also completed the VHI. The authors reported that the acoustic measures were not predictive of the overall VHI score, and individual VHI items were not significantly correlated with the acoustic measures. Factors such as patient personality, rate of disease progression, past experiences with vocal function, occupation, and social status can influence the individual's perception of handicap, so that a person with more abnormal acoustic results may not necessarily perceive this as a handicap. Wheeler et al. (2006) cautioned that acoustic measures and patient perception of disability should be addressed individually as equally important but entirely separate measures. Eadie and Doyle (2005) had listeners rate speech samples of adult speakers with vocal pathology in terms of overall severity and pleasantness, and calculated acoustic parameters from the same samples. Reportedly, only moderate correlations were found between multiple acoustic measures and voice pleasantness and overall severity. Thus, acoustic measures should be used in conjunction with auditory-perceptual evaluation in order to be clinically meaningful.

ELECTROGLOTTOGRAPHY

Electroglottography (EGG, also called electrolaryngology) is an indirect way of visualizing and assessing vocal fold vibration by taking advantage of human tissue electrical characteristics. A pair of surface electrodes is held in place at each side of a person's thyroid cartilage with a Velcro band. A weak high-frequency current is passed through the electrodes. Human tissue is a relatively good electrical conductor, whereas air is not. Therefore when the vocal folds are abducted, the resistance to the electrical current increases as it passes through the air-filled glottis; conversely, when the vocal folds are adducted, the resistance decreases. During vocal fold vibration a characteristic pattern of increases and decreases in electrical voltage occurs and is displayed on a monitor as a waveform (Lx waveform). As the vocal folds approximate, the resistance to the electrical current decreases and the amplitude of the waveform increases; as the vocal folds separate, the increased resistance to the electrical current results in decreased amplitude of the waveform. Different from an acoustic waveform, which shows pressure changes over time, the Lx waveform reflects the opening and closing of the vocal folds and changes in vocal fold contact area (Herbst, Howard, & Schlomicher-Thier, 2010). One cycle of the Lx waveform represents one cycle of vocal fold vibration (Figure 4.3).

As depicted in Figure 4.3, point A on the waveform signals the start of the closing phase as the inferior margins of the vocal folds begin to close. Between points A, B, and C the inferior

FIGURE 4.3 **Lx Waveform**

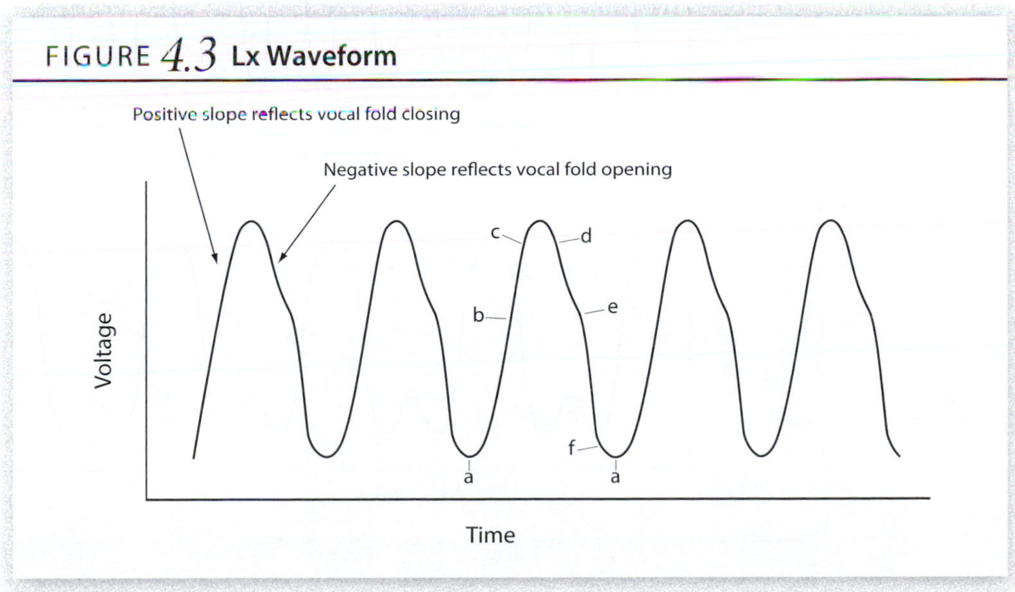

and superior margins of the vocal folds continue to close. Point C reflects maximum vocal fold contact, and the interval between points C and D indicates the closed phase of the vibratory cycle. At point D the inferior margins of the vocal folds begin to separate, and the separation continues in an upward direction between points D, E, and F. Point F reflects minimal contact (i.e., maximum separation) between the vocal folds (Baken, 1992). The cycle then begins again. Falsetto and pulse registers show different features of the waveform. In falsetto the shape becomes almost sinusoidal, reflecting the high rate of vibration and the more equal closing and opening phases (Chernobelsky, 2002). In pulse register the waveform shows characteristic

FIGURE 4.4 **Lx Waveforms of Vocal Registers and Qualities**

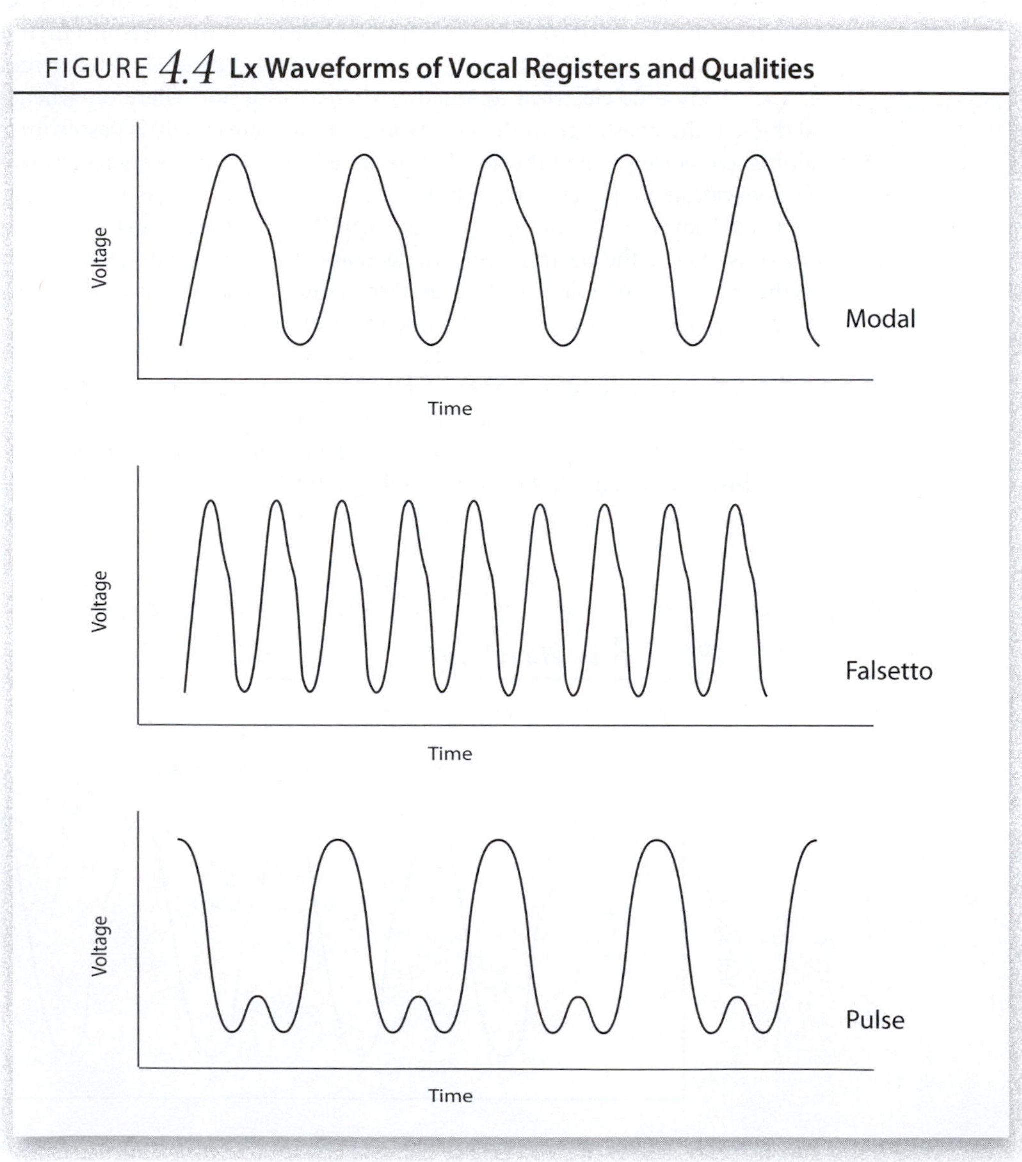

FIGURE 4.4 (Continued)

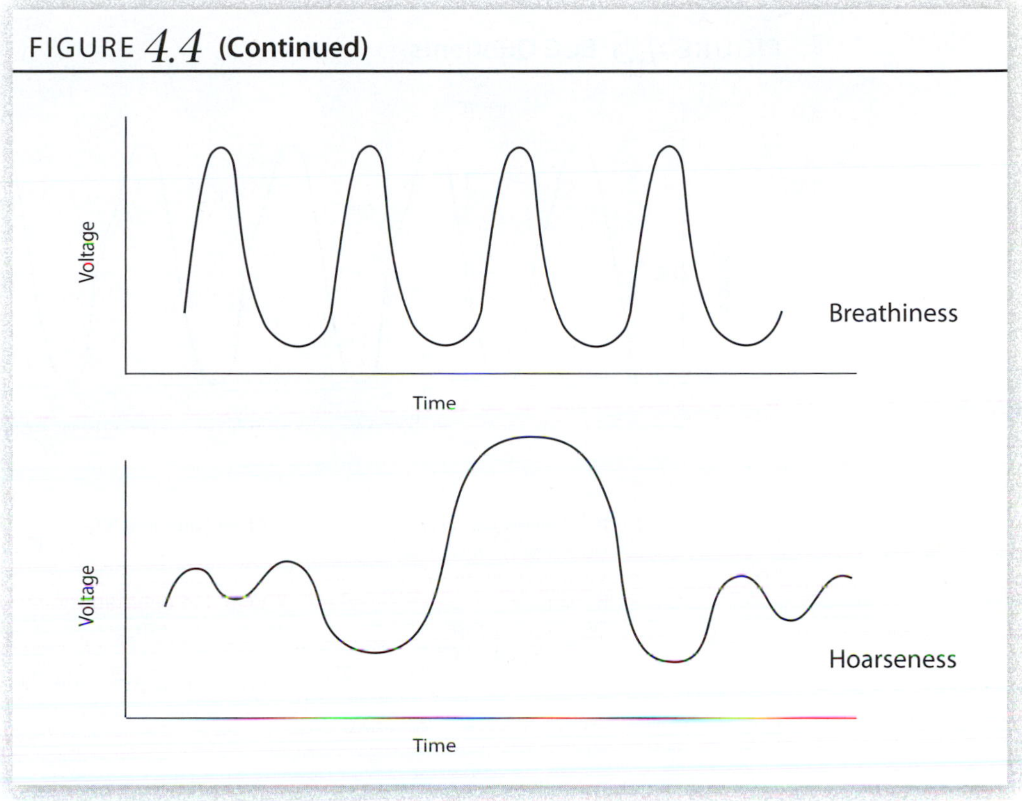

biphasic or multiphasic closure patterns of the vocal folds. Lx waveforms can also represent aperiodic and breathy patterns of vocal fold vibration (Figure 4.4).

The Lx waveform is interpreted by evaluating its shape, as well as by calculating ratios between the opening, closing, and total duration of phases of vocal fold vibration. For example, the closed quotient (CQ) compares the duration of the closed phase to the entire glottal cycle and is correlated with degree of medial compression. In modal register the CQ typically ranges from approximately 0.50 to 0.60 (Nair, 1999). The higher the CQ, the longer is the closed phase of vibration. The closed-to-open ratio (C/O ratio) compares the relative durations of the closed and open phases of vibration. A higher ratio indicates a longer closed phase and may indicate hyperfunctional vocal fold adduction (Figure 4.5).

EGG is also used to derive acoustic measures such as F0, jitter, shimmer, and noise, and it bypasses some of the problems in obtaining valid acoustic signals from dysphonic voices. Because the Lx waveform shows individual cycles of vibration, acoustic measures can be calculated more reliably and can be used to derive acoustic information from both sustained vowels and conversational speech (Kazi et al., 2008). As such, it can be useful in tracking a patient's therapeutic progress and treatment outcomes.

Although not as popular as the other types of acoustic instrumentation, EGG is quite often used clinically as a noninvasive method of obtaining information about groups of

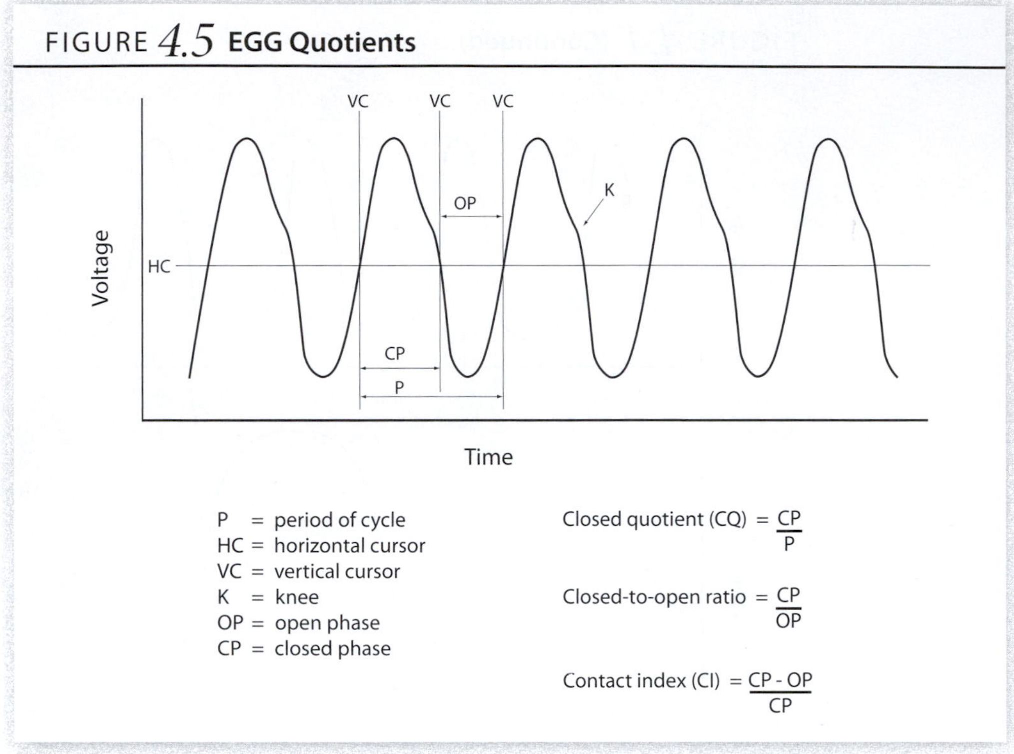

FIGURE 4.5 **EGG Quotients**

dysphonic speakers (Herbst & Ternstrom, 2006). For example, Zagolski and Carlson (2002) reported that women with vocal fold paralysis showed a delay in achieving maximum vocal fold contact during phonation, resulting in a prolonged closing phase. In a later study it was found that EGG parameters normalized with spontaneous recovery of function in the speakers with paralysis (Zagolski, 2009). Lim et al. (2006) used EGG to obtain jitter, shimmer, HNR, mean F0, and SDF0 in connected speech of patients with **Reinke's edema**. They reported that when the edema was more severe the closed quotient was higher than normal, and there were significant differences in jitter, shimmer, and HNR. Contact patterns of the vocal folds improved following surgery. EGG has also been used as a form of visual feedback to treat deaf adolescents with puberphonia. Speakers were able to visualize differences in shape between modal and falsetto registers, which provided a clear model to follow (Chernobelsky, 2002).

There are some disadvantages of EGG, primarily in interpretation of the waveform shapes. The waveform does not provide information about the width of glottal opening or the degree of closure. Thus, while the vocal folds may have reached their maximum closure as indicated on the Lx waveform, there could still be space between them resulting from conditions such as a posterior glottal gap (Herbst, Howard, & Schlomicher-Thier, 2010). Another disadvantage is that there are no specific norms for interpretation of the Lx waveform, and no standardization of waveform shapes.

AERODYNAMIC MEASURES

Aerodynamic measures quantify airflows and air volumes used for voice production purposes. Vocal fold vibration results from the interaction between muscular and elastic forces as well as subglottal, transglottal, and supraglottal pressures. Measurements of air volumes and airflows therefore reflect an individual's ability to use the laryngeal mechanism effectively in regulating the flow of air for phonation. Most current clinical aerodynamic approaches are designed to obtain indirect estimates of average glottal airflow rates (ml/sec) and average subglottal air pressures (cm H_2O) together with simultaneous acoustic measures of frequency and intensity (Mehta & Hillman, 2007).

Air Volume. Two measures of lung volume are relevant to voice production, including vital capacity (VC) and tidal volume (TV). VC refers to the total amount of air that an individual is able to use voluntarily. The measurement involves inhaling the maximum amount of air possible and then exhaling maximally into a spirometer. VC varies widely according to age, sex, and build, but an average value that is used for convenience is around 5,000 ml. TV refers to the amount of air inhaled and exhaled per breath. For normal quiet breathing TV is around 10% of VC, that is, approximately 500 ml. Normal conversational speech typically falls within 20% of VC, or 1,000 ml per breath for speech. Because normal speech requires only a small percentage of VC, patients with a somewhat limited VC may not be affected in terms of voice. However, a patient with a greatly reduced vital capacity may demonstrate short maximum phonation times, short speech phrases, and a weak voice with reduced intensity due to difficulty achieving adequate subglottal pressure during speech (Koschkee & Rammage, 1997).

Airflow Rate. Airflow rate refers to the rate at which air passes through the glottis during phonation and is measured with a pneumotachograph in ml/sec. The procedure involves the patient phonating a vowel into a face mask attached to a pressure sensor. The airflow exiting the individual's oral and/or nasal cavity is converted into an electrical signal and displayed on a monitor. The larynx is an important regulator of airflow for voice production. If too much air flows through the glottis during vocalization, airflow rates will be high, and the patient's voice may be perceived as breathy. Excessively tight glottal closure prevents the easy flow of air through the glottis, and the resulting voice is likely to be perceived as tense and strained.

There is a large amount of variation in airflow rates both within and between individual speakers, which limits the usefulness of the measure (Holmberg, Oates, Dacakis, & Grant, 2009). Further, there are currently no widely agreed-on norms for airflow (Mehta & Hillman, 2007). Nonetheless, average airflow rates of approximately 80–200 ml/sec have been reported as normal (Stemple et al., 2000), with most adult airflow rates averaging between 100–150 ml/sec (Case, 2002). Patients with glottal incompetence due to problems such as vocal fold paralysis may generate average airflow rates as high as 400–600 ml/sec (Stemple et al., 2000). Patients with severely hyperfunctional voice or glottal fry demonstrate markedly reduced airflow rates, as low as 10–15 ml/sec. Average airflow rate is reportedly most useful and reliable as an indicator of relatively large changes in vocal function (e.g., comparing vocal function before and after medialization for vocal fold paralysis), but less useful for tracking relatively small changes (Mehta & Hillman, 2007).

Subglottal Air Pressure. Subglottal air pressure (Ps) is usually not measured directly, because to do so involves inserting a measurement device into the trachea. Rather, pressure is indirectly estimated from a patient's production of a stop sound such as /p/. The rationale for this procedure is that for the voiceless stop sound, the lips are closed and the vocal folds are open, so that the pressures in the oral cavity and subglottal area are approximately equal. A tube in the patient's mouth is attached to a pressure transducer, and he or she produces a series of /pi/ syllables. Thus, pressure can be obtained orally, reflecting the pressure within the trachea. Subglottal pressure is correlated to laryngeal resistance. The greater the laryngeal resistance (i.e., greater medial compression), the greater is the phonation threshold pressure. Pressure requirements are higher to produce a louder voice, and also vary depending on F0. Higher frequencies require increased vocal fold tension, and thus have a higher phonation threshold pressure. Lower frequencies require less Ps to initiate vibration. Subglottal air pressure is also highly correlated with the sound pressure level of the voice (Mehta & Hillman, 2007). For normal conversational speech, the phonation threshold pressure is around 5–10 cm H_2O. Jiang et al. (1999) measured subglottal pressure in patients with Parkinson's disease. The authors reported that the patients demonstrated significantly greater pressures than healthy subjects to produce similar flows and intensity levels. The higher subglottic pressures imply a significantly greater laryngeal resistance during phonation, which is consistent with the increased rigidity of the vocal folds and lower intensity levels that are characteristic of Parkinson's disease.

LARYNGEAL ELECTROMYOGRAPHY

Laryngeal **electromyography** (LEMG) is a method of assessing the integrity of laryngeal nerves and muscles (Sataloff et al., 2010). The procedure is done by inserting needle electrodes into selected muscles in order to measure their electrical activity (Ysunza et al., 2007). Although it is safe and reliable (Ysunza et al., 2007), LEMG is not performed routinely because it is an invasive procedure. The procedure can only be performed by a neurologist, physiatrist, or laryngologist skilled in electrodiagnostic medicine. LEMG can be useful in distinguishing between causes of vocal fold immobility such as paralysis versus cricoarytenoid joint problems (e.g., Ysunza et al., 2007) and can help to differentiate between unilateral vocal fold paresis, bilateral paresis, muscle tension dysphonia, tremor, myoclonus, and presbylaryngis (Heman-Ackah & Barr, 2006; Sataloff et al., 2010; Stager & Bielamowicz, 2010). LEMG is also valuable in identifying the presence or absence of CT muscle involvement in patients with abductor spasmodic dysphonia, and for needle guidance for **Botox** injections.

Table 4.21 presents a list of indications for LEMG.

THE DIAGNOSTIC REPORT

The end result of the assessment process is a report that combines data from all team members to form evidence that provides the basis for the recommendations for the patient. The diagnostic report typically includes the individual's demographic information, a statement of the problem, background information, observations and assessment results, summary of findings, prognosis, and recommendations. Ideally, a team meeting is conducted with the patient and/or parents and caretakers at which the findings of the evaluation are discussed. An example of a portion of a diagnostic report is presented in Figure 4.6, followed by questions relating to the evaluation.

TABLE 4.21 Indications for Laryngeal EMG

Immobile Vocal Fold

Differentiates vocal fold paralysis from vocal fold fixation

Determines prognosis for recovery following traumatic or surgical neural injury

Determines presence or absence of tone (e.g., partial reinnervation or synkinesis in the paralyzed muscle)

May be useful for assessment of reinnervation procedure

Hypomobile Vocal Fold

Diagnosis of neuromuscular disorders

Motor neuron disease

Neuromuscular junction disorders

Focal peripheral neuropathies

Normal Mobility with an Abnormal Voice

Diagnosis of laryngeal movement disorders

Dystonias

Tremor

Myoclonus

Cerebral palsy

Parkinsonism

Chorea

FIGURE 4.6 Portion of a Diagnostic Report and Related Questions

UNIVERSITY SPEECH-LANGUAGE-HEARING CLINIC

Diagnostic Evaluation

Name: AB	Date of Evaluation: 8/3/10
Address: 10 High Street	Date of Birth: 5/16/33
Pleasantville, OH	Chronological Age: 77
Telephone: 555-832-6873	

AB, a 77-year-old male, was seen for a speech-language evaluation at the university's Speech and Language Center on August 3, 2010. Mr. B provided the following background information himself. His primary concern was with his voice. Mr. B reported hoarseness, throat dryness, and low volume. He has not received any prior voice, speech, or language therapy and feels that his voice problems have worsened since onset.

(continued)

FIGURE 4.6 Portion of a Diagnostic Report and Related Questions (Continued)

Background Information

Mr. B initially described his vocal concerns as feeling as if his voice is "caught in his throat" and very hoarse. He reported the problem first began approximately one year ago and has gotten worse since onset. Mr. B described the onset as gradual and recounted some periods of normal voice throughout the day. He has observed that after increased vocal use, stress, and fatigue, his vocal conditions appear to worsen. Mr. B did not report any further speech or language concerns other than a minor difficulty recalling words, which he believes to be due to his age. He has not had any previous voice, speech, or language therapy and had no significant familial history of voice, speech, language, or hearing difficulties.

Mr. B did not describe any significant emotional or psychological symptoms accompanying his vocal difficulty. He has not received any prior counseling services and has not experienced any unusual changes in mood within the past year. His last hearing test occurred five years ago when he was diagnosed with tinnitus.

Mr. B currently is employed part time as adjunct associate professor of market research at the university. He teaches two courses per semester. When teaching, he does not use an amplification device. He remarked that his voice worsens after each class due to the excessive use of his voice. Mr. B commented that he often feels dryness in his throat, especially in the evenings. Mr. B estimated that he drinks 5–7 8-oz glasses of water and one and a half glasses of a caffeinated beverage daily. He did not report any significant air quality conditions or excessive noise in his home or work environment.

Medical History

Mr. B was seen by an otolaryngologist, Dr. EM, on July 16, 2010, regarding concerns about his voice quality. Dr. M used a CT scan and nasoendoscopy to conclude that Mr. B exhibited "swelling of one false vocal fold." It was reported by Mr. B that another doctor has credited his "current blood pressure medicine, Simvastatin," to be a possible cause for his voice problem. Upon further research it was discovered that Simvastatin is a medication used to treat high cholesterol. Mr. B reported that he has been prescribed a new blood pressure medication, Cozaar, which he has not yet begun to take. Mr. B's daily medication intake also includes baby aspirin, Quinapril (20 mg), Atenolol (12.5 mg), Levothyroxine (88 mcg), and Furosemide (20 mg).

Mr. B reported a number of surgeries including two heart bypass surgeries, two hip replacement surgeries, and a gall bladder removal surgery. He also reported that he is scheduled for knee replacement surgery and experiences severe arthritis in his joints. Mr. B recalled no health concerns at the onset of his voice problem and noted that he was in good health on the day of the evaluation. Mr. B informed the clinicians of excessive coughing throughout the day and attributed this to extreme dryness in his throat. He further stated that the dryness gets worse in the evening and results in a "raspy" voice. He denied symptoms of gastroesophageal reflux disease (GERD) or laryngopharyngeal reflux (LPR). The client indicated that he has a habit of throat clearing when his voice "starts to go." He did not report any difficulties with swallowing or any recent instances of weight loss. Mr. B recalled that he was seen by an audiologist for a complete audiological evaluation 5 years prior to this evaluation. He was diagnosed with tinnitus, but did not feel that the condition has any impact on his hearing or vocal volume.

FIGURE 4.6 (Continued)

Auditory-Perceptual Evaluation

The Consensus Auditory-Perceptual Evaluation of Voice (CAPE-V) was used to evaluate Mr. B's voice quality, pitch, and loudness. Mr. B's overall severity was judged to be mildly to moderately deviant (26/100). Pitch range and loudness levels were evaluated as mildly to moderately deviant (30/100 and 29/100, respectively). Roughness and strain were judged to be mildly deviant (22/100 and 23/100, respectively). Pitch and loudness levels were consistently deviant throughout the evaluation; roughness and strain were intermittently present.

Voice Handicap Index (VHI) and Vocal Behavior Rating Scale

The Voice Handicap Index (VHI) was administered to score Mr. B's perception of his voice and how it affects him physically, functionally, and emotionally. Mr. B scored 16 on the "P Scale" (physical), 5 for the "F Scale" score (functional), and 9 for the "E Scale" score (emotional). Mr. B reported that his voice quality was inconsistent throughout the day, and it seemed to be worse in the evening even if he does not use his voice much during the day. He also reported that his voice quality was affected after prolonged periods of speaking (i.e., after lecturing in the classroom). Mr. B further reported that his vocal quality annoys and upsets him.

The client also completed a vocal behavior rating scale in which he was asked to report how often he partakes in activities that can affect his vocal quality. Situations included excessive talking, shouting, talking in presence of noise, phone use, singing, making noise, forceful whispering, and coughing/throat clearing. Mr. B rated talking in the presence of noise and coughing/throat clearing to be the most frequent vocally damaging behaviors.

Acoustic Analysis

The Visi-Pitch was used to evaluate Mr. B's habitual pitch, pitch range, and intensity. Data were obtained for mean speaking fundamental frequency (SFF), F0 for sustained vowel /a/, maximum phonational frequency range, standard deviation of F0 (F0SD), average vocal intensity, and dynamic range (minimum dB and maximum dB). The MDVP program was used to collect jitter and shimmer values.

Mr. B obtained the following values:

Conversational speech:	
Mean Speaking Fundamental Frequency (SFF)	*100.08 Hz*
Standard Deviation of F0 (F0SD)	*5.29 Hz*
Average Intensity	*53.59 dB*
F0 Sustained /a/	*109.54 Hz*
Maximum Phonational Frequency Range	*97.14 Hz–210 Hz*
Dynamic Range	*16.54 dB SPL*
Jitter	*0.71%*
Shimmer	*4.798 dB*
Maximum phonation time	*20 seconds*
s/z ratio	*0.80*

(continued)

FIGURE 4.6 Portion of a Diagnostic Report and Related Questions (Continued)

Observations

In summary, Mr. B's results indicate that he is within normal limits for measurements of mean speaking fundamental frequency, jitter, maximum phonation time, and the s/z ratio. However, Mr. B's results reveal abnormalities in frequency variability (pitch range), standard deviation of frequency variability, average vocal intensity, dynamic range, and shimmer. Values for mean F0 were within normal limits for conversational speech and sustained /a/; however, F0SD for conversational speech was reduced, supporting the perceptual impression of reduced pitch range and monotone voice quality. Maximum phonational frequency range and dynamic range were also reduced and support the perceptual impression of reduced loudness.

Throughout the evaluation, it was observed that Mr. B's voice decreased in volume over the span of a single sentence. In addition, his voice was intermittently hoarse and he coughed and cleared his throat often after speaking. Mr. B was visibly tense in his face and shoulders, and prolonging vowels appeared to be effortful. Although results for the s/z ratio task were within normal limits, facial tension and hand clenching were observed during production of the voiced /z/. This was not seen during productions of the voiceless /s/. It was also noted that the volume of his voice was very low and he was often difficult to hear. For the majority of the evaluation the client's posture was "slumped" in the chair and he spoke with his eyes directed downward.

Hearing

A pure tone screening was performed. The tone was presented at 25 dB through earphones. Mr. B did not respond to the 3,000 Hz and 4,000 Hz frequency in both the left and right ears.

Impressions

Mr. B, a 77-year-old male, was evaluated on August 3, 2010, at the University Speech-Language-Hearing Clinic. The reason for this evaluation was to assess his vocal quality and to provide additional information following a previous otolaryngological evaluation that revealed "swelling of one false vocal fold." Mr. B expressed concerns with his voice, stating that he felt as if his voice was "caught in his throat." Objective acoustic results supported the perceptual observations of reduced pitch variation and reduced loudness levels. It was also noted that Mr. B presented with tension in the upper body and face upon phonation of voiced sounds.

Questions

1. *Based on the data provided in the report, what other professionals should be involved in the evaluation? Provide a rationale for each professional.*
2. *Are there any other procedures that could be performed during the evaluation that might yield useful information? Provide examples and rationales.*
3. *Identify and explain all potential causes that may be contributing to Mr. B's vocal problems.*
4. *Based on the observations provided in the report, what is the prognosis for Mr. B?*
5. *What recommendations would be appropriate to include in the report?*

chapter SUMMARY

THE PRIMARY AIMS of the voice evaluation are to determine the existence of a problem; discover the cause of the problem; describe the symptoms of the problem; assess the severity of the problem; investigate the effects of the problem on the patient's life; and determine the most effective ways to treat the problem. The voice evaluation is typically divided into several components including the patient interview and case history, laryngeal examination, perceptual and instrumental assessment of voice, interpretation of test results, prognosis, and recommendations for treatment. The interview process provides an excellent opportunity for the clinician to informally evaluate the patient's voice in a conversational setting. Aspects to be noted include the overall level of severity of dysphonia, the presence of specific voice qualities such as hoarseness, roughness, breathiness, strain, tension, weakness, hyper- or hyponasality, stridor, hard glottal attacks, and so on. The individual's perception of the impact of the voice disorder on his or her life is obtained using an appropriate quality of life measure.

Auditory-perceptual measures require the clinician to make a subjective judgment of aspects of the person's voice, such as the overall level of severity, the appropriateness of the pitch and loudness levels, and the quality of the voice. The patient is asked to perform various vocal activities designed to assess aspects of vocal production such as respiratory-phonatory efficiency, vocal endurance, reflexive laryngeal function, and presence of musculoskeletal tension. The patient's performance is charted on a scale such as the GRBAS or CAPE-V.

Instrumental measures such as indirect and direct laryngoscopy, endoscopy, and videostroboscopy allow examination of the structure and function of the larynx. Acoustic analysis of the patient's vocal output permits inferences to be made about vocal fold vibration. Acoustic analysis provides visual and quantifiable information that can be used as a baseline measure, as a form of biofeedback in treatment, for documentation of the patient's progress in therapy, and as an outcome measure. Aerodynamic measures quantify airflows and air volumes used for voice production purposes and reflect an individual's ability to use the laryngeal mechanism effectively in regulating the flow of air for phonation.

Laryngeal electromyography is a method of assessing the integrity of laryngeal nerves and muscles. This is an invasive procedure that can only be performed by a neurologist, physiatrist, or laryngologist.

The end result of the assessment process is a report that combines data from all team members to form evidence that provides the basis for the recommendations for the patient. The diagnostic report typically includes the individuals' demographic information, a statement of the problem, background information, observations and assessment results, summary of findings, prognosis, and recommendations.

review QUESTIONS

1. Explain why the case history is an integral component of the evaluation process.
2. Which of the several quality of life instruments do you prefer? Why?
3. Discuss why auditory-perceptual evaluation of voice is considered the "gold standard" of evaluation. Do you agree with this position? Why or why not?
4. Identify and define the vocal fold vibratory characteristics examined during videostroboscopy.
5. Discuss the contribution of acoustic measures in a voice evaluation, noting both advantages and disadvantages.
6. Explain the ratios that are obtained from electroglottography and how these may be used to evaluate voice.
7. Identify aerodynamic measures used in vocal function assessment. How could these data be used to supplement perceptual and acoustic measures?
8. Describe advantages and disadvantages of laryngeal electromyography in distinguishing between causes of vocal fold immobility.

Appendix 1: Preferred Practice Patterns for the Profession of Speech-Language Pathology

34. VOICE ASSESSMENT

Voice assessment is provided to evaluate vocal structure and function (strengths and weaknesses), including identification of impairments, associated activity and participation limitations, and context barriers and facilitators.

Assessment is conducted according to the Fundamental Components and Guiding Principles.

INDIVIDUALS WHO PROVIDE THE SERVICE(S)

Voice assessments are conducted by appropriately credentialed and trained speech-language pathologists.

EXPECTED OUTCOME(S)

Consistent with [the] World Health Organization (WHO) framework, assessment is conducted to identify and describe—

- underlying strength and deficits related to a voice disorder or a laryngeal disorder affecting respiration and communication performance;
- effects of the voice disorder on the individual's activities (capacity and performance in everyday communication contexts) and participation;
- contextual factors that serve as barriers to or facilitators of successful communication and participation for individuals with voice disorders or laryngeal disorders affecting respiration.

Assessment may result in the following:

- Diagnosis of a voice disorder or laryngeal disorder affecting respiration.
- Description of perceptual phonatory characteristics.
- Measurement of aspects of vocal function.
- Examination of phonatory behavior.
- Identification of a communication difference possibly co-occurring with a voice or laryngeal disorder.
- Prognosis for change (in the individual or relevant contexts).
- Recommendations for intervention and support.

Source: American Speech-Language-Hearing Association (2004). *Preferred Practice Patterns for the Profession of Speech-Language Pathology [Preferred Practice Patterns]*. Available from www.asha.org/policy.

- Identification of the effectiveness of intervention and supports.
- Referral for other assessments or services.

CLINICAL INDICATIONS

Voice assessment services are provided to individuals of all ages as needed, requested, or mandated or when other evidence suggests that individuals have voice or laryngeal disorders affecting body structure/function and/or activities/participation.

Assessment is prompted by referral, by the individual's medical status, or by failing a speech screening that is sensitive to cultural and linguistic diversity.

CLINICAL PROCESS

All patients/clients with voice disorders are examined by a physician, preferably in a discipline appropriate to the presenting complaint. The physician's examination may occur before or after the voice evaluation by the speech-language pathologist.

Comprehensive assessments are sensitive to cultural and linguistic diversity and address the components within the WHO's International Classification of Functioning, Disability, and Health (2001) framework including body structures/functions, activities/participation, and contextual factors.

Assessment may be static (i.e., using procedures designed to describe functioning within relevant domains) or dynamic (i.e., using hypothesis testing procedures to identify potentially successful intervention and support procedures) and includes the following:

- Review of auditory, visual, motor, and cognitive status.
- Relevant case history, including vocal use history, medical status, education, vocation, and cultural and linguistic backgrounds.
- Standardized and nonstandardized methods:
  - Perceptual aspects of vocal production/behavior
  - Acoustic parameters of vocal production/behavior
  - Physiological aspects of phonatory behavior
  - Patient's/client's ability to modify vocal behavior
  - Emotional/psychological status
  - Medical history and associated conditions
  - Observation or review of articulation, fluency, and language
  - Functional consequences of the voice disorder
  - Use of perceptual and/or instrumental measures, including—
    - perceptual ratings
    - acoustic analysis
    - aerodynamic measures
    - electroglottography
    - imaging techniques such as endoscopy and stroboscopy (these procedures may be conducted and interpreted in collaboration with other professionals).

- Selection of standardized measures for voice assessment with consideration for documented ecological validity;
- Follow-up services to monitor voice status and ensure appropriate intervention and support for individuals with identified voice disorders.

SETTING, EQUIPMENT SPECIFICATIONS, SAFETY AND HEALTH PRECAUTIONS

Setting: Assessment is conducted in a clinical or educational setting, or other natural environment conducive to eliciting a representative sample of the patient's/client's voice production. The goals of the assessment and the WHO framework are considered in selecting assessment settings. Identifying the influence of contextual factors on functioning (activity and participation) requires assessment data from multiple settings.

Equipment Specifications: All equipment is used and maintained in accordance with the manufacturer's specifications. Instrumental measures may be used to assess voice production and/or laryngeal function. Instrumental techniques ensure the validity of signal processing, analysis routines, and elimination of task or signal artifacts.

Safety and Health Precautions: All services ensure the safety of the patient/client and clinician and adhere to universal health precautions (e.g., prevention of bodily injury and transmission of infectious disease).

Laryngeal imaging techniques and selection/placement of tracheoesophageal prostheses are conducted in settings that have access to emergency medical treatment, if needed.

Decontamination, cleaning, disinfection, and sterilization of multiple-use equipment before reuse are carried out according to facility-specific infection control policies and procedures and according to the manufacturer's instructions.

DOCUMENTATION

Documentation includes pertinent background information, results and interpretation, prognosis, and recommendations. Recommendations may include the need for further assessment, follow-up, or referral. When treatment is recommended, information is provided concerning frequency, estimated duration, and type of service (e.g., individual, group, home program) required.

Documentation addresses the type and severity of the voice disorder or difference and associated conditions (e.g., medical diagnoses).

Documentation includes summaries of previous services in accordance with all relevant legal and agency guidelines.

The privacy and security of documentation are maintained in compliance with the regulations of the Health Insurance Portability and Accountability Act (HIPAA), Family Educational Rights and Privacy Act (FERPA), and other state and federal laws.

Results of the assessment are reported to the individual and family/caregivers, as appropriate. Reports are distributed to the referral source and other professionals when appropriate and with written consent.

Chapter 5
Clinical Management

LEARNING OBJECTIVES

1. Identify and discuss the major components in a typical vocal hygiene program.
2. Discuss the use of relaxation and massage techniques for vocal fold hyperfunction.
3. Define biofeedback and explain its effectiveness in changing specific respiratory and/or laryngeal behaviors.
4. Explain how increasing respiratory support can facilitate speech production.
5. Identify the common themes underlying the holistic therapy approaches of the accent method, confidential voice therapy, resonant voice therapy, semi occluded vocal tract, and vocal function exercises.
6. Describe motivational interviewing and its application to voice therapy.
7. Compare and contrast the provision of voice therapy for children versus adults.
8. Describe vocal fold medialization techniques including thyroplasty, arytenoid adduction, injection, and laryngeal reinnervation.
9. Understand the rationales for various airway widening procedures.
10. Appreciate the role of lasers in laryngeal surgery.

Clinical management of an individual with a voice problem ideally should be a team effort with each professional on the team taking responsibility for different aspects of treatment and communicating with one another in order to provide the patient with an integrated and intelligent plan of treatment. For example, an otolaryngologist or other medically qualified physician, such as an allergist, pulmonary specialist, or endocrinologist, recommends and provides medical, surgical, or pharmacological treatment. Teaching the patient strategies to modify incorrect singing or acting techniques is usually the domain of the singing teacher or acting coach. Teachers of singing focus on developing the singer's full pitch and dynamic range, artistic quality, and vocal endurance (ASHA, 2005a). Voice and speech trainers, teachers, and coaches work to develop optimum resonance, range, clarity, expressiveness, and endurance for performance, public address, and teaching (ASHA, 2005a). Voice difficulties related to psychological problems may necessitate the services of a counselor or psychotherapist.

For children, the team includes educational personnel and the child's parents/caregivers. The speech-language pathologist has the responsibility of working with the patient and/or caregivers to develop the most efficient and effective ways of using the laryngeal mechanism, facilitating carryover of adaptive voice techniques to the individual's everyday life, and documenting rehabilitation progress and vocal outcomes.

Clinical management strategies for voice disorders can be broadly divided into two categories: medical and behavioral. Medical treatments include pharmacological regimens and surgical procedures. Behavioral voice therapy focuses on such areas as educating patients about laryngeal structure and function, instituting programs of vocal hygiene, and teaching patients strategies for altering aspects of voice production. Medical and behavioral voice treatments are complementary to each other. For instance, patients who undergo surgical removal of vocal polyps need to be taught a less damaging way of using the vocal mechanism in order to prevent the recurrence of the problem. Or, children whose vocal folds are scarred from frequent removals of **papillomas** must be encouraged to make the most efficient use of the vocal mechanism. The type of clinical management strategy that is chosen depends on the cause (or causes) and symptoms of the disorder, as well as on the patient's motivation, vocal needs, and lifestyle.

This chapter addresses both behavioral voice therapy techniques and medical/surgical procedures. The chapter begins with a description of direct versus indirect therapeutic methods. Commonly used behavioral techniques are presented and treatment efficacy and outcomes research is included for each therapeutic method where available. Factors that influence therapy outcomes, such as patient adherence, compliance, and therapy dropout, are explored. The topic of voice treatment in children is discussed. The focus then turns to an array of medical/surgical procedures that are commonly utilized to treat different voice disorders.

Behavioral Voice Therapy Techniques

Behavioral voice techniques can be used to address symptoms of the voice problem such as hoarseness, breathiness, tension, and inappropriate pitch; laryngeal mechanics such as hypo- or hyperadduction; and the cause of the problem, such as phonotrauma and/or lifestyle issues. Some techniques follow specified procedures, while others are based around loosely organized principles, and some use a combination of strategies (Pannbacker, 1998).

Behavioral voice techniques have traditionally been classified as indirect or direct (Table 5.1). Indirect techniques are based on the assumption that the voice disorder results from excessive vocal demands, phonotraumatic behaviors, lack of knowledge about healthy voice production, and personal factors such as stress, conflict, and anxiety (Carding, Horsley, & Docherty, 1998). Indirect techniques, therefore, are designed to help the patient to understand relevant aspects of voice production, and to encourage modifications of surroundings and lifestyle in order to facilitate healthy voice production and improved vocal performance (Rattenbury, Carding, & Finn, 2004; Thomas & Stemple, 2007). Therapy focuses on managing the contributing and maintaining aspects of the voice problem and typically involves vocal hygiene, voice rest, vocal fold hydration, relaxation techniques, and patient education (Branski, Murry, & Rosen, 2005). Direct techniques are designed to modify unhealthy methods of voice production and laryngeal pathophysiology by focusing on specific ways to increase vocal efficiency and improve voice quality (Branski et al., 2005; Carding et al., 1998, Rattenbury et al., 2004). Patients are taught specific laryngeal movements aimed at reducing the disordered pattern of phonation (Rattenbury et al., 2004). Direct approaches include those designed to promote less forceful vocal fold function in cases of hyperfunction, and

TABLE 5.1 Examples of Direct and Indirect Therapy Techniques

Direct	Indirect
Laryngeal massage	Voice rest
Yawn-sigh	Vocal hygiene
Chewing	Patient education
Altering tongue position	Counseling
Abdominal breathing	Auditory training
Coordinating breathing and phonation	Eliminating damaging vocal behaviors
Pitch variation and control	Voice diary
Regulating vocal loudness	Avoidance of irritants
Eliminating hard glottal attack	Modifying the environment
Establishing optimal pitch	Hydration
Forward placement of tone	Eliminate gastric reflux
Developing optimal resonance	
Effort closure techniques	
Optimizing vocal fold coordination and endurance	
Biofeedback	

those aimed at increasing the force of vocal fold adduction in cases of hypofunction. Many direct intervention models are holistic in nature and focus on facilitating the appropriate balance between the speech subsystems of respiration, phonation, and resonance. These approaches also aim to improve the balance, strength, tone, and stamina of the laryngeal muscles and to develop a healthy mucosal covering of the vocal folds (Thomas & Stemple, 2007). Most voice therapists use a combination of indirect and direct approaches, and this combination has been shown to be effective in most cases (Branski et al., 2005).

INDIRECT APPROACHES

The most common indirect approach is a vocal hygiene program that incorporates the identification and elimination of unhealthy vocal and lifestyle behaviors and facilitation of a healthier manner of phonation.

Vocal Hygiene Program. A primary focus of vocal hygiene programs is identifying and reducing phonotraumatic behaviors such as excessive amounts of talking, talking over noise, shouting, singing with poor vocal technique, and excessive coughing and throat clearing. Other damaging behaviors such as smoking and excessive alcohol consumption are also targeted. In the case of children, play vocalizations (e.g., animal and car/truck noises) are identified. The clinician and patient (and/or caregivers) work collaboratively to identify such behaviors. One strategy to identify phonotraumatic behaviors is to systematically review with the patient a typical day beginning from when he or she first awakes to bedtime. This can be done for a work/school day as well as a weekend day. The therapist can get a very good idea of the patient's communicative behaviors, as well as his or her eating and exercise habits, school or work behaviors, and social factors. The clinician and patient together can identify those aspects that may be contributing to the voice problem and that may be amenable to change. Once they have been identified, the patient (and/or caregiver) is encouraged to keep a daily record of targeted behaviors. This record is reviewed at the beginning of each therapy session, and goals and objectives can be modified as necessary. This type of exercise provides both a baseline and a record of progress, and can be very motivating for the client. A detailed example of a vocal hygiene program is shown in Table 5.2.

TABLE 5.2 Example of a Vocal Hygiene Program

A. Clearing your throat or coughing habitually might damage the vocal fold tissues. Instead, try some of these substitute behaviors:
   1. Yawn to relax your throat.
   2. Swallow slowly and deliberately.
   3. Sip water, let your throat relax for a second, and then resume speaking.
   4. Use the "silent cough" technique.
   5. Hum: concentrate on vocal resonance sensations.
   6. If necessary, suck on candy (*not* cough drops with menthol or mint).
   7. Be particularly aware of the throat-clearing habit during lecturing.

B. Speaking loudly, yelling, cheering, or screaming might damage the vocal fold tissues. Instead:
   1. Use gestures, nonvocal sounds, or instruments to attract attention from a distance (e.g., clap, whistle, ring a bell, blow a horn).
   2. Set up a system of nonvocal signals with students to get their attention and maintain discipline. If you must speak to students who are behaving undesirably, walk up to them and speak to them quietly (this is sometimes more effective than yelling). Apply these principles to your own children and pets.

C. Speaking over loud noise for a long period of time can cause vocal fatigue or increased laryngeal tension. Noisy situations include classroom noise, loud music, television, parties, restaurants, cars, buses, airplanes, and so on. Instead:
   1. Try to reduce background noise during conversations (e.g., turn off loud music or television).
   2. Wait until students/audience are quiet and attentive.
   3. Choose quiet restaurants, booths, or tables in the corner.
   4. Face your conversational partner.
   5. Reduce the distance between you and your conversational partner so you can be heard without yelling.
   6. Position yourself so your face is well lighted.
   7. Overarticulate.
   8. Practice your listening.

D. Prolonged use of unconventional vocal sounds—whispering, growls, squeaks, imitating animals, or machine noises—can harm vocal fold tissues. Instead:
   1. If you must produce special vocal effects for performance, make sure you are using a technique that minimizes muscle tension and vocal abuse.
   2. Be especially aware to avoid using such unconventional sounds during oral reading to your students.

TABLE 5.2 **(Continued)**

E. If you sing, you should know that singing beyond your comfortable pitch and loudness range can irritate the vocal folds. Instead:
   1. Know your limits for pitch and loudness.
   2. Avoid forcing your voice to stay in a register beyond the comfortable pitch range. Don't force your "chest voice" too high; and don't force your "head voice" high into falsetto range. Allow vocal registers to change with pitch.
   3. Avoid singing all parts if you teach choral music; use instrumental demonstrations instead.
   4. Seek professional voice training.
   5. Never sing a high note that you can't sing quietly; don't push beyond comfortable pitch in any register.

F. Talking with a low-pitched monotone voice and allowing vocal energy to drop so low that the voice becomes rough and gravelly (glottal fry) can be potentially harmful to your voice. Instead:
   1. Keep your voice powered by breath flow so the tone carries, varies, and rings.
   2. Try not to speak beyond the natural breath cycle by squeezing out the last few words without sufficient breath.
   3. Speak slowly, pause at natural phrase boundaries, and take another breath before running out of air.
   4. Allow pitch to vary freely and expressively; keep pitch comfortable.

G. Holding your breath as you're planning what to say can lead to hard glottal attacks (sudden tense initiation of voice) or aggressive or low-pitched fillers, such as "um" or "ah," and should be avoided. Instead:
   1. Initiate voice gradually and easily.
   2. Keep the shoulders, upper chest, neck, and throat relaxed as you begin speaking.
   3. Use the breathing muscles and airflow to start speech phrases.
   4. Avoid tightening upper chest, shoulders, neck, or throat to push the voice out.
   5. Let your abdomen and rib cage move freely.
   6. Avoid clenching your teeth or tensing your jaw or tongue during speech.

H. Speaking extensively during strenuous physical exercise is not recommended. Instead:
   1. After aerobic exercise, wait until your breathing system can accommodate optimal voice production.
   2. Avoid loud and aggressive vocal "grunts" while exercising.

I. Your general health can affect your voice. Maintain a healthy lifestyle and a healthy environment.
   1. Do not smoke. If you smoke, see your family doctor about ways to stop smoking—seek a referral to a smoking cessation clinic. Avoid spending large amounts of time in dry, smoke-filled environments.
   2. Avoid recreational drugs.
   3. Avoid caffeinated beverages such as coffee, tea, and colas.
   4. Monitor/reduce alcohol intake. Alcohol can have a drying effect on vocal fold tissues.
   5. Maintain a well-balanced diet.
   6. Get adequate sleep: 7–8 hours per night.
   7. Maintain proper humidity. A small portable vaporizer at the bedside is often helpful at night. Purchasing a room humidifier may be an option, especially if your home or work environment is extremely dry or dust-filled. Environmental levels of humidity should be at least 30%.
   8. Maintain proper hydration. Drink 8–10 glasses of decaffeinated fluids per day. Water is the preferred fluid. Have it handy at all times and sip it throughout the day, especially while teaching.
   9. Some medications, including antihistamines and decongestants, can cause increased dryness of tissues, causing a dry scratchy feeling in the throat. Be aware of this and compensate with increased hydration (i.e., fluid consumption). If possible, reduce the use of such medications.

TABLE 5.2 Example of a Vocal Hygiene Program (Continued)

J. Reduce your total amount of voice use.
   1. Rest your voice when you are tired or have an upper respiratory infection (i.e., cold or flu-like symptoms). Do not force your voice when it is hoarse because of a cold.
   2. Rest your voice before it becomes fatigued—before tightness, dryness, or hoarseness is noted. Schedule your day so that there are periods of voice rest interspersed. If you don't have to, don't schedule your classes back to back. Don't spend your lunch talking with other teachers; use that time to be quiet and rest your voice. Curtail your voice use socially.
   3. When getting involved in extracurricular activities, consider how much voice use will be required. If it is great, you may want to consider choosing another activity or becoming involved in another capacity.
   4. Change your style of teaching. Make use of audiovisual materials, desk-work, student presentations, and small group formats to reduce the amount of constant talking. Make use of student teachers, teaching assistants, and volunteer parents whenever possible.

Source: From "An Evaluation of the Effects of Two Treatment Approaches for Teachers with Voice Disorders: A Prospective Randomized Clinical Trial," by N. Roy, S.D. Gray, M. Simon, H. Dove, K. Corbin-Lewis, and J.C. Stemple, 2001, *Journal of Speech, Language, and Hearing Research, 44*, pp. 294–295. Copyright 2001 by the American Speech-Language-Hearing Association. Reprinted with permission.

Efficacy of Vocal Hygiene Programs. Investigations of vocal hygiene programs have been inconclusive regarding their efficacy. Roy et al. (2001) conducted a well-controlled study to determine effects of a vocal hygiene program for teachers with voice disorders. They reported that this approach alone, without a direct component included, may not be effective in producing the desired results. By contrast, based on a questionnaire and acoustic measures in teachers without voice problems, Pasa, Oates, and Dacakis (2007) concluded that a program of vocal hygiene for teachers is likely to be effective in preventing the occurrence of voice problems. Behrman, Rutledge, Hembree, and Sheridon (2008) provided either vocal hygiene education or resonant voice therapy to two groups of women with phonotraumatic lesions. The authors reported that six weeks of resonant voice therapy was more effective than a similar amount of vocal hygiene education. Williams and Deem (2000) surveyed 305 teachers regarding the likelihood that they could modify their lifestyles to incorporate vocal hygiene practices to prevent voice problems. Only 4 of 23 vocal hygiene strategies were rated as being very likely to be performed. Holmberg, Hillman, Hammarberg, Sodersten, and Doyle (2001) implemented a systematic vocal hygiene program with 11 women with nodules. The program included vocal education, reduction/elimination of identified vocal abuses, and various voice-facilitating approaches. No improvement was noted in a battery of perceptual and physiological assessments before and after treatment.

Vocal hygiene programs may be more effective if they are considered only as one part of a larger, more comprehensive voice program that also includes direct treatment approaches (Pasa et al., 2007; Roy et al., 2001; Thomas & Stemple, 2007). This was demonstrated by Amir, Dukas, and Shnaps-Baum (2005), who utilized both indirect and direct strategies for teachers with and without voice disorders. A traditional vocal hygiene approach was combined with techniques to support abdominal breathing and reduced respiratory effort for speech. Other direct strategies included reducing hard glottal attacks and facilitating soft vocal onsets using chant, yawn-sigh, open mouth, and chewing techniques. Perceptual and acoustic results after the conclusion of therapy showed that both groups exhibited improvement in vocal function, with the vocally disordered teachers benefiting to a greater degree.

In order for vocal hygiene programs to be effective, strategies need to be devised that are consistent with the individual's lifestyle. Expecting a person to change his or her lifestyle is not usually a realistic goal. This has been demonstrated in several studies. For example, Roy et al. (2002) compared two treatment programs to reduce **vocal hyperfunction** in teachers. One group used a portable vocal amplification (VA) device to increase their loudness levels, while another group participated in a traditional vocal hygiene (VH) program. Those in the VA program demonstrated significant lowering of their degree of voice handicap and voice disorder severity after the 6-week program, confirmed by objective acoustic analysis of pre- and posttreatment audio recordings. The group who underwent the VH program did show some changes in the desired direction, but not to the same degree as the VA group. Those in the VA group reported more overall voice improvement, clarity of speaking and singing voice, and greater ease of production after treatment. However, the VA group was also more compliant with the treatment program than the VH group, and this factor might explain the results. For many patients, it might be more difficult to adhere to a VH program that is predicated on the adoption of basic lifestyle changes, compared to a program that only requires wearing a portable voice amplifier during the workday. Roy et al. (2002) commented that most vocal hygiene programs are the equivalent of a vocal diet, involving constant monitoring and restrictions in voice use patterns that often conflict with the individual's vocal usage demands.

Patient Education. Educating the patient and/or caregiver(s) regarding normal laryngeal anatomy and physiology is essential to foster understanding of the voice problem and motivation to change selected target behaviors. When carried out in the context of the endoscopic evaluation, this can be particularly effective in providing concrete visualizations of normal versus abnormal structure and function. Even without endoscopy a patient's understanding and appreciation of normal structure and function can be enhanced by clear descriptions and illustrations, and his or her laryngeal function can be compared to the healthier version. Explanations can be geared toward adults or children, depending on the terminology used and the level of sophistication of the anatomical/physiological descriptions.

Hydration. Adequate hydration is central to healthy vocal fold function, and level of hydration has been shown to influence the viscoelastic properties of the vocal folds. Patients are often counseled to drink 8 glasses of water per day. This amount, however, should be adjusted for individual cases. Some patients may not benefit from drinking large amounts of water, for instance, one who has kidney problems. Another way to maximize laryngeal tissue hydration is to breathe through the nose whenever possible. Nasal breathing warms and humidifies inhaled air. Patients should be encouraged to avoid drying conditions and agents such as dry environments, smoke, alcohol, caffeine, diuretics, antihistamines, nasal sprays, and decongestants (Pannbacker, 1998). In some cases it may be beneficial for the individual to inhale steam or vapor from a humidifier to directly lubricate the surface of the vocal folds. Additionally, medications such as the mucolytics Humibid, Mucinex, and Robitussin thin out bodily secretions and make them less viscous. Other suggestions include decreasing or eliminating citrus juices (these contain a great deal of acid, which may be harsh to the laryngeal tissues), avoiding juices containing aspartame or saccharin, and drinking low-sugar juices such as apple, grape, and cranberry (Adler, 2006). Hydration treatment has been reported to be effective in improving voice quality and laryngeal appearance, and it may play a role in reducing phonatory effort and vocal fatigue (Leydon, Wroblewski, Eichom, & Sivasankar, 2010; Solomon & Di Mattia, 2000; Thomas & Stemple, 2007; Verdolini-Marston, Sandage, & Titze, 1994; Yiu & Chan, 2003).

Eliminate Gastric Reflux. Gastroesophageal reflux disease (GERD) and/or **laryngopharyngeal reflux** (LPR) are very commonly associated with voice disorders, and reflux treatment has become an essential component of many voice treatment regimens. Patients are encouraged to modify their eating habits in order to reduce GERD/LPR. For example, fatty and spicy foods should be avoided, and individuals should wait at least half an hour to exercise after eating. Individuals may also benefit from sleeping with their head slightly raised in order to prevent refluxate from entering the pharynx. In cases where diet and lifestyle changes are not sufficient to eliminate the reflux, H2 blockers such as Tagamet and Zantac prevent acid formation in the stomach. However, acid blockage is not 100% with these drugs. Proton pump inhibitors such as Nexium, Prilosec, and Prevacid block the formation of acid secretions completely. Also available are drugs that increase lower esophageal sphincter tone and increase gastric emptying, so acids are less likely to be moved onto the vocal folds. See Chapter 6 for a detailed discussion of GERD/LPR.

Voice Rest. Voice rest is often prescribed by a physician following laryngeal surgery, as well as encouraged in vocal hygiene programs. Voice rest can be relative or absolute. Relative voice rest refers to decreasing the amount of talking and the loudness of the patient's voice. Absolute voice rest requires the patient to not use his or her voice at all for a prescribed period of time. Absolute voice rest is typically recommended when a patient has undergone laryngeal surgery, in order to prevent scarring and to promote mucosal healing (Ishikawa & Thibeault, 2010). The topic of voice rest is somewhat controversial, as there is no established standard protocol and type and duration of voice rest varies among clinicians (Ishikawa & Thibeault, 2010). Behrman and Sulica (2003) examined opinions on voice rest among 1,208 otolaryngologists in the United States. They evaluated preference for absolute voice rest versus relative voice rest as well as the duration of voice rest after vocal fold surgery for nodules, polyps, and **cysts**. Roughly half of the physicians preferred absolute voice rest; 15% never recommended any type of voice rest. For those doctors who did prescribe voice rest the most common duration was 7 days with a range of 0–14 days for absolute voice rest, and 0 to more than 21 days for relative voice rest. There is some emerging evidence in the literature to support the use of relative voice rest in promoting healthy vocal fold function. Van der Merwe (2004) developed a formal program of voice conservation called the Voice Use Reduction Program. Reportedly, patients who completed the program demonstrated improvement in vocal fold appearance and voice quality, as well as a reduction in vocal fatigue.

Relaxation and Massage. Relaxation techniques are often used to reduce muscular tension in and around the laryngeal area that may be contributing to the voice problem. Progressive muscle relaxation (PMR) is a widely used technique that has been shown to be effective in the treatment of many conditions (e.g., Cheung, Molassiotas, & Chang, 2003; Ghafari et al., 2009; Knowlton & Larkin, 2006; Suhr, Anderson, & Tranel, 1999). The technique is deceptively simple, but has been shown to be highly effective in inducing desirable behaviors and reducing undesirable behaviors. The procedure involves slowly tensing and then relaxing specific muscle groups. The tense posture is held for 4–5 seconds, and the muscles are then allowed to relax. The individual is directed to focus on the difference between states of muscle tension versus relaxation and to become more aware of physical sensations associated with each (de Paula, de Carvalho, & dos Santos, 2002). PMR is used commonly as a component of voice therapy, focusing on facial, neck, chest, and shoulder muscles. Very few studies, however, have investigated the effectiveness of relaxation in a controlled manner. In one of the only published reports, Andrews, Warner, and Stewart (1986) compared two methods of relaxing laryngeal musculature in adults with hyperfunctional dysphonia. One group received progressive relaxation training, and one group received laryngeal EMG biofeedback. Patients were assessed pretreatment, posttreatment, and at three-month follow-up. Both groups showed significant improvement in all measures, which was maintained at follow-up.

More specific techniques involving laryngeal massage (LM) can be used for any voice condition involving tension in or around the larynx. The muscle effort involved in laryngeal hyperfunction can affect the entire vocal tract including the articulatory muscles and the extrinsic and intrinsic laryngeal muscles (Mathieson et al., 2009). The primary aim of massaging the perilaryngeal and laryngeal area is to relax the excessively tense musculature, which inhibits normal phonatory function (Mathieson et al., 2009). Laryngeal massage should help to reduce laryngeal tension for the same reasons that massage helps to reduce muscular tension in other areas of the body. If a muscle is too tense, it is contracted. Massaging the muscle helps it to lengthen and relax. Massage may also help to loosen joints that hold muscles too taut, thereby facilitating the easier function of the structure (Verdolini, 1998). Thus the aim of laryngeal massage is to relax the tight vocal tract muscles and to improve the range of movement of the laryngeal joints (Van Lierde, De Ley, Clement, De Bodt, & Van Cauwenberge, 2004).

There are several variations on the basic massage technique. The two most commonly used are manual circumlaryngeal therapy (MCT) and laryngeal manual therapy (LMT). Both involve applying pressure in a circular motion over the hyoid bone, within the thyrohyoid space, and into the suprahyoid sling. The massage begins superiorly at the level of the hyoid bone and progresses inferiorly to the thyroid cartilage (Thomas & Stemple, 2007). As the clinician does the massage, he or she can also exert slight downward pressure on the larynx and gently move the larynx from side to side. This helps to reduce laryngeal height and stiffness, thus increasing laryngeal mobility (Dromey, Nissen, Roy, & Merrill, 2008). The massage generally begins at a superficial level, with the depth increasing depending on the degree of tension and the patient's tolerance for the procedure (Ford & Bless, 1996). During or after the massage the patient begins to vocalize using humming and vowel prolongation, and the clinician points out any improvements in voice quality. Vocalizations are extended gradually as the degree of tension diminishes. The patient is also asked to note any reductions in pain and tenderness around the laryngeal area. The individual is trained to use the improved quality in vowels, syllables, words, phrases, and conversational speech while maintaining the more relaxed state of the laryngeal and supralaryngeal musculature.

The main differences between MCT and LMT consist of whether the palpatory evaluation is conducted before or during the procedure, the massage itself is carried out using one or both hands, the thyrohyoid space is or is not massaged, and the patient is asked to vocalize during or after the massage (Van Lierde, Ded Bodt, D'haeseleer, Wuyts, & Claeys, 2010). The two techniques are very similar, but laryngeal manual therapy focuses first on relaxing the sternocleidomastoid muscles (SCM), and then progresses to the supralaryngeal area (Mathieson et al., 2009). The rationale for working on the SCM early on in the process is that it helps to relax the person and prevent any discomfort, thus facilitating the later massage of the suprahyoid muscles (Table 5.3).

Laryngeal massage has been used by itself or in combination with other approaches to successfully target hyperfunctional voice use. For example, Van Lierde et al. (2004) used LM in combination with a focus on posture and abdominal breathing, as well as chant talk to treat persistent vocal hyperfunction in 4 professional voice users. All subjects showed

TABLE 5.3 **Laryngeal Manual Therapy (LMT) and Manual Circumlaryngeal Therapy (MCT)**

Feature	LMT	MCT
Palpatory evaluation	Before LMT	During the process of intervention
Manual intervention	Bimanual and unimanual Pads of index, middle, and third finger Working from areas of least muscle resistance to areas of greatest muscle resistance, guided by patient's tolerance of the intervention More prolonged attention to areas of greater muscle resistance	Unimanual Thumb and index finger Working from areas of of least muscle tension to areas of greatest muscle tension, guided by patient's tolerance of the intervention Sites of focal tenderness, nodularity, or tautness given more attention
Order of structures targeted	SCMs Supralaryngeal area Hyoid bone Larynx	Hyoid bone Thyrohyoid space Larynx Medial and lateral suprahyoid musculature as necessary
Methods	Circular massage of SCMs (bimanual) Kneading of supralaryngeal area (unimanual) Massage of hyoid bone (unimanual massage from one side to the other) Bimanual depression of the larynx with fingers on the superior border of the thyroid cartilage Larynx moved laterally by alternate application of bimanual digital pressure	Circular pressure to hyoid bone (unimanual) Procedure repeated within the thyrohyoid space Repeated over posterior borders of thyroid cartilage Larynx pulled down with fingers over the superior border of the thyroid cartilage and moved laterally occasionally
Patient vocalization	Vocalization is not requested from the patient during LMT until after the larynx responds easily to lateral digital pressure in the final stage of intervention. Counting, paragraph recitations, days of the week, vocal glides, and spontaneous speech are then encouraged. Rationale: The client's phonatory patterns are hyperfunctional and the muscle postures associated with the dysphonia have become habituated. Waiting until maximum relaxation of the laryngeal musculature has been achieved allows phonation to be attempted with optimum muscle tone and reduced/eliminated discomfort.	Patient is asked to sustain vowels or to hum during the manual procedures. Improved voice is shaped from vowels to words phrases, sentences, and to conversation. Rationale: The clinician is able to monitor changes in vocal quality during treatment and, as a result, can modify intervention as it progresses.

Source: From "Laryngeal Manual Therapy: A Preliminary Study to Examine Its Treatment Effects in the Management of Muscle Tension Dysphonia," by L. Mathieson, S. P. Hirani, R. Epstein, R. J. Baken, G. Wood, and J. S. Rubin, 2009, *Journal of Voice, 23,* pp. 363–364. Copyright 2009 by the Voice Foundation. Reprinted with permission.

improvements in perceptual vocal quality, with decreases in strain and hoarseness. Acoustic measures confirmed these improvements. The authors reported that the speakers' complaints of laryngeal pain on palpation, globus pharyngeus (sensation of a lump in the throat), and singing difficulties were diminished or disappeared. In a later study, Van Lierde and colleagues (2010) used the same approach in 10 patients with muscle tension dysphonia. Acoustic analysis demonstrated significant improvements after treatment. Mathieson et al. (2009) used LMT in 10 patients with muscle tension dysphonia. The authors reported that the frequency and severity of throat dryness, tickling, soreness, tightness, and irritability changed significantly after therapy. Significant acoustic changes also were evident after therapy.

Laryngeal massage has been shown to be effective for children as well as adults. Russell (2008) treated a 5-year-old girl with muscle tension dysphonia. After 12 sessions the girl showed significant improvements in acoustic and perceptual measures, and these improvements were maintained at a one-year follow-up. In a larger study, Lee and Son (2005) used a combination of manual circumlaryngeal massage, respiration training, and vocal hygiene in children aged 4–12 years with muscle tension dysphonia. Therapy was successful in improving perceptual symptoms and acoustic values, and improvement was maintained after more than two years in all but one of the children.

DIRECT APPROACHES

Direct approaches focus on modifying specific aspects of an individual's vocal production.

Biofeedback. Biofeedback provides information to an individual regarding some aspect of his or her physiological behavior and can be obtained via auditory, visual, tactile, or kinesthetic channels. Biofeedback has been used to alter physiologic parameters associated with speech production such as subglottal air pressure, degree of excursion of the abdomen and rib cage, and sound pressure level (Yorkston, Spencer, & Duffy, 2003). Biofeedback modalities include auditory information from tape recorders, visual information displayed on a Visi-Pitch, visual information from endoscopic viewing of the larynx, and laryngeal EMG.

Several recent reviews have demonstrated the effectiveness of different forms of biofeedback in improving vocal function (e.g., Allen, 2007; Maryn, De Bodt, & Van Cauwenberge, 2006; Yorkston et al., 2003). Most studies reported positive results in terms of decrease of laryngeal tension, improvement of voice quality, and/or resolution of dysphonia.

For example, Rattenbury et al. (2004) conducted a randomized controlled trial of patients with muscle tension dysphonia using indirect and direct therapy techniques. One group also received biofeedback from flexible nasoendoscopy. The authors reported that both groups of patients demonstrated significant improvements in perceptual voice ratings and in voice-related quality of life. However, the treatment that included endoscopic feedback was more efficient in terms of time taken to achieve the therapy goals. Leonard and Kendall (2005) used rigid endoscopy as a central component of a therapy program to address vocal process **granuloma** that was resistant to reflux treatment and/or behavioral or surgical treatment. The endoscopic protocol included patient education regarding proper and improper laryngeal function. Thereafter the visual feedback was utilized to help the individual to produce the vowel /i/ while maintaining a slight separation between the posterior portions of the folds. The patient was also asked to focus on the sound and feel that were associated with the correct production, so that the desired behavior could be maintained when the visual feedback was removed. Eight of the 10 patients demonstrated complete or significant resolution of the granuloma at the conclusion of therapy. Wong, Ma, and Yiu (2010) used surface EMG over the neck muscles as a voice training tool to provide augmented feedback for participants to reduce muscle tension during phonation and to learn a more relaxed phonatory style. Results revealed a significant decrease in muscle tension at both the orofacial and thyrohyoid sites. Participants also showed a reduction of severity in their scores on the Voice Activity and Participation Profile.

Increase Respiratory Support and Respiratory-Phonatory Coordination. An important component of many voice therapy programs is modification of respiratory patterns in order to increase the level of breath support for speech. A common strategy is teaching the person to use abdominal muscle patterns (sometimes called diaphragmatic or abdominal-diaphragmatic patterns) rather than thoracic or clavicular patterns for speech breathing. Use of the abdominal musculature is a more efficient way to breathe and imposes less strain on the intrinsic and extrinsic laryngeal muscles. Teaching the client to use the abdominal muscles can be facilitated by increasing his or her awareness of the different muscle patterns involved. Adler and Van Borsel (2006) described such a respiratory program. Initially, the client lies supine on a mat on the floor or in a recliner lounge chair and places one hand on the stomach area and the other hand on the chest area. He or she is instructed to inhale through the nose and slowly exhale through the mouth. In the supine position the individual should feel more movement of the hand on the abdomen than on the chest. The client should feel the hand being passively raised on inhalation as the abdomen expands and lowered on exhalation as the abdomen contracts. This technique helps the person to obtain tactile/kinesthetic feedback that facilitates establishing abdominal breathing patterns. The patient is encouraged to practice this technique at home while reclining on a couch, floor, or lounge chair. When the individual is able to consistently use this pattern while supine, he or she then uses the same pattern when sitting upright or standing up. Speech is introduced beginning with isolated vowels and progressing to longer and more complex utterances, while maintaining the target breathing pattern.

Biofeedback can be helpful in increasing respiratory support. Murdoch, Pitt, Theodoros, and Ward (1999) reported on a 12-year-old child with persistent dysarthria resulting from a traumatic brain injury. The child's dysarthria was characterized by a severe lack of respiratory support for speech, including incoordination of the chest wall and incoordination between expiration and phonation. The authors aimed to improve the child's breath support by increasing his control of inhalation and exhalation using a hierarchy of tasks including quiet breathing, deep breathing, prolonged vowels, syllable repetitions, and phrases. With the biofeedback, the child was able to adjust his speech breathing pattern to facilitate better coordination between expiration and phonation and to reduce air wastage. These strategies helped him to sustain phonation for a longer period of time on one breath.

Patients with neurological problems affecting the respiratory musculature may benefit from prosthetic devices to increase the force of expiration. The two primary forms are expiratory boards/paddles and **abdominal trussing**. Expiratory boards or paddles provide a stationary object for the patient to lean into, thus increasing expiratory force while speaking (Spencer, Yorkston, & Duffy, 2003). Trussing is the process of fixing the abdomen inward relative to its rest position using abdominal binders or corsets, abdominal wraps, and pneumobelts (Watson & Hixon, 2001). Poor posture can have an adverse effect on respiration, laryngeal height, perceived phonatory effort, and vocal fold vibratory behavior (Gilman, 2010). Supporting and stabilizing weak abdominal muscles can enhance posture and enable more efficient speech breathing. Watson and Hixon (2001) used trussing with three men with cervical spinal cord injury and reported that inspiratory capacity was significantly increased, which in turn allowed the subjects to increase the duration of their utterances. Further, the participants reported less effort to speak in the trussed versus the untrussed condition. Trussing should, however, be used with caution, as it can restrict inhalation and cause pneumonia (Spencer et al., 2003). Spencer et al. (2003) noted that medical approval and supervision are essential when abdominal trussing techniques are used, and extended use should be limited.

Some individuals with hyperfunctional vocal behavior may benefit from improving respiratory/phonatory coordination. Many researchers have noted that dysphonic speakers initiate and terminate utterances at significantly lower lung volumes than do vocally healthy speakers (e.g., Lowell, Barkmeier-Kraemer, Hoit, & Story, 2008; Schaeffer, Cavallo, Wall, & Diakow, 2002). Relaxation pressures are negative below resting expiratory level (REL), necessitating greater muscular force to control them. Smaller lung volumes used during speech require greater expiratory muscle force and are associated with a more constricted larynx, increased force of vocal fold adduction, and a pressed and effortful voice quality (Lowell et al., 2008). The increased expiratory effort may contribute to the frequent complaints of vocal effort and vocal fatigue reported by many dysphonic speakers (Lowell et al., 2008). One strategy to improve respiratory-phonatory coordination is to reduce the number of syllables per breath in order to prevent speech breathing below REL (Schaeffer et al., 2002). By reducing the length of each breath group and replenishing the air supply more frequently, patients are more likely to remain within the mid range of lung volume.

An approach to facilitating more efficient speech breathing was described by Spencer et al. (2003). The first step focuses on helping patients to become aware of the optimal breathing pattern for speech. This involves a quick inhalation and extended exhalation. An easy way to achieve this pattern is by having the individual sniff, which requires a quick inhalation, and then blow the air out slowly, which involves a controlled exhalation. As the patient becomes more adept, he or she increases the pace of the sniffing and blowing systematically to facilitate coordination between inspiratory and expiratory phases of the respiratory cycle. Speaking tasks can then be introduced, beginning with a few syllables per exhalation and increasing the length of phrases and sentences on a single breath group (Spencer et al., 2003).

Chant Therapy. The word "chant" comes from the French *chanter*, meaning to sing. Chanting refers to the rhythmic speaking or singing of words or sounds, primarily on one or two pitches called *reciting tones*. Chants may range from a simple melody involving a limited set of notes to highly complex musical structures. When used as a therapy approach, chant is characterized by a raised pitch, prolonged vowels, lack of syllable stress, and a softening of glottal attack (Van Lierde et al., 2004). These factors contribute to a more relaxed mode of phonation. Once the patient is able to perform the chant consistently, he or she alternates chant voice and regular voice while maintaining the easy, relaxed phonation (Boone, McFarlane, & Von Berg, 2005). The chant quality is faded gradually. This manner of voice production is more efficient and can therefore be helpful in reducing vocal fatigue (McCabe & Titze, 2002). While many voice programs mention the use of chant talk as one component, only one study by McCabe and Titze (2002) reported that chant therapy was effective in reducing vocal fatigue in four teachers.

Effort Closure Techniques. Effort closure techniques refer to methods of increasing the force of vocal fold adduction in patients with glottal incompetence. The original pushing method was promoted by Froeschels, Kastein, and Weissin (1955) and involves the patient pressing down hard on a surface while he or she vocalizes. The rationale is that forcefully contracting one set of muscles facilitates the contraction of other groups of muscles (Thomas & Stemple, 2007). Similar techniques include pulling upward on a chair, squeezing the palms of the hands together as hard as possible, interlacing the hands and pulling outward, pushing down on the speaker's raised arms, pushing against a firm surface, and grunting/coughing (Spencer et al., 2003). While these methods can be effective in enhancing laryngeal function, they are by their nature hyperfunctional. It is important, therefore, to prevent these hyperfunctional behaviors from becoming habituated. Thus, effort closure techniques should be used for the least possible amount of time and should always be combined with relaxation procedures (Spencer et al., 2003).

Although effort closure techniques are widely used as a clinical tool, very few efficacy studies have been published on these techniques. In one of the few studies, Yamaguchi et al. (1993) used pushing to treat clients with glottal incompetence. Pre- and posttreatment measures based on perceptual and acoustic analysis and stroboscopy supported the efficacy of the technique in some of the patients. However, the authors cautioned that other approaches may provide equally good or better results than pushing because complete glottal closure is not always necessary for normal voice. In addition, they noted that overcompensation could result in undesirable strain and trauma to the vocal folds, and pushing is inappropriate for individuals who have vocal fold hemorrhage or adequate closure of the posterior glottis.

Yawn-Sigh, Easy Onset, Chewing. Techniques that have been used extensively to reduce laryngeal hyperfunction and hard glottal attack include yawn-sigh, easy onset, and chewing. Individuals with vocal hyperfunction often demonstrate an elevated position of the larynx within the neck. This position tends to increase the adductory force of the vocal folds (Xu, Ikeda, & Komiyama, 1993). In the yawn-sigh technique the patient breathes in on a yawn and exhales gently on a sigh. Yawning widens the pharynx and lowers the larynx (Boone & McFarlane, 1993). The laryngeal lowering has been shown to continue through the initial part of the sigh (Xu et al., 1993). As the patient yawns and then sighs, he or she is encouraged to focus on the proprioceptive sensations of the more relaxed vocal tract posture. Phonation is gradually introduced and extended as the individual becomes more comfortable with the technique. The yawn and sigh are faded as the patient becomes able to monitor the vocal tract without these strategies. Patients can monitor the lowered laryngeal position manually. If the larynx is raised the individual again goes through the yawn-sigh maneuver to lower the larynx. For the patient with severe hyperfunction, the sighed voice may be his or her first attempt at producing, feeling, and hearing a relaxed voice (Xu et al., 1993). Phonation is introduced when the individual is able to consistently maintain the larynx in the lowered position, and extends systematically to longer utterances.

Easy onset utilizes a similar approach to the sigh portion of the yawn-sigh technique. The speaker allows a slight exhalation to occur prior to initiating phonation, preventing the vocal folds from adducting too forcefully. Some therapists ask the patient to insert the /h/ sound before the target utterance, which has the same effect of softening the glottal attack. As with the yawn-sigh, attention is focused on the differences in sensation between a more and less tense vocal tract posture. The chewing technique introduced by Froeschels in 1952 has long been a mainstay of therapy for reducing hyperfunctional phonation. Based on the assumption that the natural act of chewing is incompatible with a tense vocal tract the patient practices vocalizing while engaging in chewing motions. The chewing is gradually faded as the speaker becomes more adept at producing relaxed phonation.

While these techniques are commonly used, there are no studies investigating their effectiveness or efficiency in achieving the goal of less hyperfunctional phonation.

Establishing a New Pitch. Sometimes individuals with voice disorders use a conversational pitch level that is perceptually too low or too high. In the 1960s, 1970s, and 1980s, the concept of optimum pitch was endorsed by many clinicians, and pitch modification toward this theoretical optimum was commonly advocated and utilized. Optimum pitch was defined as the pitch range most suited to the individual's laryngeal mechanism, where phonation was produced with the least amount of muscular effort for the most amount of vocal output. Koufman and Blalock (1988) used pitch modification as a component of voice therapy for professional voice users with laryngeal musculoskeletal tension. Reportedly, most of the participants, both male and female, used a noticeably low pitch. Optimal pitch was determined by comparing the patient's speaking fundamental frequency (SFF) to the lowest note he or she could sustain. If the SFF was within 30 Hz of the lowest note, the speaking voice was judged to be too low. The optimal SFF was determined to lie between 10–50% of the individual's vocal range. Once the SFF was established, the patient used auditory and visual biofeedback to stabilize the new pitch level. In conjunction with progressive muscle relaxation, the authors reported that symptoms resolved in 71% of patients. Current thinking holds that pitch problems related to lesions on the vocal folds or to laryngeal tension should not be directly addressed, but treatment should rather be directed to the underlying problem. Once the underlying pathology is resolved, the patient's pitch level is likely to normalize (Thomas & Stemple, 2007). Results from a study by Roy and Hendarto (2005) support this position. The researchers used manual circumlaryngeal massage in 40 women with **functional dysphonia** (FD) and disordered pitch and reported that vocal improvement was accompanied by a change in SFF of one semitone or more for 80% of subjects. Roy and Hendarto (2005) argued that their results support the hypothesis that abnormal pitch in FD results from laryngeal muscle tension, and reducing the tension facilitates the pitch change. In cases where the pitch level is truly problematic, for instance, in individuals with **mutational falsetto** or male-to-female transsexual voice, direct pitch modification is the appropriate approach. Chapter 10 presents a detailed description of pitch modification techniques for these cases.

HOLISTIC APPROACHES

Holistic approaches focus on the coordination of respiration, phonation, and resonation in the production of voice. These approaches include the accent method (Smith & Thyme, 1976), confidential voice therapy (Colton, Casper, & Leonard, 2006), resonant voice therapy (Roy et al., 2003; Verdolini,1998), semioccluded vocal tract (Titze, 2006), and vocal function exercises (Stemple, 2005; Stemple, Lee, D'Amico, & Pickup, 1994).

Accent Method. The accent method was developed in Denmark and is popular in Europe for both voice and stuttering therapy. It is becoming increasingly utilized in the United States. The method integrates respiratory and phonatory function by focusing on abdominal breathing patterns to help patients produce a well-supported, easy voice with a relaxed throat, in conjunction with rhythmic movements of the whole body. The body movements are faded as therapy progresses (Table 5.4).

The program begins with the patient producing a voiceless fricative (e.g., /s/) using a rhythmic pattern (short/weak segment followed by an accentuated longer and stronger segment). The same pattern is then practiced using voiced fricatives and vowels. At the vowel level different rhythms are practiced, and the patient continues to maintain optimal breath support and a resonant quality (Kotby & Fex, 1998). Initially the vowels are produced in a breathy and soft quality to eliminate hyperfunction and hard glottal attacks. Good body posture is also targeted. During the exercises the patient engages in rhythmic arm and body movements that match the phonatory rhythms, following the therapist's model.

TABLE 5.4 **Stages of the Smith Accent Method**

Stage	Name	Activities
1	Rest breathing	Optimize inspiration for speech (hand on abdomen to feel outward movement with inhalation and inward movement with exhalation).
2	Abdomino-phonatory accents	Practice control of rhythm, strength, and speed of abdominal muscle contraction, going from a slow largo rhythm to a 4-beat andante rhythm and finally to a fast allegro rhythm. Exercises are practiced first with voiceless fricatives, and phonation is gradually introduced while maintaining optimal breathing patterns. Different rhythms are practiced as the clinician and client take turns with the exercises.
3	Stabilization	Client uses variable rhythms and stress patterns, loudness, and intonation contours to increase the flexibility and range of the voice using the three basic rhythms.
4	Transfer to connected speech	Client focuses on optimal phrase length, pause location, duration, and speech rate. This is practiced in normal conversational speech mode, a performance speech, or song, according to the patient's needs.

Source: Information from Khidr (2010).

Khidr (2003) used the accent method for 3 patients with unilateral vocal fold paralysis and evaluated the results using voice recordings, aerodynamic testing, stroboscopy, and the VHI. The author reported improved auditory perceptual and aerodynamic parameters, and a notable reduction in the size of the glottal gap with concomitant improvements in vocal fold vibratory characteristics. Additionally, patients rated their degree of voice handicap on the VHI as decreased after therapy. Older studies have also demonstrated positive results. For example, Kotby, El-Sady, Abou-Rass, and Hegazi (1991) evaluated the effects of the accent method on subjects with a variety of voice disorders using patient interviews, auditory-perceptual ratings, stroboscopic ratings, and aerodynamic measures. The authors reported improvements in almost 90% of subjects. Furthermore, stroboscopic examination revealed a reduction in nodule size in all subjects with nodules. Fex, Fex, Shiromoto, and Hirano (1994) similarly reported significant positive changes on acoustic and perceptual measures in subjects with functional voice disorders. Bassiouny (1998) conducted a well-controlled study in which subjects with voice disorders were randomly assigned to a vocal hygiene plus accent group or a vocal hygiene only group. The accent group demonstrated significantly greater gains on perceptual, acoustic, and stroboscopic parameters.

Resonant Voice Therapy. Resonant voice has been defined as a vocal quality that projects well, is easy to produce, and involves a sensation of vibration in the area of the face around the nose and mouth called the *mask* (Smith, Finnegan, & Karnell, 2005; Titze, 2001). Resonant voice is typically produced with extremely gentle onset of vibration, with the vocal folds just barely touching or barely separated during vibration. This phonatory posture allows for efficient conversion of exhaled air into voiced sound, resulting in vibrations that are distributed all over the head, neck, and thorax (Barrichelo-Lindstrom & Behlau, 2009; Chen, Hsiao, Hsiao, Chung, & Chiang, 2007). Resonant voice therapy (RVT) is a systematic program developed by Verdolini (1998) based on earlier work by Arthur Lessac to train actors. The goal of RVT is to achieve the strongest and clearest possible voice with the least effort and impact stress between the vocal folds (Chen et al., 2007). RVT targets both vocal hygiene and neuromuscular retraining of laryngeal function. Hygiene goals focus primarily on hydration and the management of reflux (Verdolini-Marston, Burke, Lessac, Glaze, & Caldwell, 1995). Therapy sessions begin with a series of stretching and breathing exercises, after which the patient practices the "basic training gesture." The basic training gesture involves gliding on the /m/ sound from a high to low pitch. The individual is instructed to focus the sound in the facial bones using abdominal breath support. Patients are encouraged to feel the sensation of resonance in the facial area during this maneuver, as well to continually be aware of and reduce any excessive muscular effort. Once the patient is able to achieve the basic training gesture, practice continues with different variations of rhythm, pitch, and loudness. As the individual becomes more comfortable with the desired laryngeal behavior, the new manner of vocal production is extended into voiceless sounds, phrases, reading, and conversation (Hirsch, 2006). The patient is provided with home exercises to reinforce the targets.

Resonant voice therapy has been demonstrated to be effective in reducing phonatory effort and enhancing voice quality. For example, Chen et al. (2007) implemented a program of RVT with teachers with voice disorders. The authors reported that, based on videostroboscopy, acoustic analysis, and the VHI, the program had positive effects on participants' voice quality, vocal fold vibration, vocal fold closure, speaking flexibility, phonatory effort, and functional communication. Hard glottal attacks were almost eliminated. The mucosal wave and amplitude of vocal fold vibration returned toward normal after therapy, and speaking F0 increased to normal levels for females. There was also an increased range of speaking F0 and increased maximum intensity. VHI scores improved, particularly on the physical scale. Roy et al. (2003) conducted a randomized clinical trial comparing the efficacy of voice amplification, resonant therapy, and respiratory muscle training in teachers with voice problems. Voice amplification and resonant therapy were shown to result in a significant decrease of voice handicap as indicated on the VHI, as well as significant reduction in voice disorder severity as perceived by the subjects.

Confidential Voice Therapy. A "confidential" voice is one that is produced softly, with a slightly breathy quality that prevents the vocal folds from colliding with excessive force. Most people understand intuitively how to produce a confidential voice, so it is easy to teach patients this technique and have them carry it over to conversation without much further training. This approach has been reported to reduce factors that can be damaging to the vocal folds, such as excessive muscular tension, high vocal fold collision forces, high intensity levels, and strained or tight breathing patterns (Thomas & Stemple, 2007). Patients are also instructed in appropriate vocal hygiene and are taught a resonant method of producing voice to be used once the confidential voice is discontinued.

Use of the confidential voice is helpful when a patient needs to talk but the vocal folds need to be used gently, for example, after a recent vocal fold injury or surgery. However, pitch and loudness flexibility are decreased in this type of phonation, so confidential voice therapy is usually used for only a few weeks following an acute injury. Very little literature support exists to document the efficacy of this type of therapy. However, in one, Verdolini-Marston et al. (1995) compared confidential voice therapy and resonant voice therapy in women with nodules. Both treatment approaches were beneficial in terms of phonatory effort, auditory-perceptual status of voice, and laryngeal appearance. The authors reported that compliance with the therapy program appeared to be more important than the type of therapy provided.

Semioccluded Vocal Tract. When the vocal tract is narrowed air pressure increases within the vocal tract above the vocal folds. The increased air pressure keeps the vocal folds slightly separated during phonation, which helps to reduce the force of vocal fold collision (Titze, 2006). Based on this principle, individuals with hyperfunctional voice disorders can be taught to produce normal vocal intensity with less mechanical trauma to tissues (Titze, 2006). Methods to semiocclude the vocal tract include lip trills, bilabial fricatives, raspberries, tongue trills, humming, and phonating into tubes or straws (Titze, 2006). The degree of resistance can be manipulated by narrowing or widening the vocal tract to various degrees. Titze (2006) suggested that the exercises be structured from most to least resistant. Thus the initial exercise is phonating through a highly resistant (small diameter) stirring straw, followed by a less resistant (larger diameter) drinking straw. Therapy could then progress to phonating labiodental voiced fricatives (/v/), followed by lip or tongue trills, nasal consonants, and the high vowels /u/ and /i/. These activities can be performed with nonspeech and then speech activities. Nonspeech exercises usually consist of repeated pitch glides, gradually increasing the frequency range until two octaves or more can be produced easily (Titze, 2006). Titze also suggested creating more variety by extending the pitch glides to the melody of a simple song, and then using the intonation and stress patterns of spoken sentences.

A variant of the semioccluded vocal tract technique was described by Simberg and Laine (2007). In this method the patient phonates a vowel-like sound into a tube that has one end in water. The resistance felt by the patient as he or she phonates is controlled by the depth of the tube in the water. When the exercise is done correctly, the patient usually feels distinct vibrations in the larynx, face, and sometimes even in the chest (Simberg & Laine, 2007). As with resonant voice training, clients are encouraged to feel the sensations in the face and mask area.

Vocal Function Exercises. The program of vocal function exercises (VFE) was developed by Stemple and his colleagues based on the earlier work of Briess (1957, 1959). The rationale of these exercises is that laryngeal muscles can be exercised like any other muscles of the body to increase their strength, endurance, and coordination. The approach is straightforward and easy, involving four specific exercises that are practiced twice each, two times per day. The exercises include maximum vowel prolongations and pitch glides (Table 5.5).

The patient is instructed to produce all phonations as softly as possible and with a forward focus in which vibrations are felt in the facial area. In order to maximally prolong a vowel, the vocal folds must close with the right amount of muscular force and must work in coordination with the respiratory muscles. Similar to RVT, the target laryngeal position calls for barely adducted vocal folds, which facilitates a clear and easy voice production (Verdolini, 1998). The rationale for practicing pitch glides is that high pitches exercise the cricothyroid muscles, and low pitches exercise the thyrovocalis muscles. By practicing pitch glides the strength, bulk, and endurance of these muscles should be increased. The exercises consist of four steps including warm-up, stretching, contraction, and adductory power exercises. The warm-up involves sustaining the vowel /i/ as long as possible at a comfortable frequency. Stretching involves the speaker gliding from the lowest to the highest note in his or her frequency range on the word 'knoll' (/o/ vowel). Contraction is similar to stretching, but involves the patient gliding on the /o/ vowel from the highest to the lowest note in the frequency range. The fourth step, adductory power exercises, requires the patient to sustain the musical notes C, D, E, F, and G

TABLE 5.5 Vocal Function Exercise Program

These 4 exercises are performed 2 times each, twice daily (morning and evening) for 6 weeks.

Exercise 1:	Warm-up exercise
	Sustain vowel /i/ as long as possible
	Women on musical note F above middle C
	Men on musical note F below middle C
	Extreme forward focus "almost but not quite nasal"
Goal: sustained /i/ equal to length of maximum sustained /s/	
Exercise 2:	Stretching exercise
	Glide upward from lowest to highest note on the word "knoll"
	May also use tongue or lip trills, or the word "whoop"
	Emphasis is on forward placement, open pharynx, sympathetic vibration on lips
Goal: no voice breaks during upward pitch glide	
Exercise 3:	Contracting exercise
	Glide downward from highest to lowest note on the word "knoll"
	Focus on half-yawn in the throat with the pharynx open
	May also use a lip trill, tongue trill, or the word "boom"
Goal: no voice breaks during downward pitch glide	
Exercise 4:	Low-impact adductory power exercise
	Sustain the musical notes (C-D-E-F-G) for as long as possible on the word "knoll" minus the "kn"
	Middle C for women, octave below middle C for men
	Focus on open pharynx and constricted vibrating lips
Goal: same as exercise 1 (i.e., as long as maximum sustained /s/ production).	

Important Principles of Vocal Function Exercises:

1. All exercises are produced as softly as possible, but the voice is engaged, not breathy. No hard glottal attack at initiation of phonation.
2. It is very important that the placement of the tone is forward (constricted, sympathetically vibrating lips) and pharynx is open (i.e., inverted megaphone shape).
3. Specific speech stimuli are selected to help achieve placement of the tone and pharyngeal opening (i.e., "knoll," "oll").
4. The tone should not be muscled at the larynx; rely on interaction between abdominal contraction and breath support.
5. Practice consistency is encouraged; the individual charts progress on a graph or voice record sheet and audiotapes are provided to guide practice sessions.

Source: From "An Evaluation of the Effects of Two Treatment Approaches for Teachers with Voice Disorders: A Prospective Randomized Clinical Trial," by N. Roy, S. D. Gray, M. Simon, H. Dove, K. Corbin-Lewis, and J. C. Stemple, 2001, *Journal of Speech, Language, and Hearing Research, 44*, p. 295. Copyright 2001 by the American Speech-Language-Hearing Association. Reprinted with permission.

(still using /o/) as long as possible. Females are instructed to use the middle C range, and males use the range one octave below. Exercises should be practiced twice each, as softly as possible but without breathiness, using easy onset of voice and keeping the tone focused frontally.

There is some support in the literature for the efficacy of vocal function exercises. For example, Roy et al. (2001) compared vocal hygiene and vocal function exercises in teachers with voice problems. Subjects in the VFE group demonstrated significantly greater symptom improvement and reported greater vocal clarity and ease of voice production than those receiving vocal hygiene alone. Other studies have demonstrated positive effects of VFE in healthy speakers, singers, and elderly individuals with dysphonia resulting from presbylaryngis (e.g., Sabol, Lee, & Stemple, 1995; Sauder, Roy, Tanner, Houtz, and Smith, 2010; Stemple et al., 1994).

Voice Therapy Boot Camp. Patel, Bless, and Thibeault (2010) developed a new approach to voice therapy, which they termed "voice therapy boot camp." The approach is designed to facilitate vocal behavior change using intensive short-term voice therapy and concentrated practice with a large number of clinicians (3–7). Therapy utilizes a variety of techniques and lasts from 1–4 days with 4–7 hours of therapy per day. According to the developers, this approach provides numerous options in which the variety and intensity of practice can be manipulated to meet the patient's needs to bring about change most efficiently and effectively. For example, if a patient has difficulty achieving the appropriate vocal training gesture used in VFE, he or she can take advantage of different strategies such as drilling the gesture multiple times, or increasing practice variability by working with different therapists until the target production is achieved. Goals such as reducing vocal hyperfunction can be targeted using a variety of approaches such as RVT, VFE, and so on. An advantage of this model is that clinicians are able to observe and work with patients over an entire day of vocalizing and are not limited to "snapshots" of voice obtained in a single session. Another advantage is that carryover practice can be incorporated into the sessions. The authors report that the approach is particularly beneficial for patients with long-term dysphonia (greater than one year); those who have recalcitrant dysphonia where voice therapy has not been successful and continues to be indicated; those who have reached a plateau with traditional voice therapy but have potential for further change; those who have upcoming vocal performances; those who have an inability to schedule weekly therapy sessions; and/or those who live at great distances from a voice center.

Patient Compliance

It has been known clinically for a long time that a patient's motivation for and compliance with behavioral voice therapies is a major factor in the successful outcome of such treatment. In fact, patient adherence to the treatment has been shown to play a greater role in voice rehabilitation than the specific therapy approach (Hapner, Portone-Maira, & Johns, 2009). Adherence was defined by Behrman (2006) as the extent to which a patient follows through with agreed upon or prescribed actions and does what the therapist expects him or her to do. This includes regular attendance in therapy sessions and consistent practice of the learned vocal behaviors (Behrman, 2006). Unfortunately, the rate of nonadherence to programs of behavioral change is high, and clinicians often complain of clients who miss appointments or who drop out of therapy (Portone, Johns, & Hapner, 2008). Dropout has been reported to range from 16% to 25% over 6-week sessions, with an additional 10% dropout rate at 12–14 weeks (Behrman, 2006). Van Leer and Connor (2009) cited a dropout rate of 18–65%.

Hapner et al. (2009) examined the records of 147 patients at two voice centers. The authors reported that only around one-third completed therapy and two-thirds dropped out. There was no significant difference between "completers" and "dropouts" on gender, age, race/ethnicity, otolaryngology diagnosis, severity of QOL handicap, and severity of dysphonia (Hapner et al., 2009). Portone et al. (2008) noted that 38% of patients who were referred by a physician for voice treatment did not adhere to the physician's recommendation. Of those who did, almost half did not return after the initial speech-language pathology evaluation. Reasons reported for dropout and/or nonattendance include, among others, insurance denials, resolution of the problem, distance to the clinic, loss of interest, negative effects of the treatment, and unrealistic therapy demands (Portone et al., 2008; Roy et al., 2003) (Table 5.6).

Smith, Kempster, and Sims (2009) reviewed the medical charts of 100 patients seen for voice care and assigned these to successful versus unsuccessful outcome groups in order to determine whether specific patient characteristics influenced therapy outcomes. Fifty-six percent of these patients attended therapy on a regular basis. Of this number, 21% made some improvement in their voice, and 73% achieved normal or near normal voice quality. Forty-four percent of patients for whom therapy was recommended did not attend. Based on their review, the authors concluded that patients with successful outcomes were younger, employed, in good health, had mild voice impairments at the start of therapy, and had lower scores on the VHI. Patients with less successful outcomes (including those who did not attend therapy) and/or who required more clinician support and guidance tended to be older, with lower employment rates, more health issues, more severe voice and laryngeal diagnoses, and higher VHI scores.

TABLE 5.6 Reported Reasons for No-Show and/or Noncompliance with Voice Therapy Recommendations

Clinician/Clinic-Related Factors	Patient-Related Factors
Lack of training/experience in voice	Lack of understanding of the role of voice therapy
Lack of clinician empathy	Difficulty in transportation
Lack of awareness of patient readiness for change	Difficulty arranging time off work
Lack of follow-up support	No insurance coverage
Lack of communication between physician and speech pathologist	Mobility issues
Inflexible scheduling	Lack of readiness for change
Lack of reminder calls	Employment status
Inconvenient clinic location	Voice/laryngeal diagnosis
	Severity of voice problem
	General health
	Age

Source: Information from Andrews & Schmidt (1995); Behrman (2005); Hapner et al. (2009); Harvey (1997); Portone et al. (2008); Roy et al. (2003); Sims, Smith, & Johnson (2007); Smith et al. (2009); Stemple (2000); Van Leer et al. (2008).

Behavioral voice therapy, like any other kind of program that requires behavioral and lifestyle changes (e.g., weight loss, smoking cessation, etc.) necessitates a readiness of the participant to change, as well as a commitment to carry out time-consuming therapy and homework sessions. Behavioral voice therapy also requires patients to self-monitor their laryngeal function and vocal output, and to resist reverting to habitual maladaptive vocal patterns and behaviors (Van Leer & Connor, 2009). A patient's level of compliance depends on the interplay between barriers to change and facilitators of change. Van Leer and Connor (2009) identified barriers as lack of motivation, forgetting to practice or self-monitor, fatigue or pain during exercises, and low self-efficacy (described in the following paragraphs). Facilitators include a high level of motivation, perceived improvement, and the ability to plan strategies to organize oneself and one's environment to create an optimal situation for change.

In an effort to determine specific barriers to and facilitators of voice therapy adherence, Van Leer and Connor (2009) interviewed patients undergoing voice therapy. Analysis of the interview transcripts revealed that patients found voice therapy to be difficult for a multitude of reasons. These included the attention and awareness required for change, difficulty finding time to practice, managing loud environments, finding the exercises silly, feeling unmotivated, forgetting to practice, feelings of embarrassment, and fear of ridicule by family members. Many patients noted that voice therapy tasks were difficult to understand and execute independently outside the clinic. Despite these obstacles, however, all participants perceived their vocal goals as very important and were therefore motivated to continue their participation in therapy. An important facilitator reported by Van Leer and Connor (2009) was patient-perceived clinician support. Specific clinician behaviors that participants noted as helpful included the use of a variety of analogies and strategies to demonstrate voice techniques; individualization of exercises to the needs and level of understanding of the patient; provision of specific feedback to reinforce the individual's accuracy in producing the target vocal behavior; and provision of explicit strategies to manage connected speech. The authors reported that overall, patients perceived vocal rehabilitation as an effective but demanding process that required difficult motor learning and active self regulation, and that was facilitated by a good match with the clinician. The authors concluded that adherence may be improved when the therapist and the client together identify barriers and facilitators and discuss ways of dealing with the barriers. This kind of collaborative problem-solving approach may be more useful than the traditional approach to adherence, which involves the therapist identifying for the client the behaviors that need to be changed and emphasizing the importance of these changes (Behrman, 2006).

MOTIVATIONAL INTERVIEWING

A systematic approach to increasing patient motivation and compliance is exemplified by a client-centered program called **Motivational Interviewing** (MI). This psychotherapeutic approach was developed by Rollnick and Miller (1995), who defined MI as "a directive, client-centered counseling style for eliciting behavior change by helping clients to explore and resolve ambivalence" (p. 326). As its name implies, the central theme of MI is to increase a client's motivation to engage in change. The approach has been widely used in programs for alcohol addiction, drug abuse, smoking cessation, weight loss, adherence to treatment and follow-up for asthma and diabetes, and increasing physical activity (Rubak, Sandbaek, Lauritzen, & Christensen, 2005). Rollnick and Miller (1995) identified the principles that characterize the approach (Table 5.7).

The central principle is that motivation to change is elicited from the client, not imposed from an outside source. Direct persuasion is not effective in resolving ambivalence,

TABLE 5.7 Principles and Strategies in Motivational Interviewing

Principles

1. Motivation to change comes from the patient.
2. It is the patient's responsibility to resolve his or her ambivalence about change.
3. Trying to persuade the individual to change is not effective.
4. The clinician maintains a quiet and nonconfrontational approach.
5. The therapist's focus is to help the client in the process of resolving his or her ambivalence.
6. Resistance to and/or denial of the need to change are not stable client traits but fluctuate depending on the client/clinician interaction.
7. The therapeutic relationship is a collaborative partnership.

Strategies to Facilitate Change

1. Understand the client's perspective by using reflective listening techniques.
2. Accept and affirm the individual's feelings and perceptions.
3. Help the individual to recognize the problem.
4. Monitor the client's readiness to change.
5. Avoid jumping ahead of the client in terms of his or her readiness to change.
6. Affirm the individual's freedom of choice and self-direction.

Sources: Information from Behrman (2006); Rollnick & Miller (1995).

so an individual who is ambivalent about change has the responsibility to articulate and resolve his or her own ambivalence. The style of interviewing is quiet and nonconfrontational, as the clinician helps the client to examine and resolve his or her ambivalence and resistance to change. It is emphasized that the individual's readiness to change fluctuates depending on the interaction between the client and clinician. Thus resistance and denial are not seen as client traits, but as feedback regarding therapist behavior. Finally, the therapeutic relationship is conceptualized as a dynamic partnership rather than expert/recipient roles. Through these principles MI aims to increase the patient's perception of the importance of change as well as to increase his or her confidence in bringing about such change (Treasure, 2004).

Specific clinician strategies to facilitate change include using reflective listening techniques to understand the client's frame of reference; accepting and affirming the individual's feelings and perceptions; helping the patient to recognize the problem; monitoring his or her readiness to change; avoiding "jumping ahead" of the client in terms of readiness; and affirming the individual's freedom of choice and self-direction (Rollnick & Miller, 1995). The MI approach has been shown to facilitate behavior change in approximately 80% of outcomes studies, compared to traditional advice giving (Rubak, Sandbaek, Lauritzen, & Christensen, 2005).

Behrman (2006) adapted MI as a viable means of increasing patient motivation to change their vocal behaviors in a program of voice therapy. Based on Rollnick and Miller's model, Behrman (2006) outlined four principles used to achieve the objectives of voice change.

These include expressing empathy for the patient's perspective, developing discrepancy, rolling with resistance, and supporting self-efficacy. Expressing empathy involves the therapist acknowledging the patient's ambivalence about changing vocal behaviors and letting the individual know that this is normal and expected. To develop discrepancy the therapist helps the client to become aware of differences between his or her current vocal behavior and future goals. Rolling with resistance involves the notion that resistance is a natural and anticipated reaction to change. Self-efficacy refers to an individual's belief in his or her ability to change a specific behavior. Self-efficacy is a vital component of behavioral change, because it influences the goals an individual chooses and the lengths to which he or she will go to achieve the goal (Van Leer, Hapner, & Connor, 2008). MI can help a patient to achieve self-efficacy by having him or her recognize and express his or her own reasons for the importance of changing, and by helping the person develop the confidence to do so (Treasure, 2004). A patient's confidence can be fostered by structuring therapy tasks that are likely to lead to success as well as by focusing on positive changes the individual has made in the past (Behrman, 2006; Van Leer et al., 2008).

TRANSTHEORETICAL MODEL OF BEHAVIOR CHANGE

MI is often conducted within the framework of the Transtheoretical Model of behavior change (TTM). This model, developed by Prochaska and Velicer (1997), addresses the issue of a patient's readiness to make behavioral changes. TTM has been applied across a variety of health behaviors including physical exercise, nutrition and diet, and HIV prevention (Van Leer et al., 2008). TTM identifies five stages of change, including precontemplation, contemplation, determination, action, and maintenance (Table 5.8).

In the first stage individuals are not seriously considering behavioral change. In the second stage individuals are ready to think about change, but they are ambivalent as they weigh the advantages and disadvantages of changing. At this stage patients in voice therapy are unlikely to have the motivation necessary to adhere to the therapy program (Van Leer et al., 2008). The determination stage sees a reduction in ambivalence as the patient becomes more committed to change. At this stage the individual is ready to set goals for voice therapy in collaboration with the clinician (Van Leer et al., 2008). The last two stages involve the patient actively working to modify vocal behaviors and to integrate target behaviors into everyday life. Although these stages are discussed in terms of a hierarchy, patients may move back and forth between stages and may even relapse, depending on their level of mastery of objectives (Van Leer et al., 2008). The clinician's role also changes depending on the patient's stage. At the initial stages the clinician may take more of a counseling or coaching role, while at later stages the focus is more on teaching the patient vocal techniques and strategies.

TABLE 5.8 Stages of the Transtheoretical Model of Behavior Change

Stage	Description
Precontemplation	No serious consideration of change
Contemplation	Ambivalence as to the advantages and disadvantages of change
Determination	Reduction in ambivalence and increasing commitment to change
Action	Implementation of behavioral changes
Maintenance	Habituating and integrating changes into everyday life

Treatment of Children

A large number of children have voice disorders, with estimates of prevalence ranging between 6–9% (Hooper, 2004). Between 45–80% of childhood dysphonias involve vocal nodules related to phonotraumatic behaviors such as yelling, screaming, play vocalizations of animals and cars, and so on. Connelly, Clement, and Kubba (2009) identified phonotrauma in 45% of children who presented to a tertiary care center with dysphonia. Of these, more than half had nodules. There appears to be a relationship between the age of the child and the type of voice disorder. In the Connelly et al. (2009) study, most of the children aged 2 years and older presented with phonotrauma, although other conditions were also seen including webs, cysts, congenital vocal fold paralysis, inflammatory conditions, and intubation trauma. Children aged younger than 2 years showed a wide range of pathologies including papilloma, cysts, webs, RLN injury, reflux, and intubation trauma. Voice problems in adolescence can include functional (conversion) aphonia and mutational falsetto (Hooper, 2004). Voice disorders in children, if left untreated, may persist for many years (Hooper, 2004).

Many children are seen in clinics and outpatient hospital settings. Some children are treated in a school setting. School services are regulated by the Individuals with Disabilities Education Act (IDEA) Amendments of 1997, which was further amended in 2004 to align with the No Child Left Behind Act. The amended act is now called Individuals with Disabilities Education Improvement Act (IDEIA). Under this act a child is eligible for services if the impairment adversely impacts educational performance. Ruddy and Sapienza (2004) identified many adverse effects of voice impairment on a child's educational performance (Table 5.9).

A child's eligibility for services is determined by a team that includes the child's parents, at least one regular education teacher (if the child participates in regular education), at least one special education teacher or provider, a representative of the school, the speech-language pathologist, and possibly an otolaryngologist (Ruddy & Sapienza, 2004). Children

TABLE 5.9 Potential Adverse Effects of Voice Impairment on a Child's Educational Performance

Difficulty being heard or communicating in educational environments inside or outside the classroom
Limited participation in public speaking activities
Fear of participating in oral reading activities
Limited participation in classroom discussions
Fear of conversing in interpersonal interactions
Limited participation in regular physical education routines due to compromised laryngeal structure and/or function
Limited participation in music education due to a compromised upper airway
Reluctance to participate in activities such as school plays, cheerleading, and debate
Negative attention from peers, teachers, and other school personnel

Source: Information from Ruddy and Sapienza (2004).

are eligible for services only if they satisfy criteria on standardized speech and language tests. Standardized criteria for dysphonia are not available, so it is difficult for a child with vocal problems to qualify for services. Thus, children who need voice therapy may not be eligible for treatment (Hooper, 2004). Some school districts have developed their own criteria to determine a child's eligibility for voice therapy. For example, the Oxford Public Schools in Massachusetts published Entry and Exit Criteria for School-Based Therapy Services on their website (http://special-services.osd.schoolfusion.us). This document, adopted by the district in August 2009, specifies criteria for voice disability and provides guidelines regarding adverse effects on educational performance and eligibility for services. Evidence of voice disability is evaluated based on voice measurement(s), attitude/self-perception measures, speech sample(s), structured observation, oral classroom participation, other curriculum/academic results, teacher report/interview, child report/interview, and parent report/interview. Adverse effect on educational performance is described in terms of the child's oral participation in class, oral reading, social/emotional adjustment/behavior, and reactions of the child him- or herself, peers, teachers, and parents. The child is considered to be eligible for voice services if he or she exhibits chronic or persistent impairment (at least 6 weeks' duration) in connected speech in phonation, resonance, or prosody, with accompanying adverse effect on educational performance.

The speech-language pathologist often serves as the team coordinator in providing a link between the physician and the parents, educating the team and other staff members about voice, and providing parents with resources available in their community as well as providing materials that parents can use at home (Ruddy & Sapienza, 2004). Providing materials and strategies for home use is particularly important in helping the child's parents to understand the need to change the home environment and to participate fully in facilitating the child's target vocal behaviors in the home setting (Middendorf, 2007).

The same direct and indirect approaches that are used in treating adults with voice disorders can be adapted for use with children. Some children are not aware of their voice problem, and therapy in these cases typically begins with strategies to help the child become aware of his or her vocal behaviors. Other children may be aware of and concerned about their voices (Connor et al., 2008; Verduyckt et al., 2010). In both cases the child can learn to identify phonotraumatic behaviors by identifying these in cartoon characters, TV characters, family members, and so on (Middendorf, 2007). Once the child is familiar with these behaviors, he or she can then identify similarities in his or her own vocal behaviors. The therapist can produce models of desirable versus undesirable vocal behaviors and voice qualities, and the child learns to distinguish between these. The therapist can then ask the child to produce similar qualities and help the child to focus proprioceptively and auditorily on differences in modes of production.

Treatment for children often includes a focus on pragmatic behaviors associated with voice, such as interrupting, turn taking, and appropriate loudness levels (Hooper, 2004). A program of vocal hygiene may be appropriate to identify and eliminate harmful vocal and lifestyle behaviors and to substitute more desirable behaviors. Patient education is targeted to the child and his or her caregivers regarding normal voice production as well as the child's structural and/or functional limitations for voice (Woodnorth, 2006). Some children and teens may benefit from counseling focusing on interpersonal relationships, academic concerns, and so on. Voice production can be addressed using the same techniques as those discussed for adults, such as the accent method, chant talk, confidential voice, chewing, resonant voice, vocal function exercises, and yawn-sigh. As noted in the section on patient compliance, these techniques may seem silly to children and their caregivers, and it is important to provide an environment where the child feels comfortable trying new things with his or her voice (Trani, Ghidini, Bergamini, & Presutti, 2007; Woodnorth, 2006).

Phonosurgery

Phonosurgery is the name given to a group of different types of surgical procedures that have as their aim the preservation or restoration of the patient's best possible voice. Phonosurgery differs from older concepts of laryngeal surgery, in which the primary concern was the removal of the disease, and the voice was of secondary importance. Phonosurgical techniques have been facilitated by two interrelated developments over the past several decades. One is the dramatic increase in knowledge about the complex structure and function of the vocal folds. This has been facilitated by technological advances such as the electron microscope, which enables finely detailed examination of structures at the cellular level. The increased understanding has led to the realization of the crucial importance of avoiding damage to the cover of the vocal folds and preservation of the mucosal wave. Hand-in-hand with this expanded knowledge, technological developments such as binocular microscopes that attach to the laryngoscope have greatly refined the surgical procedures. The binocular operating microscope permits detailed visualization of the laryngeal tissues, as well as the insertion of appropriate instruments (long-handled forceps, scalpels, and scissors) into the patient's pharynx and larynx. Other advances include better lasers, enhanced delivery systems, and multichannel flexible scopes, allowing many endolaryngeal phonosurgical procedures to shift from the operating room to the office (Zeitels, Blitzer, Hillman, & Anderson, 2007). Phonosurgical procedures include thyroplasty, arytenoid adduction, airway widening procedures, laser microsurgery, injection laryngoplasty, Botox injection, and laryngeal reinnervation.

THYROPLASTY

Thyroplasty refers to a group of surgical procedures designed to modify the position and tension of the vocal folds by altering the relationships between the thyroid and other laryngeal cartilages. As first described by Dr. Isshiki and his colleagues in 1974, there are four types of thyroplasties, numbered from I to IV. Type I involves medialization of the vocal folds, Type II lateralizes the folds, Type III relaxes the vocal folds, and Type IV stretches and tenses the vocal folds. For all four procedures, the surgeon accesses the vocal folds through a window cut into the thyroid cartilage. Type I is the most common. The surgery is performed typically for cases of glottal insufficiency resulting from unilateral vocal fold paralysis as well as from other conditions such as vocal fold bowing in elderly individuals (Linville, 2001; Postma, Blalock, & Koufman, 1998; Slavit, 1999). The other types of thyroplasties are not as common, although Type IV (cricoarytenoid approximation) is used in situations where a higher pitch is desired, such as transsexual voice treatment. Thyroplasty Type IV involves moving and suturing the thyroid and cricoid cartilages toward each other in order to achieve the stretching and tensing of the vocal folds that normally occur for a higher pitch (Zeitels, Hillman, Desloge, & Bunting, 1999).

Type I Thyroplasty. Type I thyroplasty is designed to medialize the paralyzed vocal fold by inserting a synthetic implant behind the fold. The surgeon cuts a small window into the thyroid cartilage and places the implant behind the immobile vocal fold (Figure 5.1). This has the effect of pushing the fold toward the midline, thus facilitating glottal closure during phonation. This procedure is useful for patients who have a large gap (greater than 3 mm) in the midportion of the vocal folds (Baylor, Yorkston, Eadie, Strand, & Duffy, 2006).

The surgery is usually done under local anesthetic, so that the patient is able to phonate during the procedure. By manipulating the degree of medialization different voice qualities

FIGURE 5.1 Medialization Thyroplasty

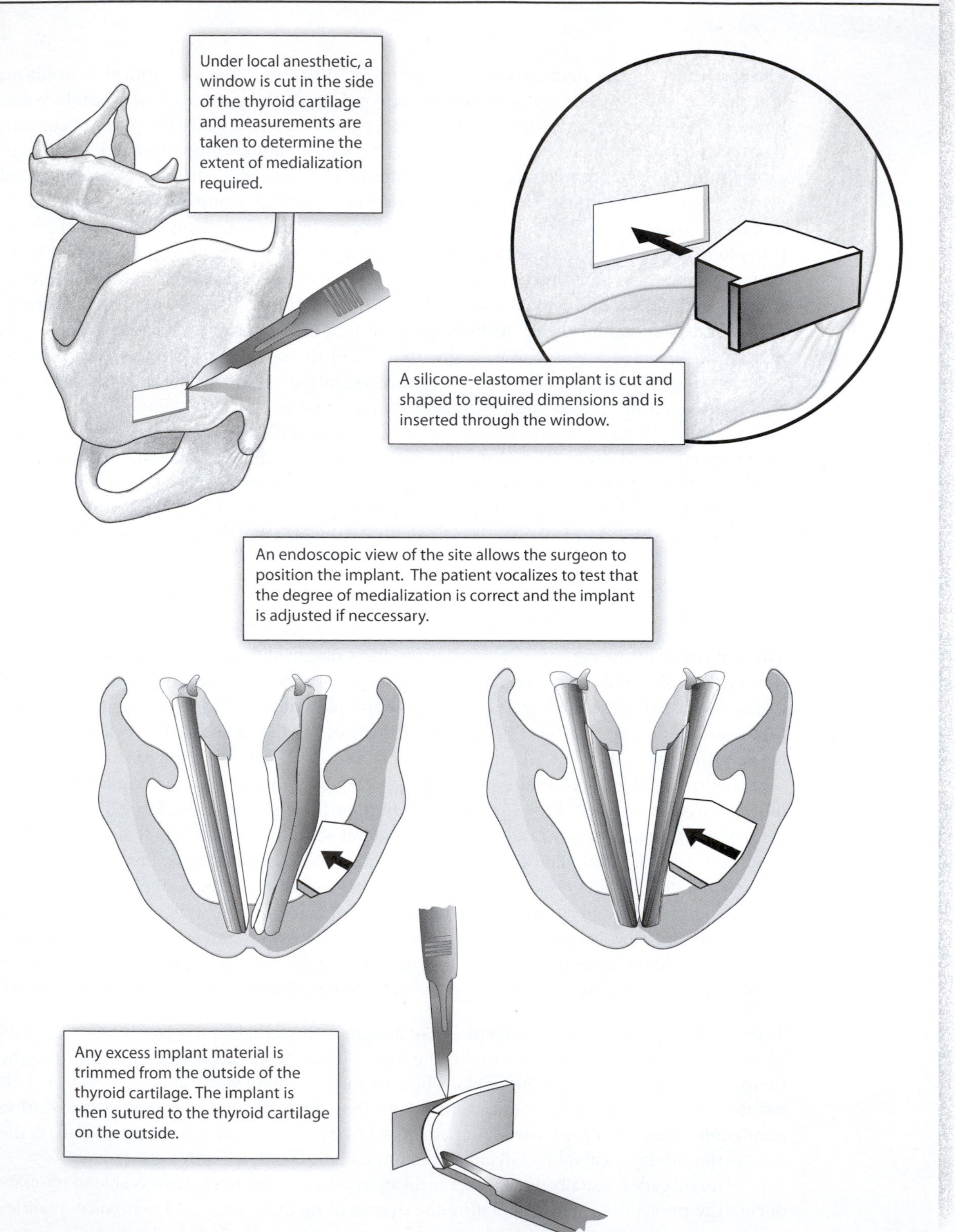

are obtained, and the speech-language pathologist and patient decide on the optimal voice quality. The implant is then sutured in place, and the larynx is closed (Blaugrund, Isshiki, & Taira, 1992).

Implant materials. Implant materials include Silastic, Gore-Tex, and titanium (Figure 5.2). Silastic has a soft, pliable consistency that is easy to mould into any required shape (Abrahams & Caceres, 1998). The disadvantage of Silastic is the necessity for the surgeon to position the implant, listen to the patient's voice, remove the implant, and make adjustments accordingly (Suehiro, Hirano, Kishimoto, Tanaka, & Ford, 2009). Because of the need to remove and reshape the implant, surgery time is increased, and the procedure is difficult to standardize (Witt et al., 2010). Gore-Tex implants have several advantages. The first is the flexibility of this material, which allows the degree of medialization to be distributed differentially along the length of the vocal fold (Buckmire, Bryson, & Patel, 2010; Selber, Sataloff, Spiegel, & Heman-Ackah, 2003). Another advantage is its ease of adjustment and high degree of biocompatibility (Suehiro et al., 2009). In contrast to a Silastic implant, adjustments to achieve the patient's best voice are done in vivo, rather than inserting and removing the implant (Suehiro et al., 2009). In addition, the procedure requires a shorter incision and takes considerably less time than using Silastic (Suehiro et al., 2009). Titanium is a recent addition to available implant materials. Reportedly, use of this implant significantly reduced the width of the glottal gap (Witt et al., 2010). Witt et al. (2010) reported that the use of a preformed titanium implant decreased operation time, resulting in reduced swelling and hematoma during and after surgery. Implant size and shape are standardized, but titanium is malleable and can be adapted to individual patients (Witt et al., 2010). Videostroboscopic, perceptual, and acoustic measures have shown significant improvements in voice quality and vocal efficiency with titanium medialization (Friedrich, 1999; Schneider, Denk, & Bigenzahn, 2003; 2003b).

Advantages and Disadvantages of Medialization Thyroplasty. The primary advantage of medialization thyroplasty is that the medial edges of the vocal folds that make contact during phonation are unaffected, facilitating smooth glottal closure and good voice quality. The procedure provides a great deal of flexibility because it is reversible, and revision or adjunctive procedures (including injection) can be performed if necessary. The technique may also be done in conjunction with other surgical procedures to enhance the patient's voice quality. Finally, thyroplasty can be performed under local anesthetic, so the patient is able to phonate during the process. This facilitates active participation with the speech-language pathologist and surgeon in the determination of the patient's optimal voice quality. In order for the patient

FIGURE 5.2 **Additional Types of Vocal Fold Medialization Implants**

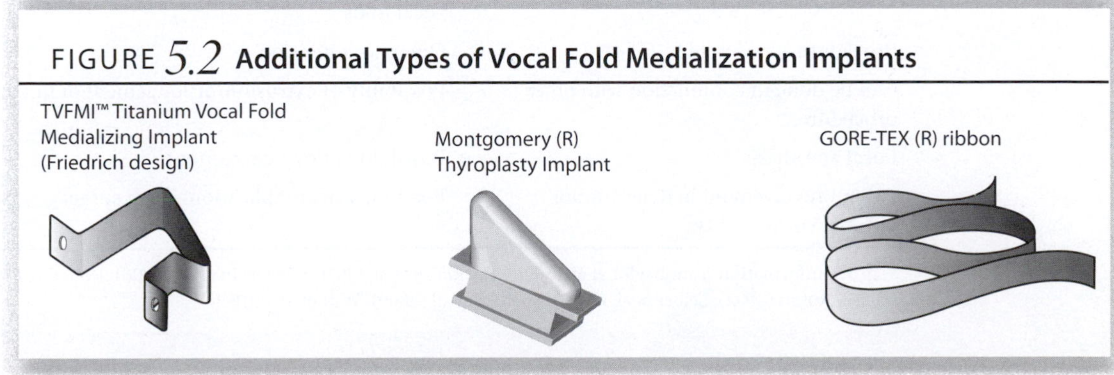

to achieve his or her best possible voice, the vocal fold must be positioned appropriately in three planes: medial-lateral, superior-inferior, and anterior-posterior (Rosen, 2002). Usually, the speech-language pathologist monitors both the position of the vocal folds and the patient's voice quality, using nasoendoscopy and auditory-perceptual techniques.

A disadvantage of medialization thyroplasty is that the surgery does not address differences in the vertical positions of the paralyzed and intact vocal folds. Additional disadvantages include inability of the procedure to close large posterior gaps; an open neck incision and possibility of wound infection; the possibility of improper positioning of the implant; extrusion or dislodgement of the implant material; insufficient amount of the implant material; possibility of overcorrection of the glottal defect; or complications from the implant itself (Dworkin, Shah, Stachler, & Meleca, 2006; Franco & Andrus, 2008; Rontal & Rontal, 2003) (Table 5.10).

Outcomes Studies. Despite the potential disadvantages, many outcomes studies have demonstrated the effectiveness of medialization thyroplasty. Sridhara et al. (2003) reported an increase in mean maximum **phonation time** (MPT) from 4.87 seconds preoperatively to 12.07 seconds postoperatively. This increase reflects improved laryngeal resistance and laryngeal valving. Franco and Andrus (2008) used a combination of arytenoid adduction and Gore-Tex medialization and reported increases in maximum phonation time and intensity and decreases in glottal airflow. Selber et al. (2003) also utilized Gore-Tex and evaluated patients using videostroboscopy, aerodynamic and acoustic analysis, perceptual evaluation (GRBAS), patient self-evaluation, and EMG where appropriate. The authors noted that patient satisfaction with voice improvement was high, and stroboscopic analysis indicated that vocal fold vibratory parameters improved after thyroplasty. Positive outcomes have been reported even when the thyroplasty has been performed many years after the initial recurrent laryngeal nerve injury (Billante, Clary, Sullivan, & Netterville, 2002).

TABLE 5.10 **Advantages and Disadvantages of Medialization Thyroplasty**

Advantages	Disadvantages
Vibratory edges of vocal folds unaffected	Not suitable for large posterior gaps
No inflammation	Does not address vertical level differences between vocal folds
Procedure is reversible	Open neck incision
Can be done in conjunction with other procedures	Possibility of extrusion/dislodgement of implant
Local anesthesia	Possibility of overcorrection
Patient involvement in determining optimal voice quality	Possibility of complications from surgery

Sources: Information from Baylor et al. (2006); Buckmire et al. (2010); Dworkin et al. (2006); Rontal & Rontal (2003); Rosen (2002); Selber et al. (2003); Suehiro et al. (2009); Witt et al. (2010).

There is some evidence that thyroplasty affects the neural control of phonation. Galgano et al. (2009) performed fMRI (an imaging technique that measures brain function) on a patient before and after Type I thyroplasty for unilateral vocal fold paralysis. They found correlations between improvements in voice function following surgery and changes in neural activations. The authors noted that acoustic and aerodynamic measurements associated with voice improvements after surgery positively correlated with changes in activations in many areas of the central nervous system (CNS), including frontal, temporal, and parietal cortices, the cerebellum, and the thalamus. This led these researchers to suggest that the central nervous system changes reflect an increasingly efficient way of producing voice, possibly due to the ability of the CNS to process new sensory information that results from regained function after surgery.

ARYTENOID ADDUCTION/ARYTENOPEXY

Sometimes medialization thyroplasty by itself is not enough to produce an optimal voice quality for a patient with unilateral vocal fold paralysis. If the paralyzed fold is shorter than the intact fold, or if the affected arytenoid cartilage is rotated outward, then effective vocal fold closure cannot be achieved, even with medialization (Linville, 2001). **Arytenoid adduction** involves suturing the muscular process of the arytenoid of the affected fold to another point in the larynx. The tension of the suture is adjusted to stretch and medialize the fold (Rammage et al., 2001). The vocal process is rotated medially, thus allowing a closer approximation of the posterior portion of the vocal folds (Figure 5.3). This procedure allows the vocal folds to be adjusted in different planes to create the best possible voice for the patient. This technique is also helpful in closing posterior glottal gaps (Baylor et al., 2006).

It is important for the surgeon to avoid overrotation of the affected vocal process, which can result in less than optimal vocal fold position and negatively affect voice quality. The adduction arytenopexy avoids the possibility of overrotation by positioning the arytenoid on the medial aspect of the cricoid articular facet in a way that is closer to its normal adduction during phonation (Zeitels, Hochman, & Hillman, 1998). Thus, the normal synergistic action of the vocal fold adductors and abductor muscles is facilitated. Zeitels et al. (1998) reported that the adduction arytenopexy procedure resulted in greater lengthening of the affected vocal fold, higher vocal fold positioning, and a more normally contoured arytenoid, compared to the classic procedure.

AIRWAY WIDENING PROCEDURES

Airway widening procedures include total **arytenoidectomy**, medial arytenoidectomy, and transverse cordotomy (Figures 5.4, 5.5). These procedures are used in situations requiring increased glottal opening to prevent airway compromise. Although the term *total arytenoidectomy* implies the complete removal of the arytenoid cartilage, in some "total arytenoidectomy" surgeries only a portion of the cartilage is removed (Rosen & Simpson, 2008). The procedure is done under general anesthetic using a **CO_2 laser** (e.g., Aubry et al., 2010). Once the arytenoid cartilage (or portion thereof) is removed, the posterior portion of the vocal fold is sutured in an appropriate position. This results in a widening of the posterior glottis. **Medial arytenoidectomy** creates a concavity along the glottic edge of the body of the arytenoid cartilage, which increases the size of the airway by 1–2 mm (Bosley, Rosen, Simpson, McMullin, & Gartner-Schmidt, 2005). This procedure preserves more of the laryngeal structure in comparison to the total arytenoidectomy (Buckmire, 2006). The advantage of medial arytenoidectomy is that it allows the membranous (anterior) portion of the vocal folds to adduct for phonation, while widening the posterior third of the glottis for breathing.

FIGURE 5.3 **Arytenoid Adduction**

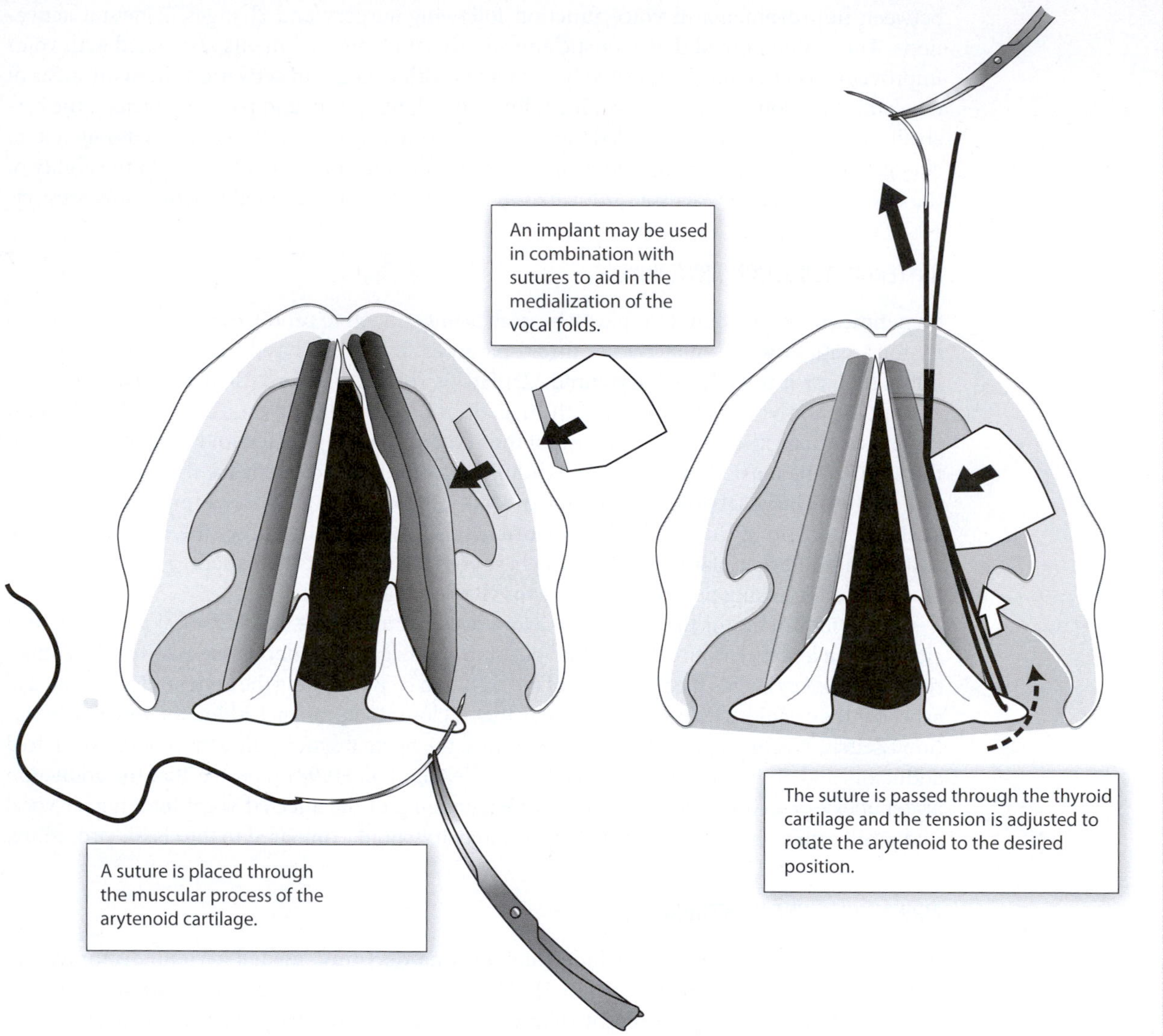

Transverse cordotomy involves using a laser to create a transverse cut in the membranous vocal fold immediately anterior to the vocal process. This results in a wedge-shaped opening in the posterior glottis while maintaining the ability of the vocal folds to make contact along their anterior portion (Lagier, Nicollas, Sanjuan, Benoit, & Triglia, 2009). Advantages of this procedure are that the magnitude of the posterior glottic enlargement does not depend on arytenoid position and mobility; the procedure is technically easy; and there is minimal

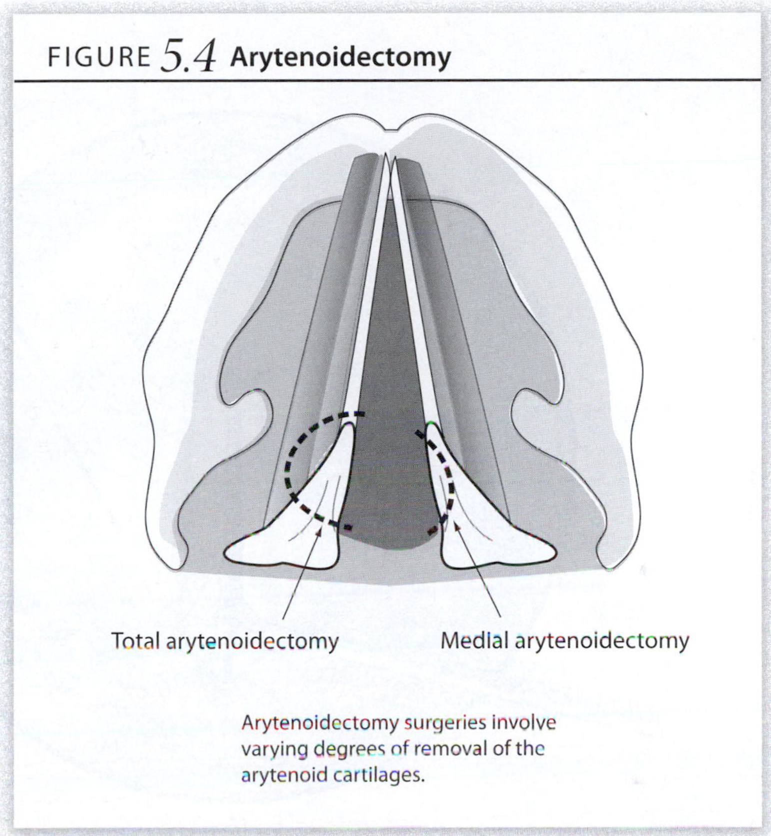

FIGURE 5.4 Arytenoidectomy

Arytenoidectomy surgeries involve varying degrees of removal of the arytenoid cartilages.

tissue destruction (Buckmire, 2006). In addition, the procedure can be unilateral or bilateral (Bajaj et al., 2009), and it can be done in conjunction with other procedures. Furthermore, if the surgery is not effective, it is possible to perform a second operation either on the same or opposite side. Other advantages of transverse cordotomy are that the procedure is short, thus reducing the time of anesthesia; easy to perform; minimally invasive; and can be used even if the patient later recovers vocal fold function spontaneously (Lagier et al., 2009). A potential complication of all the airway enlarging procedures is postoperative aspiration. In addition, while these surgeries are designed to preserve the patient's ability to phonate, vocal quality may be affected depending on the extent of tissue alteration and/or destruction.

Outcomes Studies. Several outcomes studies suggest that airway widening surgeries are very successful in reducing airway symptoms and maintaining the patient's functional voice (Bosley et al., 2005). Worley, Bajaj, Cavalli, and Hartley (2007) performed surgery to improve the airway in children with bilateral vocal fold paralysis. The authors removed the vocal process of one arytenoid and a small part of the anterior body of the arytenoid, while leaving the anterior two-thirds of the vocal fold undisturbed. All six children rated both the airway and their voices as better, and four of the children who had been tracheotomized were successfully decannulated. Hans, Vaissiere, Crevier-Buchman, Laccourreye, and Brasnu (2000) reported outcomes of patients with bilateral vocal fold paralysis who were treated with CO_2

FIGURE 5.5 **Transverse Cordotomy**

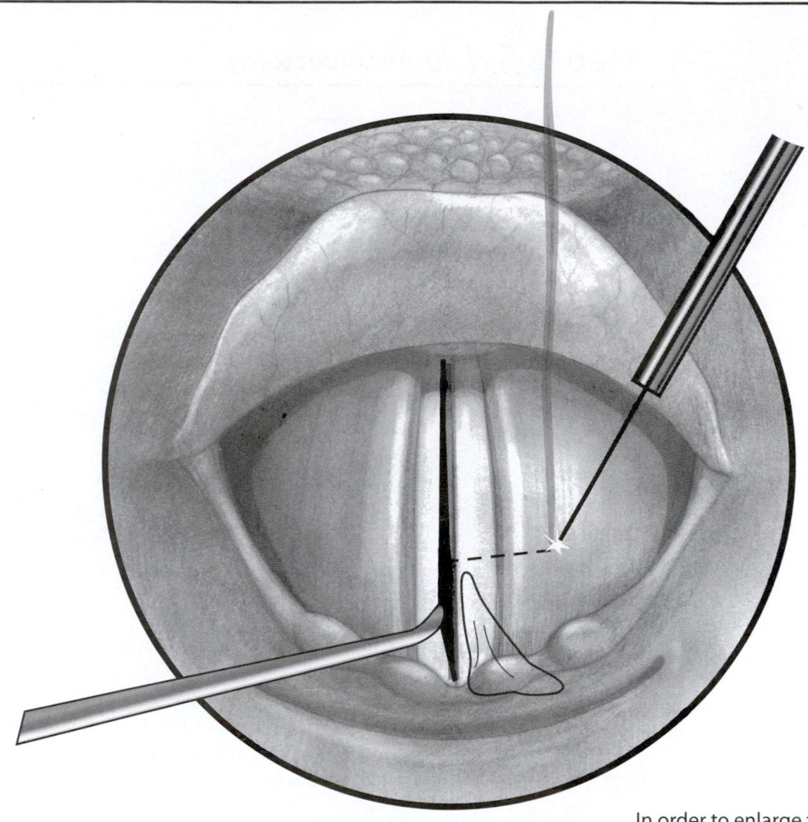

In order to enlarge the glottic airway, a laser is used to cut through both the true and false vocal folds just anterior to the arytenoid cartilage.

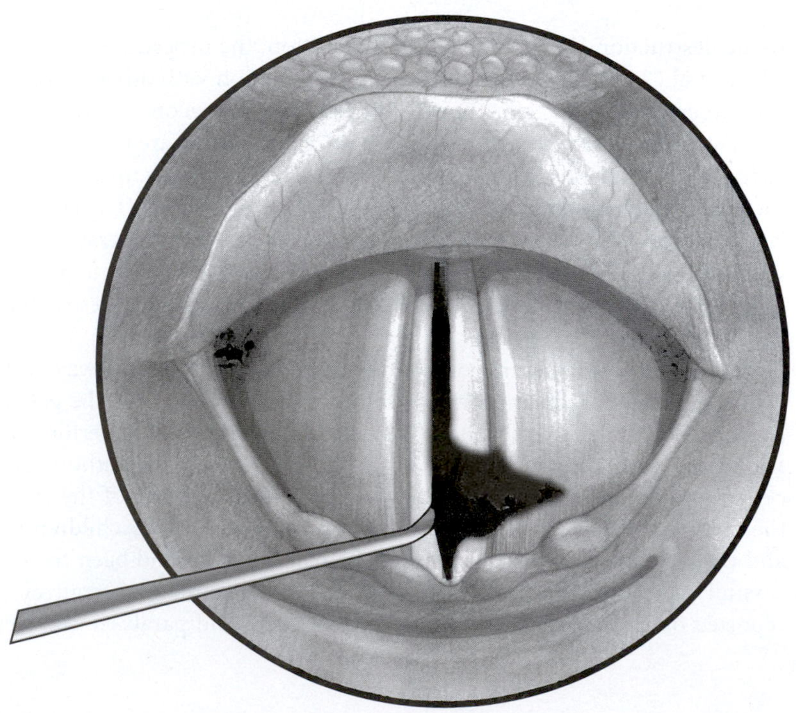

laser posterior transverse cordotomy. The airway was improved and was stable 2 years postoperatively. Acoustic and aerodynamic parameters improved 6 months postoperatively and continued to improve to the 2-year mark. Olthoff, Zeiss, Laskawi, Kruse, and Steiner (2005) treated patients with bilateral vocal fold paralysis with bilateral posterior cordectomy. Outcome measures included assessment of dyspnea and voice quality. They reported excellent results in terms of improved respiratory function. Voice quality was mildly dysphonic in terms of hoarseness, roughness, and breathiness, but was reported to nonetheless be excellent. Segas, Stavroulakis, Manolopoulos, Yiotakis, and Adamopoulos (2001) performed partial posterior cordectomy on 20 patients with bilateral vocal fold paralysis. Eighteen of the 20 patients achieved good to excellent results, while two patients continued to require tracheotomy with a speaking valve.

LASER MICROSURGERY

Lasers are used to treat pathologies such as stenoses, **recurrent respiratory papillomatosis, leukoplakia**, nodules, malignant laryngeal disease, Reinke's edema, and granulomas (Yan et al., 2010). The development of laser technology has benefited laryngeal surgery immensely by reducing bleeding and avoiding swelling and scarring of tissue during and after surgery. The laser is used in conjunction with an operating microscope, which allows detailed inspection of laryngeal structures, and very precise and delicate removal of lesions and diseased tissue. There are two major types of lasers: photoangiolytic lasers such as the 585 nm pulsed-dye laser (PDL) and CO_2 lasers. Photoangiolytic lasers obliterate blood vessels, while CO_2 lasers are primarily used for cutting and/or ablating tissue (Halum & Moberly, 2010; Yan et al., 2010). CO_2 lasers have been the most commonly used in laryngeal surgery for many years, but angiolytic lasers are becoming increasingly popular (e.g., Zeitels et al., 2009). CO_2 laser surgeries are typically performed in the operating room under general anesthesia. Recently, however, a flexible CO_2 laser has been developed, allowing some procedures to move from the operating room to the surgeon's office (Halum & Moberly, 2010; Yan et al., 2010). Halum and Moberly (2010) used both types of lasers on patients with various lesions in a nonsedated manner in the office. All patients tolerated both types of laser treatment without difficulty.

Angiolytic lasers are useful in treating lesions that have aberrant and/or excessive microvasculature, such as recurrent respiratory papillomatosis, ectasia, varices, and hemorrhagic polyps (Mouadeb & Belafsky, 2007; Zeitels et al., 2009). Angiolytic lasers can be used in an office setting because the energy is delivered though thin glass fibers, which can easily be transmitted through the port of a flexible nasoendoscope (Halum & Moberly, 2010). Angiolytic lasers such as the PDL target blood vessels and have been shown to spare the vocal fold epithelium (Mouadeb & Belafsky, 2007).

The use of office-based laser surgery has many advantages. First, it avoids the risks inherent in general anesthesia (Koufman et al., 2007; Zeitels et al., 2009). Second, office-based procedures are less expensive, because they do not have the costs associated with the preoperative evaluation and procedural intervention (Koufman et al., 2007; Zeitels et al., 2009). Because of the reduced morbidity associated with local anesthesia, it is easier to treat older patients, particularly those with cardiovascular and pulmonary disease, while there is less disruption to younger working individuals (Koufman et al., 2007; Mouadeb & Belafsky, 2007; Zeitels et al., 2009). Office-based procedures are particularly beneficial for patients who require multiple surgeries such as those to treat recurrent respiratory papillomatosis (Koufman et al., 2007). However, office based treatment can require multiple staged procedures, which is not appropriate for lesions that are typically resolved with one operation, such as nodules or cysts (Zeitels et al., 2009).

Koufman et al. (2007) performed 443 procedures using lasers with different wavelengths. Following treatment, there were no cases of airway obstruction, web formation, vocal fold scarring, or granuloma formation. Four hundred six **pulsed dye laser** (angiolytic) procedures were performed for RRP, glottal **dysplasia**/leukoplakia, and granuloma. Fifteen percent of the patients required subsequent operating room–based surgery after initial PDL treatments, usually because the disease was too bulky for office-based treatment.

Advantages and Disadvantages of Laser Surgery. Advantages of laser surgery include decreased costs, decreased complications and morbidity, precision of lesion removal, and minimal bleeding (Yan et al., 2010). The advantages of PDL include its excellent safety record; its effectiveness; ability to be used as an office-based procedure, low risk of web formation at the anterior commissure, low risk of scar formation, and possibility for earlier intervention because of its ease of use and safety (Mouadeb & Belafsky, 2007). There are, however, some disadvantages to the CO_2 laser. Laser heat can increase scarring and cause damage to adjacent tissue. There is potential for endotracheal explosion, facial burns, mucosal burns, vocal fold webs, fibrosis of the superficial layer of the lamina propria, stenoses, and glottal incompetence (Yan et al., 2010; Zeitels et al., 2009). Therefore, CO_2 laser use is not suitable for treating lesions of the membranous vocal folds (Zeitels et al., 2009). Further, it is not possible to treat nodules, polyps, and cysts with CO_2 laser because the epithelium would be vaporized (Zeitels et al., 2009). CO_2 lasers are best used for epithelial lesions and/or whenever preservation of the superficial lamina propria is either not necessary (i.e., most supraglottic lesions) or when it is impossible (already lost from disease or prior surgery) (Zeitels et al., 2009).

INJECTION LARYNGOPLASTY/VOCAL FOLD AUGMENTATION

A treatment approach that has been in use for many years for glottal incompetence resulting from unilateral paralysis and other vocal fold conditions is the injection of a substance such as gelfoam paste, fat, collagen, or synthetic compounds into the affected fold. Injection laryngoplasty is typically used for three reasons: as a permanent solution for glottic insufficiency; as a temporary method when recovery of the recurrent laryngeal nerve is possible; or in the treatment of vocal fold scar (Carroll & Rosen, 2009; Rosen & Simpson, 2008). The rationale for use in glottic insufficiency is that the injected material (injectate) increases the bulk of the fold, thereby decreasing the width of the glottal gap and facilitating improved glottal closure. The increased approximation results in a stronger and less breathy voice quality. The substance is injected either via the mouth (transoral) or through the skin (transcutaneous). Transoral injections may be done using a laryngeal mirror or a direct laryngoscope. Transcutaneous injections are inserted through the cricothyroid membrane. The procedure is done under local anesthetic with specially designed needles (Figure 5.6).

Materials used for injection. Many different substances have been used for injection, and new injectibles continue to be developed as researchers look for materials that have similar viscoelastic properties to the vocal folds. Each type of injectate is associated with advantages and disadvantages (Table 5.11). Some materials are designed to be temporary, while others are designed to be long-lasting or permanent. The ideal material should be biologically inert to avoid tissue reactions, available "off the shelf," contain no risk of infectious disease transmission, be a good match with the host tissue, and be able to be delivered with a fine-gauge needle (Carroll & Rosen, 2009).

FIGURE 5.6 **Vocal Fold Injection**

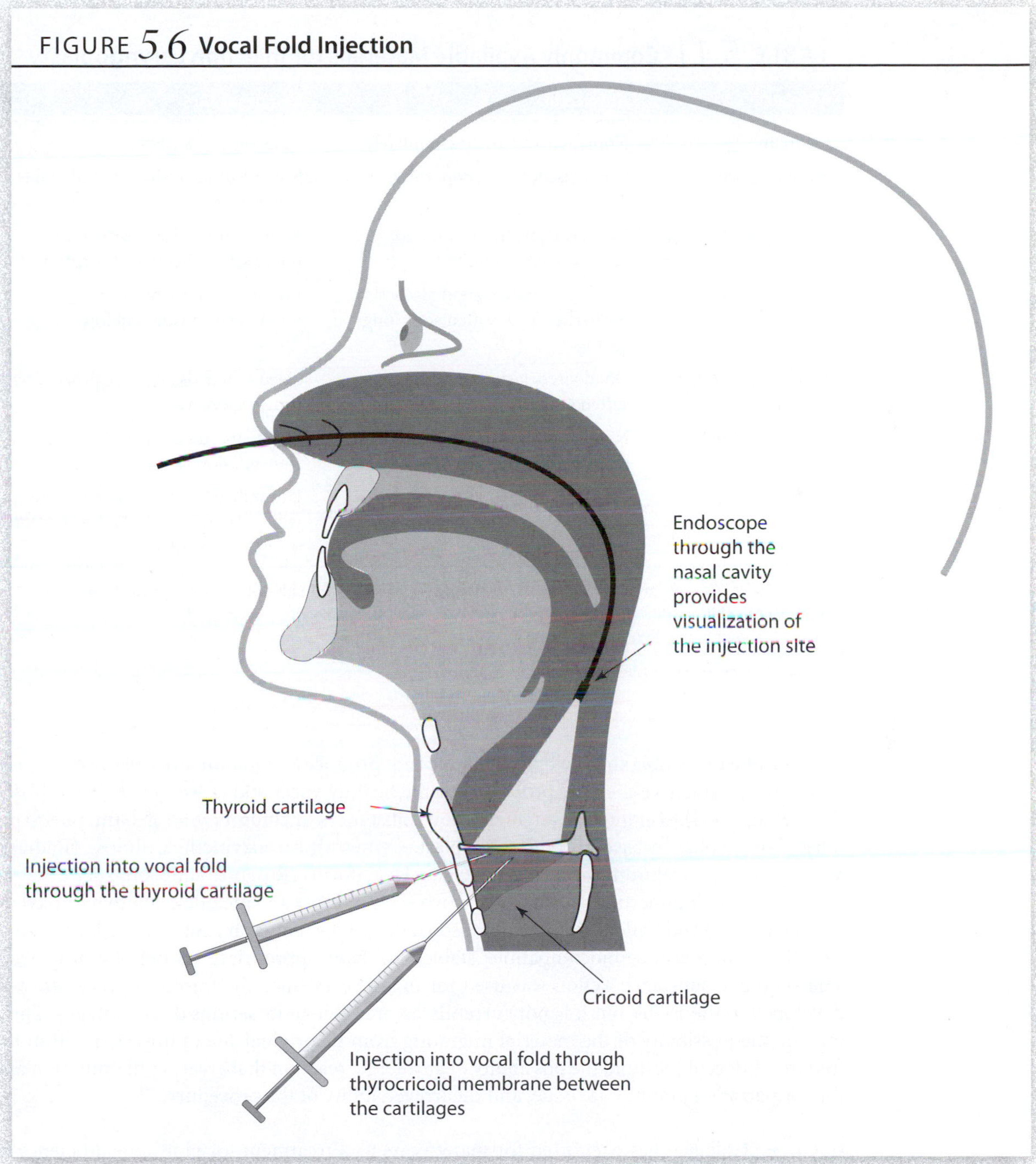

Temporary substances are used when there is a possibility that the paralyzed vocal fold may regain function, or used on a trial basis to determine the likely outcome of a more permanent material (Kwon, Rosen, & Gartner-Schmidt, 2005). Effects typically last from 2–6 months (Rosen & Simpson, 2008). Temporary material should completely dissolve in the vocal

TABLE 5.11 Commonly Available Materials for Injection Laryngoplasty

Material	Advantages	Disadvantages
Gelfoam	Nonreactive, resorbs completely	Lasts only 6–8 weeks
Autologous fat	Good viscoelastic properties	Second surgical site, unpredictable absorption
Autologous fascia	No hypersensitivity, does not require overinjection	Second surgical site, difficult to inject, unpredictable absorption
Bovine collagen	Readily available, good viscoelastic properties, may soften scar, long lasting	Hypersensitivity reactions, need for skin test 4 weeks before using
Human autologous collagen	Good viscoelastic properties, may soften scar	Need donor tissue, long processing time, expensive
Human dermal collagen	No hypersensitivity, good visco-elastic properties, may soften scar	Expensive, theoretical disease transmission risk
Teflon	Permanent	Unpredictable immune reactions with granuloma, implant migration, not recommended

Source: From "Complications of Collagen Injection of the Vocal Fold: Report of Several Unusual Cases and Review of the Literature," by T. D. Anderson and R. T. Sataloff, *Journal of Voice, 18*, p. 395. Copyright 2004 by the Voice Foundation. Reprinted with permission.

folds, be biocompatible and biologically stable (not produce an inflammatory tissue response), and possess similar viscoelastic properties to the healthy vocal fold (Kwon et al., 2005; Rosen & Thekdi, 2004). Temporary augmentation substances include bovine gelatin (Gelfoam, Surgifoam), collagen-based products (Zyplast, Cymetra), carboxymethylcellulose (Radiesse Voice Gel), and hyaluronic acid gel (Restylane, Hyalaform) (Rosen & Simpson, 2008).

Effects of long-lasting substances last two years or more and include calcium hydroxylapatite (Radiesse) and Teflon (Rosen & Simpson, 2008). Like temporary substances, long-lasting varieties should also be biocompatible, stable, and have appropriate viscoelastic properties. The synthetic substance Teflon was used for many years since the injection procedure was developed in the 1970s, but it is not currently favored due to its serious disadvantages. These include the possibility of the material migrating from its original site of injection within the fold to a different location, the possibility of an allergic reaction that creates inflammation and the formation of granuloma tissue, and the irreversibility of the procedure.

Collagen. Collagen has been used for many years as a treatment for glottic insufficiency as well as for vocal fold scar. Collagen can soften stiff scar tissue and thus restore the pliability of the vocal fold cover (Dailey & Ford, 2006; Linville, 2001; Stemple et al., 2000). The advantages of collagen are that it is readily available and can last for several months up to years. Collagen is also advantageous because it is gradually colonized by vocal fold fibroblasts and new blood vessels. This facilitates the synthesis of new proteins and the remodeling process of the extracellular matrix (Kimura, Nito, Imagawa, Tayama, & Chan, 2008). Collagen is similar in its cellular structure to vocal fold tissues, which increases its compatibility to the host tissue. This in turn decreases the risk of an allergic response and **granulation** formation.

Both autologous human collagen and bovine collagen have been used. Autologous collagen is harvested from the patient and thus has the advantage of not causing an immune system reaction. The disadvantages are that considerable preparation is necessary to harvest the substance, the procedure has risks because the collagen is injected under general anesthetic, and more side effects are expected (Luu, Tsai, Mangunta, Berke, & Chhetri, 2007). The most popular current material is cross-linked bovine or human collagen. Cross-links are bonds that link chains of proteins to one another and thereby change the properties of the resulting material. The substance used for cross-linking of the collagen is glutaraldehyde, which is an agent that reacts with proteins to produce a less soluble material. This is important because collagen that has not been cross-linked is absorbed rather quickly into the host tissue.

Current forms of injectable collagen include Zyplast, Cymetra, and Dermologen. Zyplast is a bovine dermal collagen that is highly purified and cross-linked with glutaraldehyde. With this substance the vocal folds are typically overinjected because some absorption of the material will occur. This type of collagen has been shown to be more stable, have a longer duration, and provide more predictable results than noncross-linked collagen. Luu et al. (2007) reviewed medical records of patients from 1997 to 2006 and reported that 83% of Zyplast injections were successful in improving dysphonia associated with glottic insufficiency. Other researchers have reported adverse effects with cross-linked bovine collagen, such as stiffness of the mucosal layers, which interferes with the mucosal wave (Remacle, Lawson, Keghian, & Jamart, 1999). In addition, some people may be hypersensitive to bovine collagen, with reported reactions ranging from erythema and itching of the injection or test site to massive induration (soft tissues becoming extremely firm but not as hard as bone) and erythema of both the test and injection site (Anderson & Sataloff, 2004). Another concern is the development of autoimmune collagen vascular diseases. According to Anderson and Sataloff, approximately 30% of patients who are exposed to bovine collagen develop anti–bovine collagen antibody reactions.

Zyplast has been used since the 1980s. Cymetra and Dermologen are newer products that use banked human collagen (not autologous), elastin, and proteoglycans (Anderson & Sataloff, 2004). Welham, Rousseau, Ford, and Bless (2003) used Dermologen in the treatment of a patient with **sulcus vocalis** in conjunction with excision of the sulcus. Measures of phonation threshold pressure and F0 showed progressive improvement over a 6-month period.

Hyaluronic Acid. A high level of hyaluronic acid (HA) in tissues is associated with less scarring because HA suppresses collagen synthesis from fibroblasts (Finck et al., 2009; Hirano, Bless, Massey, Hartig, & Ford, 2003). Thus increasing HA levels can lessen scar formation. However, pure HA has a short half-life, so investigators have tried many ways of increasing the duration and quantity of HA available in injured tissue. One way is by cross-linking the HA with other chemicals. Hylaform is a cross-linked HA gel that has been shown to be available for a longer time in vocal fold tissue (Hansen & Thibeault, 2006). However, while cross-linking is beneficial in increasing HA duration, the possibility also exists of undesirable changes such as increased **viscosity** of the resulting material (Rousseau et al., 2006). Another version of cross-linked HA is Restylane, which was the first version of HA to be approved by the FDA (in December 2003) (Perazzo, Duprat, & Lancellotti, 2008). The advantages of this preparation are that it is biocompatible, easy to store, and not too expensive.

Researchers have tried to stimulate the production of HA by combining the substance with different agents. HA is broken down in the body by an enzyme called hyaluronidase. Echinacoside is an antihyaluronidase that prevents the breakdown of HA. Rousseau, Sohn,

Montequin, Tateya, and Bless (2004) used echinacoside to increase HA levels in an animal model. They reported that injured vocal folds treated with echinacoside had levels of HA that were similar to uninjured controls. Further, the treated vocal folds had less accumulation of collagen compared with untreated vocal folds.

Several investigators have examined the effects of hepatocyte growth factor (HGF) on increasing levels of HA. HGF has been shown to stimulate HA production and to reduce collagen production, and may promote appropriate lamina propria viscosity and improved mucosal wave (Hirano et al., 2003; Krishna Rosen, Branski, Wells, & Hebda, 2006). Branski et al. (2006) reported that HGF treatment in a rabbit model decreased vocal fold stiffness, improved mucosal wave propagation, and also improved phonation threshold pressure, vocal efficiency, and glottal closure. Krishna et al. (2006) used both HGF and decorin to increase the amount of HA in vocal fold fibroblasts. They noted that HGF alone and decorin alone did not have a major impact on collagen synthesis, but the combination of HGF and decorin did decrease the concentration of collagen compared with control skin and vocal fold fibroblasts.

Another biomaterial that is based on HA is called Extracel-LG. This is a synthetic form of extracellular matrix that links a network of a chemically modified derivative of hyaluronan with a type of gelatin (Thibeault & Duflo, 2008). The advantage of this substance is that it has viscoelastic properties similar to those of human vocal fold extracellular matrix, which can help to restore the biomechanical properties of the vocal fold layers.

Autologous Fat. Autologous fat (fat that is harvested from the patient's own body) has been advocated as an excellent option because of its low viscosity, which is similar to that of the intermediate layer of the lamina propria (Schweinfurth & Ossoff, 2006). Canine studies have shown that vocal folds injected with autologous fat demonstrate improved vibratory activity, with resulting lower PTPs, increased sound intensity, and increased glottal efficiency (Neuenschwander et al., 2001). Advantages of autologous fat include reduced invasiveness compared with thyroplasty, reduced inflammation, less granulation tissue formation, and good physiological performance with favorable viscoelastic properties (Umeno, Chitose, Sato, & Nakashima, 2009). Reportedly, fat provides comparable acoustic results to medialization thyroplasty for up to two years (Hartl, Hans, Crevier-Buchman, Vaissiere, & Brasnu, 2009). A disadvantage of fat is that the procedure involves harvesting the fat from the patient's abdomen through liposuction or an open incision, which requires general anesthesia (Andrews et al., 2008; Hartl et al., 2009; Rosen, 2002). Further, it is not possible to determine the quantity of fat to inject, and some investigators report overinjecting fat to compensate for the absorption (Hartl et al., 2009; Umeno et al., 2009). Other disadvantages include the necessity for repeated injections due to rapid fat resorption, and the possibility of inconsistent voice quality because of limited control over vocal fold positioning (Kieff & Zeitels, 1996).

Results of fat injection for vocal fold scar and sulcus vocalis have demonstrated good results. Neuenschwander et al. (2001) did a retrospective review of 8 patients who received autologous fat implantation for vocal fold scar. The authors created "pockets" in various locations of the scar and inserted the fat into these pockets. This technique allows the low viscosity characteristics of fat to restore the normal cover-body relationship of the vocal folds. The patients demonstrated significant improvements in glottal closure, mucosal wave, and vocal fold stiffness, and the resulting vocal quality was also improved. Zhang, Sprecher, Wei, and Jiang (2010) used autologous fat to fill in the sulcus defect in 12 patients. Laryngoscopy after 6 months showed improved glottal closure and vocal fold morphology, as well as increased maximum phonation times for all patients.

Autologous Cellular Therapy. An evolving technique called **autologous cellular therapy (ACT)** has promise in the treatment of vocal fold scars. ACT is based on taking cells from an individual, expanding those cells in the laboratory, and then injecting them back into the same individual to repair defects (Chhetri et al., 2004). There are many advantages to this technique. First, obtaining and culturing fibroblasts by biopsying the laryngeal mucosa is an easy procedure. Second, injection of autologous fibroblasts replenishes the lamina propria layer, resulting in the return of the mucosal wave. Third, the injected fibroblasts do not migrate, but tend to remain more or less within the injection site. Fourth, to date no adverse effects have been reported (Chhetri et al., 2004). Chhetri et al. reported that histologic data of treated scars in an animal model showed that normal lamina propria components were present after replacement therapy, and the lamina propria was able to provide adequate viscoelasticity to the scarred vocal fold. They suggested that this kind of treatment may be superior to fat injections because ECM components are continuously replenished by the injected fibroblasts, thus bypassing the resorption problem inherent in fat injection.

Calcium Hydroxylapatite. A long-lasting substance that has been used recently is **calcium hydroxylapatite (CaHA)**. CaHA is a compound of phosphate and calcium, which are found in teeth and bone, making this material extremely compatible with the vocal fold tissues. The substance is inert and biologically stable, does not create an inflammatory response, and has been found to remain intact at the injection site up to five years after the procedure (Rosen & Thekdi, 2004). CaHA has been used under the trade names Radiesse and Bioform. In this form the CaHA is mixed with a gel. Once it has been injected the gel is absorbed and the vocal fold tissues replace the gel. This creates a stable and long-lasting augmentation (Hughes & Morrison, 2005). Dursun, Boynukalin, Ozgursoy, and Coruh (2008) used CaHA and reported significant differences in patients' levels of hoarseness, roughness, and breathiness pre- and postsurgery for sulcus vocalis. They noted that CaHA produced better and more long-lasting perceptual results in severity, roughness, and breathiness than fat injection.

Outcomes Studies. Numerous outcomes studies have demonstrated the beneficial effect of injection laryngoplasty using a variety of injectates. For example, Kwon, Rosen, and Gartner-Schmidt (2005) used CaHA in a gel carrier with patients who demonstrated glottal insufficiency resulting from paralysis, paresis, scar, and atrophy. Eight of 10 patients had very good voice quality after injection, and stroboscopy revealed normal mucosal vibration at each follow-up visit. Effects lasted approximately 2–3 months depending on the volume of the injection. Bergamini et al. (2010) evaluated patients before surgery, a day or two after the injection procedure, after 3 months, and then every 6 months. Outcome measures included acoustic voice analysis as well as perceptual evaluation using the GRBAS scale. Patients demonstrated an improvement in breath support for speech and a greater pitch range. The authors reported that the average MPT before injection was 6.8 seconds, the postoperative value was 11.1 seconds, and further improvement to 12.8 seconds was seen during follow-up. Preoperatively the mean pitch range was 10 semitones, which increased to 19 semitones after surgery, and 20 semitones on follow-up. Videolaryngoscopy after the injection showed that all but one patient obtained medialization with good glottic closure, resulting in normalization of vibration and the mucosal wave. Rosen and Thekdi (2004) evaluated patients in terms of mean flow rate of expelled air during phonation. They reported that the mean volume of air expelled while speaking was cut nearly in half after injection. Stroboscopic examination showed improved vocal fold vibration due to improved vocal fold closure patterns. In addition, patients reported positive changes in their emotional, physical, and functional lives as assessed by the VHI. Hertegard et al. (2004)

examined treatment outcomes using videostroboscopy, acoustic analyses, and maximum phonation time. While 75% of the patients demonstrated significant improvements, approximately 25% required either an additional injection or thyroplasty due to unsatisfactory voice quality. Umeno et al. (2005) reported significant improvement in most of their patients immediately following injection, and the improvements were maintained over a 2-year follow-up period. Karpenko, Dworkin, Meleca, and Stachler (2003) reported improvements in MPT, glottal competency, and voice quality in their patients who received injection laryngoplasty. Kimura et al. (2010) used high-speed digital imaging to assess the results of collagen injection in patients with unilateral vocal fold paralysis and hoarseness, breathiness, restricted pitch range, reduced loudness range, and vocal fatigue. High-speed digital imaging showed significantly improved vocal function following injection, with vocal fold vibratory patterns becoming more symmetrical.

BOTOX INJECTION

Injection of Botox into the vocal folds is used for patients with spasmodic dysphonia. Botox is the medical form of a toxin related to botulism. As a disease botulism is often fatal, because it is a toxin that paralyzes muscles. However, when used medically, the toxin reduces muscle spasms, and it has been used extensively and successfully to treat focal dystonias such as **blepharospasm, oromandibular dystonia**, and **spasmodic torticollis** (Case, 2002). The substance prevents the transmission or release of acetylcholine at the myoneural junction, essentially creating a flaccid paralysis or paresis. The human dosage is approximately 2.5 Us. A "U" is a so-called mouse unit, based on the amount of toxin that can kill 50% of injected mice. The lethal dosage for humans is probably around 3,500 times that needed to cause paralysis and death in mice (Case, 2002). For the first week or two after the injection the patient's voice may be weak and breathy, and he or she may have some slight difficulty in swallowing. Thereafter the voice stabilizes, and the individual is able to talk with much less effort and strain. The positive effects last between two to four months, and the person's voice starts to revert to the pre-injection level. Most patients are re-injected every few months. Many clinicians have reported that behavioral voice therapy in conjunction with Botox lengthens the time between injections.

For the adductor form of spasmodic dysphonia the Botox is usually injected through the cricothyroid membrane into the thyrovocalis muscle, under local anesthetic. For the **abductor** version the drug is injected into the posterior cricoarytenoid muscle.

LARYNGEAL REINNERVATION

Medialization techniques position the affected fold closer to the midline. However, the fold may atrophy and become increasingly flaccid. Laryngeal reinnervation techniques can be beneficial in preventing atrophy of the affected fold. Laryngeal reinnervation (LR) refers to any method that attempts to reestablish neural pathways to the vocal fold. This includes nerve-muscle pedicle, muscle-nerve-muscle pedicle, and donor nerve-recurrent laryngeal nerve anastomosis (Lorenz et al., 2008). The nerve supply to the healthy transplanted pedicle is transferred to the paralyzed muscle, providing an alternate source of innervation. A nerve that is often used in LR is the **ansa cervicalis**. This is a loop of nerves in the neck, attached to the hypoglossal nerve and to the first two to three cervical spinal nerves. Branches of the ansa cervicalis innervate the **infrahyoid muscles**. The ansa cervicalis has several characteristics that make it ideal as a donor nerve, including its closeness to the larynx and its similarity in size and diameter to the RLN (Lorenz et al., 2008). The ansa cervicalis-RLN **anastomosis** technique involves surgically connecting (anastomosis) the ansa cervicalis to the RLN.

Other donors aside from nerves may be used to reinnervate the damaged laryngeal nerve. Debnath, Rich, and Paniello (2008) used muscle-nerve-muscle (MNM) neurotization. In this procedure a nerve **graft** is placed between a healthy donor muscle on one end to a target denervated muscle on the other end. The rationale is that nerve axons will grow or regenerate into this nerve conduit. With this technique, the intact CT muscle (innervated by the SLN) can be used as the donor and connected through the nerve graft to the impaired RLN without sacrificing function of the CT muscle.

Outcomes of LR have reportedly been very good. Lorenz et al. (2008) reported improved glottic closure with resulting decreased severity of dysphonia, roughness, breathiness, and strain. Smith, Roy, and Stoddard (2008) reported an increase in MPT from 6.5 seconds to 13.2 seconds in adolescents and young adults with severe dysphonia. In addition, voice quality ratings improved, pitch range expanded, and the speakers' self-assessment ratings improved by around 50%.

LR procedures can be used in conjunction with other medialization techniques. In fact, Tucker (1999) noted that combining nerve-pedicle reinnervation with surgical medialization would appear to meet most of the short- and long-term needs of patients with unilateral paralysis.

chapter SUMMARY

BEHAVIORAL VOICE TECHNIQUES are classified as indirect or direct. Indirect techniques are designed to help the patient to understand relevant aspects of voice production, and to encourage modifications of surroundings and lifestyle in order to facilitate healthy voice production and improved vocal performance. Therapy focuses on managing the contributing and maintaining aspects of the voice problem, and typically involves vocal hygiene, voice rest, vocal fold hydration, relaxation techniques, and patient education. Direct techniques are designed to modify unhealthy methods of voice production and laryngeal pathophysiology by focusing on specific ways to increase vocal efficiency and improve voice quality. Patients are taught specific laryngeal movements aimed at reducing the disordered pattern of phonation. Direct approaches include those designed to promote less forceful vocal fold function in cases of hyperfunction and those aimed at increasing the force of vocal fold adduction in cases of hypofunction. Increasing respiratory support and facilitating respiratory-phonatory coordination is often targeted in direct approaches. Many direct intervention models are holistic in nature and focus on facilitating the appropriate balance between the speech subsystems of respiration, phonation, and resonance.

A patient's motivation for and compliance with behavioral voice therapies is a major factor in the successful outcome of such treatment. High rates of drop-out and noncompliance have been reported. Behavioral voice therapy necessitates a readiness of the participant to change, as well as a commitment to carry out time-consuming therapy and homework sessions. A patient's level of compliance depends on the interplay between barriers to change and facilitators of change. An approach called Motivational Interviewing has been widely used in behavioral programs for alcohol addiction, drug abuse, smoking cessation, weight loss, and others. This approach has been modified for voice therapy and is often conducted within the framework of the Transtheoretical Model of behavior change, which addresses the issue of a patient's readiness to make behavioral changes.

A large number of children have voice disorders, with estimates of prevalence ranging between 6–9%. A large percentage of childhood dysphonias involve vocal nodules related to phonotraumatic behaviors such as yelling, screaming, play vocalizations of animals and cars, and so on. Many children are seen in clinics and outpatient hospital settings. Some children are treated in a school setting. School services are regulated by the Individuals with Disabilities Education Act (IDEA) Amendments of 1997, which was further amended in 2004 to align with the No Child Left Behind Act. The amended act is now called Individuals with Disabilities Education Improvement Act (IDEIA). Under this act a child is eligible for services if the impairment adversely impacts educational performance. The same direct and indirect approaches that are used in treating adults with voice disorders can be adapted for use with children. Treatment for children often includes a focus on pragmatic behaviors associated with voice, such as interrupting, turn taking, and appropriate loudness levels.

Phonosurgery is the name given to a group of different types of surgical procedures that have as their aim the preservation or restoration of the patient's best possible voice. Phonosurgical procedures include thyroplasty, arytenoid adduction, airway widening procedures, laser microsurgery, injection laryngoplasty, Botox injection, and laryngeal reinnervation. Thyroplasties are a group of surgical procedures designed to modify the position and tension of the vocal folds by altering the relationships between the thyroid and other laryngeal cartilages. Airway widening procedures are used in situations requiring increased glottal opening to prevent airway compromise. Lasers are used to treat pathologies such as stenoses, recurrent respiratory papillomatosis, leukoplakia, nodules, malignant laryngeal disease, Reinke's edema, and granulomas. Glottal incompetence is often treated by injecting a substance such as gelfoam paste, fat, collagen, or synthetic compounds into the affected fold.

review QUESTIONS

1. Explain the differences between, and rationales for, direct and indirect behavioral voice therapy techniques.
2. What is the rationale for maintaining adequate hydration of the vocal folds?
3. Discuss the advantages and disadvantages in implementing a vocal hygiene program.
4. Describe the two major laryngeal massage techniques. Do you think one is better than the other? Why or why not?
5. Explain why biofeedback is effective in changing motor behaviors related to voice and speech production.
6. Discuss the role of respiratory support in the production of voice.
7. Which of the holistic behavioral therapy approaches do you like the most? Which the least? Why?
8. What might be some difficulties encountered by a speech-language professional in using motivational interviewing?
9. If you had a client with unilateral vocal fold paralysis, would you feel comfortable describing and recommending available surgical procedures? Why or why not?
10. Compare and contrast the use of angiolytic versus $C0_2$ lasers for various vocal fold pathologies.

Appendix 1: The Use of Voice Therapy in the Treatment of Dysphonia

The overall goal for the patients with dysphonia is optimal long-term voice quality and communication function with minimal recurrence. Diagnosis and treatment should be both efficient and effective. Voice therapy is an integral component of intervention and contributes to both its efficacy and efficiency. Evidence from clinical trials documents the efficacy of voice therapy for a spectrum of voice disorders in both adults and children. Even in patients with a long history of dysphonia, voice therapy can be highly effective. Efficiency includes cost effective and prompt intervention provided over a time period most suitable for achieving optimal outcome.

Voice therapy is the treatment of choice for muscle tension dysphonia and there is evidence to support its utility in these cases. In complex disorders, such as paradoxical vocal fold motion, voice therapy prevents long-term costs of treatment by helping reduce expensive emergency room visits and hospitalizations.

Benign vocal fold lesions are a common cause of dysphonia. Most laryngologists consider voice therapy, often together with medical management, the initial treatment of choice for benign lesions. Many studies have documented excellent outcomes after voice therapy in patients with a variety of benign lesions. Increasingly, otolaryngologists are using response to voice therapy to help differentiate among benign mucosal lesions, inform the treatment decision for surgery, and optimize surgical outcome. In cases in which surgery is necessary, pre- and postoperative voice therapy may shorten the postoperative recovery time, allowing faster return to work and limiting scar tissue and permanent dysphonia.

Most laryngologists consider voice therapy essential for patients with unilateral vocal fold paralysis as definitive treatment or as adjunctive to surgery. Evidence suggests that preoperative voice therapy improves voice outcomes for greater than 50% of patients with unilateral vocal fold paralysis and may render surgery unnecessary. In other neurological-based dysphonia, such as Parkinson's disease, voice therapy has yielded significant improvements in overall communication.

In conclusion, research data and expert clinical experience support the use of voice therapy in the management of patients with acute and chronic voice disorders. Voice therapy contributes to increased effectiveness and efficiency in the treatment of voice disorders. When surgery is necessary, adjuvant voice therapy can improve surgical outcomes, prevent additional injury, and limit additional treatment costs.

Source: American Speech-Language-Hearing Association. (2005). *The Use of Voice Therapy in the Treatment of Dysphonia* [Technical Report]. Available from www.asha.org/policy.

Chapter 6
Inflammatory Conditions of the Larynx

LEARNING OBJECTIVES

1. Understand the inflammatory process and potential effects of inflammation on laryngeal health and vocal function.
2. Identify components of wound healing and scar remodeling.
3. Become familiar with symptoms and signs of vocal fold scar and sulcus vocalis.
4. Appreciate the roles of voice therapy and surgical management in the treatment of sulcus vocalis and scar.
5. Discuss the relationship between laryngopharyngeal reflux and laryngitis.
6. Describe diagnostic and treatment techniques in the management of laryngopharyngeal reflux (LPR).
7. Recognize laryngeal signs and symptoms of autoimmune inflammatory diseases such as systematic lupus erythematous, relapsing polychondritis, and rheumatoid arthritis.
8. Appreciate the need for differential diagnosis and treatment of cricoarytenoid joint fixation and vocal fold paralysis.

Inflammation is a regulatory process in which cellular and chemical reactions occur in blood vessels and connective tissues in response to injury and defense against harmful stimuli (Scheff, Calvano, Lowry, & Androulakis, 2010; Vodovotz et al., 2009). **Laryngitis** is an umbrella term for any inflammation of the larynx from any cause. Because various forms of laryngitis and laryngeal inflammatory conditions are extremely common, it is important for speech-language pathologists to have a thorough understanding of the inflammatory process and potential effects on laryngeal health and vocal function. This chapter begins with a discussion of wound healing and the inflammatory process, followed by an explanation of how vocal fold scarring may result from laryngeal inflammation. The relationship between sulcus vocalis, an indentation of the mucosal cover of the vocal fold, and scar is described. Information regarding treatment for vocal fold scars and sulcus vocalis is presented. Discussion then turns to acute and chronic forms of laryngitis, including laryngopharyngeal reflux (LPR), inflammation resulting from the backflow of stomach acid and pepsin into the laryngopharyngeal area. The close relationship between behavioral and medical management of LPR is emphasized. Other inflammatory laryngeal conditions that are discussed include those resulting from autoimmune diseases such as systemic lupus erythematosus, relapsing polychondritis, and rheumatoid arthritis.

Wound Healing

Wound healing refers to the repair of a tissue that has been injured or damaged through infection, trauma, neoplasms, or illness. Wound healing is a complex physiological mechanism encompassing three major stages: inflammation, extracellular matrix (ECM) cell proliferation, and scar remodeling.

INFLAMMATION

Inflammation is the response of the immune system to injury. The inflammatory process begins when the blood vessels in and around the wound constrict (vasoconstriction) in order to stop the bleeding (Figure 6.1). Shortly thereafter the vessels dilate, allowing plasma to leak into the tissue, with resulting edema and swelling (Branski, Verdolini, Sandulache, Rosen, & Hebda, 2006; Thibeault & Gray, 2004). The inflamed tissues are **erythematous** (red) and may feel warm and tender to the touch (Dworkin, 2008). During this phase **macrophages** (a type of white blood cell that ingests foreign material) and other cells help to clean the wound by destroying and removing dead and damaged tissue and bacteria. Also during this phase chemical agents such as cytokines and other inflammatory mediators are released. **Cytokines** are small protein molecules that regulate the inflammatory process by facilitating communication between different types of cells and by influencing cell behavior and interactions (Lim, Tateya, Tateya, Munoz-del-Rio, & Bless, 2006; Thibeault & Duflo, 2008; Welham, Lim, Tateya, & Bless, 2008). Cytokines function to summon immune cells to the wound site, initiate the migration of cells to close the wound, and signal the beginning of extracellular matrix synthesis (Welham et al., 2008).

EXTRACELLULAR MATRIX PROLIFERATION

The extracellular matrix (ECM) proliferation phase involves the migration of epithelial cells and fibroblasts from surrounding undamaged areas into the damaged tissue in order to repair the epithelium and ECM (Branski et al., 2006; Thibeault & Gray, 2004). Fibroblasts are connective tissue cells that produce fibrous and interstitial proteins such as collagen, hyaluronic acid (HA), fibronectin (FN), and decorin. These proteins have specific functions in the wound healing process. For example, collagen is produced in order to fill in the tissue defect. FN promotes migration of fibroblasts into the wound (Hirano et al., 2008). Decorin helps to regulate the formation and organization of collagen fibers. Too high or too low levels of these proteins can have a negative impact on the wound healing process. For example, increased levels of FN can result in excessive inflammatory cell and fibroblast migration to the wound, while decreased levels of decorin may result in the formation of disorganized networks of collagen (Hansen & Thibeault, 2006).

In addition to fibrous and interstitial proteins, the fibroblasts produce granulation tissue. This is a specialized tissue that contains many myofibroblasts. **Myofibroblasts** are cells

FIGURE 6.1 Wound Healing

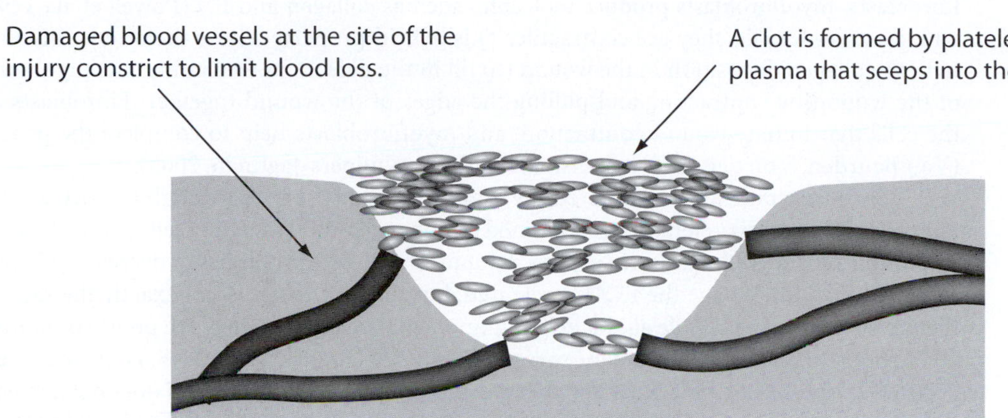

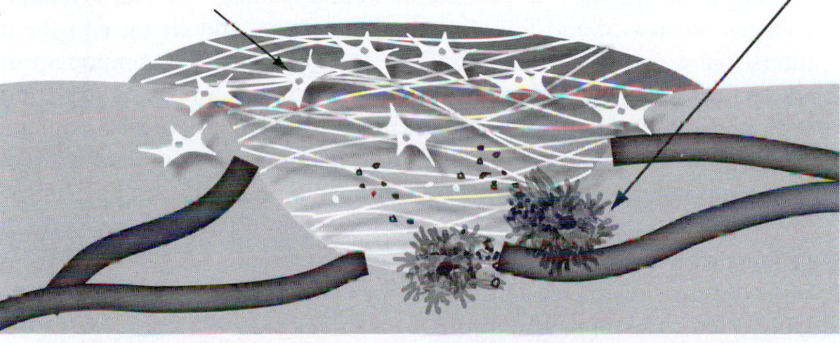

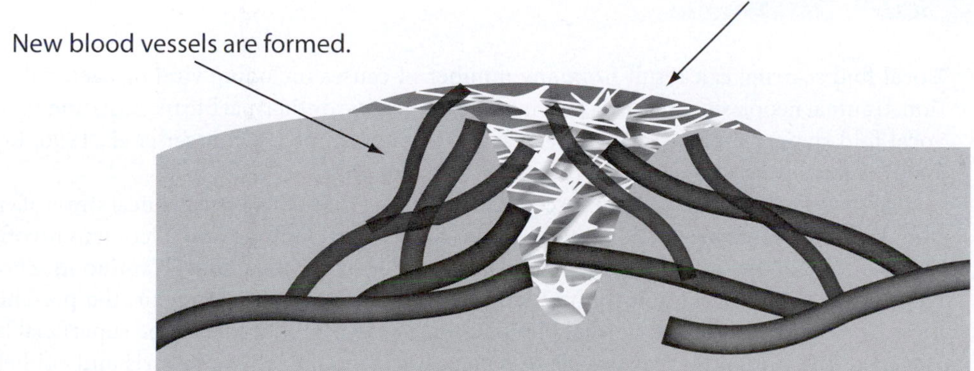

that have characteristics of both fibroblasts and smooth muscle cells (myo = muscle). Like fibroblasts, myofibroblasts produce molecules such as collagen and FN (Powell et al., 1999), and like muscle cells, they are contractile. This hybrid property allows them to be involved in both collagen deposition in the wound (to fill in the defect), as well as in reducing the size of the wound by contracting and pulling the edges of the wound together. Fibroblasts are the cells that initiate wound contraction, and myofibroblasts help to complete the process (Van Beurden, Von den Hoff, Torensma, Maltha, & Kuijpers-Jagtman, 2005).

Once the epithelium is repaired the granulation cells resolve through a process called **apoptosis**. Apoptosis refers to programmed (as opposed to traumatic) cell death. With the resolution of the granulation tissue, the amount of FN within the tissue decreases (Hirano et al., 2008). At this stage the ECM is repaired, but the new tissue is not exactly the same as the pre-wound tissue. While all the ECM components are present, they are poorly organized, and the region is less pliable than the surrounding tissue (Branski et al., 2006; Hapner & Klein, 2009). If apoptosis does not occur and the granulation tissue persists, the FN does not decrease. Persistence of FN in the ECM may contribute to the fibrosis and excessive collagen that are major components of scar tissue (Hansen & Thibeault, 2006).

REMODELING

A scar represents the end product of wound healing. Scars are characterized by increased collagen, decreased and fragmented elastin fibers, and changes in the proportion of other interstitial proteins (Thibeault & Gray, 2004). The major component of a scar is collagen, which makes up 50% of the scar protein and which is thickly bundled and disorganized (Lim et al., 2006; Thibeault & Gray, 2004). Therefore, the new tissue has a different texture and quality than the surrounding tissue. As the scar matures it continues to change, a process known as **scar remodeling**. In this phase ECM components continue to be deposited and reorganized. For example, Type III collagen, a weaker form, is largely replaced by the stronger Type I. The production of collagen becomes stable at approximately 21 days after the injury. However, the scar continues to change and mature for up to 12 months (Branski et al., 2006; Thibeault & Gray, 2004). The immature scar tissue is stiff and thick, whereas mature scar tissue is thinner and more pliable, and the collagen fibers become better organized (Branski et al., 2006).

Vocal Fold Scar

Vocal fold scarring can result from any number of causes including viral or bacterial infection, trauma, neoplasms, endotracheal intubation, caustic or thermal burns, radiation therapy, vocal fold surgery, inflammatory diseases, and phonotrauma (Benninger et al., 1996; Rosen, 2000). Table 6.1 lists possible causes of vocal fold scarring.

The vocal folds may be both susceptible and yet resistant to the mechanical stress of vibration. Reportedly, normal adult vocal folds (see color insert photos 1 and 2) contain myofibroblasts located in the superficial layer of the lamina propria (Catten, Gray, Hammond, Zhou, & Hammond, 1998). Because myofibroblasts are associated with ECM repair, the presence of these elements suggests that normal phonation may cause mild injury in the superficial layer. However, the vocal folds may be able to repair damage to the lamina propria and epithelium without a full-scale wound healing process until a threshold of damage is reached (Branski et al., 2006). Ongoing damaging vocal fold behaviors may result in a relatively permanent state

TABLE 6.1 Potential Causes of Vocal Fold Scarring

- Traumatic
  - Blunt trauma (with or without fracture)
  - Penetrating injury (e.g., knife, bullet, dog bite)
- Neoplastic
  - Carcinoma of the vocal cord
    - Prior radiation therapy
    - Prior surgical treatment
- Iatrogenic
  - Prior Teflon injection
  - Injudicious vocal cord surgery
  - Prolonged endotracheal intubation
  - Prolonged nasogastric intubation
  - Tracheotomy
- Inflammatory
  - Gastroesophageal (laryngopharyngeal) reflux disease
  - Acute (thermal) inhalation injury
  - Rheumatoid arthritis
  - Relapsing polychondritis
  - Bacterial laryngotracheitis
  - Other acute necrotizing infections
  - Chronic granulomatous disorders
- Miscellaneous
  - Sulcus vocalis
  - Congenital webs
  - Radiation injury (e.g., fibrosis)
  - Intracordal cysts

Source: From "Vocal Fold Scarring: Current Concepts and Management," by M. S. Benninger, D. Alessi, S. Archer, R. Bastian, C. Ford, J. Koufman, R. T. Sataloff, J. R. Spiegel, 1996, *Otolaryngology—Head and Neck Surgery, 115,* pp. 479–480. Copyright 1996 by Elsevier. Reprinted with permission.

of tissue repair, which may eventually manifest as a benign vocal fold lesion and/or scar (see color insert photos 3 and 4) (Branski et al., 2006).

One of the major causes of vocal fold scar is surgery for benign and malignant disorders (Chhetri et al., 2004). While new techniques to prevent or reduce scarring are becoming more widespread, vocal fold scarring following surgery is not uncommon (Schweinfurth & Ossoff, 2006). The most important predictors of scar formation are the depth of the surgical incision and the damage to surrounding tissues. Damage to the vocal ligament is particularly likely to result in scarring because of the high concentration of fibroblasts. When the intermediate and deep layers of the lamina propria are injured, the fibroblasts are stimulated, which promotes scar formation. The biomechanical properties of the vocal folds are determined largely by the relationship, density, and organization of the ECM components (Hansen & Thibeault, 2006). Therefore, scar tissue in the lamina propria changes the viscoelastic and vibratory characteristics of the vocal folds and disrupts the mucosal wave. The disorganized collagen and loss of essential ECM elements results in contraction of the vocal fold cover as well as loss of vocal fold pliability (Dailey & Ford, 2006).

Sulcus Vocalis

Vocal fold scar is often associated with a condition called *sulcus vocalis* (see color insert photo 5). A sulcus is any type of groove, furrow, or depression (Figure 6.2). Sulcus vocalis refers to a groove on the medial surface of one or both vocal folds. The groove may be shallow, in which case it is confined to the cover of the folds, or deep, extending into the vocal ligament. The longitudinal extent also varies. In exceptionally deep cases the furrow seems to divide the vocal fold in half (Hsiung, Kang, Pai, Su, & Lan, 2004). The groove has the effect of tethering the epithelium to the vocal ligament (Dailey & Ford, 2006).

FIGURE 6.2 **Sulcus Vocalis**

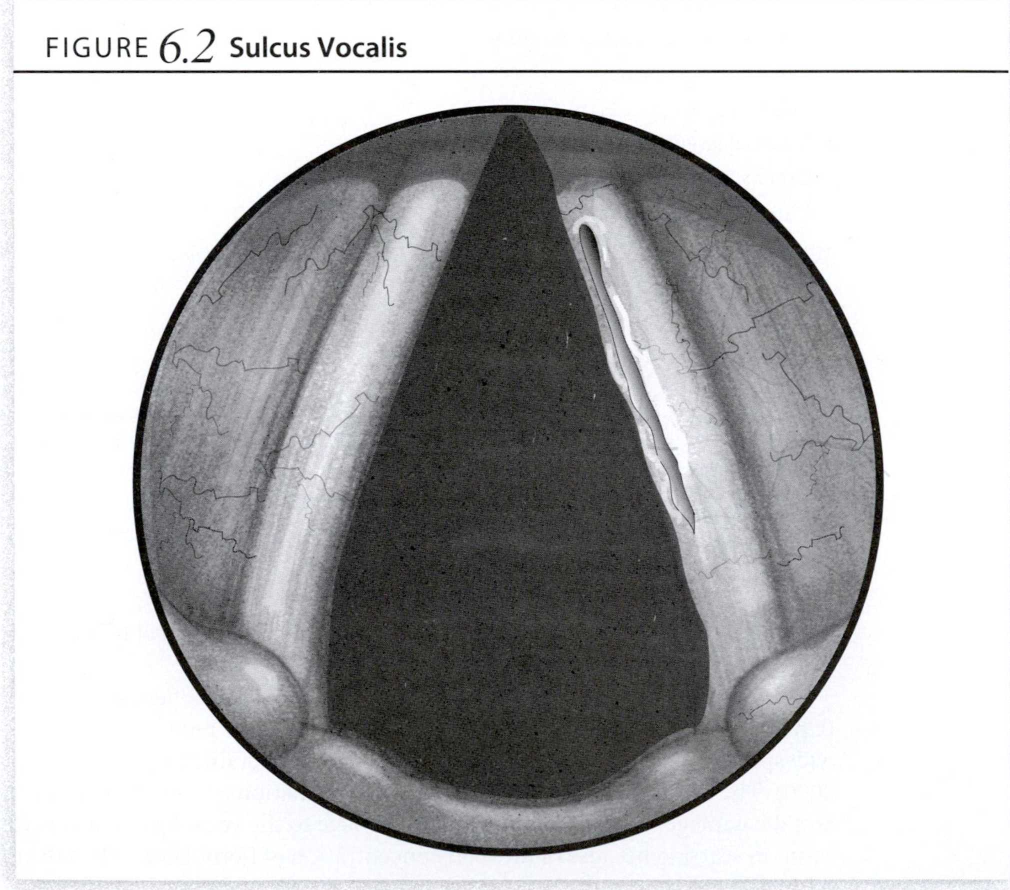

Sulci have been classified into three types: **physiological sulcus** (Type 1), **sulcus vergeture** (Type II), and sulcus vocalis (Type III) (Ford, Inagi, Khidr, Bless, & Gilchrist, 1996). Type 1 sulcus may be a consequence of the aging process. When the vocalis muscle is thin and weak, the upper and lower edges of the folds are drawn toward each other, creating a groove between them. In Type I the lamina propria is normal and there is minimal disturbance of the mucosal wave. Voice quality is essentially normal and does not call for any kind of voice treatment (Eller, Hawkshaw, & Sataloff, 2006; Hsiung et al., 2004). This type of mild defect is present in approximately 10% of people (Eller et al., 2006). Type 2 shows loss of the superficial layer of the lamina propria with a linear depression or vergeture along the free edge of the fold. The result is an abnormally thin layer of tissue between the epithelium and the vocal ligament (Eller et al., 2006; Hsiung et al., 2004). Dysphonia results from the disruption to the mucosal wave in the vicinity of the sulcus. Type 3 refers to a pit in the vocal fold epithelium, with severe loss of lamina propria tissue that extends into the vocal ligament or even into the thyroarytenoid muscle (Hsiung et al., 2004). Histologic examination of Type 3 sulci has demonstrated the presence of diffuse fibrosis and inflammation (Dailey & Ford, 2006). Loss of the superficial layer of the lamina propria results in the epithelium adhering directly to the vocal ligament (Eller et al., 2006; Pinto et al., 2007). This tethering effect results in an inward concavity of the medial edge of the vocal fold, which contributes to the glottal insufficiency associated with sulcus vocalis (Hapner & Klein, 2009).

The cause of sulcus vocalis has not been conclusively established, but may be either congenital or acquired. Congenital sulcus may be the result of abnormal maturation of the vocal fold cover in embryologic development (Stemple et al., 2000). Patients with congenital sulci typically have a lifelong history of disordered voice (Schweinfurth & Ossoff, 2001). Causes of acquired sulcus include aging changes, vocal fold paralysis, infection, degeneration of benign lesions, laryngeal surgery, and repeated chronic inflammation (Hsiung et al., 2004; Kandogan & Ziya, 2007; Schweinfurth and Ossoff, 2001). Vocal fold scar and sulcus vocalis have been characterized as distinct but related conditions, as the sulcus is characterized by loss of tissue in conjunction with the replacement of normal tissue with disorganized fibrous material (Welham, Dailey, Ford, & Bless, 2007).

SYMPTOMS AND SIGNS OF VOCAL FOLD SCAR AND SULCUS VOCALIS

The dysphonia resulting from vocal fold scar and sulcus vocalis is characterized by symptoms of glottal insufficiency including breathiness, roughness, loss of pitch range, loss of volume, and vocal fatigue (Dailey & Ford, 2006; Hapner & Klein, 2009; Kishimoto, Hirano, Kojima, Kanemaru, & Ito, 2009; Welham et al., 2003). Speakers may also lack the ability to project the voice and may experience irregular vocal breaks, effortful phonation, diplophonia, and aphonia (Zeitels, Mauri, & Dailey, 2003).

Individuals may use the false vocal folds to phonate, which results in a strained, low-pitched voice. If the scarring or sulcus is severe, patients may complain of shortness of breath caused by excessive loss of air with phonation (Rosen, 2000). In less severe cases the individual's voice may sound essentially normal, with the main symptoms being vocal fatigue or a decreased pitch range (Schweinfurth & Ossoff, 2001).

Videostroboscopy has shown that scarring and sulcus vocalis can result in a loss of the mucosal wave, lack of approximation of the medial edges of the folds, a spindle-shaped glottic closure pattern, different vertical vocal fold levels, asymmetrical amplitude of vibration, decreased amplitude, and an adynamic segment of the vocal folds (Dailey & Ford, 2006; Neuenschwander et al., 2001; Rosen, 2000; Schweinfurth & Ossoff, 2006;

Zhang et al., 2010). Other findings include compensatory behaviors such as ventricular phonation (Neuenschwander et al., 2001). Scarring can give the vocal fold cover an opaque or white appearance (Dailey & Ford, 2006).

TREATMENT

Treatment for scar and/or sulcus vocalis may be behavioral, surgical, or a combination. Voice therapy may be the primary mode of treatment or may be used in conjunction with surgical intervention (Hapner & Klein, 2009).

Voice Therapy. Rosen (2000) emphasized that surgical intervention for vocal fold scar should not be performed without the patient first undergoing voice therapy. Patients often try to compensate for the vocal difficulties created by the scar or sulcus by tensing the intrinsic and/or extrinsic laryngeal muscles, increasing the subglottal air pressure, or changing the shape of the supraglottic resonators (Benninger et al., 1996). Excessive laryngeal tension in patients with scar or sulcus is characterized by a high laryngeal position with elevated pitch, tension in the base of the tongue that prevents the vocal output from being projected, breath holding with poor coordination of respiration and phonation, effortful voice onset, or a generalized decrease in vocal loudness (Hapner & Klein, 2009). Voice therapy including a program of vocal hygiene in conjunction with laryngeal massage, resonant voice therapy, and/or vocal function exercises can be extremely helpful in promoting a more efficient and effective manner of voice production (Dailey & Ford, 2006; Hapner & Klein, 2009; Neuenschwander et al., 2001). Any underlying factors that may contribute to the problem should be identified and eliminated or reduced. Laryngopharyngeal reflux may induce or perpetuate inflammation and edema, so it is critical to control this condition (Dailey & Ford, 2006). Other factors that can affect the larynx such as smoking and allergies also need to be addressed. Whatever approach is taken, therapy for vocal fold scar and/or sulcus vocalis is a long-term process, and improved outcomes may not be apparent for six months to one year (e.g., Kishimoto et al., 2009; Welham et al., 2003). Thus patients should be counseled early in the therapeutic process about the need for patience and persistence in order to maximize clinical benefits. Depending on the severity of the scar or sulcus and the patient's vocal needs, voice therapy may be the only method of treatment required (Rosen, 2000).

Surgical Treatment. In cases where voice therapy alone is not adequate, surgical intervention may be necessary. Surgical strategies for vocal fold scar and sulcus vocalis are similar as both conditions are characterized by glottal insufficiency (Kishimoto et al., 2009). Current treatments are aimed at manipulating the histologic properties of the vocal folds by means of various bioinjections and implantations of substances such as bovine and human collagen, hyaluronic acid, autologous fat, and autologous fibroblasts (Figures 6.3 and 6.4). Surgery for sulcus vocalis also involves removing the adhesion between the mucosa and vocal ligament (Zhang et al., 2010).

Hsiung and Pai (2006) used autologous fat injection to treat sulcus vocalis. The fat was harvested from the patient's lower abdomen and injected into the lateral portion of the middle third of the vocal fold at the level of the thyroarytenoid muscle. Hsiung and Pai (2006) concluded that autologous fat alone may not be suitable for patients with sulcus vocalis, because it cannot solve the problem of lesions of the vocal fold cover. For these cases, transplantation of fascia (sheet of fibrous tissue that surrounds muscles) may be helpful. This procedure is similar to the transplantation of stem cells to regenerate other organs (Hsiung et al., 2004). However,

FIGURE 6.3 **Superficial and Deep Vocal Fold Injections for Scarring**

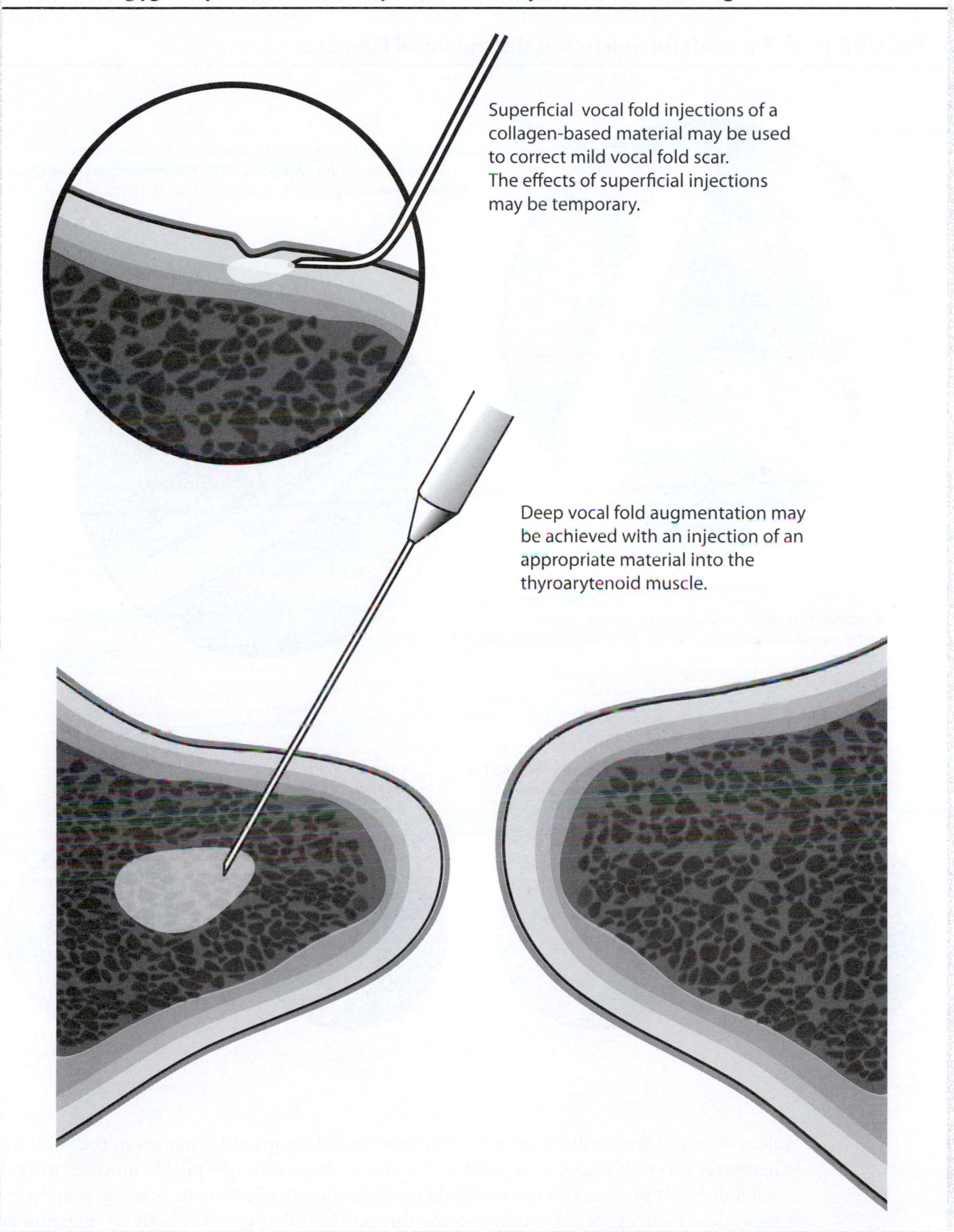

FIGURE 6.4 Fat Graft for Sulcus Vocalis and Vocal Fold Scar

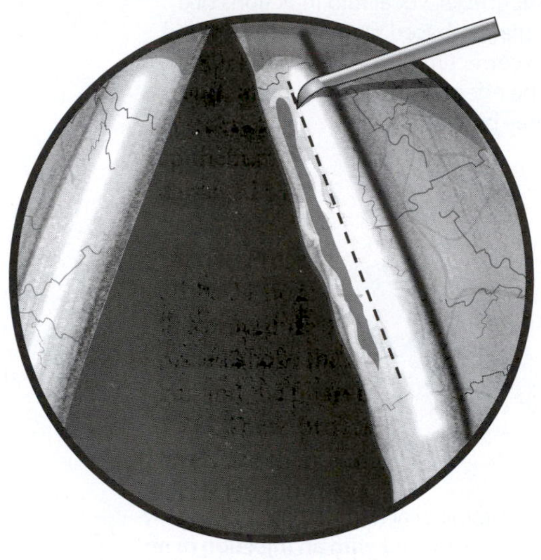

Both sulcus vocalis and vocal fold scarring are sometimes corrected with a surgical procedure that uses a fat graft from the patient's own body to fill in or reshape the affected vocal fold.

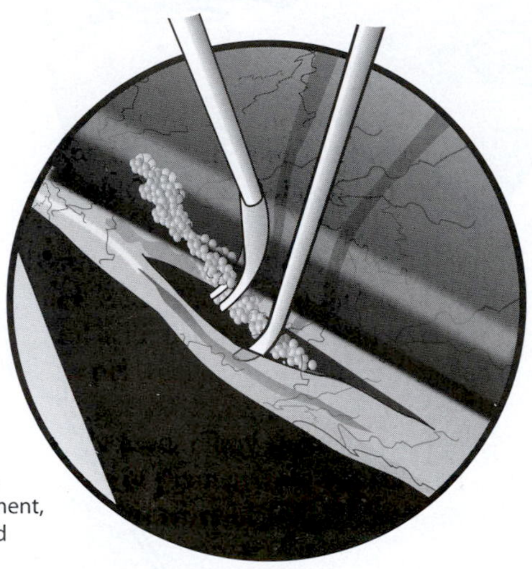

An incision is made and scar tissue may be removed if present. A pocket is created by elevating the mucosa off the vocal ligament, and the pocket is then packed with fat and the incision sutured closed.

Sulcus in true vocal fold

Incision and creation of pocket between the mucosa and the vocal ligament

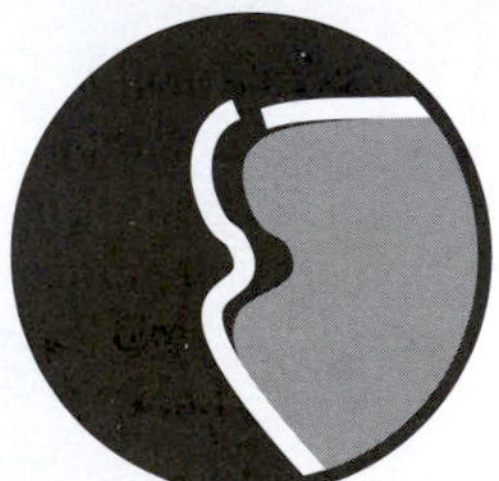

Implantation of autologous fat in the pocket.

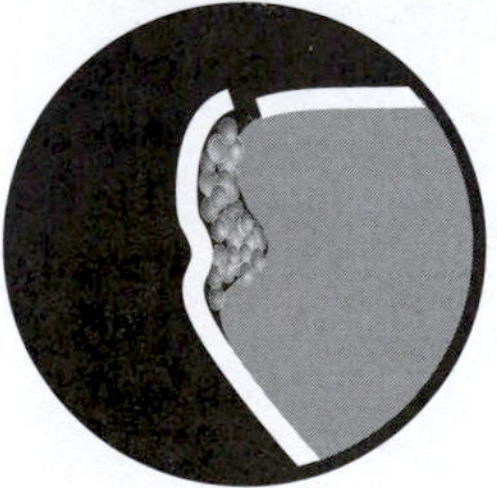

Sutures close the incision in the now reshaped vocal fold.

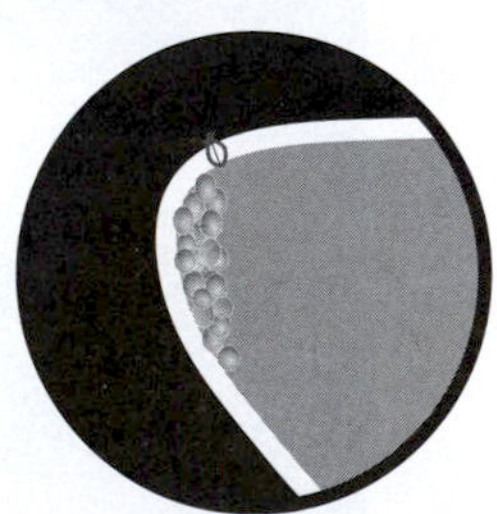

sulcus vocalis is frequently associated with bowing and/or atrophic changes in the vocal fold. Therefore, although fascial transplant is effective in regenerating a pliable mucosal wave, by itself it does not provide enough vocal fold medialization to alleviate the bowing. Hsiung et al. (2004) described a procedure to overcome this problem that involves both fat injection and fascia transplantation (FIFT). In this procedure the area of adhesion between the sulcus and the vocal ligament is separated, and the fascia is inserted into the pocket between the cover and the body of the vocal fold. The pocket is sutured closed and the fat is injected into the soft tissue to medialize the vocal fold. With this combination of techniques Hsiung et al. (2004) reported that their patients' phonation times increased, and overall severity of dysphonia, roughness, and breathiness all improved. Seventy-two percent of patients reported satisfactory voice results.

Laryngitis

Laryngitis is an umbrella term covering any inflammation of the larynx. Normally the inflammatory response is activated only when necessary and subsides when healing is complete (Scheff et al., 2010). However, inflammation can persist and cause damage to healthy tissues (Scheff et al., 2010). Inflammation can be acute, lasting for a few days; subacute, persisting for up to 3 weeks; or chronic, with a duration longer than 3 weeks. Persistent inflammation is implicated in a wide variety of diseases.

There are innumerable causes of laryngitis, including viral infections (influenza, measles, mumps, chicken pox), bacterial and fungal infections, phonotrauma, smoking, allergies, acid reflux, radiation treatment for head and neck tumors, autoimmune problems (rheumatoid arthritis, lupus), and parasitic infections (trichinosis and leishmaniasis). See Table 6.2.

Often, however, there is more than one cause. An individual can have a viral respiratory infection that causes laryngitis, and the person may also smoke, use improper vocal technique for singing, and suffer from laryngopharyngeal reflux. The most common cause of laryngitis in infants and children is acute infection, whereas noninfectious, chronic causes are more typical of adults (Koufman, 1996). In adults, laryngopharyngeal reflux is probably the most common cause of laryngitis, followed by smoking. Laryngitis affects individuals of all ages, but it is often more of a problem in infants and young children than it is in adults, because of the much smaller pediatric larynx. Swelling of the laryngeal tissues may create airway obstruction in a small larynx, while the same amount of swelling in a larger larynx would have minimal effects.

TABLE 6.2 Some Causes of Acute and Chronic Laryngitis

Acute	Chronic
Phonotrauma	Phonotrauma
Environmental irritants	Laryngopharyngeal reflux
Laryngotracheitis	Smoking and alcohol
Supraglottitis	Autoimmune diseases
Viral infections	Allergies
Bacterial infections	Regular steroid inhaler usage
Fungal infections	Immunocompromise
Intubation	Chronic cough/throat clearing

ACUTE LARYNGITIS

Acute laryngitis most often results from infection. Refer to color insert photos 6 and 7. The condition begins abruptly, and typically the infection is self-limiting, lasting up to around 10 days (Koufman, 1996). Acute infection results in swelling and edema of the vocal folds, leading to hoarseness and even aphonia.

Patients may also complain of **odynophonia** (pain on talking), dysphagia, **odynophagia** (painful swallowing), and dyspnea. Visual examination of the vocal folds typically shows erythema and edema, secretions, irregularities of the vocal fold, asymmetrical vibration, reduced mucosal wave, and incomplete vocal fold closure (Shah & Shapshay, 2006). Ulcers on the membranous portions of the vocal folds have been reported in some cases of acute laryngitis (Hsiao, 2011).

While most types of acute laryngeal infections are relatively benign, some are more dangerous, particularly in the case of infants and very young children. Acute laryngotracheitis, commonly called **croup**, is a disease affecting very young children. The subglottal area tends to be most severely inflamed, and the child develops the characteristic "barky" cough, as well as hoarseness and inspiratory stridor. The disease can be life-threatening depending on how severely the airway is obstructed. Another serious form of laryngitis is **acute supraglottitis** (epiglottitis). Both adults and children can be affected, although the disease is more common in young children. This disease is associated with severe throat pain, difficulty swallowing, and drooling. There is a high fever, and the epiglottis and aryepiglottic folds are very swollen and red. It is important to get medical help as soon as possible, because the airway can become seriously obstructed in a matter of hours, resulting in death.

Treatment. Antibiotics are not indicated for most cases of acute laryngitis (Reveiz, Cardona, & Ospina, 2007). Strategies to lessen the intensity of the laryngitis include inhaling humidified air to keep the upper airway lubricated, avoiding speaking as much as possible, speaking in a soft, "confidential" voice, and avoiding, to the extent possible, antihistamines and corticosteroids, which tend to dry the mucosa. Mucolytics such as guaifenesin may be helpful in thinning and clearing secretions.

CHRONIC LARYNGITIS

Laryngitis that lasts for more than 3 weeks is classified as chronic (Shah & Shapshay, 2006). The ongoing inflammatory process may damage the vocal fold epithelium resulting in **hyperkeratosis** (thickening of the mucous membrane), fibrosis, and scarring (Berliti, Omidi, & Wenig, 2005; Dworkin, 2008).

Chronic laryngitis is often seen in individuals who smoke, drink alcohol, and overuse their voices. Chronic laryngitis resulting from phonotraumatic behaviors can lead to the formation of polyps, nodules, and vocal fold scarring (Dworkin, 2008). A person with chronic laryngitis may also cough habitually, clear his or her throat to try to get rid of the irritation, and have gastric reflux. Some individuals may be exposed to environmental pollutants and toxic products in their workplaces, and these can cause or exacerbate the problem. In addition, allergies often contribute to chronic laryngitis. Chronic laryngitis can also occur in patients who are immunocompromised, because fungal infections are very common in these individuals. Other potential causes include fumes, dust, prescription or OTC medications that can cause local drying and/or mucosal injury (e.g., diuretics, antihypertensives, psychotropics, antihistamines, decongestants), intubation, neck trauma; and ingestion of caustic substances (Berliti et al., 2005).

The laryngoscopic signs of chronic laryngitis include thick sticky mucus and thickening of the vocal fold epithelium. The soft pliant epithelium may become replaced by fibrosis, and when this happens, the initial pain of the irritation dissipates. The person's voice is typically low pitched, hoarse, and breathy, and may be weak in volume.

Treatment should focus on identifying and eliminating the laryngeal irritants. A program of vocal hygiene can be helpful, as well as voice therapy to minimize vocal hyperfunction such as resonant voice treatment, accent method, or other holistic approaches.

GASTROESOPHAGEAL REFLUX DISEASE AND LARYNGOPHARYNGEAL REFLUX

Gastroesophageal reflux (GER) refers to the movement of stomach contents into the esophagus through the lower esophageal sphincter (LES). The LES regulates the opening and closing of the junction between the stomach and the esophagus. GER is a normal physiologic process occurring mostly after meals. However, sometimes excess reflux or increased occurrences of reflux can cause gastroesophageal reflux disease (GERD). GERD refers to a broad array of diseases associated with injury to the esophagus or adjacent organs from the highly acidic gastric contents (called *refluxate*) into the esophagus or above into the pharynx and oral cavity (Sataloff, Castell, Katz, & Sataloff, 2006). Reflux that enters the pharyngeal area and comes into contact with the posterior larynx is called *laryngopharyngeal reflux (LPR)*. See color insert photos 8 and 9.

There are several important differences between GERD and LPR (Table 6.3). First, patients with GERD often have **esophagitis** (inflammation of the esophagus), while those with LPR typically do not. Second, most patients with GERD have lower esophageal sphincter problems, while those with LPR seem to have upper esophageal sphincter problems. Third, most GERD patients have nocturnal symptoms that occur in the supine position, whereas LPR patients have more symptoms during the daytime in the upright position. Heartburn is a common symptom in GERD, and less common in LPR. Some individuals, however, suffer from both GERD and LPR.

GERD/LPR can occur for a wide variety of reasons (Table 6.4). These include decreased pressure within the lower and/or upper esophageal sphincter, delayed gastric emptying, decreased esophageal motility, and increased acid production and secretion. It is well known that certain foods and behaviors contribute to GERD, such as eating spicy foods, eating close to bedtime, smoking, and alcohol consumption. Medications such as calcium channel blockers, nitrates, beta-blockers, and progesterone may cause predisposition to GERD by decreasing

TABLE 6.3 **Differences between GERD and LPR**

GERD	LPR
Esophagitis	No esophagitis
Lower esophageal sphincter problems	Upper esophageal sphincter problems
Nocturnal symptoms in supine position	Daytime symptoms in upright position
Heartburn very common	Heartburn less common

TABLE 6.4 Causes of GERD/LPR
Decreased pressure in the lower and/or upper esophageal sphincter
Delayed gastric emptying
Decreased esophageal motility
Increased acid production and secretion
Dietary and lifestyle factors
Medications

the tone and pressure of the LES. Tobacco and alcohol have a negative impact on almost all of the body's antireflux mechanisms. For example, they delay gastric emptying, decrease LES pressure, decrease esophageal motility, decrease mucosal resistance, and increase gastric acid secretion (Koufman, 1995; Qadeer, Colabianchi, Strome, & Vaezi, 2006). Smoking can also decrease salivary secretions, which are important in neutralizing acid.

GERD/LPR has been shown to be the cause of or to contribute to many laryngeal and nonlaryngeal problems (Table 6.5).

There are two mechanisms by which the laryngeal injuries are caused. The first is direct injury to the laryngeal tissues caused by the refluxate. As the pharynx is situated directly behind the larynx, the highly acidic refluxate can easily reach the posterior portions of the larynx. The delicate and sensitive tissues are washed in acid, resulting in inflammation (Edmunds, Mudd, Jailwala, Shaker, & Amirlak, 2007; Sataloff et al., 2006). This is particularly likely to happen at night, when the tone of the upper esophageal sphincter is diminished. Eating late at night is known to cause reflux, and because of the lack of upper esophageal sphincter protection, the larynx is directly exposed to the refluxate (Kahrilas, 2000).

The second mechanism is indirect and is hypothesized to occur when the vagus nerve is stimulated by irritation of the lower esophagus. Recall that the vagus nerve innervates not only the intrinsic muscles of the larynx, but many other visceral organs including the stomach. Thus, stimulation of the vagus nerve in the stomach and esophageal areas can result in reflexive coughing or throat clearing. The traumatic coughing and throat clearing may eventually lead to injury of the laryngeal mucosa such as vocal fold hemorrhage or vocal fold scarring (Edmunds et al., 2007; Sataloff et al., 2006).

GERD/LPR in Children. The occurrence of LPR is widespread in infants and children. However, the diagnosis may be more difficult to establish in children, because infants, with their immature digestive systems, have considerable physiological regurgitation. This makes it difficult to differentiate between normal and pathological reflux (Eckley, 2000). The incidence of reflux in all infants has been estimated at around 18%, but is thought to be as high as 70% in infants who have conditions such as tracheoesophageal fistula, neurological impairment, or dysphagia (Karkos, Leong, Apostolidou, & Apostolidis, 2006). This high incidence may be partly explained by differences in the digestive systems of infants and adults. Infants are predisposed to reflux due to a shorter esophagus and an immature lower esophageal sphincter. Children are also more at risk for nocturnal reflux than adults, because at night they have a reduced rate of swallowing and less esophageal acid neutralization by the alkaline saliva that

TABLE 6.5 **Reported Laryngeal and Nonlaryngeal Problems Associated with LPR**

Laryngeal Problems	Nonlaryngeal Problems
Posterior laryngitis	Xerostomia
Cricoarytenoid joint arthritis	Sinusitis
Subglottic stenosis	Otitis media
Cancer of the larynx	Sleep apnea
Laryngeal webs	Aspiration pneumonia
Chronic cough	Choking sensation
Persistent hoarseness	Pain in neck and jaw
Vocal fatigue	Asthma
Voice breaks	Bronchitis
Excessive throat mucus	Sudden infant death syndrome
Chronic sore throat	
Intermittent or chronic airway obstruction	
Wheezing	
Reinke's edema	
Contact ulcers and granulomas	
Posterior glottic stenosis	
Laryngospasm	
Globus pharyngeus	
Vocal nodules	
Laryngomalacia	
Recurrent leukoplakia	

Sources: Information from Carrau et al. (2004); Chung et al. (2009); Kelchner et al. (2007); Koufman et al. (2002); Pribuisiene, Uloza, Kupcinskas, & Jonaitis (2006); Sataloff et al. (2006).

counteracts the high acid present in refluxate (Karkos, Yates, Carding, & Wilson, 2007). Other reasons for the higher infantile reflux include the higher liquid intake (100–120 ml/kg/day) compared to adults (30–50 ml/kg/day) and an increased number of transient lower esophageal relaxations (Stavroulaki, 2006). As with adults, LPR in children may result in various respiratory and otolaryngological conditions, including asthma, chronic cough, recurrent bronchitis, **laryngomalacia**, laryngospasm, subglottic stenosis, otitis media, apnea, recurrent infections such as spasmodic croup or recurrent laryngotracheitis, and sinusitis (Karkos et al., 2007; Megale, Scanavini, Andrade, Fernandes, & Anselmo-Lima, 2006; Stavroulaki, 2006).

Diagnosis and Evaluation. Diagnosis and evaluation of LPR is based on a variety of measures including clinical signs and symptoms, laryngoscopy, and pH monitoring. The classic laryngeal signs of LPR are edema and erythema along the membranous glottis and in the posterior glottis on the arytenoids or in the interarytenoid space. Ulcerations or granuloma may also occur. The arytenoids appear reddish and swollen, and there are often layers of thickened granulation tissue between the arytenoids (Belafsky, Postma, & Koufman, 2001; Dworkin, 2008; Mesallam, Stemple, Sobeih, & Elluru, 2007; Sataloff et al., 2006). The edema present in the glottal and supraglottal areas can obscure the laryngeal ventricles, a condition called *ventricular obliteration*. With partial ventricular obliteration the ventricular space is reduced and the false fold edge is indistinct. With complete obliteration the true and false folds appear to touch and there is no true ventricular space (Belafsky et al., 2001; Dworkin, 2008). Additional laryngoscopic signs that have been reported include pseudosulcus (a longitudinal groove extending below the medial margin throughout the length of the vocal fold, including the cartilaginous portion), Reinke's edema, nodules or other masses, and laryngeal stenosis. However, these signs are not specific to LPR, and have been reported in individuals who do not have subjective symptoms of LPR (e.g. Belafsky, Postma, Amin, & Koufman, 2002).

Clinical signs and symptoms can include chronic rhinitis, chronic sinusitis, chronic cough, throat clearing, globus pharyngeus, chronic sore throat, referred otalgia, recurrent croup, and respiratory symptoms such as stridor (Block & Brodsky, 2007; Reichel, Dressel, Wiederanders, & Issing, 2008). These symptoms occur because the ciliated respiratory epithelium of the posterior larynx that normally functions to clear mucus from the airway is damaged by the refluxate, with a resulting buildup of mucus (Ford, 2005).

Double-Probe 24-hour Ambulatory pH Monitoring. Over the past 15 years the use of double-probe 24-hour ambulatory pH monitoring has become the gold standard to diagnose LPR. In this procedure one probe is placed slightly above the lower esophageal sphincter and another is placed above the upper esophageal sphincter, which forms the boundary between the esophagus and the pharynx (Figure 6.5).

These probes sample the acid levels at these two locations for a 24-hour period, and levels are then compared with normal values. Acid is measured on the pH scale, which has levels from 0–14. A level of 7 indicates neutral acid; the lower the acid level, the higher is the pH value. Normally the esophagus has a higher pH (that is, lower acid levels) than the stomach. The target level for stomach pH is 4 or higher.

While double probe monitoring is widely used, many specialists have noted problems with the procedure. One problem is that results of pHmetry are not sufficiently sensitive or specific to conclusively establish or rule out the presence of LPR. Small amounts of LPR are often present even in individuals who do not have symptoms, making it hard to define the boundary between physiological and pathological reflux (Karkos et al., 2007). Another problem is that the criteria used to diagnose GERD do not apply in LPR, because baseline pH values for the hypopharynx are still unknown (Karkos et al., 2007). Based on a systematic review of the literature, Joniau, Bradshaw, Esterman, and Carney (2007) reported that the clinical diagnosis of LPR is not confirmed by 24-hour pH monitoring in the majority of patients, leading to significant overdiagnosis of this disorder. Ford (2005) also stressed that the current heightened awareness of LPR can lead to overdiagnosis because the typical symptoms of excessive throat clearing, cough, hoarseness, and globus are also indicative of other conditions such as infection, phonotrauma, allergies, smoking, and inhaled environmental irritants.

There are other reasons why diagnosis of LPR can be challenging. First, the condition can be occult, meaning that an individual can have the disease without being aware of it (Connor, Palazzi-Churas, Cohen, Leverson, & Bless, 2007). Reulbach, Belafsky, Blalock, Koufman, and Postma (2001) found that almost two-thirds of 100 people over the age of 40 without any

FIGURE 6.5 pH Monitoring

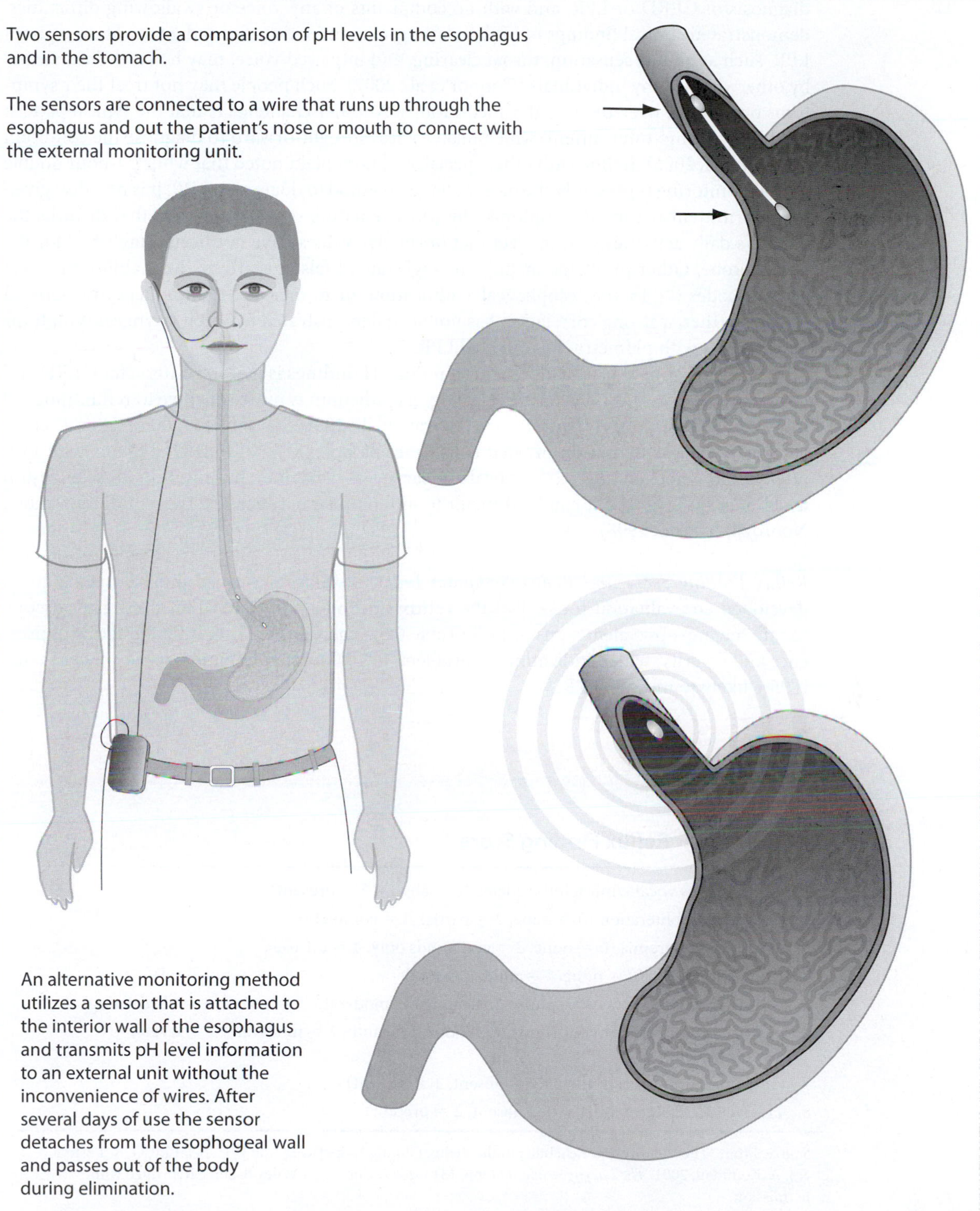

diagnosis of GERD or LPR, and with no complaints of any voice or swallowing difficulties, demonstrated clinical findings of LPR on laryngeal examination. Second, many of the signs of LPR, such as globus sensation, throat clearing, and impaired voice, may be viewed as normal by otherwise healthy individuals (Connor et al., 2007). Such people may not treat their symptoms or may use over-the-counter medications. Another challenge is that the typical pattern of LPR is chronic-intermittent, which makes it less straightforward to diagnose the condition (Stavroulaki, 2006). In line with other specialists, Stavroulaki noted that while 24-hour double probe monitoring is presently the most accepted method to document LPR, it is not ideal given the intermittent nature of symptoms, the invasive nature of the procedure that disturbs the patient's daily activities, and the fact that normative values have not been established for the upper probe. Other problems include the high rate of false negatives, the inability to detect brief episodes (> 15 s) of esophageal acidification, or to measure the frequency of nonacid reflux. Further, a strong correlation has not been demonstrated between laryngeal symptoms and/or signs with pHmetry documented LPR.

Complicating the difficulty in interpreting pH findings is that the criteria for GERD and LPR are different. This is because the laryngeal epithelium is more sensitive to reflux-induced injury than the esophageal epithelium (Carrau et al., 2005; Stavroulaki, 2006). Thus, there is currently no clear definition of what constitutes pathologic LPR. Finally, patients with LPR often demonstrate compensatory vocal and laryngeal behaviors that result in muscle tension dysphonia (MTD), and it can be difficult to differentiate between the two conditions (Ross, Noordzji, & Woo, 1998).

Reflux Finding Score and Reflux Symptom Index. Belafsky, Postma, and Koufman (2001) developed an evaluation tool called the **reflux finding score (RFS)** that uses laryngoscopy to rate the most prevalent signs of LPR (Table 6.6). The signs are quantified in terms of presence and severity, with 0 indicating no problem, to 26 (worst possible). A score greater than 7 is 95% likely to indicate LPR.

TABLE 6.6 Reflux Finding Score

1. Pseudosulcus vocalis/infraglottic edema (0 = absent, 2 = present)
2. Ventricular obliteration (0 = none, 2 = partial, 4 = complete)
3. Erythema/hyperemia (0 = none, 2 = arytenoids only, 4 = diffuse)
4. Vocal fold edema (0 = none, 1 = mild, 2 = moderate, 3 = severe, 4 = polypoid)
5. Diffuse laryngeal edema (0 = none, 1 = mild, 2 = moderate, 3 = severe, 4 = obstructing)
6. Posterior commissure hypertrophy (0 = none, 1 = mild, 2 = moderate, 3 = severe, 4 = obstructing)
7. Granuloma/granulation tissue (0 = absent, 2 = present)
8. Thick endolaryngeal mucus (0 = absent, 2 = present)

Source: From "The Validity and Reliability of the Reflux Finding Score (RFS)," by P. C. Belafsky, G. N. Postma, & J. A. Koufman, 2001, *The Laryngoscope, 111,* pp. 1313–1317. Copyright Wiley & Sons. Reprinted with permission.

Belafsky, Postma, and Koufman (2002) also developed a questionnaire, the Reflux Symptom Index, that probes the types and degree of severity of patient-perceived symptoms (Table 6.7). Symptoms are scored on a 5-point scale where 0 equals never and 5 represents a severe problem. An RSI greater than 13 is considered to be abnormal based on the authors' statistical analysis.

These two scales have been used extensively to document symptoms and signs of LPR. Kelchner et al. (2007) examined interrater reliability between otolaryngologists and speech-language pathologists in rating symptoms of LPR using the RFS. Reliability between the speech-language pathologists was high, but decreased when the otolaryngologists' ratings were included in the evaluation. Items receiving highest agreement were ventricular obliteration, vocal fold edema, and granuloma. The authors concluded that even under ideal practice conditions where close ongoing collaboration between professionals is standard care, variability exists in interpretation of the presence, degree, or absence of physical findings. Musser, Kelchner, Neils-Strunjas, and Montrose (2010) compared scores on the RSI and RFS in healthy individuals and in patients with suspected LPR who underwent 24-hour dual pH monitoring. Only the RSI differentiated between experimental and control subjects. The RFS and RSI were not significantly associated. There was a relationship between RSI scores and LPR, yet 70% of participants who were symptomatic for LPR had normal pH scores. The authors suggested that the RSI may be overidentifying patients for whom upper respiratory complaints are common and not exclusively secondary to LPR. Conditions such as allergies, asthma, postnasal drip, chronic nasal congestion or sinusitis, upper respiratory infections, phonotrauma, or alcohol/tobacco use could result in similar symptoms and inflated RSI scores. The authors also found a lack of agreement between RFS and physical evidence of LPR. They suggested that a range of normal anatomic variations may be falsely positive for LPR.

The RSI has been used as a parent proxy instrument for children (Simons et al., 2008). LPR is a common cause of dysphonia in children, and the symptoms are the same as those

TABLE 6.7 **Reflux Symptom Index**

Within the last month, how did the following problems affect you?

Circle the appropriate response. 0 = no problem; 5 = severe problem

1. Hoarseness or a problem with your voice
2. Clearing your throat
3. Excess throat mucus or postnasal drip
4. Difficulty swallowing food, liquids, or pills
5. Coughing after you ate or after lying down
6. Breathing difficulties or choking episodes
7. Troublesome or annoying cough
8. Sensation of something sticking in your throat or a lump in your throat
9. Heartburn, chest pain, indigestion, or stomach acid coming up

Source: From "Validity and Reliability of the Reflux Symptom Index (RSI)," by P. C. Belafsky, G. N. Postma, & J. A. Koufman, 2002, *Journal of Voice, 16,* pp. 274–277. Copyright 2002 by the Voice Foundation. Reprinted with permission.

TABLE 6.8 Health-Related Quality of Life in Individuals with LPR

Voice/Hoarseness

Rated on a 7-point scale

1. Difficult to work
2. Satisfied with sound
3. Hard to communicate
4. Others uncomfortable
5. Cannot sing
6. What others think
7. Sound upset when not
8. Strain is tiring
9. Embarrassed by voice
10. Avoid talking
11. Difficult to do job
12. Fear permanent voice loss
13. Overall voice/hoarse effect

Cough

Rated on a 7-point scale

14. Cough embarrassing
15. Avoid social events
16. Need to leave room
17. Perceived as sick
18. Hear me in the halls
19. Worry about timing
20. Overall cough effect

Throat Clearing

Rated on a 7-point scale

21. People notice
22. Disrupts sex life
23. Friendships affected
24. Makes it hard to talk
25. Frustrating frequency
26. Avoid social events
27. Overall clear throat effect

Swallowing

Rated on a 7-point scale

28. Hard to swallow
29. Avoid public eating
30. Fear choking in sleep
31. Burning in throat
32. Awaken gasping
33. Overall swallow effect

Overall Impact

Rated on a 10-point scale

34. Effect on energy
35. Job productivity effect
36. Social relations effect
37. Intimate relations effect
38. Sexual relations effect
39. Sleep effect
40. Lying down problems
41. Self-perception effect
42. Lifestyle effect
43. Affects ability to enjoy

Source: From "The Impact of Laryngopharyngeal Reflux on Patient-Reported Quality of Life," by R. L. Carrau, A. Khidr, J. A. Crawley, E. M. Hillson, J. K. Davis, C. L. Pashos, 2004, *The Laryngoscope, 114,* pp. 670–674. Copyright 2004 by Wiley & Sons. Reprinted with permission.

reported for adults (Block & Brodsky, 2007; Karkos et al., 2006; Shah, Woodnorth, Glynn, & Nuss, 2005). In addition to parental interviews, it is important to ask children directly about reflux-related symptoms using child-friendly terms, because their parents are often unaware of the condition (Theis & Heatley, 2009).

Quality of life may be affected in individuals with LPR. Four major complaints have been identified that affect LPR patients: voice problems, chronic cough, throat clearing, and swallowing difficulties (Lenderking et al., 2003). Carrau et al. (2004) developed and validated a tool to measure health-related quality of life in patients with LPR (LPR-HRQL). The instrument measures five domains including voice quality/hoarseness, cough, throat clearing, swallowing, and overall impact of the disorder (Table 6.8). The first four domains are measured on a 7-point scale; the last domain is measured on a 10-point scale. The higher the score obtained by the patient, the more his or her quality of life is affected by the LPR.

Treatment. Treatment of GERD and/or LPR is multifaceted and is aimed at reducing acid levels by behavioral changes in diet and lifestyle, by pharmacological means such as antireflux medications or prokinetic agents, or by surgery in severe cases. Because LPR involves multiple anatomic sites and causes a wide spectrum of signs and symptoms, it is important that the patient be treated with a multidisciplinary team approach including a laryngologist, internist, gastroenterologist, speech-language pathologist, pulmonologist, psychologist and nutritionist. Voice therapy is critical, since patients with LPR commonly have dysphonia for which they try to compensate by using hyperfunctional voice patterns that can result in muscle tension dysphonia.

Changes in Diet and Lifestyle. It is well known that many foods can create or contribute to both GERD and LPR. Examples include fats, alcohol, chocolate, citrus, tomato-based foods, and spicy foods. These foods, as well as tobacco smoke, affect the pressure of the lower esophageal sphincter, making it easier for stomach contents to escape. Behavioral habits such as eating late at night just before going to bed, exercising vigorously shortly after eating, and smoking also contribute to GERD. Eating late at night and then lying down to sleep means that gravity does not help to keep the stomach contents contained within the stomach. Changes in diet and lifestyle are typically advised as the initial or primary step in reflux control (Table 6.9).

While dietary and lifestyle changes are widely advised in the treatment of GERD and LPR, they have not been supported by strong research evidence, as shown by recent systematic literature reviews (e.g., Kaltenbach, Crockett, & Gerson, 2006; Meining & Classen, 2004). The exceptions are weight loss and raising the head of the bed, which were reported to improve patients' pH profiles and symptoms (Kaltenbach et al., 2006). Wo, Goudy, Winstead, and Mohiuddin (2003) examined the efficacy of lifestyle and diet modifications in patients who were newly diagnosed with LPR. Data were obtained on alcohol use, smoking, secondhand smoke, caffeine and chocolate consumption, eating late at night, and vocally traumatic behaviors. Each patient kept a diary recording symptoms of globus sensation, cough, sore throat, hoarseness, throat clearing, and throat mucus. Thirty-five percent of patients had greater than 50% improvement in total symptom scores; another 35% had some improvement but less than 50%. No changes were noted for globus and sore throat, and there was no improvement in laryngeal scores. Nonetheless, the authors concluded that with proper lifestyle and dietary counseling, many LPR patients can obtain some symptomatic improvement without pharmacotherapy.

TABLE 6.9 **Dietary and Lifestyle Modifications in the Treatment of GERD and/or LPR**

Foods/Drinks to Restrict	Lifestyle Factors
Caffeine	Stop smoking
Tomato-based foods	Avoid secondhand smoke
Citrus	Avoid eating 2–3 hours before bedtime
Chocolate	Wait at least 1 hour to exercise after eating
Carbonated drinks	Raise the head of the bed
Red wine	Lose weight if necessary
Fatty foods	Avoid medications such as anticholinergics, calcium channel
Spicy foods	blockers, antibiotics, aspirin, NSAIDs
Mint	Modify vocally damaging behaviors

Sources: Information from Ford (2005); Khan, Hashmi, Elahi, Tariq, & Ingrams (2006); Sataloff et al. (2006).

Antireflux Medications. Antireflux medications include H2 blockers, proton pump inhibitors (PPIs), and prokinetic agents. These drugs either reduce the amount of acid produced in the stomach, or increase the rate at which the esophagus moves food through the system. Antireflux medications are prescribed very commonly for individuals with GERD and/or LPR, usually in conjunction with advice on diet and lifestyle changes. It is also very common for individuals to self-medicate with OTC versions of H2 blockers and PPIs.

H2 Blockers. H2 blockers are histamine receptor antagonists. They function to block histamine receptors found on the acid-producing cells in the stomach. This decreases but does not entirely eliminate the production of acid. These medications have been used since the 1970s and have no known serious side effects. They are available over the counter and include cimetidine (Tagamet), famotidine (Pepcid), nizatadine (Axid), and ranitidine (Zantac). These agents can be helpful in controlling mild or moderate cases of GERD, but they are less effective in controlling more severe cases. H2 blockers are often used in conjunction with PPI therapy to prevent nocturnal acid breakthrough, or as a means of weaning the patient from PPIs (Stavroulaki, 2006).

Proton Pump Inhibitors. The term *proton pump* refers to a molecule in the acid-producing cells of the stomach. PPIs work to prevent the cell from discharging the acid. There are many PPIs available both OTC and by prescription, including esomeprazole (Nexium), lansoprazole (Prevacid), omeprazole (Prilosec), pantoprazole (Protonix), and rabeprazole (Aciphex).

PPI therapy is the treatment of choice for patients with LPR (Sataloff et al., 2006). While symptoms of GERD typically respond to PPI treatment within 2–3 months, patients with LPR often require longer treatment periods of at least 6 months to achieve symptom resolution (Sataloff et al., 2006). In addition to the PPI, an H2 blocker may be added at bedtime to prevent gastric acid breakthrough. Despite PPI therapy, 30% of patients with asthma, cough, or LPR continue to have abnormal acid exposure, and the dose may need to be increased (Sataloff et al., 2006).

PPIs have been found to be safe for long-term use. However, there are several issues to keep in mind. First, while two PPIs (omeprazole and lansoprazole) are approved by the FDA for use in children, they are not approved for children younger than 1 year of age (Stavroulaki, 2006). Second, some patients are omeprazole resistant, and resistance can also develop in patients who respond well initially (Sataloff et al., 2006). Third, many patients are young and will require prolonged or lifetime use of high doses of antireflux medications. The long-term effects over a long period of time are unknown (Sataloff et al., 2006). Fourth, the drugs are expensive, and for some individuals the cost and financial strain may result in poor compliance with the treatment regimen. Fifth, while the medications control the symptoms by suppressing acid production and neutralizing the acidity of the reflux material, they do not cure the disease. Some patients may continue to experience a degree of reflux and aspirate the neutralized fluid and bile salts. This can result in a continuation of symptoms such as throat clearing, excess phlegm, or cough (Sataloff et al., 2006). Finally, treatment for LPR often needs to be more aggressive and prolonged than for GERD, because the larynx is more susceptible to reflux injury than the esophagus (Koufman, Aviv, Casiano, & Shaw, 2002). The majority of patients with LPR require at least twice daily dosing with PPIs, because none of the PPIs exert acid suppression for more than 16.8 hours (Koufman et al., 2002).

PPI Outcome Studies. Omeprazole has been the most thoroughly investigated PPI with regard to LPR (Edmunds et al., 2007). Kamel, Hanson, and Kahrilas (1994) evaluated patients with LPR who had failed to respond to initial treatment with dietary and lifestyle measures. After 6 weeks of PPI therapy the patients' laryngeal and esophageal symptom scores improved significantly. By contrast, symptoms reoccurred within 6 weeks in all patients after therapy was stopped. Hanson, Kamel, and Kahrilas (1995) studied patients with mild (posterior laryngeal erythema), moderate (marked erythema, secretions, and mucosal granularity), or severe (ulceration, granulation tissue, or hyperkeratosis) laryngeal symptoms of LPR. Patients were treated with an H2 blocker. Those who did not respond to the famotidine were given a PPI. Hanson et al. found that patients with mild symptoms and minimal laryngeal changes responded to conservative doses of the H2 blocker, whereas those with severe laryngitis required PPI treatment for symptom resolution. Selby, Gilbert, and Lerman (2003) collected perceptual and acoustic data from patients with LPR. Immediately following the pretreatment evaluation the examining physician prescribed an antireflux treatment program lasting a minimum of 8–10 weeks. Treatment consisted of dietary and lifestyle modifications, PPI, and behavioral voice therapy to eliminate patterns of vocal hyperfunction (easy onset, decreased muscular tension, improved respiratory support). While acoustic data were essentially unchanged after treatment, the patients' overall levels of hoarseness decreased. Reichel et al. (2008) conducted a well-controlled study using the RSI to assess the efficacy of PPI therapy compared to a placebo. The authors noted a significant placebo effect within the first 6 weeks of therapy. After three months of treatment, only those patients who took the PPI showed a significant decrease in the total RSI score.

Prokinetics. **Prokinetics** are agents that enhance the muscular function of the esophagus (esophageal motility) and thus increase the movement of food and liquid through the gastrointestinal tract (Edmunds et al., 2007). However, these medications also increase heart rate and can therefore have serious cardiac side effects. One such medication, Cisapride, has been discontinued because of side effects of ventricular arrhythmia. Another one, Tegaserod, has side

FIGURE 6.6 **Fundoplication**

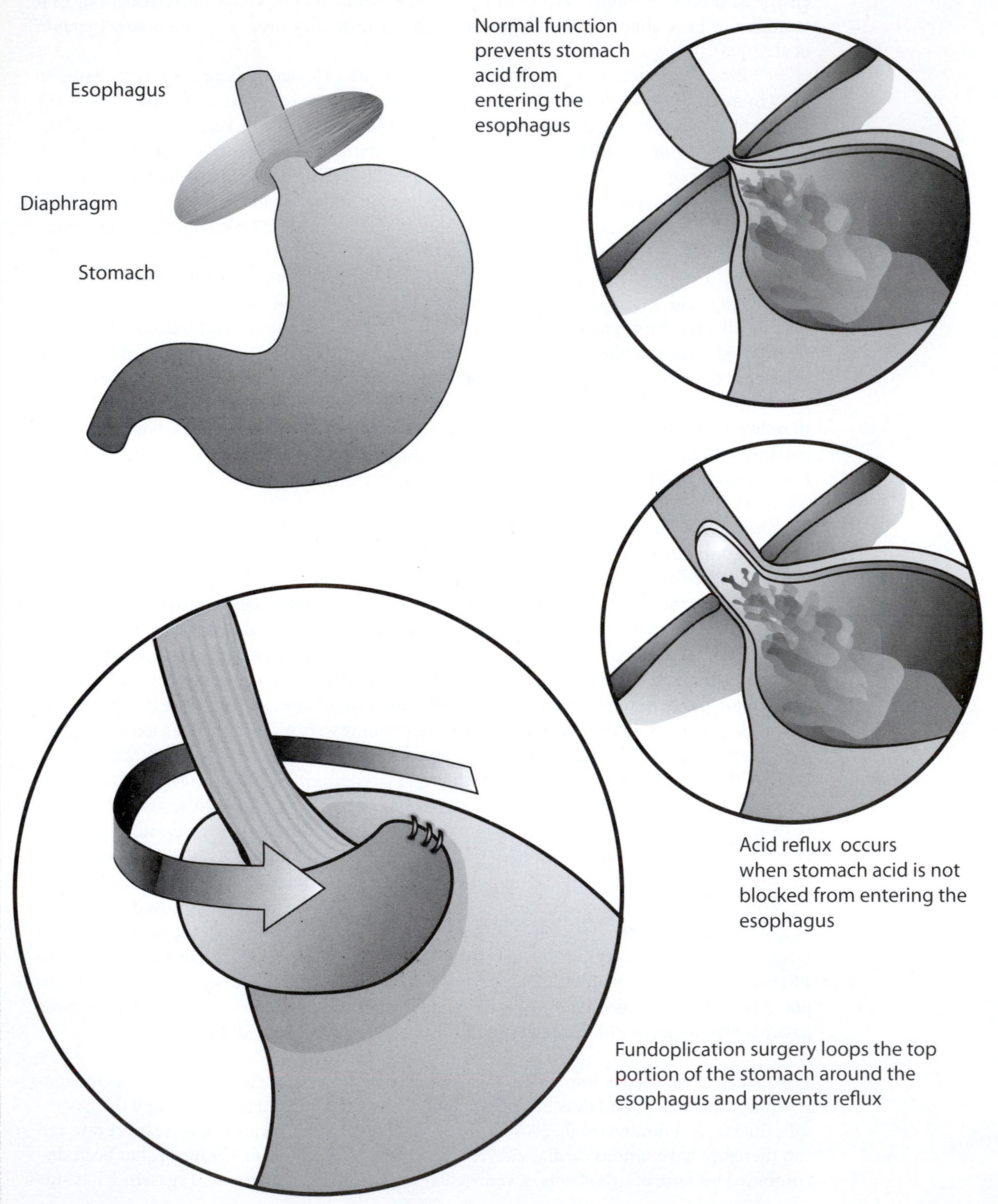

effects including angina, myocardial infarction, and stroke and was temporarily withdrawn from the U.S. market in March 2007. However, as of July 2007 it is now permitted for restricted use in irritable bowel syndrome or chronic idiopathic constipation in women younger than 55 who are in critical need with no heart disease.

Surgery. Surgery is the only option for completely eliminating gastric reflux. Laryngopharyngeal manifestations of reflux disease are more resistant to conservative treatment and often require more surgical therapy (Stavroulaki, 2006). The surgical procedure of choice for GERD/LPR is **Nissen fundoplication**, named after the doctor who first performed it in the 1950s. The procedure, which can be done laparoscopically or with an open approach, involves wrapping (plicating) the gastric fundus (upper part of the stomach) around the inferior portion of the esophagus and suturing it in place. Thus, whenever the stomach contracts it also blocks off the esophagus, preventing the backflow of contents (see Figure 6.6).

Reportedly, around 80–90% of patients are asymptomatic or have minimal symptoms following either conventional open or laparoscopic fundoplication (Edmunds et al., 2007). Westcott et al. (2004) reported that patients with LPR who presented with a variety of laryngeal disorders and who did not respond to other forms of medical treatment demonstrated improved postsurgery RSI, RFS, and quality of life scores.

In addition to fundoplication, other endoscopic techniques have become available since 2000. These techniques attempt to tighten or thicken the area near the gastroesophageal junction. FDA-approved therapies include EndoCinch (endoscopic suturing of the junction), the Stretta procedure (delivery of radiofrequency energy to the junction), and Enteryx (injection of a substance into the junction). Enteryx, however, has been recalled because complications have been reported such as the injection going through the esophageal wall and penetrating into the chest cavity.

Inflammatory Autoimmune Diseases

Autoimmune diseases are those caused by the body's aberrant response to its own cells. There are several autoimmune inflammatory diseases that affect the larynx, including systemic lupus erythematosus, relapsing polychondritis, and rheumatoid arthritis.

SYSTEMIC LUPUS ERYTHEMATOSUS

Systemic lupus erythematosus (SLE) is a progressive disorder that damages connective tissues, blood vessels, and mucous membranes (Ozcan et al., 2007). Around one-third of individuals with this disease have been reported to show laryngeal involvement including inflammation, infection, subglottic stenosis, and epiglottitis (Teitel, Mackenzie, Stern, & Paget, 1992). As the disease progresses the vocal fold mucosa may become thickened and scarring may result from the inflammation (Smith, Ward, & Berci, 1978). Cricoarytenoid arthritis occurs relatively commonly in conjunction with SLE, and recurrent laryngeal nerve damage with resulting vocal fold paralysis has also been reported (Schwartz & Grishman, 1980). Laryngeal symptoms range in severity from mild hoarseness to life-threatening airway obstruction (Ozcan et al., 2007; Tsunoda & Soda, 1996). Treatment is usually administration of systemic corticosteroids, which have been reported to be effective in reducing laryngeal symptoms (e.g., Ozcan et al., 2007; Tsunoda & Soda, 1996).

RELAPSING POLYCHONDRITIS

Relapsing polychondritis (RP) is characterized by recurring episodes of inflammation of connective tissues, particularly affecting the cartilages of the ears, nose, larynx, trachea, eyes, heart valves, kidneys, and blood vessels (Bandi, Munnur, & Braman, 2002). This disorder occurs often in conjunction with rheumatoid arthritis and other connective tissue diseases. When the larynx, trachea, and bronchi are involved, the disease can be very serious, because the supporting cartilages of these structures collapse, causing respiratory problems. In fact, the death rate after five years of suffering from this illness is close to 30% (*The Merck Manual*, 2005, www.merck.com/pubs/mmanual/section5/chapter50/50d.htm).

RP is more prevalent in females than males, and its peak onset is in the middle years, although younger and older individuals have been reported as having it. Fifty percent of individuals with this disease have laryngeal symptoms that result in hoarseness and even aphonia, and can also lead to airway problems (Shirley, 1999). Other laryngeal symptoms include tenderness and swelling over the thyroid cartilage, cough, dyspnea, wheezing, and choking (Bandi et al., 2002; Shirley, 1999). The most serious aspect of the disease is airway obstruction, which can result due to subglottic edema, laryngeal and tracheal ring collapse, or tracheomalacia. It has been reported that 50% of related deaths occur from airway complications. Treatment is typically corticosteroids and immune system suppressants (Bandi et al., 2002).

RHEUMATOID ARTHRITIS

Rheumatoid arthritis (RA) is a relatively common chronic inflammatory autoimmune disease that affects around 1% of the population in North America (Segebarth & Limbird, 2007). The disease disrupts the normal structure and function of synovial joints by infiltrating the joints with immune and inflammatory cells (Tanoue, 1998). The cricoarytenoid and cricothyroid joints are true synovial joints and are therefore also subject to arthritis (Koufman, 1996; Kumai, Murukami, Masuda, & Yumoto, 2007; Stemple et al., 2000). Cricoarytenoid arthritis is fairly common, but it may not be recognized because the symptoms are nonspecific, typically are subclinical, and tend to manifest only with increased exertion or with an upper respiratory infection (Bandi et al., 2002; Berjawi et al., 2009; Brunner & Chirayath, 2010). Only around 12–33% of patients with RA demonstrate overt clinical signs of laryngeal involvement. Laryngeal signs include posterior laryngeal inflammation, decreased arytenoid mobility, and dysphonia (Koufman, 1996; Speyer et al., 2008). Kumai et al. (2007) reported that the presence of laryngeal involvement in RA has ranged from 13–75% in various clinical studies and between 45–88% in postmortem reports. However, in some patients with RA the CA joint is the most severely involved, and CA joint involvement may occur early in the course of the disease while other joints are not yet affected (Tanoue, 1998).

Cricoarytenoid joint arthritis usually goes through acute and chronic phases. In the acute phase, the vocal folds are inflamed, the synovial membrane is thickened, and the arytenoid cartilages look swollen and red (Brunner & Chirayath, 2010; Buckmire, 2006; Stemple et al., 2000; Tanoue, 1998). Pain is common during this stage of the disease, accompanied by the sensation of a foreign body in the throat, possible dysphagia and stridor, and hoarseness (Bandi et al., 2002; Segebarth & Limbird, 2007; Woo, Mendelsohn, & Humphrey, 1995). These symptoms may be exacerbated by speaking (Woo et al., 1995). As the disease progresses and becomes chronic, the articular surfaces of the joints (the locations where the joints articulate) are destroyed, and the joint space becomes filled in with vascular, fibrous, and fatty tissue (Buckmire, 2006). The arytenoid mucosa look rough and thickened, but pain is not usual at this stage and the individual may be asymptomatic (Segebarth & Limbird, 2007). The soft tissues surrounding the joint may also exhibit rheumatoid signs, including rheumatoid nodules or bamboo nodes (Speyer et al., 2008). These nodes or nodules are not uniform, but may appear as white submucosal nodules, polypoid lesions, or as ill-defined masses deep within the vocal folds (Buckmire, 2006; Koufman, 1996).

The symptoms of CA joint difficulties depend on whether the problem is unilateral or bilateral, the degree of joint fixation, and the position of the immobilized vocal fold or folds. Symptoms may range from mild dysphonia to aspiration and even acute airway compromise. The individual may be hoarse, may complain of a laryngeal fullness feeling, and may describe pain associated with inflammation of the joint. In more severe cases the joint may be completely fixed (**ankylosed**) and imitate the appearance of a vocal fold paralysis.

While considerable attention has been paid to the cricoarytenoid joints in rheumatoid arthritis, the cricothyroid (CT) joints have received less attention. This joint is also a true synovial joint, making it susceptible to rheumatoid changes (Berjawi et al., 2009). Involvement of the CT joint can result in a loss of pitch range with limited ability to project the voice (Berjawi et al., 2009). Berjawi et al. (2009) reported a prevalence of CT joint involvement in more than 90% of their patients with rheumatoid arthritis.

Diagnosis and Evaluation. Accurate diagnosis of cricoarytenoid arthritis is critical, because joint fixation resulting from RA can mimic vocal fold paralysis. Direct laryngoscopy is the standard for clinical assessment and definitive diagnosis as it allows evaluation of the vocal fold mucosal lining and laryngeal biomechanics (Berjawi et al., 2009; Buckmire, 2006). One laryngoscopic sign that helps to differentiate between joint fixation and vocal fold paralysis is lateral bowing of the vocal folds on inspiration in joint fixation. This is an uncommon finding in laryngeal paralysis (Buckmire, 2006). High-resolution CT scanning can be helpful in evaluating the integrity of the laryngeal cartilages and joints (Berjawi et al., 2009). However, CT scanning may be limited depending on the extent of ossification of the laryngeal cartilage and the plane and thickness of the CT sections (Buckmire, 2006). In addition, electromyography of the thyroarytenoid, cricothyroid, and posterior cricoarytenoid muscles can help to clarify whether the immobility is due to paralysis or joint fixation. Patients with a normal pattern of laryngeal muscle activation and recruitment are likely to have CA joint fixation rather than vocal fold paralysis.

Treatment. Acute CA rheumatoid arthritis is typically treated medically with anti-inflammatory and pain medications (Tanoue, 1998). Systemic steroid therapy or local steroid injections may also be prescribed. Vocal rest, local heat, and humidification may give the patient some temporary relief. Surgery may also be an option. If the CA joint is dislocated rather than fixed, the surgeon can relocate the displaced arytenoid in a manner similar to the treatment for a dislocated knee or shoulder (Buckmire, 2006). If the joint is completely fixed and immovable, surgical techniques are designed to improve the patient's airway. Standard surgical approaches include transverse laser cordotomy, partial cordectomy, arytenoidectomy, lateralization procedures, and tracheotomy.

chapter SUMMARY

WOUND HEALING REFERS TO the repair of a tissue that has been injured or damaged through infection, trauma, neoplasms, or illness. Wound healing is a complex physiological mechanism encompassing three major stages: inflammation, extracellular matrix (ECM) cell proliferation, and scar remodeling. The end of the wound healing process may be a scar. Vocal fold scarring can result from any number of causes including viral or bacterial infection, trauma, neoplasms, endotracheal intubation, caustic or thermal burns, radiation therapy, vocal fold surgery, inflammatory diseases, and phonotrauma. Vocal fold scar is often associated with sulcus vocalis, which is a groove on the medial surface of one or both vocal folds. The groove may be shallow, confined to the cover of the folds, or deep, extending into the vocal ligament. The groove has the effect of tethering the epithelium to the vocal ligament. The dysphonia resulting from vocal fold scar and sulcus vocalis is characterized by symptoms of glottal insufficiency including breathiness, roughness, loss of pitch range, loss of volume, vocal fatigue, inability to project the voice, irregular vocal breaks, effortful phonation, diplophonia, and aphonia. Treatment for scar and/or sulcus vocalis may be behavioral, surgical, or a combination.

Laryngitis refers to any inflammation of the larynx. Inflammation can be acute or chronic. Causes of laryngitis include viral, bacterial and fungal infections, phonotrauma, smoking, allergies, acid reflux, radiation treatment for head and neck tumors, autoimmune problems and parasitic infections. Gastroesophageal reflux disease (GERD) and laryngopharyngeal reflux (LPR) are common causes of laryngeal inflammation and have been shown to be the cause of or to contribute to many laryngeal and nonlaryngeal problems. Diagnosis and evaluation of LPR is based on a variety of measures including clinical signs and symptoms, laryngoscopy, and pH monitoring. The reflux finding score and reflux symptom index are widely used evaluation tools for laryngopharyngeal reflux. Treatment of GERD and/or LPR is aimed at reducing acid levels by behavioral changes in diet and lifestyle, by pharmacological means such as antireflux medications or prokinetic agents, or by surgery in severe cases.

There are several autoimmune inflammatory diseases that affect the larynx, including systemic lupus erythematosus, relapsing polychondritis, and rheumatoid arthritis (RA). RA disrupts the normal structure and function of synovial joints including the cricoarytenoid and cricothyroid joints by infiltrating the joints with immune and inflammatory cells. The symptoms of CA joint difficulties depend on whether the problem is unilateral or bilateral, the degree of joint fixation, and the position of the immobilized vocal fold or folds. Symptoms may range from mild dysphonia to aspiration and even acute airway compromise. In more severe cases the joint may be completely fixed (ankylosed) and imitate the appearance of a vocal fold paralysis. Direct laryngoscopy allows evaluation of the vocal fold mucosal lining and laryngeal biomechanics. Electromyography of the thyroarytenoid, cricothyroid, and posterior cricoarytenoid muscles can help to clarify whether vocal fold immobility is due to paralysis or joint fixation. Acute CA rheumatoid arthritis is typically treated medically with anti-inflammatory and pain medications as well as steroids. Vocal rest, local heat, and humidification may provide some temporary relief. If the joint is completely fixed and immovable, surgical techniques are designed to improve the patient's airway.

review QUESTIONS

1. Describe the three primary stages involved in wound healing.
2. Explain how inflammation may result in a vocal fold scar and/or sulcus vocalis.
3. Discuss the various behavioral and surgical techniques used to treat vocal fold scar/sulcus vocalis.
4. Differentiate between acute and chronic forms of laryngitis.
5. Compare and contrast the causes, signs and symptoms, and diagnostic and treatment approaches for GERD and LPR.
6. Describe the clinical signs and symptoms of cricoarytenoid arthritis.
7. Explain the importance of differential diagnosis and treatment of cricoarytenoid joint fixation and vocal fold paralysis.

Chapter 7
Structural Lesions of the Larynx

LEARNING OBJECTIVES

1. Identify causes, symptoms, and treatment of laryngomalacia.
2. Compare the causes and symptoms of congenital versus acquired subglottic stenosis.
3. Describe surgical techniques for subglottic stenosis and understand the effects of surgery on voice quality.
4. Appreciate different degrees of laryngeal webbing and their effects on respiratory and vocal function.
5. Differentiate between laryngoceles and laryngeal cysts.
6. Understand the viral nature of recurrent respiratory papillomatosis.
7. Distinguish between juvenile and adult onset of papillomatosis in terms of severity and recurrence.
8. Describe surgical and adjuvant treatments for recurrent respiratory papillomatosis.

Structural lesions of the larynx can occur in any of the tissues of the larynx and vocal folds. These lesions have a wide variety of causes including congenital conditions, injury, systemic disease, infectious and inflammatory conditions, and phonotrauma. Lesions can interfere with phonation by affecting the mass of the vocal folds, their stiffness characteristics, the mucosal wave, and vocal fold approximation. Some structural disorders interfere more with respiration than with phonation, and some affect both functions. Feeding and swallowing can also be affected. This chapter considers the disorders of laryngomalacia, subglottic stenosis, glottic stenosis/laryngeal web, laryngoceles, cysts, and recurrent respiratory papillomatosis. These conditions may be congenital or acquired in later life through trauma, infection, illness, and/or systemic disease. Other structural tissue changes such as nodules, polyps, Reinke's edema, leukoplakia, ulcers, and granulomas are typically associated with vocal behaviors related to lifestyle and personality factors, and they are discussed in Chapter 8.

Laryngomalacia

Laryngomalacia is a relatively common, usually congenital laryngeal disorder, making up 75% of all congenital laryngeal abnormalities (Andrews, 1995). The condition is characterized by pathologically soft and flexible supraglottic cartilages, particularly the epiglottis. Three structural abnormalities are typically associated with this condition (Figure 7.1). First, the epiglottis tends to be elongated and omega-shaped, rather than broad and flat (Sesterhenn et al., 2009). Second, the aryepiglottic folds are unusually short, pulling the epiglottis toward the laryngeal lumen (Sesterhenn et al., 2009; Valera, Tamashiro, De Araujo, Sander, & Kupper, 2006). Third, the arytenoid cartilages may appear enlarged due to an excessive amount of overlying bulky tissue (Fajdiga, Beden, Krivec, & Uglic, 2008; Kuo-Sheng, Bo-Nien, Cheng-Chien, & Yu-Chun, 2007; Manning, Inglis, Mouzakes, Carron, & Perkins, 2005; Rye, 2000; Sesterhenn et al., 2009; Valera et al., 2006).

The excessive tissue may cause the arytenoid cartilages to collapse downward and anteriorly (Manning et al., 2005). The vocal folds themselves are not affected, and the primary problem is respiratory in nature. Because the aryepiglottic folds do not have enough firmness to withstand the negative pressures created by inspiration, they are sucked inward and collapse as the child inhales (Fajdiga et al., 2008). This causes the airway to be obstructed.

FIGURE 7.1 **Laryngomalacia**

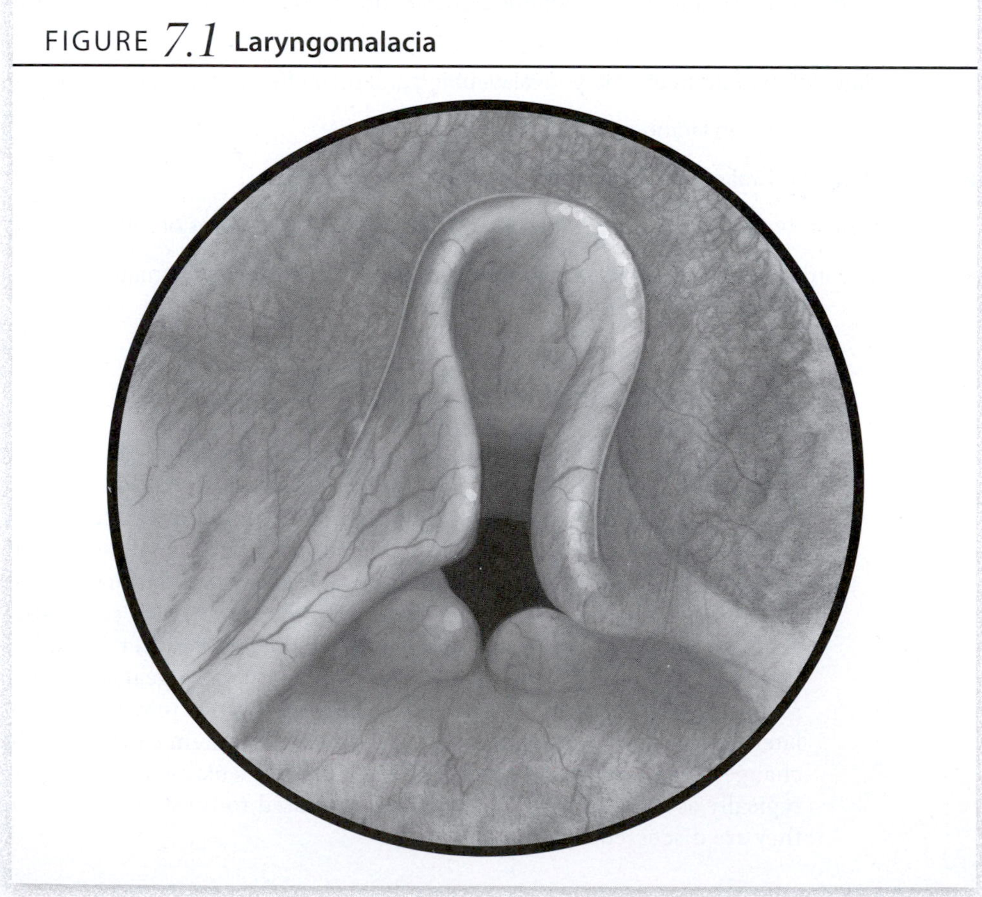

CAUSE

The cause of laryngomalacia is not known with certainty, but proposed explanations include structural anomalies of the laryngeal cartilages and aryepiglottic folds, lack of neuromuscular coordination, and gastroesophageal reflux disease (GERD) (Manning et al., 2005). Laryngomalacia and GERD both may result from low muscle tone in the upper aerodigestive tract (Manning et al., 2005). Other associations between laryngomalacia and GERD may also exist. For example, if the child's airway is significantly obstructed, the resulting difficulty in breathing can create a high amount of abdominal pressure, which can either cause reflux or worsen existing reflux. Conversely, existing reflux can worsen the airway obstruction, because the acidic contents of the refluxate can further irritate and inflame the laryngeal tissues and increase the amount of secretions and mucus that is already present. GERD has been documented in around 80% of patients with laryngomalacia (Richter & Thompson, 2008). It is important to take into account the link between laryngomalacia and GERD, because if the reflux is not treated and persists or recurs after surgery, the child's condition will not be alleviated.

Laryngomalacia has also been related to brain injury, seizure disorder, and cerebral palsy (Manning et al., 2005). In around 17–47% of cases the disorder occurs in conjunction with other problems such as **tracheomalacia** (collapse of the tracheal walls), vocal fold paralysis, weakness of the pharyngeal muscles, and subglottic stenosis (Valera et al., 2006). Isolated laryngomalacia is usually self-limiting and resolves spontaneously by age 2 or 3 years (Fajdiga et al., 2008; Rawlings, Derkay, Chu, & John, 2009; Sesterhenn et al., 2009; Unal et al., 2006).

SYMPTOMS

The symptoms of laryngomalacia depend on the degree of airway obstruction. Symptoms range from a slight amount of stridor (noisy breathing) on inhalation to cyanosis (a condition in which the skin turns blue or purplish due to a lack of oxygen), retraction of the chest wall, choking, regurgitation after feeding, failure to thrive, and even heart failure (Kuo-Sheng et al., 2007). Swallowing symptoms occur because severe respiratory distress interferes with the infant's ability to feed properly (Richter, Wootten, Rutter, & Thompson, 2009). The primary symptom is inspiratory stridor, which has a high-pitched, harsh quality (Rawlings et al., 2009; Richter & Thompson, 2008). The stridor typically becomes apparent within a few days to months of the infant's life. It becomes worse when the child cries, exerts him- or herself in any way, is laid on his or her back, is feeding, is excited, or has an upper respiratory infection (Fajdiga et al., 2008; Rawlings et al., 2009; Sesterhenn et al., 2009; Valera et al., 2006). It is often worst when the child is around 6 months of age, and then gradually starts to improve.

While most cases of laryngomalacia do resolve spontaneously, the condition occasionally persists to an older age, particularly in children with neuromuscular disorders such as cerebral palsy (Hitchings, Crampsey, & Kubba, 2007). The older child may not show any symptoms until he or she becomes more active and needs to inhale a larger volume of air.

EVALUATION AND TREATMENT

Flexible laryngoscopy is the best way to diagnose and determine the degree of severity of laryngomalacia. Flexible laryngoscopy can also be helpful to assess the infant's feeding (Richter & Thompson, 2008). In more severe cases rigid laryngoscopy or bronchoscopy may be necessary (Richter & Thompson, 2008). For a child with severe GERD and/or LPR, swallowing studies may be indicated (Richter & Thompson, 2008).

As the larynx matures and the cartilages become more stable, most children grow out of this condition and typically, no formal therapy is necessary (Kuo-Sheng et al., 2007; Sesterhenn et al., 2009). For a child with mild stridor there are a few simple strategies that parents may use to help the child breathe more easily. For example, children with this condition often do better if they lie on their stomach rather than their back. Feeding should also be done in an upright position, and some otolaryngologists suggest holding the child upright for half an hour after feeding. In mild cases, what Goberman and Robb (2005) termed "watchful waiting" is the treatment of choice as long as the child continues to thrive. However, an estimated 5–20% of children with laryngomalacia show severe or progressive worsening of airway difficulties (Manning et al., 2005; Rawlings et al., 2009). Such difficulties may include dyspnea (difficulty breathing) that is present either at rest and/or during effort; obstructive sleep apnea syndrome (episodes when the child stops breathing during sleep, associated with frequent awakening and daytime sleepiness); **hypoxia** (abnormally low oxygen levels) or **hypercapnia** (abnormally high carbon dioxide levels); pulmonary hypertension; difficulty in swallowing; failure to thrive; and general delay in neurological maturation and motor development. For these children, surgical treatment is necessary (Rawlings et al., 2009; Valera et al., 2006).

Supraglottoplasty. Until the 1980s, the standard procedure for severe laryngomalacia was tracheostomy (O'Donnell et al., 2007). Since that time a variety of techniques known collectively as **supraglottoplasty** have been developed. These are endoscopic techniques that may involve fixating the epiglottis to prevent it from being pulled inward (called **epiglottopexy**), and/or removing excess tissue to enlarge the airway (O'Donnell, Murphy, Bew, & Knight, 2007; Rawlings et al., 2009; Valera et al., 2006). A technique that is currently popular is the CO_2 laser supraglottoplasty. In this procedure the aryepiglottic folds are divided and the excess arytenoid tissue is vaporized (e.g., Rawlings et al., 2009; Sesterhenn et al., 2009). Cold steel microinstruments such as microscissors or microdebriders may also be used to remove the excess arytenoid tissue (Groblewski, Shah, & Zalzal, 2009; Rawlings et al., 2009; Valera et al., 2006; Whymark, Clement, Kubba, & Geddes, 2006).

Supraglottoplasties have been shown to be safe and effective in relieving stridor and other airway symptoms, as well as swallowing problems such as aspiration (e.g., Groblewski et al., 2009; Richter et al., 2009; Sesterhenn et al., 2009). In the case of isolated laryngomalacia, most patients are able to return home the day following the procedure. However, as with any type of laryngeal surgery, complications may occur. These include **synechias** (adhesions between the margins of the vocal folds, particularly at the anterior commissure), granulomas, scarring, and supraglottic stenoses (Rawlings et al., 2009). When successful, the surgery can prevent the necessity for a tracheotomy, help to resolve feeding problems, and overcome the child's failure to thrive (Whymark et al., 2006). However, the procedure is less likely to be effective when the child has coexisting neurological or structural deficits, or when the procedure is necessary earlier than two months of age (Hoff, Schroeder, Rastatter, & Holinger, 2010).

In order to maximize the chances of a successful outcome, it is recommended that all patients undergoing surgery be treated for GERD both prior to the procedure and in the immediate postoperative period as well (Richter & Thompson, 2008).

Subglottic Stenosis

Stenosis refers to the narrowing or constricting of an orifice. The airway can be narrowed along any point, but stenosis is most common in the subglottic cricoid area because that is the narrowest and least expandable point of the airway in both adults and children. Subglottic stenosis, thus, is defined as a narrowing of the airway between the glottis and the first tracheal ring (Figure 7.2).

The condition can be either congenital or acquired through various causes, such as infection, GERD, abnormal tissue growth, chronic illness, chronic inflammatory disease, radiation therapy, external trauma, and, most commonly, endotracheal intubation. There is also an idiopathic form of the condition that affects adult women, characterized by inflammation, scarring, and dense fibrosis of the lower larynx and upper tracheal rings (Liberman & Mathisen, 2009; Valdez & Shapshay, 2002; Wright, 2008). Approximately 5% of cases are idiopathic (Damrose, 2008). Regardless of the cause of the stenosis, some type of injury to the delicate epithelial lining of the airway is the precipitating factor (Eaton & Murray, 2006; Rahbar, Valdez, & Shapsay, 2000). Any type of injury to this lining can result in edema, ulcerations, tissue erosion, scarring, and ultimately subglottic stenosis (Baker et al., 2006).

The degree of stenosis is categorized in a staging system called the **Myer-Cotton system** (Myer, O'Connor, & Cotton, 1994). The staging uses rigid endoscopy to evaluate the vertical and radial extent of the airway narrowing (Baker et al., 2006). The percent obstruction is calculated and assigned a grade level (Table 7.1). The Myer-Cotton system is widely used in the pediatric community (Monnier, Ikonomidis, Jaquet, & George, 2009) as well as for adults.

FIGURE 7.2 **Subglottic Stenosis**

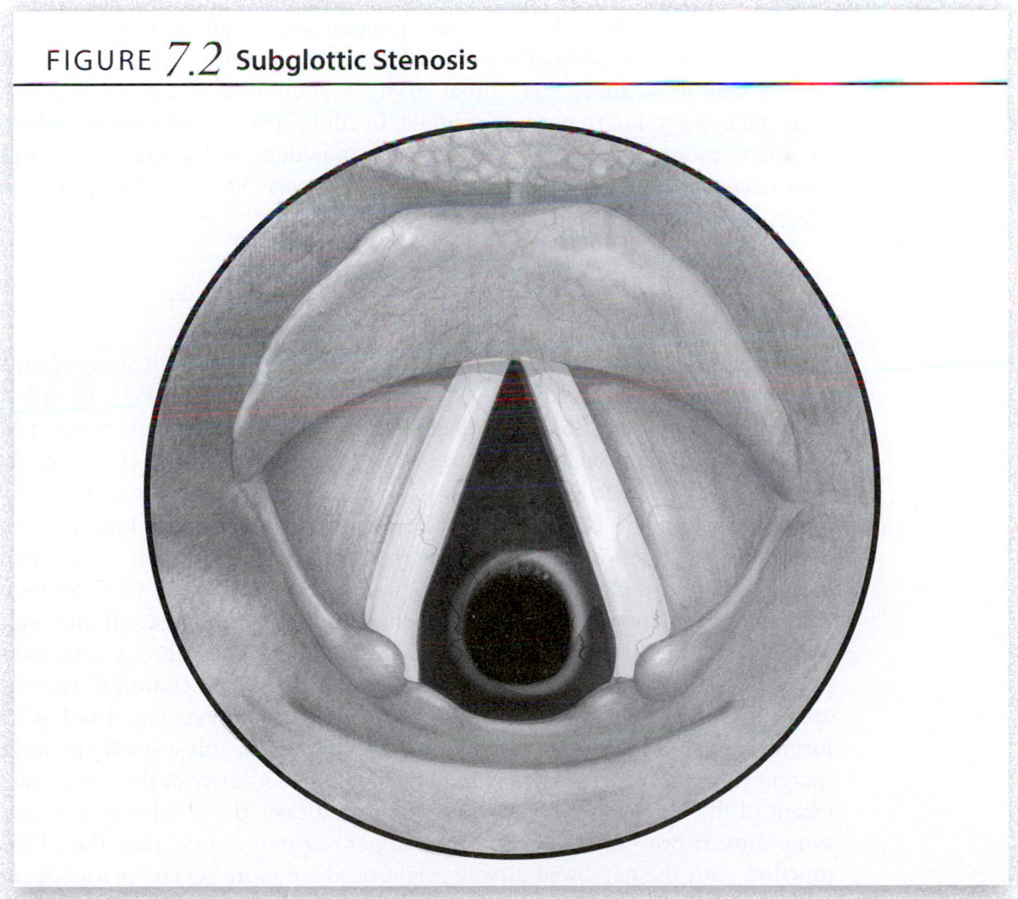

TABLE 7.1 Percentages of Obstruction in Subglottal Stenosis

Grade	Percentage of Obstruction
I	0–50
II	51–70
III	71–99
IV	100

SYMPTOMS

The symptoms of subglottic stenosis are primarily those that indicate airway compromise, although laryngeal symptoms may also be present. Respiratory symptoms include dyspnea, which may occur at rest or on exertion, **tachypnea** (rapid breathing), apnea (absence of breathing), cyanosis, stridor, recurrent pneumonia, cough, recurrent aspiration, and failure to thrive (Baker et al., 2006; Garnett, 2005; Lee, Zhou, Rahn, Wang, & Jiang, 2008; Zawadzka-Glos & Chmielik, 2006). Perceptual laryngeal symptoms in infants may include a weak or high-pitched cry, hoarseness, or aphonia. In adults, perceptual symptoms have been reported as mild to moderate dysphonia, particularly in patients with multiple site stenoses and those who have undergone prior surgery for the stenosis (Ettema, Tolejano Thielke, Toohill, & Merati, 2006).

CONGENITAL SUBGLOTTIC STENOSIS

Subglottic stenosis is considered to be congenital if there is no history of intubation or other acquired causes such as infection or trauma (Garnett et al., 2005). In order for **congenital subglottic stenosis (CSS)** to be diagnosed, the subglottic diameter must be 4 mm or less in a full-term infant or 3.0–3.5 mm or less in a preterm infant (Baker et al., 2006; George, Ikonomidis, Jaquet, & Monnier, 2009). CSS occurs from some kind of problem in embryological development. During normal development the laryngeal lumen is established by the tenth week of gestation (Eaton & Murray, 2006). If for any reason the lumen fails to develop, various degrees of glottic and subglottic stenosis are the result. CSS can be membranous or cartilaginous (George et al., 2009). In **membranous stenosis**, the soft mucosal tissue that lines the inside of the cartilage is thickened due to an increase in fibrous connective tissue, hyperplasia of the mucus glands, or presence of granulation tissue (Eaton & Murray, 2006; Garnett, 2005). **Cartilaginous stenosis** occurs when the cricoid cartilage itself is thickened or deformed, creating a shelf-like plate of cartilage that leaves only a small opening at the posterior margin (Eaton & Murray, 2006; Garnett, 2005). The severity of the condition depends on the extent of the narrowing. For instance, in a mild case, the child may not usually exhibit any symptoms. However, if the child has an upper respiratory infection, the added edema in conjunction with the narrowed airway might produce more severe airway obstruction. A child with a more severe case will present with more symptoms, such as stridor on both inhalation and exhalation, and a hoarse or weak voice. Most children outgrow the condition. However, depending on the cause and whether or not there are any related problems, some individuals will need surgical and/or pharmacological treatment with antibiotics, corticosteroids, and reflux medication.

CSS is often associated with other congenital head and neck problems, such as a small larynx in a patient with Down syndrome (Rutter, 2006). It should also be kept in mind that if a child with a congenital problem requires intubation, there is a high risk of developing an acquired SGS in addition to the underlying congenital anomaly. However, less than 50% of children with CSS need surgical intervention (Lesperance & Zalzal, 1998).

ACQUIRED SUBGLOTTIC STENOSIS

Acquired subglottic stenosis (ASS) may result from numerous causes. Many decades ago, the major causes of ASS were infectious diseases such as syphilis, tuberculosis, typhoid fever, and diphtheria (McClay, 2001). These days, the most prevalent cause of ASS is endotracheal intubation. Intubation occurs whenever an individual undergoes general anesthetic, or in cases of respiratory distress. The subglottic area is vulnerable to intubation trauma because it is the narrowest part of the larynx, and the only portion completely surrounded by cartilage that does not allow for expansion of the airway (Brigger & Hartnick, 2009; Duynstee, De Krijger, Monnier, & Verwoerd, 2002). The endotracheal tube presses against the airway lining, which can result in swelling and irritation. In severe cases the epithelium can become ulcerated with subsequent growth of granulation tissue. The tissues surrounding the cricoid cartilage and the cartilage itself can become inflamed and eventually collapse. When the tissue damage starts to heal it can result in scarring, which, together with the weakened cartilage, narrows or completely closes the lumen. It has been reported that endotracheal intubation is the cause of 90% of ASS cases (Garnett, 2005). One reason for this high number is that increasing numbers of premature infants are surviving. More of these infants need long periods of intubation because of their underdeveloped respiratory systems (Johnson, Rutter, Cotton, Vijayasekeran, & White, 2008). However, while endotracheal intubation is a major source of ASS, the incidence has been decreasing over the past three decades. This is due to improvements in the management of the endotracheal tube, as well as advances in obstetric, neonatal, and pediatric services (Leung & Berkowitz, 2007). The use of synthetic surfactant rather than long-term intubation for premature infants has also contributed to the decrease, as has the use of nasopharyngeal continuous positive airway pressure (Bluestone, 2005; Gustafson et al., 2000). Despite these advances, it has been reported that approximately 25,000 premature babies per year suffer from respiratory distress syndrome and may require some period of prolonged intubation (Kelchner et al., 2010). The most important factor in the development of stenosis in infants is the length of time the child is intubated. **Prolonged intubation** typically refers to a time period greater than 14 days, but injury to the tracheal epithelium has been reported to occur less than 17 hours after intubation (Baker et al., 2006; Garnett, 2005). Other risk factors include the size of the endotracheal tube; increased motion of the tube, which can cause abrasion and trauma to the mucosa; repeated or traumatic intubations; birth weight less than 1,500 g; infection; compromised immune status; presence of nasogastric tubes; and reflux (Zawadzka-Glos & Chmielik, 2006). Because the size of the tube can impact the respiratory epithelium, it is important that the tube be as small in diameter as possible, while still allowing the infant to breathe properly (Rutter, 2006).

EVALUATION

When the child with severe subglottic stenosis is very young, the initial evaluation focuses on the extent of the stenosis and airway obstruction, determined by means of x-rays, MRI scans, and videostrobolaryngoscopy. Both flexible and rigid endoscopic evaluation, as well as laryngoscopy and bronchoscopy under general anesthesia may be necessary (Zawadzka-Glos & Chmielik, 2006; Zur, 2006). The endoscopy is important to identify specific areas of obstruction, the degree of narrowing, the length of the narrowed segment, and any associated pathologies that may be present in addition to the stenosis (Zur, 2006). Pulmonary testing may also be done to determine how the stenosis affects inspiratory and expiratory airflow (Baker et al., 2006). This is important not only for respiration, but also in terms of vocal function. Information regarding restrictions on the child's breathing can help to determine whether the child has adequate respiratory support for speech, including the ability to generate normal loudness levels.

Once the child's airway has been stabilized, an additional evaluation should be conducted to determine the status of the child's vocal function. This process should be a team approach that includes collaboration between speech-language pathologists and pediatric otolaryngologists (De Alarcon et al., 2009). Children with SGS often use supraglottic structures as the primary source of vibration (Baker et al., 2006; Kelchner, de Alarcon, Weinrich, & Brehm, 2009). Therefore an important part of the assessment is to identify the specific vibration source and vibratory patterns used by the child (Table 7.2).

Other compensatory strategies should also be noted, such as inspiratory phonation. This is not uncommon in patients who have been tracheotomized, as is quite often the case in children with severe subglottic stenosis. With a tracheotomy tube in place, vocal fold vibration occurs on inhalation rather than exhalation. Once the child has been decannulated, this pattern may persist as a learned motor behavior (Baker et al., 2006). If the child has a tracheotomy

TABLE 7.2 **Vibratory Sources and Patterns of Supraglottic Compression in Children with Subglottal Stenosis**

Vibratory Source
True vocal folds only
False vocal folds only
True and false vocal folds
False vocal folds and prolapsed arytenoid cartilages against epiglottic petiole
Arytenoid cartilage to contralateral false vocal fold
Arytenoid cartilage to epiglottic petiole and contralateral vocal fold
Arytenoid cartilage to epiglottis
Patterns of Supraglottic Compression
Lateral-medial
Anterior-posterior
Mixed

Sources: Information from Baker et al. (2006); Kelchner et al. (2009); Krival et al. (2007).

at the time of the evaluation, the assessment should also determine whether he or she is able to phonate with the tracheotomy tube covered, the child's ability to tolerate and phonate with a Passy-Muir valve, and use of any form of alternative communication (Baker et al., 2006). The presence of stridor during crying, breathing, or babbling should also be documented. An important part of the evaluation process is to identify any handicapping effects of the child's voice on his or her daily functioning, using a validated quality of life instrument such as the pVHI.

SURGICAL TREATMENT

Surgery is the primary treatment for subglottic stenosis, whether congenital or acquired. Treatment initially focuses on establishing a functional airway, safe swallowing, and some kind of voicing if possible. In severe cases, the child may need a tracheotomy while the otolaryngologist and other professionals determine the best type of treatment. The type of treatment depends on the severity of the obstruction. Milder cases (e.g., Grades I and II) can usually be treated endoscopically with CO_2 laser, while more severe obstruction will more likely be treated with open surgical techniques (Bakthavachalam & McClay, 2008). Laser treatment (Figure 7.3) has the advantage of improving the airway without causing significant bleeding or edema.

Endoscopic treatment is not indicated when there is excessive scar tissue more than 1 cm in length, exposed perichondrium or cartilage after previous laser treatment, previous attempts at endoscopic repair, loss of cartilage, or severe infection (Eaton & Murray, 2006; Zawadzka-Glos & Chmielik, 2006). In these cases, open surgery is necessary. Whether endoscopic or open, surgical techniques focus on removing the obstruction, enlarging the airway, and maintaining a functional voice.

The degree of stenosis in ASS tends to be more severe than that in CSS (Zawadzka-Glos & Chmielik, 2006), and treatment therefore needs to be more aggressive. In fact, many more children require a tracheotomy for ASS, as well as endoscopic removal of granulation tissue. It is very important that any underlying and/or coexisting conditions be treated in conjunction with endoscopic or open surgery. In particular, gastric reflux can exacerbate the problem (Eaton & Murray, 2006). Many otolaryngologists feel that the reflux should be treated before surgery is attempted. Halstead (cited in http://www.utmb.edu/otoref/Grnds/Subgot-sten-9904/Subglot-sten-9904.htm) showed that when antireflux therapy was used, several children whose previous surgeries had not been successful were successfully operated on and decannulated.

Laryngotracheal Reconstruction. Surgical procedures include an array of techniques collectively known as **laryngotracheal reconstruction (LTR)** (Table 7.3). These are highly complex techniques that include resection (cutting or excising) of various portions of cartilage, with or without the incorporation of grafts and stents (Syal, Tyagi, & Goyal, 2006). Techniques are classified as splits, augmentations, and resections (Eaton & Murray, 2006). Because the surgical procedures are so complex, LTR requires a team approach and close collaboration of pediatric specialists including the otolaryngologist, intensive care specialist, anesthetist, gastroenterologist, respiratory physician, dietician, and speech-language pathologist, as well as strong parental understanding and support (Agrawal, Black, & Morrison, 2007).

Anterior Cricoid Split. The **anterior cricoid split (ACS)** is designed to widen the cricoid cartilage by making an incision through the first two tracheal rings, cricoid cartilage, and the bottom one-third of the thyroid cartilage. To stabilize and maintain the wider lumen, an endotracheal tube is inserted to act as a stent for 7–14 days postoperatively. The ACS technique is most often used in cases of congenital SGS due either to a small cricoid ring or to localized

FIGURE 7.3 **Laser Treatment for Subglottic Stenosis**

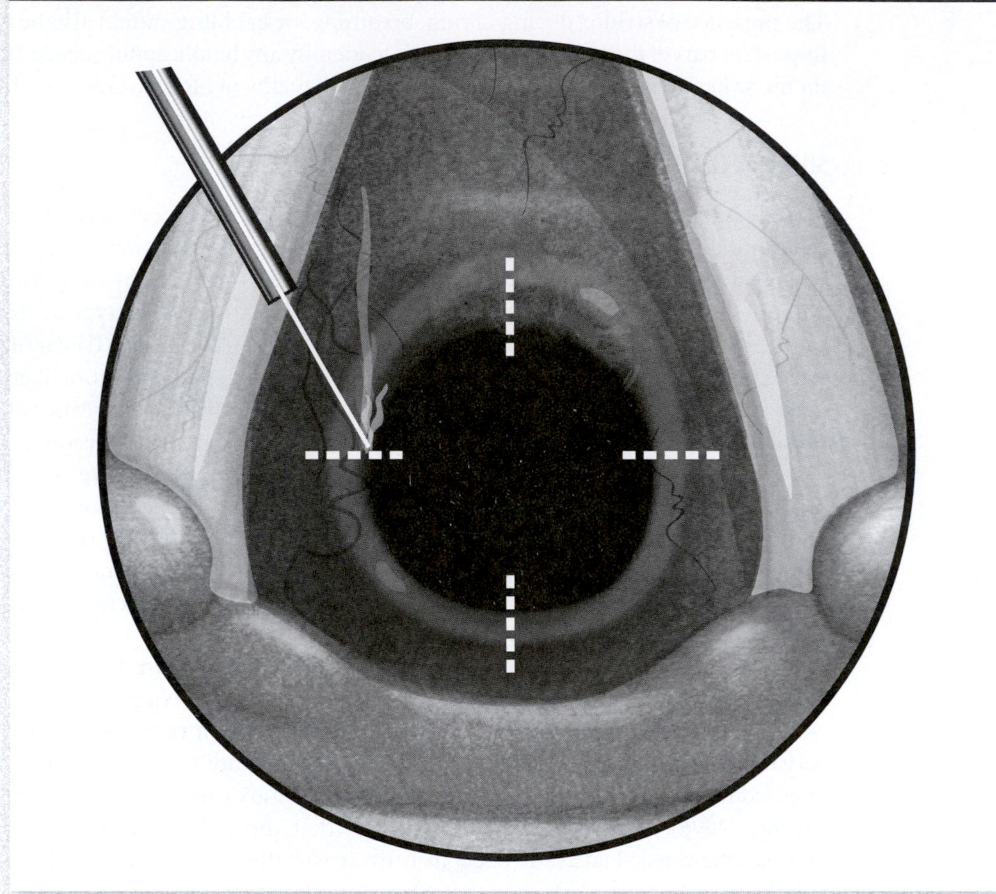

TABLE 7.3 **Types of Laryngotracheal Reconstruction Techniques**

Anterior cricoid split
Augmentation
Anterior cricoid
Posterior cricoid
Anterior and posterior cricoid
Single stage
Staged
Cricotracheal resection

fibrosis with a normal cartilage in infants who have not been able to be extubated (Eaton & Murray, 2006). The success of this procedure may depend on the length of time the child has been intubated. Rotenberg and Berkowitz (2006) found that patients who had successful ACS procedures had an average of 4.1 weeks of prior intubation, whereas those whose procedures failed had a longer duration of around 11 weeks. In addition, they reported higher numbers of failures in infants with concomitant complex medical conditions.

Augmentation Procedures. **Augmentation procedures** are necessary when the laryngeal framework requires widening greater than 3 mm (Eaton & Murray, 2006). The technique involves splitting the laryngotracheal framework and expanding the narrowed segment using various combinations of grafts and stents (Agrawal et al., 2007). For the graft, cartilage is taken from elsewhere in the patient's body such as the rib, hyoid bone, thyroid cartilage, or auricular cartilage (Rizzi, Thorne, Zur, & Jacobs, 2009). Synthetic materials such as titanium have also been used successfully (e.g., Daneshi, Mohammadi, & Hassannia, 2009). A split is created surgically in the anterior and/or posterior cricoid (Krival et al., 2007), and the grafted cartilage or synthetic material is inserted between the split. When costal cartilage is used, a 4-cm section of the fifth rib is typically obtained (Fayoux, Vachin, Merrot, & Bernheim, 2006). The larynx may be augmented anteriorly, posteriorly, or both, but the most common is anterior (Eaton & Murray, 2006). When the stenosis is very narrow, a laryngofissure may be done in conjunction with the anterior split. **Laryngofissure** is another type of surgical split that separates the vocal folds at the anterior commissure (Krival et al., 2007). The risk in this procedure is that the vocal folds can be damaged, and any inaccuracy in the procedure can result in the vocal folds being misapproximated with resulting dysphonia. In most cases, however, the graft can be achieved without manipulating the attachment of the vocal folds to the thyroid cartilage (Baker et al., 2006).

Augmentation procedures can be done in one or two stages. A staged augmentation requires the patient to be tracheotomized, and the tracheostomy is maintained postoperatively while the graft is stabilized with an indwelling stent (Agrawal et al., 2007). A further surgical procedure is required to remove the stent once the graft is stable. Currently it has become more common for the surgery to be performed without the postoperative tracheostomy (Agrawal et al., 2007). Instead of an indwelling stent, the child remains intubated with a nasotracheal or orotracheal tube for 5–7 days, and the tube itself acts as a stent that provides stability to the reconstructed airway (Eaton & Murray, 2006; Saunders, Thirlwall, Jacob, & Albert, et al., 1999). This eliminates the necessity for a tracheotomy and subsequent stent removal. However, the prolonged period of intubation can create a risk of complications such as the growth of granulation tissue. The patient may need several endoscopic procedures to remove any such growths (Agrawal et al., 2007). The single-stage procedure is reported to be successful for grades I and II, and selected short-segment grades III (Liew, Blaney, & Morrison, 2003). The staged procedure is recommended for other grade III and IV stenoses. Staged procedures are typically performed when children have more significant and complex medical problems (Agrawal et al., 2007; Saunders et al., 1999). Outcomes for these children are often not as successful, regardless of whether they undergo a single stage or staged procedure, and such patients may require further surgery or even tracheotomy. Agrawal et al. (2007) reported that patients in their study who required both anterior and posterior cartilage grafts had a higher rate of intubation and were more likely to require a tracheotomy than those with a single graft. Depending on the grade of stenosis and the child's medical status, the single-stage procedure is currently one of the best accepted techniques for airway augmentation (Fayoux et al., 2006).

Cricotracheal Resection. **Cricotracheal resection (CTR)** (Figure 7.4) involves cutting away the anterior cricoid arch and the narrowed portion of the subglottic/tracheal region, and connecting the remaining healthy trachea to the thyroid lamina (Baker et al., 2006; Krival et al., 2007). CTR by itself is used for reconstruction of higher grade stenoses (III or IV) when the narrowing is well below the vocal folds (Baker et al., 2006). If the stenosis extends upward and/or includes the vocal folds, the CTR can be combined with an augmentation procedure. For extremely complex airway reconstructions, CTR is often performed as one of many steps toward decannulation, particularly in children with vocal fold dysfunction in addition to the stenosis. Successful outcomes in terms of decannulation have been reported to be as high as 96% with CTR in the United States, England, Mexico, and France (e.g., Ahn, Sung, & Kim, 2004; Alvarez-Neri et al., 2005; Garabedian et al., 2005; White, Cotton, Bean & Rutter, 2005). Thus, CTR has become a preferred method of treatment for high-grade SGS in children, including children under the age of 2 years (e.g., Johnson et al., 2008).

Despite the high success rate, complications may occur after CTR, including destabilization and prolapse of the arytenoids, destabilization of the cricoarytenoid joint, and damage of the PCA ligament resulting from a posterior cricoid split (Baker et al., 2006).

Balloon Dilation. A balloon catheter is a soft hollow tube with an inflatable "balloon" at its tip. This type of device is used to enlarge or dilate/stretch a narrow opening or passage within the body. The deflated balloon catheter is positioned within the target location, and then inflated to perform the desired enlargement. Once the procedure is complete the balloon is deflated and removed. **Balloon dilation** is a less invasive method to treat mild cases of subglottic stenosis, with demonstrated good results (e.g., Axon, Hartley, & Rothera, 1995; Edmondson & Bent, 2010; Lee & Rutter, 2008). This procedure can be used as a preliminary step before open surgery, as an adjunct immediately postsurgery (Brigger & Hartnick, 2009), or may even provide an alternative to cricotracheal resection (Lee & Rutter, 2008).

Vocal Quality Following Surgery. While laryngotracheal reconstruction procedures are very successful in alleviating airway problems, the patient is usually left with a less than desirable voice quality. Some children reportedly demonstrate a normal or near normal voice quality after surgery (e.g., Bailey, Clary, Pengilly, & Albert, 1995). However, most children are left with a voice quality that may be breathy, weak, hoarse, low-pitched, with reduced pitch range, reduced vocal intensity, and abnormal resonance (e.g., Francois, Dumont, & Narcy, 1997; Kelchner et al., 2010; Krival et al., 2007; Smith, Marsh, Cotton, & Myer, 1993; Zalzal, Loomis, Derkay, Murray, & Thomsen, 1991). There are many reasons for the poor voice quality. First, the surgery itself can change the position and movement of the vocal folds. For instance, pitch regulation may be affected by a graft in the anterior portion of the cricoid, which inhibits the action of the cricothyroid muscles; a cricotracheal resection can damage the cricothyroid muscle and obliterate the cricothyroid space (De Alarcon et al., 2009; Krival et al., 2007). A graft in the posterior cricoid region widens the posterior glottis. This can affect the functioning of the interarytenoid muscles, resulting in glottal incompetence. Second, complications of the surgery may occur, such as vocal fold paralysis if the recurrent laryngeal nerve is damaged, prolapse of the base (petiole) of the epiglottis, re-stenosis of the airway, vocal fold fibrosis and scarring, different vertical levels of the vocal folds, blunting of the anterior commissure, cricoarytenoid joint fixation, and anterior or posterior glottal gap (Bailey et al., 1995; Kelchner et al., 2009; Krival et al., 2007). Third, some children use supraglottic structures for phonation both prior to and following surgery, probably as a compensatory strategy (e.g., Bailey et al., 1995; Clary et al., 1996; Rizzi et al., 2009). This seems to be particularly prevalent in patients with

FIGURE 7.4 Cricotracheal Resection

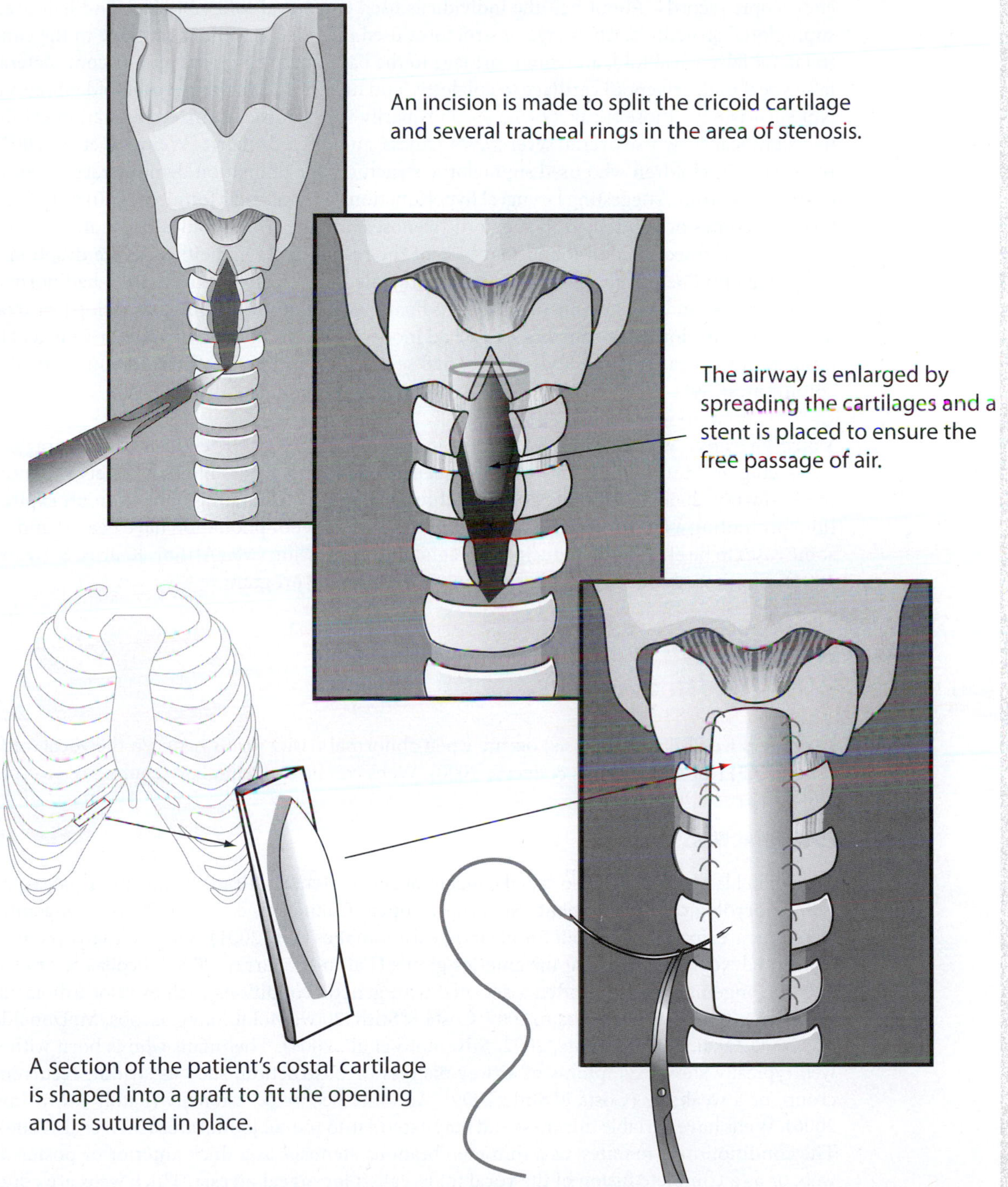

An incision is made to split the cricoid cartilage and several tracheal rings in the area of stenosis.

The airway is enlarged by spreading the cartilages and a stent is placed to ensure the free passage of air.

A section of the patient's costal cartilage is shaped into a graft to fit the opening and is sutured in place.

a higher grade of SGS prior to the laryngotracheal reconstruction (Rizzi et al., 2009). Krival et al. (2007) investigated the records of 16 individuals who had received LTR as children. They assessed the taped voices perceptually and acoustically, as well as analyzing videonaso-endoscopic records. About half the individuals used true vocal fold vibration, and half used supraglottal structures. The range of structures used included arytenoid cartilage to the contralateral false vocal fold, arytenoid cartilage to the base of the epiglottis and/or contralateral false vocal fold, arytenoid cartilage to epiglottis, and mixed true and false vocal fold vibration. Not surprisingly, those speakers who used primarily supraglottic or mixed phonation exhibited significantly worse overall severity, roughness, and pitch deviance. Weinrich et al. (2007) reported that children who used supraglottic structures for phonation demonstrated significantly more strain, suggesting laryngeal hyperfunction. George and Monnier (2010) examined voice outcomes of children with subglottic stenoses ranging from Grades II–IV after partial cricotracheal resection and found that 95% of the respondents had either severe dysphonia or aphonia preoperatively. The questionnaire revealed that postoperatively, 18% had normal voice; 64% had mild dysphonia (described as hoarse voice with some difficulty being heard or understood in a loud environment); 13% had moderate dysphonia (weak voice or ventricular phonation with easy fatigability); and 5% had severe dysphonia (breathy voice and difficulty communicating).

Voice Therapy. Voice therapy is essential in order to minimize the child's use of supraglottic voicing and improve his or her voice quality to the extent possible (e.g., Theis, Connor, & McMurray, 2006; Rizzi et al., 2009). Techniques such as facilitating phonation on expiration, promoting a frontal focus, and encouraging easy onset of phonation have been found in some cases to be effective in reducing supraglottal compression (MacArthur, Kearns, & Healy, 1994). Children should also be involved in a vocal hygiene program.

Laryngeal Web/Glottic Stenosis

Laryngeal web (glottic stenosis) occurs when abnormal tissue forms between the vocal folds (Figure 7.5) (Milczuk, Smith, & Everts, 2000). Webs can be congenital or acquired.

CONGENITAL WEBS

Congenital laryngeal web, also called congenital glottic stenosis, results from abnormal laryngeal embryological development (Men, Ikis, Topcu, Cakmakci, & Ecevit, 2006). Congenital webs are rare, making up about 5% of laryngeal anomalies (Lee, 2001). Seventy-five percent of congenital webs are located at the anterior glottis (Eaton & Murray, 2006; Nicollas & Triglia, 2008). Congenital webs are often associated with genetic conditions such as velocardiofacial syndrome (Cheng & Beckenham, 2009; Costa & Stith, 2009; McElhinney, Jacobs, McDonald-McGinn, Zakai, & Goldmuntz, 2002; Miyamoto et al., 2004). The infant who is born with a web typically shows symptoms of airway distress or obstruction, such as stridor, recurrent croup, or a weak cry (Costa & Stith, 2009). Aphonia occurs occasionally (Eaton & Murray, 2006). Webs have variable thickness and may extend into the subglottal area (Men et al., 2006). The condition may manifest as a thin membranous stenosis, as a thick anterior or posterior web, or as a complete fusion of the vocal folds, called **laryngeal atresia**. Thick webs are composed of dense connective tissue and may even contain muscle fibers and cartilaginous tissue

FIGURE 7.5 Laryngeal Web

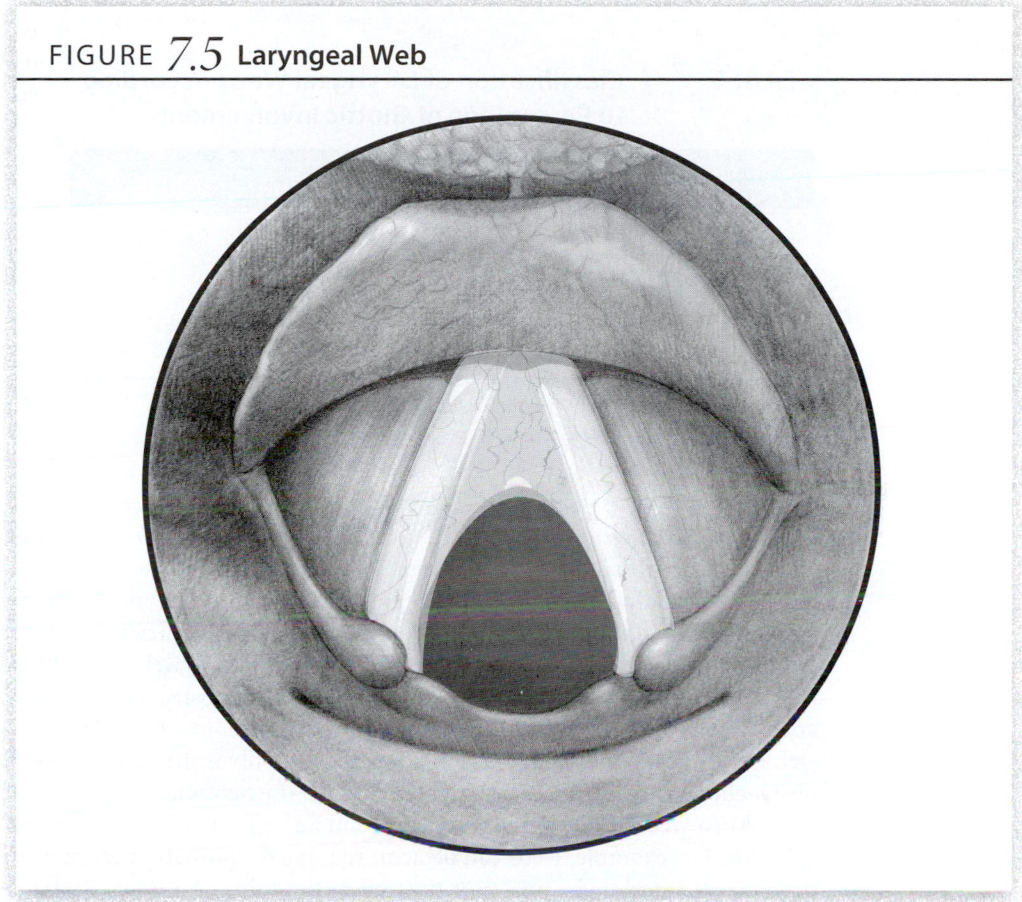

(Cheng & Beckenham, 2009). Congenital laryngeal webs, stenosis, and atresia may represent a continuum of pathology from least to most severe resulting from the failure of the airway to develop normally in the embryo (Wyatt & Hartley, 2005).

Congenital webs can be classified according to four types (Table 7.4). Types 1, 2, and 3 are considered anterior and involve 35% or less of the glottis, 35–50% of the glottis, and 50–75% of the glottis, respectively. Type 4 covers 75–90% of the glottis. In addition, Types 2, 3 and 4 extend into the subglottic space to increasing degrees, causing narrowing of the subglottis (Wyatt & Hartley, 2005). It should be noted, however, that glottic and subglottic stenosis can exist simultaneously when abnormalities of both the glottis and cricoid cartilage are present (Wyatt & Hartley, 2005).

ACQUIRED LARYNGEAL WEBS

Typically, acquired laryngeal webs are located at the anterior commissure and vary in length and thickness. A web can be so small that the person is unaware of its presence, or so extensive that it causes severe airway obstruction. Acquired webs are also classified in four categories ranging from least to most severe in terms of both airway obstruction and voice symptoms

TABLE 7.4 **Classification of Laryngeal Webs According to Percentage of Glottic Involvement**

Type	Percentage of Glottic Involvement
1	up to 35
2	35–50
3	50–75
4	75–90

Source: Information from Wyatt & Hartley (2005).

(Table 7.4). Type I webs are the mildest, involving less than 35% of the glottis. This kind of web is usually thin with a uniform thickness. The airway is adequate, and the individual may have a normal-sounding voice or a mild degree of dysphonia. A Type II web involves 35–50% of the glottis and can vary in thickness from thin to thick. The airway is relatively unobstructed. A Type III web involves 50–75% of the glottis. This kind of web is usually thicker in the front and thins out toward the back. In these cases the airway obstruction is moderate to severe, and vocal dysfunction is typical. Type IV is the most severe, involving 75–90% of the glottis. The web is uniformly thick along its entire length. Not only is the patient aphonic, but the airway obstruction is usually severe enough to require a tracheotomy.

Most webs are acquired from some kind of trauma that irritates and inflames the vocal folds. For example, webs can be acquired due to intubation trauma, and these typically occur on the middle or posterior portion of the folds (Andrews, 1995). Webs can also be acquired following laryngeal surgeries such as removal of papillomas (Holland, Koufman, Postma, & McGuirt, 2009). These webs are usually very small and are called microwebs or synechias (Stemple et al., 2000). A synechia refers to an adhesion between tissue surfaces and occurs when the anterior commissure is irritated and then heals with excess tissue. Other causes include ingestion of caustic material, infections, and foreign bodies (Gerber & Chen, 2009). Webs have also been associated with vocal nodules (Ruiz, Pontes, Behlau, & Richieri-Costa, 2006). Respiratory and vocal symptoms vary depending on the extent and location of the web. The individual may be aphonic or hoarse and stridor and/or dyspnea may be present.

POSTERIOR GLOTTIC STENOSIS

Posterior glottic stenosis (PGS) typically results from prolonged endotracheal intubation (e.g., Chitose, Umeno, & Nakashima, 2009; Liu, Bove, & Nemeth, 2010; Wolf, Primov-Fever, Talmi, & Kronenberg, 2007; Zalzal, 1999). Approximately 15% of patients who are intubated for more than 10 days develop some degree of glottic stenosis resulting from pressure from the endotracheal tube and resulting ulceration of the mucosa (Eaton & Murray, 2006; Mankekar, Eaton, & Murray, 2009). Ulceration is followed by infection, growth of granulation tissue, and formation of a scar. In some cases the individual's cricoarytenoid joint(s) may become ankylosed. Other causes of PGS include ingestion of caustic substances, infections (such as

TABLE 7.5 **Classification of Posterior Glottal Stenosis in Terms of Posterior Commissure and Cricoarytenoid Joint Involvement**

Grade	Posterior Commissure and Cricoarytenoid Joint Involvement
1	Adhesion between vocal processes; normal posterior commissure
2	Posterior stenosis and scarring
3	Posterior stenosis and scarring; unilateral cricoarytenoid joint ankylosis
4	Posterior stenosis and scarring; bilateral cricoarytenoid joint ankylosis

Source: Information from Wolf et al. (2007).

croup), external trauma, laryngeal surgery, and long-term nasogastric intubation (Mankekar et al., 2009). A four-grade classification system is also used for PGS (Table 7.5). Grade 1 is the least extensive and involves adhesion between the vocal processes but a normal posterior commissure. In grade 2 the posterior commissure is stenosed with scarring. Grade 3 includes posterior stenosis with unilateral cricoarytenoid joint ankylosis; grade 4 is the most extensive with posterior stenosis and bilateral cricoarytenoid joint ankylosis (Wolf et al., 2007). Symptoms are primarily those related to respiratory difficulty, such as dyspnea and stridor (Eaton & Murray, 2006).

TREATMENT

Small anterior webs that produce minimal or no symptoms and that are less than 2–3 mm wide do not generally require treatment.

Surgical Treatment. Webs comprising more than 50% of the glottis typically require surgical treatment (Men et al., 2006). The goals of surgery are to establish a stable airway and provide a functional voice (Nicollas & Triglia, 2008). Glottic stenosis and laryngeal webs are usually treated surgically by means of dilation or lysis, either endoscopically or with open surgery. Endoscopic procedures are suitable for thin webs, while thick webs are best treated with an open approach (Nicollas & Triglia, 2008). **Dilation** refers to enlarging an opening or the lumen of a hollow structure. **Lysis** refers to the surgical division of adhesions. Laryngeal webs can be dilated endoscopically with a bronchoscope. However, dilation by itself tends to be successful only in the case of extremely thin membranous webs (Eaton & Murray, 2006). In addition, the procedure itself can result in the formation of scar tissue (Izadi et al., 2010). Other ways of dividing the web include the use of microscissors, knife, or CO_2 laser (e.g., Chitose et al., 2009). Reportedly, however, laser is not beneficial with those patients who have thick webs. Endoscopic lysis by itself has also not been too successful in treating thick webs. A treatment that works better for thick webs is an anterior thyrotomy together with lysis. In this procedure, access to the web is via anterior laryngofissure, and the web is surgically divided (e.g., Wolf et al., 2007). A keel, usually made of silicon, is then inserted between the folds and kept in place for 3–6 weeks. This is done to keep the folds separated to prevent them from healing with a new web. However, there are a few drawbacks to this technique. First, it is an open procedure rather than an endoscopic one, which is more invasive. Second, the keel must be removed surgically once healing has occurred. Another disadvantage is that after the keel is removed, a temporary tracheotomy may be necessary to ensure that the patient has a functioning airway. Thick webs require tracheotomy in approximately 40% of patients with a subsequent open repair (Rutter, 2006).

Voice Therapy. While surgery typically results in a stable airway, the resulting voice quality is often poor, and voice therapy is important. Therapy should focus on identifying any maladaptive compensatory strategies the child is using and substituting more effective ways of voicing. Therapy employing such approaches as vocal hygiene, improving breath support, resonant voice therapy, and vocal function exercises may facilitate the child's best use of his or her laryngeal mechanism.

Laryngoceles and Laryngeal Cysts

Laryngoceles and cysts refer to sacs that are filled either with air (laryngoceles) or fluid (cysts).

LARYNGOCELES

Recall that the laryngeal ventricle is the space between the true and false vocal folds and is filled with mucous and other fluid producing glands. The anterior portion of the ventricle leads upwards into a little pouch called the saccule, and around 60–70 mucous glands open into the saccule (Moorhead, 1991). A **hernia** is the protrusion of a part or structure through the tissues that normally contain it. A **laryngocele** is a dilation or herniation of the saccule extending upward within the false vocal fold (Dursun, Boynukalin, Ozgursoy, & Coruh, 2008). Laryngoceles are usually filled with air, although mucus can also be present. There are three types of laryngoceles, classified according to their relationship to the thyrohyoid membrane: internal, external, and combination. **Internal laryngoceles** are those in which the inflated tissue does not penetrate the thyrohyoid membrane, but instead pushes against the false vocal folds and/or aryepiglottic folds, which consequently look swollen. **External laryngoceles** protrude through the thyrohyoid membrane, forming a bulge or swelling on the side of the individual's neck. A **combination laryngocele** has features of both internal and external types and has been found to be the most common type of laryngocele (Devesa, Ghufoor, & Lloyd, 2002; Thome, Thome, & De La Cortina, 2000).

The cause of laryngoceles is mostly from excessive pressure within the larynx. This can happen when a person engages in activities that require a lot of pressure, such as playing a wind instrument, weight lifting, or habitual excessive coughing due to asthma or smoking. Laryngoceles have also been reported as a possible rare long-term complication following neck surgery (Marom, Roth, & Cinamon, 2010). Most cases occur in males in their midlives, and the condition is characterized by dysphonia and/or a swelling in the neck, as well as dyspnea, cough, inspiratory stridor, dysphagia, and globus (Dursun et al., 2008). A congenital form of laryngocele is also found. Infants with the external type may show symptoms of airway obstruction such as stridor, as well as a weak cry and difficulty feeding.

Diagnosis and Treatment. The best way to diagnose laryngoceles is by CT scan followed, if necessary, by laryngoscopy. Depending on the size of the mass, and the patient's symptoms, the disorder may be left untreated except for periodic observation, or the laryngocele may be aspirated or excised by means of endoscopic CO_2 laser resection or excision by an external approach (e.g., Devesa et al., 2002; Dursun et al., 2007). If the patient is having extreme difficulty breathing, a tracheotomy may be necessary.

LARYNGEAL CYSTS

A cyst is a closed sac filled with fluid or a semisolid substance. Cysts typically occur when glandular secretions and mucus accumulate and are unable to dissipate due to blockage of the sac (Yilmaz, Yildizbas, Yaman, Guclu, & Ozturk, 2010). Cysts are classified as epidermoid or retention, and **laryngeal cysts** can be further classified as either saccular or ductal (Figure 7.6) (Moorhead, 1991). Anterior and lateral saccular cysts arise in the saccule. Ductal cysts involve any structure in the larynx where mucous glands are present, including the true and false vocal folds (Stemple et al., 2000). Epidermoid cysts are spherical in shape and are composed of **keratin** and **sebum** (an oily substance secreted by the sebaceous glands). The cyst is lined by a keratinizing epithelium that resembles the epidermis. **Retention cysts** result from some obstruction to the excretory duct of a gland and typically contain mucus. These cysts can be

FIGURE 7.6 **Laryngeal Cyst and Removal**

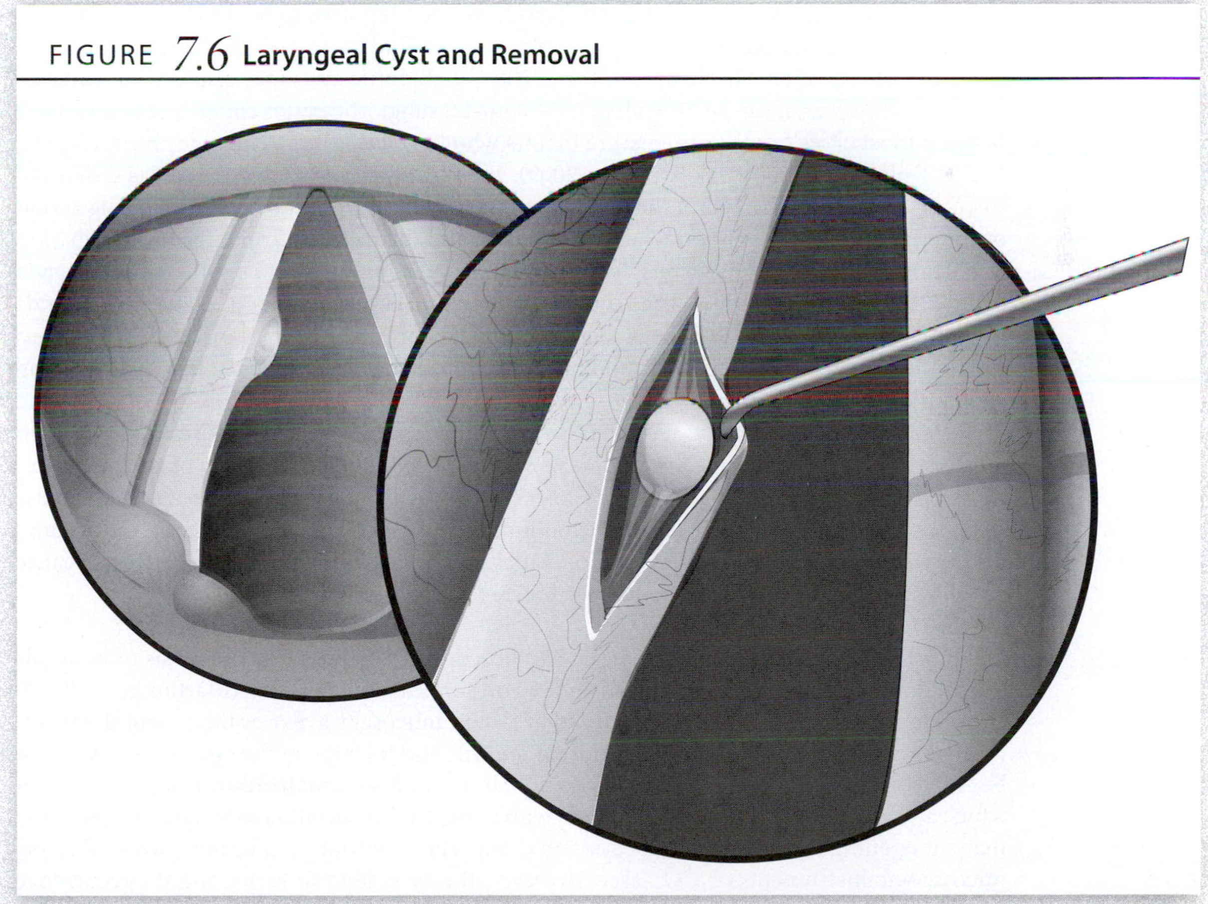

the result of phonotrauma, laryngopharyngeal reflux, or upper respiratory tract infections (Martins, Santana, & Tavares, 2011). Epidermoid cysts are the most common in the vocal folds, but retention cysts are also frequently found in the superficial layer of the lamina propria (Gallivan, Gallivan, & Eitnier, 2008). Refer to color insert photos 10, 11, and 12.

Cysts can be confined to the larynx (Type I) or extend beyond the larynx (Type II) (Forte, Fuocco, & James, 2004). The cyst may protrude onto the vibratory margin of the vocal fold, increasing the mass and stiffness of the cover (Gallivan et al., 2008). The resulting dysphonia is characterized by hoarseness, loss of pitch range, and vocal fatigue. Pain and dysphagia may also occur (Moorhead, 1991).

When a cyst occurs within the true vocal fold, it is typically firmly stuck to the underlying vocal ligament, but not to the overlying tissue of the superficial layer of the lamina propria. Cysts are usually sessile with a broad base. Vocal fold cysts are generally unilateral, although they do sometimes occur bilaterally. In some cases they are initially misdiagnosed as nodules.

Cysts may be congenital or acquired. Congenital cysts are generally epidermoid and are lined with squamous or respiratory epithelium (Gallivan et al., 2008). Acquired saccular cysts may be associated with laryngeal cancer, so it is important that the patient be referred for a laryngeal examination to rule out the possibility of malignancy.

Subglottic Cysts. While most laryngeal cysts occur at the level of the vocal folds, they may also occur subglottally. In fact, subglottic cysts have been reported to be the fourth most common laryngeal abnormality after laryngomalacia, vocal fold paralysis, and subglottic stenosis (Watson, Malik, Khan, Sheehan, & Rothera, 2007). Subglottic cysts may also be congenital or acquired. However, it can be difficult to tell whether a subglottic cyst is congenital or acquired, because most cases occur in premature infants who have been intubated since birth (Agada, Bell, & Knight, 2006; Jaryszak & Collins, 2009). The blockage of the subglottal ducts is thought to occur due to scarring within the subglottal area, resulting from the repeated pulsing action of the ventilator on the endotracheal tube, damage of the mucosa from repeated intubation or suctioning, and/or endotracheal tube movement and subsequent subglottic trauma (Agada et al., 2006). In addition, it has been found that there is a larger number of submucosal glands in premature infants, and that the mucus produced is more viscous (Watson et al., 2007). Thus premature infants are subject to a combination of factors that increases their risk of developing subglottic cysts.

Subglottic cysts may be superficial or located deeper in the submucosal tissues. When located deep in the tissue, the airway can be narrowed giving the impression of subglottic stenosis (Watson et al., 2007). The impression may be further strengthened because symptoms may be those of airway obstruction, including stridor, dyspnea, apneic periods, and feeding difficulties (Agada et al., 2006). Symptoms may not be apparent initially, however, because subglottic cysts tend to gradually increase in size (Watson et al., 2007).

Diagnosis and Treatment. Videolaryngostroboscopy is helpful in the diagnosis of cysts, although in some cases the cyst is only diagnosed on surgical manipulation (Martins et al., 2011). Videolaryngostroboscopy shows a reduced or absent mucosal wave over the area of the lesion (Martins et al., 2011). Treatment depends on the type and location of the cyst. Type I cysts can be treated by endoscopic excision or marsupialization. **Marsupialization** is a procedure in which a surgical incision is made in the cyst with a few stitches on either side. This creates a permanent opening through which the cyst can drain. The procedure can be done with cold steel microscopic instruments or CO_2 laser. However, the cysts tend to recur, and the recurrence is often located at different sites from the original (Watson et al., 2007). For larger Type II cysts an external procedure may be necessary. One such procedure is a **lateral thyrotomy**. In this procedure the thyroid cartilage is divided vertically, and the cyst is cut out through this incision. Tracheotomy may be necessary for infants with cysts that block the airway causing severe respiratory distress. Various surgical techniques have been reported as effective in treating laryngeal cysts, including CO_2 laser, cold dissection with microlaryngeal instruments, marsupialization, and microdebrider (e.g., Jaryszak & Collins, 2009; Ransom, Antunes, Smith, & Jacobs, 2009).

Recurrent Respiratory Papillomatosis

Recurrent respiratory papillomatosis (RRP) (Figure 7.7) is a disease that affects the larynx as well as other structures of the airway and can have devastating effects on both phonation and respiration. A papilloma is a benign wartlike growth of the epithelium (see color insert photos 13, 14, and 15), and papillomatosis refers to the development of numerous papillomas.

FIGURE 7.7 Recurrent Respiratory Papillomatosis

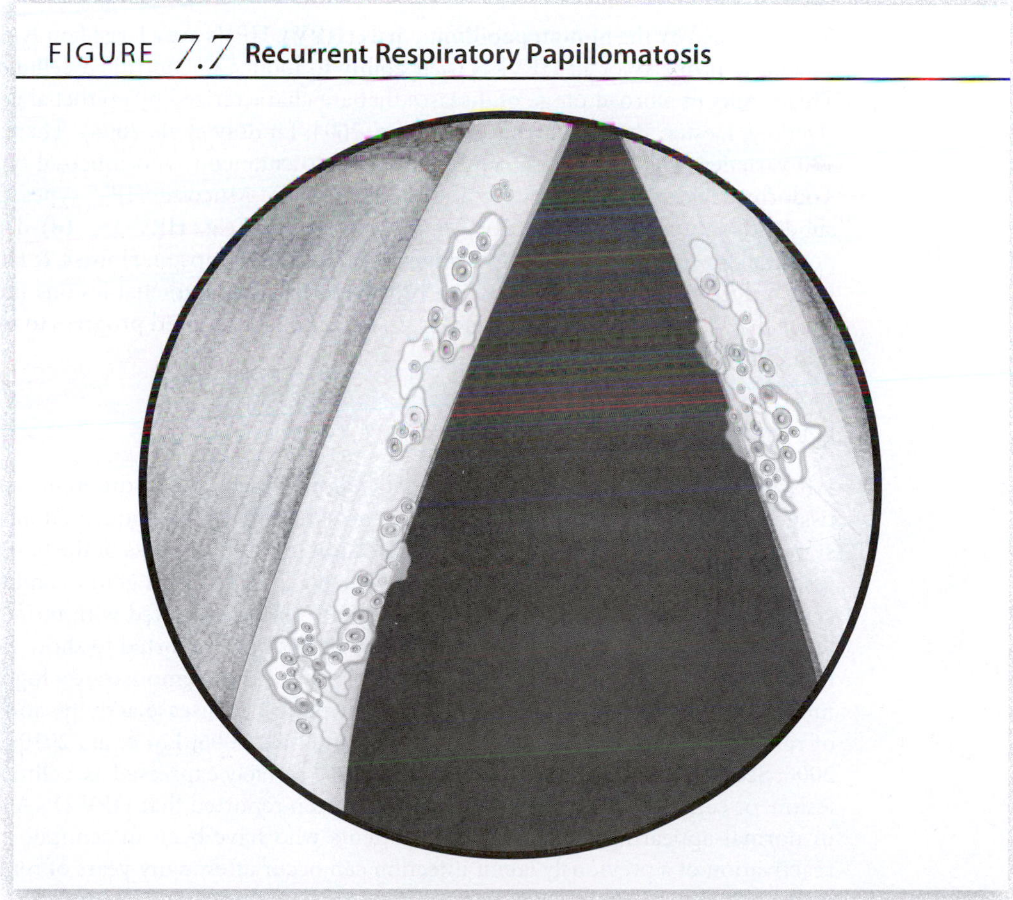

Papillomas may be sessile (broad based) or pedunculated (on a stalk). The growths are characterized by fingerlike projections and masses of nonkeratinized stratified squamous epithelium overlying the inner core of connective tissue (Lindsay, Bloom, Pransky, Stabley, & Shick, 2008; Preuss et al., 2007). Lesions are particularly prone to occur at areas of transition between different types of epithelium, such as the junction between ciliated respiratory epithelium and squamous epithelium in the larynx (Derkay & Darrow, 2006). The growth typically appears first at the anterior portion of the vocal folds, but it can then spread to cover part or all of the vocal folds, as well as spreading to the false and aryepiglottic folds, trachea, and even to the bronchi and lungs (Hammoud & El Haddad, 2009). Although they mostly occur in the epithelium, papillomas can spread deeper into the vocal ligament and even invade the thyrovocalis muscle (Stemple et al., 2000).

The disease is often extremely aggressive, both in its spread to structures of the airway and in its recurrence following treatment. The aggressiveness of the disease is what makes it so devastating in its effects on the airway.

The incidence of RRP is estimated at 4.3 per 100,000 in children younger than 14, and 1.8 per 100,000 in individuals older than 15. This roughly translates to between 1,500–2,500 new cases per year (Harmon, 2002; Lindsay et al., 2008; McClay, 2001).

CAUSE

RRP is caused by the **human papillomavirus (HPV)**. HPVs are a large family of DNA viruses. The basic property of all HPVs is their ability to induce uncontrolled cellular proliferation. This results in a broad range of diseases that are characterized by epithelial cell proliferation (Derkay, Hester, Burke, Carron, & Lawson, 2004; Lindsay et al., 2008). There are more than 130 varieties of HPVs, which can be divided into cutaneous and mucosal types (Draganov, Todorov, Todorov, Karchev, & Kalvatchev, 2006). Mucosal HPV types can be further subdivided into low-risk (e.g., HPV-6, -11) or high-risk (e.g., HPV-16, -18), depending on the potential for transformation into malignancy (Donne, Hampson, Homer, & Hampson, 2010). HPV infections are associated with a broad spectrum of epithelial lesions including benign warts that rarely progress to cancers, as well as lesions that could progress to malignant carcinomas (Torrente & Ojeda, 2007).

HPV SUBTYPES ASSOCIATED WITH RRP

HPV subtypes cause infection in different anatomic areas and in different types of epithelial tissues. Infection can result in lesions of the skin and of the anogenital and aerodigestive systems. Some HPV subtypes can cause infection in multiple areas of the body. The subtypes associated with RRP are HPV-6 and -11, which can cause both genital and laryngeal warts (Donne et al., 2010). There is evidence that HPV-11 is associated with more severe cases of RRP than HPV-6. RRP associated with HPV-11 has been reported to show worse long-term response to therapy, necessitate more surgical procedures, demonstrate a higher incidence of malignant transformation and death, a longer period of disease activity, and less likelihood of remission compared to HPV-6 (e.g., Gerein et al., 2006; Lin et al., 2010; Maloney et al., 2006; Seedat et al., 2010). The virus can either be actively expressed as a clinically observable lesion, or can exist as a latent infection. It has been reported that HPV DNA can be detected in normal-appearing mucosa in RRP patients who have been in remission for years, and reactivation of a previously latent infection can occur after many years of remission (Derkay et al., 2004).

JUVENILE ONSET RECURRENT RESPIRATORY PAPILLOMATOSIS

Juvenile onset recurrent respiratory papillomatosis (JORRP) is diagnosed in children prior to age 12 years (Johnson & Derkay, 2009). Children at most risk for JORRP are first-born babies delivered vaginally to teenage mothers who have active genital warts (Johnson & Derkay, 2009). The risk of transmitting the disease is estimated to be 200–400 times as high for women with HPV compared to a child delivered to a woman without disease (Freed & Derkay, 2006). The virus is thought to be transmitted by an infected mother to the baby either during gestation or during the birth process at the time of delivery (Freed & Derkay, 2006). However, not all babies born to infected mothers develop RRP. For every 1,000 children born to mothers with genital warts, approximately 7 cases have HPV-related diseases (Comar et al., 2006). Bitar, Baz, Fuleihan, and Muallem (2007) noted that the classic triad of firstborn child vaginally delivered by a teenage mother has been described in around a third of affected children. Other factors such as the status of the baby's immune system, length of time in the birth canal, and amount of virus in the birth canal may influence the development and course of the disease. An infant whose immune system is immature or dysfunctional may be more susceptible to developing the disease (Lindsay et al., 2008; Sedlacek et al., 1989; Stern, Felipovich, Cotton, & Segal, 2007). Women who have RRP but no genital warts have not been found to transmit the disease to their children (e.g., Gerein et al., 2006).

RRP is the most common type of laryngeal growth in children and is equally prevalent in boys and girls. RRP is most common in children younger than 5 years old. Very young children appear to be more likely to be affected by the more aggressive form of the disease related to HPV-11. Draganov et al. (2006) typed the HPV in children with RRP and identified HPV-6 in approximately 24% and HPV-11 in approximately 62% of cases. Around 15% of children were found to be positive for both HPV 6 and -11.

RRP in children often takes an extremely aggressive course in terms of spread and recurrence of the disease. Severity is measured in terms of number of surgical removals of the papilloma as well as the number of affected sites. The age at which the disease manifests may be related to the severity, with more severe disease presenting in children whose onset occurs before the age of 3 years (Draganov et al., 2006). Children diagnosed at less than 3 years old have been found to be 3.6 times more likely to have more than 4 surgeries per year, and almost 2 times more likely to have two or more anatomic sites affected than those diagnosed later than 3 years (Derkay et al., 2005). One hypothesis that has been offered to explain the age association may be the degree of maturity of the child's immune system. Older children may have a stronger immune response and be better able to withstand the virus.

There is a question as to whether or not children tend to grow out of the disease by puberty. While some clinicians have anecdotally reported disease remission by puberty, Preuss et al. (2007), noted that their patients who presented with childhood onset of RRP continued to produce papillomas in adult life. This observation does not support the theory that juvenile onset disease regresses at puberty.

ADULT ONSET RECURRENT RESPIRATORY PAPILLOMATOSIS

The incidence of adult onset recurrent respiratory papillomatosis (AORRP) is lower than in children, at 1.8 cases per 100,000, and mostly affects individuals in their 30s and 40s (Freed & Derkay, 2006; Harmon, 2002). In adults the ratio of males to females with the disease is somewhat greater (Johnson & Derkay, 2009; McClay, 2001). The disease in adults is typically less aggressive, with less spread to other airway structures and fewer surgical removals required.

In AORRP the virus may be transmitted sexually or may result from a reactivation of a latent infection (Freed & Derkay, 2006; Harman, 2002; McClay, 2001). Pregnancy in women with RRP associated with HPV-11 has been noted to increase the growth of papillomas, resulting in more frequent surgeries. In cases associated with HPV-6, RRP progression in pregnant women occurs less frequently. Gerein et al. (2006) suggested that the progress of the disease during pregnancy may be increased by hormonal changes, as well as by changes in the immune system, particularly in those women with the HPV-11 subtype of the disease.

SYMPTOMS

Symptoms depend on the location and extent of the tumors. Hoarseness is often present and may be the first indication of a problem. The child may also be breathy, or even aphonic. It is very common for the spread of the tumors to obstruct the airway, resulting in stridor and dyspnea. At first, the stridor may only occur during inspiration, but as the disease progresses the stridor may occur during both phases of breathing. The individual may also develop a chronic cough, recurrent pneumonia, and dysphagia (Rosen & Bryson, 2004). Because the disease is rare, it is often misdiagnosed as asthma, croup, tonsillitis, allergies, vocal nodules, or bronchitis (McClay, 2001).

DIAGNOSIS AND EVALUATION

Diagnosis of RRP is made using direct laryngoscopy. If the growths have spread beyond the larynx, a bronchoscopy may be necessary. To confirm the diagnosis and determine the type of HPV, a biopsy of the tumor should be taken (Lindsay et al., 2008). It is extremely important to obtain a comprehensive medical history to determine risk factors for RRP and any current or past conditions that may have a bearing on the disease. The clinician should probe the onset and duration of symptoms, any prior surgeries and intubation, medications that the patient may be taking, allergies, and evidence of reflux. Information regarding any maternal or paternal history of HPV-related diseases should be obtained. A comprehensive voice quality evaluation should be conducted, including the status of the patient's respiratory function (e.g., dyspnea, stridor).

Several staging systems are available to determine the extent of disease. Derkay et al. (2004) developed a severity/staging system that numerically grades the extent of papillomatosis at defined sites in the larynx and other aerodigestive sites and assesses clinical voice and breathing parameters. A final numeric score is assigned that reflects the patient's current extent of disease (Table 7.6). The clinical parameters include voice quality (normal, abnormal, or aphonic), urgency of intervention (elective, urgent, or emergent), and stridor (absent, present with activity, present at rest). The extent of the lesion is rated on a 4-point scale where 0 = no lesion present, 1 = surface lesion, 2 = raised lesion, 3 = bulky lesion. The functional and anatomic scores are used together to measure an individual patient's clinical course and response to therapy over time.

TREATMENT

The goals of treatment include eliminating or reducing the papilloma, creating a safe airway, improving voice quality, and increasing the time interval between surgical procedures (McClay, 2001). Surgery is the only way to remove the growths. However, even when all the lesions have been removed, the virus may remain in a latent state in surrounding tissues.

TABLE 7.6 Laryngoscopic and Clinical Assessment Scale for Recurrent Respiratory Papillomatosis

A. Clinical Score

DATE OF SURGERY ______________ SURGEON ______________

INSTITUTION ______________

1. Describe the patient's voice today:
   normal ______________ (0), abnormal ______________ (1), aphonic ______________ (2)
2. Describe the patient's stridor today:
   absent ______________ (0), present with activity ______________ (1), present at rest ______________ (2)
3. Describe the urgency of today's intervention:
   scheduled ______________ (0), elective ______________ (1), urgent ______________ (2), emergent ______________ (3)
4. Describe today's level of respiratory distress:
   none ______________ (0), mild ______________ (1), moderate ______________ (2), severe ______________ (3), extreme ______________ (4)

   Total score for questions 1–4 = ______________

B. Anatomical Score

For each site, score as: 0 = none, 1 = surface lesion, 2 = raised lesion, 3 = bulky lesion

LARYNX

Epiglottis:	Lingual surface ______________	Laryngeal surface ______________
Aryepiglottic folds	Right ______________	Left ______________
False vocal cords	Right ______________	Left ______________
True vocal cords	Right ______________	Left ______________
Arytenoids	Right ______________	Left ______________

Anterior commissure ______________

Posterior commissure ______________

Subglottis ______________

TRACHEA

Upper one-third ______________

Middle one-third ______________

Lower one-third ______________

Bronchi	Right ______________	Left ______________

Tracheotomy stoma ______________

OTHER

Nose ______________

Palate ______________

Pharynx ______________

(continued)

TABLE 7.6 **Laryngoscopic and Clinical Assessment Scale for Recurrent Respiratory Papillomatosis (Continued)**

Esophagus ____________

Lungs ____________

Other ____________

Total score for anatomical ____________

C. Total score = total anatomical score plus total clinical score ____________

Source: From "Analysis of a Staging Assessment System for Prediction of Surgical Interval in Recurrent Respiratory Papillomatosis," by C. S. Derkay, R. P. Hester, B. Burke, J. Carron, L. Lawson, 2004, *International Journal of Pediatric Otorhinolaryngology, 68,* pp. 1493–1498. Copyright 2004 by Elsevier. Reprinted with permission.

This may explain why RRP recurs so often and can spread to other aerodigestive sites (RRP Task Force Practice Guidelines for Management of Children with RRP, www.rrpf.org/rrpf/publications/TaskForceGuidelines.htm). Because of the aggressiveness of the disease, repeated surgeries are the norm, with particularly severe cases sometimes requiring removal as often as every two to four weeks. The National Registry of Children with RRP reported that on average, a child with RRP will have 19.7 surgical procedures with an average of 4.4 surgeries per year (Derkay, 1995). Another report estimated that children with RRP in the United States undergo more than 10,000 surgical procedures a year (Schraff, Derkay, Burke, & Lawson, 2004). There have been anecdotal reports of patients who have needed surgery more than 100 times. These frequent surgeries often have secondary consequences. Up to 30% of patients whose papilloma in the anterior commissure has been excised have developed anterior glottic scarring, web formation, and subglottic stenosis (McClay, 2001). In addition, the repeated hospitalizations can affect the child in terms of social, emotional, and academic development. The impact of RRP and its treatment is a burden not only on patients and their families, but on the U.S. health care system as well. An estimated $109–$123 million is spent every year on the frequent surgical procedures and hospital admissions (Leung, Hawkes, & Campisi, 2007; Tasca, McCormick, & Clarke, 2006).

Surgical Procedures. Surgical techniques are designed to maintain the patient's airway and ensure as functional a voice as possible. Techniques include cold steel dissection, laser excision, microdebrider removal, and radiofrequency ablation to excise the growths (Alexander & Fried, 2007; Timms, Bruce, & Patel, 2007).

Cold steel removal of the growths using microlaryngeal techniques may be used in cases of very extensive and bulky growth in children (Preuss et al., 2007). This technique remains a cost-effective, technology-independent, safe way of managing RRP (Alexander & Fried, 2007). The Voice Committee of the American Academy of Otolaryngology-Head and Neck Surgery stated in 2002 that cold steel excision is the preferred technique for removal of papilloma for adults (Derkay & Darrow, 2006).

CO_2 laser excision of the papilloma is extremely popular among surgeons (Schraff et al., 2004; Tasca et al., 2006). Large published series on laser excision have demonstrated its effectiveness in controlling disease when applied with appropriate frequency (Alexander & Fried,

2007). However, despite advances in laser surgery, it is still difficult to avoid damage to adjacent healthy tissues, and delayed complications can occur since most patients require multiple procedures (Timms et al., 2007). Potential complications include glottic webbing, interarytenoid scarring, and arytenoid fixation. In order to reduce the risk of complications from the CO_2 laser, some surgeons have used the 585-nm pulsed dye laser (PDL). This is an angiolytic laser that is designed to avoid damage to surrounding structures and to preserve the epithelial covering of the vocal folds (Hartnick, Boseley, Franco, Cunningham, & Pransky, 2007). The PDL has the advantage of being able to treat the anterior commissure without risk of scarring. Other advantages include a flexible delivery system that permits access to the areas that are difficult to reach, the ability to treat both vocal fold surfaces simultaneously, and its effectiveness in removing disease from scarred areas without causing more damage (Hartnick et al., 2007).

The microdebrider has become widely used by surgeons for papilloma removal. Microdebrider excision has been reported to have reduced operative time and expense, less postoperative pain, lower risk of laryngeal scarring, and greater improvement in voice quality (Alexander & Fried, 2007; Preuss et al., 2007; Roy & Vivero, 2008). Schraff et al. (2004) compared results from their most current survey of American Society of Pediatric Otolaryngology (ASPO) members with those obtained from a 1994 survey. They noted that in 1994 the preferred surgical tool was overwhelmingly the CO_2 laser. In their 2004 survey the microdebrider replaced the laser as the most preferred instrument. Perceptual and acoustic voice outcomes have been reported to be superior with microdebrider compared with CO_2 laser excision (Holler et al., 2009). This procedure is not without its disadvantages, however, which include difficulty in excising the sessile form of the papillomas, difficulty working in areas where scarring and fibrosis are present, and accessing areas such as the ventricle (Hartnick et al., 2007).

Radiofrequency Ablation. A recent technique developed to control neoplastic diseases is **radiofrequency ablation**. In this technique grounding pads are placed on the patient's skin, and a very small needle electrode with an insulated shaft and an uninsulated distal tip is inserted through the skin and directly into the tumor, guided by ultrasound or CT scanning [RadiologyInfo, www.radiologyinfo.org/en/info.cfm?pg=rfa&bhcp=1 (retrieved 8/10/07)]. The energy in the needle tip causes the tumor cells to become heated and die. The dead tumor cells are not removed, but they are gradually replaced by fibrosis and scar tissue, which shrinks over time. The heat from the radiofrequency energy also closes up small blood vessels and reduces bleeding. This procedure may be performed on an outpatient basis without general anesthesia. Timms et al. (2007) reported that there was no bleeding at any stage of the procedure, and no physical contact pressure was applied to the underlying tissues. This method makes large-volume tissue ablation more effective and safer for local control of neoplastic disease (National Institutes of Health, www.cc.nih.gov/drd/rfa/faq.html).

Airway management in most children with RRP is managed adequately with surgical procedures. Tracheotomy is avoided if at all possible, as there have been reports that this can result in even more extensive spread of the disease and malignant transformation. However, 10–15% of individuals with RRP do require a tracheotomy due to severe airway obstruction (Harmon, 2002; Schraff et al., 2004).

Nonsurgical Adjuvant Therapies. In addition to surgical removal of the growths, many patients and their families and doctors have turned to nonsurgical therapies, including antiviral, hormonal, and immunological (Table 7.7). The goal of these therapies is to reduce the spread of the disease and to lengthen the interval between surgical procedures (Craig & Derkay, 2001). The most commonly used therapies reported by ASPO members are interferon, indole-3-carbinol, cidofovir, and heat shock protein (HSP) (Schraff et al., 2004; Tasca

TABLE 7.7 **Nonsurgical Adjuvant Therapies for Recurrent Respiratory Papillomatosis**

Therapy	Agent
Interferon	Antiviral, antiproliferative
Indole-3-carbinol	Hormonal
Cidofovir	Antiviral
Heat shock protein	Immunological

et al., 2006). Schraff et al. (2004) reported that significantly more children are currently being treated with adjuvant therapies than in the past (22% compared to 10% previously reported in the literature). The criteria that practitioners have indicated for adjuvant therapies include (1) patient underwent more than 4 surgical procedures per year, (2) distal spread of disease, and (3) rapid regrowth with airway compromise. Based on these criteria, around 10% of patients require adjuvant therapy (Craig & Derkay, 2001).

Interferon. **Interferon (IFN)** is a protein that is produced naturally in the body. It has antiviral and antiproliferative actions that can also modify immune system reactions (Bitar et al., 2007; Harman, 2002). IFN blocks the ability of a virus to replicate itself using the person's RNA and DNA, and it also makes the cell less easy to be infected by the virus. There are three types of interferons produced by different cells. Interferon alpha is the most commonly used subtype. In 1994 IFN was the most widely used adjuvant therapy for RRP. It has become less popular as studies have shown mixed results regarding its effectiveness, as well as many negative side effects (Schraff et al., 2004). Reported side effects can be acute or chronic and range from fever, chills, headache, nausea, and general malaise to decreased growth rates, seizures, elevated liver functions, and thrombocytopenia (abnormally small number of platelets in the circulating blood) (Derkay & Darrow, 2006; Lindsay et al., 2008). Another disadvantage of interferon therapy is that it involves subcutaneous injections every other day, which is a difficult regimen for small children to tolerate and for their caretakers to follow (Shirley & Wiatrak, 2004).

There is some evidence that IFN is more effective for RRP associated with HPV-6 than for HPV-11. Gerein, Rastorguev, Gerein, Jecker, and Pfister (2005) conducted a 20-year follow-up of patients treated with interferon-alpha and found that patients with HPV-6 showed significantly better initial and long-term response than patients with HPV-11.

Indole-3-Carbinol. **Indole-3-carbinol (I3C)** is an FDA-approved nutritional supplement found in vegetables such as cabbage, broccoli, and cauliflower and which is also sold in health food stores. This compound acts hormonally by inducing an estrogen metabolite balance that helps to prevent the growth of papilloma (Rosen & Bryson, 2004; Stern, 2001). Clinical trials have shown cessation of growth of papilloma or reduced growth rate in approximately two-thirds of patients tested, while one-third showed no response to the substance (Derkay & Darrow, 2006). Rosen and Bryson (2004) examined the short-term and long-term effects of I3C in children and adults with RRP. Reportedly, 70% of patients had either a complete or partial response to the compound, with adults showing a stronger response than children. The authors noted that the initial response was quick, and the decreases in the recurrence rate were sustained over a long term of treatment, approximately 5 years in some patients. Reported side effects are mild and include dizziness and headache (Bitar et al., 2007).

Cidofovir. Surgeons have turned to the use of antiviral agents such as cidofovir in an attempt to neutralize the virus in its latent state. **Cidofovir** is an antiviral agent that was first approved for cytomegalovirus (CMV)-related retinitis in HIV patients. It has since been found to have antiviral activity against a number of DNA viruses. Cidofovir has been shown to lessen the severity of RRP or to increase the time between surgeries when used in conjunction with laser treatment (Chung, Akst, & Koltai, 2006). This has become the most common adjuvant medical therapy used by pediatric otolaryngologists (Bitar et al., 2007; Tasca et al., 2006). Cidofovir works by being absorbed into cells and then killing off cells with HPV, while not affecting normal cells (Stern, 2001). The drug is usually injected either directly into the lesions or into the places where the lesions were removed at the time of surgery (Harman, 2002; Stern, 2001). Numerous otolaryngologists have reported on their experiences with cidofovir. From these reports it has emerged that the drug has significant benefits for a majority of individuals with RRP. Reports of a positive response range from 40% to 89% of patients (e.g., Bielecki, Mniszek, & Cofala, 2009; Derkay, 2005; Donne, Rothera, & Homer, 2008; Lee & Rosen, 2004; Naiman et al., 2006a, 2006b; Schraff et al., 2004). Pontes, Avelino, Pignatari, and Weckx (2006) evaluated 10 adult patients who received cidofovir injections. The time interval between recurrences for the group increased from a median of 102 days before cidofovir to 239 days after cidofovir. Only 1 patient did not exhibit significant improvement. However, up to 20% of patients either do not respond to the medication or their condition worsens.

Despite the generally positive findings with cidofovir, there are some cautions. First, the clinical studies have used small numbers of participants. Second, control groups have not been used, and third, HPV typing has not been done in many of the studies (Donne et al., 2008). However, based on the overall positive patient response to cidofovir, the RRP Task Force has recommended the following guidelines (cited in Derkay, 2005):

1. Given the promising results reported in pediatric and adult patients, cidofovir should be routinely presented as a treatment option in moderately-to-severely afflicted RRP patients, i.e. those patients whose disease is not improving on surgical therapy alone or in conjunction with less potentially morbid adjuvant measures and/or requiring surgical intervention greater than three times per year. With appropriate consent, cidofovir therapy should be a viable option in patients whose disease severity is resulting in a need for frequent surgery, worsening airway compromise or severely impaired communication or those who otherwise may be considered candidates for tracheotomy.
2. Patients with more mild disease, particularly children, should be discouraged in most cases from seeking treatment with cidofovir, until a better understanding of the use of this drug has been established. With appropriate informed consent, cidofovir could still be utilized on a case-by-case basis, at the discretion of the prescribing physician, for the more mildly affected patient.
3. As with all surgical procedures, informed consent should be obtained and documented in the patient's record. At a minimum, this should include a frank discussion of the nephrotoxic and carcinogenic potential of this drug.
4. Adverse responses, particularly evidence of dysplasia or malignant transformation to squamous cell carcinoma, either locally or remotely, should be reported simultaneously to the FDA and to the RRP Task Force.

HPV Vaccines. Researchers are working on a variety of vaccines against HPV-related diseases. One such agent is **heat shock protein (HSP)**, which consists of molecules that trigger an immune response in the body. HSPE7 is a form of HSP that has been linked to another chemical. This agent is used as a broad-spectrum vaccine for HPV-related conditions by triggering an immune response that destroys infected cells. The advantages of this treatment are that it utilizes the body's own immune system, acts systemically to reach infected cells, and is administered by a short series of injections. Because it is relatively noninvasive it can be administered in the outpatient setting (Derkay et al., 2005). Reports indicate a positive response in many patients. The interval between surgeries increased, and the rate of growth of the tumors decreased (e.g., Derkay et al., 2005; Kimberlin, 2004).

Other HPV vaccines include Gardasil and Cervarix. Gardasil has recently received FDA approval. The clinical trials thus far have shown excellent safety data with no serious vaccine-related side effects. The response to the vaccine has been very good with 99.7% of those vaccinated developing an antibody response (Freed & Derkay, 2006). Gardasil could have a significant impact on the future incidence of RRP by decreasing the number of HPV-infected women who give birth to babies with the virus. However, there are as yet no data regarding the effects of HPV vaccination specifically for RRP (Chang et al., 2009).

Treatment for GERD/LPR. It is extremely important that any coexisting GERD and/or LPR be identified and treated. It has been reported that the clinical course of the RRP may be modified by treatment of coexisting LPR (McKenna & Brodsky, 2005). Further, antireflux medications have been shown to reduce soft tissue complications such as webbing and scarring in patients with RRP (Schraff et al., 2004). However, only 15% of responding physicians in the Schraff et al. (2004) survey reported routine use of reflux medications for their patients with RRP.

Voice Therapy. Voice therapy is an important factor in helping the patient to make the best possible use of his or her vocal mechanism following surgery. Vocal function exercises may reduce the stiffness of the vocal folds. Helping the patient to develop a well-coordinated pattern of breathing, phonation, and resonation through approaches such as resonant voice therapy and/or the accent method can optimize the individual's efficient and effective use of his or her vocal mechanism. Education regarding normal laryngeal function, the nature of RRP, and current surgical and medical treatments can help the patient and his or her family to understand and better cope with the disorder (Morgan, Triana, & Hertel, 2006). Such information may also motivate the patient to comply with a vocal hygiene program. The clinician can help the patient to identify any phonotraumatic behaviors and explore strategies to eliminate them. The patient should be taught to reduce any compensatory laryngeal muscle tension. If the patient is an adult, he or she should be strongly cautioned against smoking.

Support Groups. Support groups such as the RRP Foundation (www.rrpf.org) are an important resource for patients and for their families. RRP is devastating not only to the victim, but to his or her family and friends as well. Support groups can be helpful in providing current information about surgical and nonsurgical treatments, as well as emotional support for all involved.

chapter SUMMARY

STRUCTURAL LESIONS OF THE LARYNX can occur in any of the tissues of the larynx and vocal folds and have a wide variety of causes including congenital conditions, injury, systemic disease, infectious and inflammatory conditions, and phonotrauma.

Laryngomalacia is a congenital condition characterized by pathologically soft and flexible supraglottic cartilages, particularly the epiglottis. The primary symptom is inspiratory stridor resulting from airway obstruction when the aryepiglottic folds are drawn inward during inhalation. Most children grow out of this condition and typically no formal therapy is necessary. However, an estimated 5–20% of children with laryngomalacia show severe or progressive worsening of airway difficulties and require surgical intervention. Supraglottoplasties are endoscopic techniques that involve fixating the epiglottis to prevent it from being pulled inward (epiglottopexy) and/or removing excess tissue to enlarge the airway.

Subglottic stenosis is a narrowing of the airway between the glottis and the first tracheal ring. The condition can be either congenital or acquired through infection, GERD, abnormal tissue growth, chronic illness, chronic inflammatory disease, radiation therapy, external trauma, and endotracheal intubation. Respiratory symptoms can include dyspnea, tachypnea (rapid breathing), apnea (absence of breathing), cyanosis, stridor, recurrent pneumonia, cough, recurrent aspiration, and failure to thrive. The primary treatment is surgery to establish a functional airway, safe swallowing, and some kind of voicing if possible. Laryngotracheal reconstruction techniques are classified as splits, augmentations, and resections. Resections involve removing various portions of cartilage, with or without the incorporation of grafts and stents. Voice quality following surgery may be breathy, weak, hoarse, low-pitched, with reduced pitch range, reduced vocal intensity, and abnormal resonance. Voice therapy is essential in order to minimize the child's use of supraglottic voicing and improve his or her voice quality to the extent possible.

Laryngeal web (glottic stenosis) can be congenital or acquired and occurs when abnormal tissue forms between the vocal folds. Respiratory and vocal symptoms vary depending on the extent and location of the web. Causes of webs include intubation trauma, laryngeal surgery, ingestion of caustic material, infections, and foreign bodies. Webs are usually treated surgically by means of dilation or lysis, either endoscopically or with open surgery. Endoscopic procedures are suitable for thin webs, while thick webs are best treated with an open approach. Voice quality is often poor, and voice therapy should focus on identifying any maladaptive compensatory strategies the child is using and substituting more effective ways of voicing.

A laryngocele is an air-filled dilation of the saccule extending upward within the false vocal fold, resulting from excessive pressure within the larynx. Depending on the size of the mass and the patient's symptoms, the disorder may be left untreated except for periodic observation, or the laryngocele may be aspirated or excised by means of endoscopic CO_2 laser resection or excision by an external approach.

Laryngeal cysts may be congenital or acquired and typically occur when glandular secretions and mucus accumulate and are unable to dissipate. Most laryngeal cysts occur at the level of the vocal folds, but they may also occur subglottally. The resulting dysphonia is characterized by hoarseness, loss of pitch range, vocal fatigue, and possible pain and dysphagia. Subglottal cysts may create symptoms of airway obstruction including stridor, dyspnea, apneic periods, and feeding difficulties. Cysts are treated surgically by excision or marsupialization.

Recurrent respiratory papillomatosis (RRP) is characterized by wart-like growths, which typically appear first at the anterior portion of the vocal folds, but can then spread to cover part or all of the vocal folds, as well as spreading to the false and aryepiglottic folds, trachea, and even to the bronchi and lungs. The disease is often extremely aggressive, both in its spread to structures of the airway and in its recurrence following treatment. RRP is caused by the human papillomavirus, specifically types 6 and 11. There are juvenile and adult forms of the disease, with the juvenile form typically being more aggressive. Symptoms depend on the location and extent of the tumors and can include hoarseness, breathiness, aphonia, stridor, dyspnea, chronic cough, recurrent pneumonia, and dysphagia. Treatment is designed to eliminate or reduce the papilloma, create a safe airway, improve voice quality, and increase the time interval between surgical procedures. Surgical techniques include cold steel dissection, laser excision, microdebrider removal, and radiofrequency ablation. Nonsurgical adjuvant therapies are often used to supplement surgical removal and include interferon, indole-3-carbinole, cidofovir, and heat shock protein (HSP). Voice therapy is an important factor in helping the patient to make the best possible use of his or her vocal mechanism following surgery.

review QUESTIONS

1. Discuss the relationship between GERD and laryngomalacia.
2. Describe clinical management options for laryngomalacia.
3. Explain the different causes of congenital versus acquired subglottic stenosis and membranous versus cartilaginous stenosis.
4. Compare different forms of surgical intervention for subglottic stenosis. Comment on the likely voice quality following surgery.
5. Describe the staging systems for subglottic and glottic stenoses. Why is it important to stage these conditions?
6. Identify treatment options for laryngeal webs.
7. Identify the differences between laryngoceles and laryngeal cysts in terms of etiology and treatment.
8. Explain the relationship between RRP and HPV status.
9. Describe surgical and nonsurgical treatments for RRP.

PREPARING FOR THE PRAXIS

CASE STUDY 7.1: Recurrent Respiratory Papillomatosis

Directions: Please read the case study and answer the five questions that follow. The answers can be found at the bottom of the page.

Michael James is a 3-year-old boy whose mother, Courtney, is 20 years old. He has recently begun to evidence stridor when he breathes, and he often cries and says "It's hard to breathe, mommy." Courtney took him to her family doctor, who referred him to a pediatric laryngologist. The laryngologist diagnosed juvenile onset recurrent respiratory papillomatosis.

1. The severity of disease in recurrent respiratory papillomatosis (RRP) is related to
   a. type of HPV
   b. age of onset
   c. time since diagnosis
   d. a and b
   e. a, b, and c
2. One reason that makes it difficult to completely eliminate the disease in a child is that
   a. parents of young children are resistant to surgical removal of the tumors
   b. the virus may remain in a latent state in surrounding tissues even after surgical removal
   c. the occurrence of secondary laryngeal injuries such as webs and scarring stimulates further growth of the tumors
   d. all of the above
   e. none of the above
3. Removal of Michael's tumors is best done using
   a. either CO_2 or angiolytic laser
   b. cold steel dissection
   c. microdebrider
   d. radiofrequency ablation
   e. any of the above depending on the extent and location of Michael's tumors, as well as the surgeon's preference
4. Cidofovir
   a. is only indicated for adults
   b. works best for RRP caused by HPV-6
   c. is a protein produced naturally in the body
   d. is the most common adjuvant medical therapy used by pediatric otolaryngologists
   e. none of the above
5. Which of the following therapy approaches (if any) would NOT be appropriate for Michael?
   a. vocal function exercises to reduce the stiffness of the vocal folds resulting from surgery
   b. resonant voice therapy and/or the accent method to optimize Michael's efficient and effective use of his vocal mechanism
   c. education targeted to both Michael and his mother regarding normal laryngeal function
   d. identification of any phonotraumatic behaviors and exploration of strategies to eliminate them
   e. all of the above are appropriate therapeutic strategies

Answers for Case Study 7.1: 1 (d); 2 (b); 3 (e); 4 (d); 5 (e)

Chapter 8

Benign Lesions of the Vocal Fold Mucosa and Vocal Fatigue Associated with Lifestyle, Personality, and Occupational Factors

LEARNING OBJECTIVES

1. Identify occupational and personal factors that can injure the vocal folds.
2. Compare etiological, histological, and symptomological differences and similarities between nodules, polyps, ulcers, and granulomas.
3. Describe vocal fold vascular changes that can result from vocal fold trauma.
4. Discuss the role of voice therapy in the treatment of benign vocal fold lesions.
5. Understand the central and peripheral bases of vocal fold fatigue.
6. Identify factors that increase occupational risk of voice disorders for teachers.

Lifestyle, personality, and occupational factors have long been thought to play a causative or maintaining role in many benign conditions of the vocal folds including nodules, polyps, contact ulcers and granuloma, leukoplakia, vocal fold hemorrhage, and vocal fatigue. The terms *vocal abuse* and *vocal misuse* were commonly used to describe vocal behaviors that can result in structural and/or physiological changes to the vocal folds. Currently, the term *phonotrauma* has to a large degree replaced these older terms. The term was first used by Verdolini in 1998 to refer to the inflammatory response of the vocal fold mucosa to the biomechanical stresses that the vocal folds undergo during hyperfunctional phonation (Behrman et al., 2008). Vocal hyperfunction has been described as a hypertonic state of both intrinsic and extrinsic laryngeal musculature (Holmberg, Doyle, Perkell, Hammarberg, & Hillman, 2003). Phonotrauma is considered a major common factor contributing to the formation of many benign lesions of the vocal fold mucosa, as well as to vocal fatigue. Excessive talking, talking over noise, poor singing technique, excessive throat clearing, excessive coughing, and smoking can irritate and inflame the sensitive tissues of the vocal folds, resulting in swelling and edema. With continued trauma, the diffuse swelling can localize and create histological changes. Commonly, many phonotraumatic factors interact to create the voice problem. For example, people who depend on their voice for their occupation may also sing in a choir, smoke, be under stress at work, and suffer from laryngopharyngeal reflux. All these factors can combine to create the conditions for laryngeal changes to occur. The chapter begins with consideration of benign lesions of the vocal fold mucosa including nodules, polyps and Reinke's edema, leukoplakia, contact ulcers and granuloma, and vascular lesions. Discussion then turns to central and peripheral factors that can cause vocal fatigue. Finally, occupational aspects that can impact vocal function are described, using teaching as an example.

Nodules

Nodules are benign growths that develop on the epithelium of the vocal folds as a consequence of vocal hyperfunction and resulting inflammation of the folds (Figure 8.1). The increased muscular tension may be present during both adduction and abduction, and the abnormally strong collision forces that are generated result in the tissue damage (Iwarsson & Sundberg, 1999; Pontes, Kyrillos, Behlau, De Biase, & Pontes, 2002). The growths typically occur at the midpoint of the membranous glottis where vocal fold vibration is most vigorous and the collision forces between the vocal folds are strongest. Nodules tend to be bilateral, as the growth on one fold irritates the corresponding spot on the opposite fold. See color insert photos 16 and 17.

Videolaryngostroboscopy often shows that the larynx is abnormally contracted from front to back. The arytenoid cartilages are pulled forward, and there may be an open space or chink at the back of the glottis related to the increased tension of the thyroarytenoid muscle (Pontes et al., 2002).

While phonotrauma is usually the primary cause of nodules, GERD and/or LPR have also been implicated in around two-thirds of speakers with nodules (e.g., Chung et al., 2009; Kuhn et al., 1998). Other conditions that have been associated with nodules include allergies, chronic cough, dehydrated vocal folds, endocrine imbalance, infectious laryngitis, throat clearing, and upper respiratory infections (Pannbacker, 1999).

HISTOLOGY

The high collision forces generated during high effort vocal fold vibration disrupt the epithelium and basement membrane zone (Dikkers, Hulstaert, Oosterbaan, & Cervera-Paz, 1993). Increased levels of fibronectin have been found in the lamina propria, suggesting that the nodule is the end result of the wound healing process (Branski et al., 2006; Martins, Defaveri, Domingues, Silva, & Fabro, 2010). Histologically, nodules are characterized by the presence of edema with excessive fibroblast proliferation (Martins et al., 2010; Wallis, Jackson-Menaldi, Holland, & Giraldo, 2004). The lesion begins as a soft vascular growth filled with fluid. Over time and with continued hyperfunction, the nodule matures and becomes whitish due to the

FIGURE 8.1 Nodules

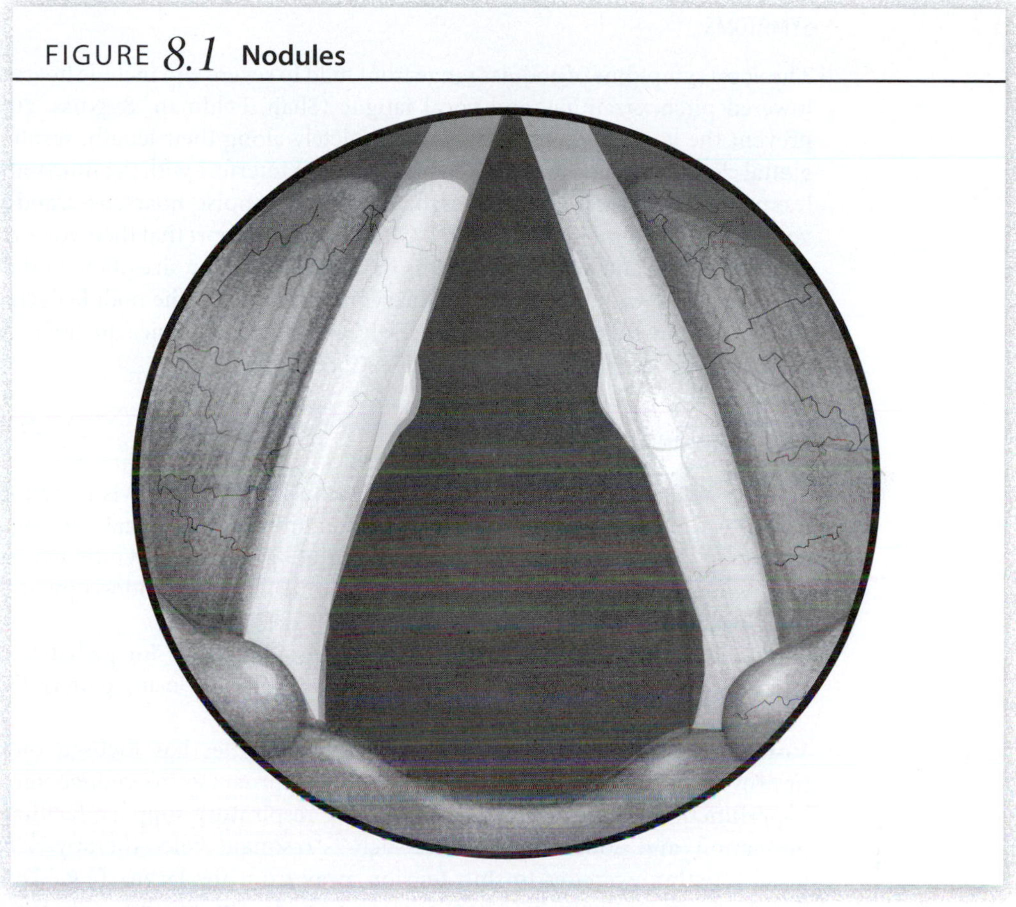

fibrosis and thickening of the epithelium (Kilic, Okur, Yildirim, & Guzelsoy, 2004; Martins et al., 2010). Reportedly, children mostly have immature nodules, whereas in adults there is a higher prevalence of mature nodules (Kilic et al., 2004).

AGE AND PERSONALITY FACTORS

It has been well established that the ratio of males to females with nodules changes depending on age. Young boys have a considerably higher incidence of nodules than young girls, with the incidence peaking between ages 5–10 years (Roy, Holt, Redmond, & Muntz, 2007; Shah et al., 2005). In the teenage and young adult years more females than males develop nodules (De Bodt et al., 2007; Shah et al., 2005).

Personality factors have been associated with the likelihood of developing nodules, particularly in young women and in prepubertal boys. Young women with nodules tend to engage in a great deal of social interaction, such as talking on the phone, socializing at clubs and bars, and participating in vocally demanding activities (cheerleading, singing, debating, etc.). Children with nodules have also been reported to be more social and highly extroverted than children with healthy vocal folds (Roy et al., 2007).

SYMPTOMS

The vocal symptoms of nodules range from mild to severe and include hoarseness, breathiness, lowered pitch, straining, and vocal fatigue (Shah, Feldman, & Nuss, 2007). The nodules prevent the vocal folds from closing completely along their length, resulting in incomplete glottal closure during vibration. The growths also interfere with the mucosal wave, resulting in less periodic vibration. This creates the perception of noise, hoarseness, and a strained/pressed vocal quality (Holmberg et al., 2003). Often, patients report that their voice quality is best early in the morning and deteriorates as the day progresses. The size of the nodule does not necessarily correlate with the severity of the symptoms. Even if the nodule decreases in size, vocal symptoms may still persist, and conversely, an individual's voice quality may improve despite persistence of the nodule (Shah, Engel, & Choi, 2008).

EVALUATION AND TREATMENT

Nodules are best diagnosed by flexible endoscopy, which allows visualization of the size of the lesion, as well as documentation of the effect of the lesion on vocal fold vibration. Ultrasound technology has also been used to assess vocal nodules in children (Bisetti et al., 2009). However, while this procedure is less invasive than flexible nasoendoscopy, it does not offer the same quality of imaging.

Shah et al. (2007) developed a 4-point grading scale for pediatric nodules based on endoscopic evaluation of the size of the lesion and glottal closure pattern (Table 8.1).

Voice Therapy. Traditionally, treatment for nodules has focused on vocal education, improved vocal usage, and direct therapy approaches to reduce muscle tension and hyperfunction. Strategies include improving respiratory support, facilitating easy onset of phonation, and holistic approaches such as resonant voice therapy, accent method, and vocal function exercises to shift tension away from the larynx (e.g., Tezcaner, Ozgursoy, Sati, & Dursun, 2009). It is also important to identify other factors that may be contributing to the patient's vocal problems, such as allergies, GERD, and prescription and/or over-the-counter medications. GERD and/or LPR have been reported as common in individuals with nodules (e.g., Kuhn et al., 1998). These factors need to be addressed in addition

TABLE 8.1 Grading Scale for Pediatric Nodules

Grade	Description
0	Normal, complete adduction, smooth vocal fold contour
1	Normal, complete adduction, nodule protrudes < 0.5 mm on vibratory edge
2	May have anterior glottic gap on adduction, nodule protrudes > 0.5–1.0 mm on vibratory edge
3	Anterior and posterior glottic gap (hourglass) always present on adduction, nodule protrudes > 1.0 mm on vibratory edge

Source: Information from Shah et al. (2007).

to the patient's vocal usage, and it may be necessary to refer the patient to an appropriate professional such as an internist, gastroenterologist, and/or allergist.

Surgery. Occasionally nodules do not resolve, even when the patient is compliant with the therapy regimen, and in that case, surgery may be necessary to remove the growth. Surgical techniques include microdissection or removal with CO_2 laser (e.g., Benninger, 2000). However, surgery should be avoided if at all possible and used only when other approaches are not effective (Murry & Woodson, 1992). A survey of members of the American Academy of Otolaryngology-Head and Neck Surgery found that 91% of respondents use voice therapy as the initial treatment for nodules (Sulica & Behrman, 2003).

Polyps

Polyps are benign growths on the vocal fold mucosa that may result from laryngeal hyperfunction as well as from other causes (Figure 8.2). While polyps and nodules may arise from similar causes, there are several differences between them (Table 8.2). Polyps are usually filled with

FIGURE 8.2 Polyp

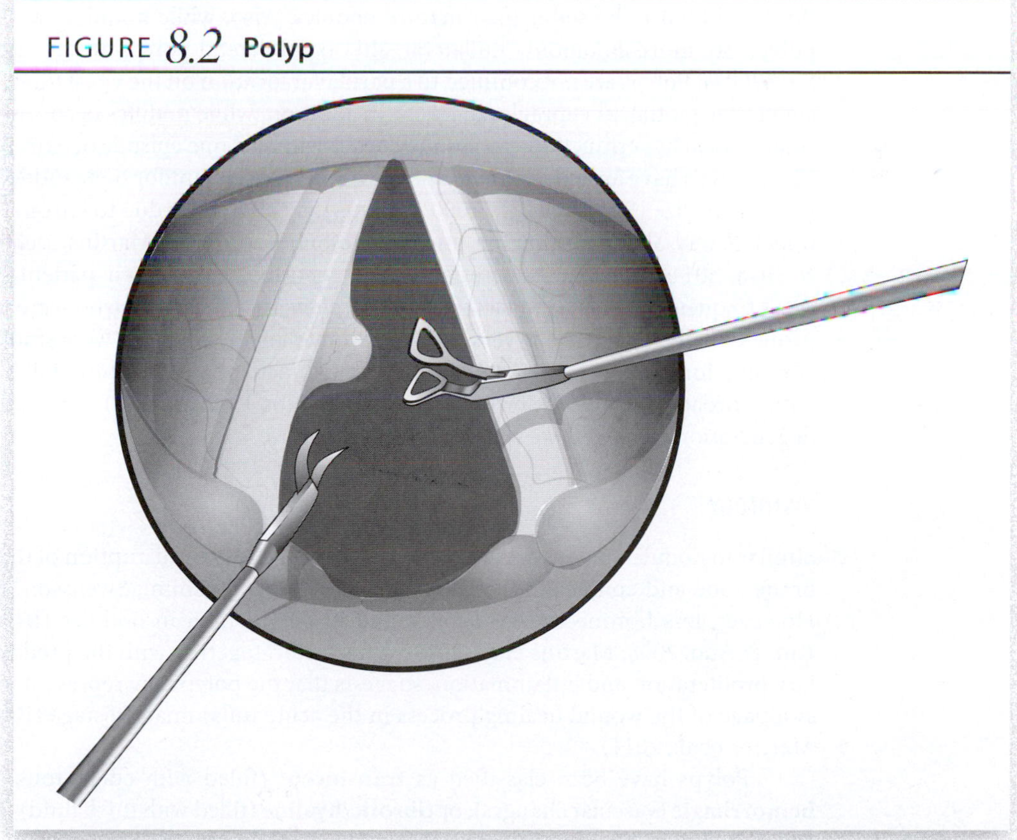

TABLE 8.2 **Differences between Nodules and Polyps**

Nodules	Polyps
Immature may be fluid-filled; mature are fibrotic	May be translucent, hemorrhagic, or fibrotic
Develop over time with continued phonotrauma	Can occur from one episode of extreme phonotrauma
Usually bilateral	Usually unilateral
Occur at the midpoint of the membranous glottis	Can occur at subglottal, glottal, or supraglottal levels
Typically sessile	May be sessile, pedunculated, or nonlocalized
Greater amounts of fibronectin	Smaller amounts of fibronectin
May be the end result of the wound healing process	May represent an interruption or stoppage of the wound healing process

fluid and tend to be softer than mature nodules. Also, while nodules are typically bilateral, polyps are more commonly unilateral, although bilateral polyps are not rare (Yun, Kim, & Son, 2007). Polyps are not confined to a particular location on the vocal folds, but may occur at subglottal, glottal, or supraglottal levels. In addition, while nodules occur over time with continued vocal hyperfunction, polyps may occur with just one episode of extreme phonotrauma. Most polyps have an active blood supply, which may account for their sudden onset and rapid increase in size (Stemple et al., 2000). Polyps may also occur due to chronic infections of the upper airway, allergies, smoking, and gastroesophageal reflux (Martins, Defaveri, Domingues, & Silva, 2011). Petrovic-Lazic et al. (2009) reported that in their patients with polyps, the most frequent predisposing factors were vocal overuse in people who were using their voices professionally (teachers, lawyers, etc.), had upper airway allergies, were smokers, and had any combination of these factors. Polyps may be pedunculated with a thin, stalklike base, or sessile with a broad, flat base. Refer to color insert photos 18 through 21. A condition of polypoid degeneration called *Reinke's edema* affects the entire vocal fold.

HISTOLOGY

Similar to nodules, polyps are characterized histologically by disruption of the basement membrane zone and epithelial thickening (Eckley, Corvo, Yoshimi, Swensson, & Duprat, 2009). However, less fibronectin has been found in polyps than in nodules (Branski et al., 2006; Kim & Auo, 2008; Martins et al., 2011). This factor, together with the predominance of capillary proliferation and inflammation, suggests that the polyp may represent an interruption or stoppage of the wound healing process in the acute inflammatory stage (Branski et al., 2006; Martins et al., 2011).

Polyps have been classified as **translucent** (filled with edematous-appearing fluid); **hemorrhagic** (vascular changes); or **fibrotic/hyaline** (filled with thick fluid) (Cohen & Garrett, 2007). Polyps may be translucent at the earliest stages of the growth (immature). Hemorrhagic polyps may represent an intermediate stage of development, and fibrotic polyps appear to be the most mature (Cohen & Garrett, 2007). Hemorrhagic polyps may occur when strong collision forces during vibration damage the basement membrane of the epithelium and the superficial layer of the lamina propria. When the damage starts to heal, the blood vessels within the newly formed tissue are prone to rupture and bleed. This results in the formation of a hematoma and, ultimately, the polyp (Klein et al., 2008). Ahmad and Soliman (2008) studied polyp specimens and reported that all were characterized by a combination of loose **myxomatous material** (benign neoplasm derived from connective tissue), **stroma** (connective tissue framework of an organ), submucosal hemorrhage, fibrosis, and acute and chronic inflammation.

Polyps have been associated with other vocal fold lesions. Eckley et al. (2009) reported that over 44% of their patients who underwent surgical excision of polyp had associated lesions including cysts, sulcus vocalis, capillary ectasias, and microwebs. They suggested that patients with these underlying deviations are more vulnerable to vocal fold damage from phonotrauma or other causes.

REINKE'S EDEMA

Reinke's edema (RE) is the name for a condition of polypoid degeneration of the vocal folds. This is a chronic inflammatory disease in which the entire membranous portion of the vocal folds becomes infiltrated with thick, gelatinous fluid (Martins, Fabro, Domingues, Chi, & Gregorio, 2009; Stemple et al., 2000). The swelling is typically bilateral, but is often more pronounced on one side. See color insert photos 22 through 24.

The condition varies in its severity, but usually it is a result of heavy smoking. RE is associated with hemorrhage, keratosis of the epithelium, increased fibrin deposition, dilated blood vessels, and thickening of the basement membrane zone (Jovanovic et al., 2008; Martins et al., 2009). Similar to a localized polyp, the condition may represent an arrest in the normal wound healing process due to prolonged exposure to inflammatory stimuli (Branski et al., 2006).

RE is also characterized by abnormal patterns of vascularization. In normal vocal folds the blood vessels run in a parallel direction to the free edge of the vocal fold. Blood vessels in the vocal folds of individuals with RE reportedly demonstrate a variety of irregular shapes, positions, and patterns, as well as an increased amount of vessel proliferation (Jovanovic et al., 2007; Martins et al., 2009). The abnormal vascular structure appears to be related to smoking. Jovanovic et al. (2009) suggested that tobacco smoke could decrease the speed at which blood flows through the vessels, which increases the possibility of thrombosis. In addition, edema can result in abnormal blood supply to tissues, which affects the ability of the vocal folds to undergo the repair and remodeling process.

SYMPTOMS

Symptoms of polyps and/or RE vary depending on the extent and location of the lesion. If the polyp interferes with vocal fold adduction and vibration, dysphonia will result. Typically the dysphonia is characterized by a hoarse and breathy quality, and a low pitch. Large polyps and RE may result in airway obstruction with stridor and dyspnea on exertion (Ahmad & Soliman, 2008). In addition, patients may complain of frequent throat clearing, throat pain, and globus sensation.

TREATMENT

Treatment may be behavioral, surgical, or a combination.

Voice Therapy. Several reports have documented resolution of polyps with behavioral voice therapy in at least a percentage of patients. Voice therapy approaches include vocal hygiene and direct techniques to improve vocal production. Yun et al. (2007) provided a systematic program of vocal hygiene and vocal education for patients prior to scheduled surgical removal of polyps. The vocal hygiene program included information regarding beneficial environmental changes, vocal behavioral habits and changes, and dietary changes. Vocal education included a review of the pathophysiology of vocal polyps, identification of vocally traumatic behaviors, and tips on how to reduce the identified behaviors. More than one-third of the patients demonstrated 50% to 100% resolution of the polyp, and they reported more stable and better voice quality, less vocal fatigue, and less throat discomfort. Based on their experience, the authors concluded that a substantial number of patients may avoid surgery when provided with behavioral strategies to change vocal behavior. Cohen and Garrett (2007) reviewed medical records of 435 patients with polyps or cysts who had received at least 2 sessions of voice therapy. The therapy approach included vocal hygiene, improving breath support, decreasing laryngeal tension, and regulating pitch. If present, allergies and GERD were treated. Improvement with voice therapy alone was achieved in around half of the patients. Individuals with translucent polyps were more likely to have improved voice after therapy than those with the other types of polyps, perhaps because these types of polyps are less mature and therefore more likely to respond to voice therapy. Klein et al. (2008) reported that voice therapy resolved 9 out of 16 polyps, roughly within 4–5 months after initial presentation. The authors suggested that patients with an acute, recent onset of symptoms and a small or medium-sized hemorrhagic polyp may respond well to nonsurgical therapy.

Surgery. When voice therapy alone is not sufficient, surgery is quite often required, particularly in the case of RE and large or persistent polyps. The polyp is excised under general anesthesia with microlaryngeal instrumentation, CO_2 laser, pulsed dye laser, or the laryngeal microdebrider (Ahmad & Soliman, 2008; Kim & Auo, 2008). A recently reported technique is excision of a pedunculated polyp under local anesthesia by means of micro tweezers through a flexible nasoendoscope (Vegas, Cobeta, Mico, & Rivera, 2010). Surgical excision has been reported to result in a smooth free edge of the operated fold, normal mucosal wave, reduced phonation threshold pressures, less effortful phonation, and normalized acoustic values (Petrovic-Lazic et al., 2009; Vegas et al., 2010; Wang, Shau, & Hsiao, 2010). In the case of RE, the excess material may be removed via laser, phonomicrosurgical excision, or laryngeal debrider (e.g., Murry, Abitbol, & Hersan, 1999; Sant'Anna & Mauri, 2010; Yonekawa, 1988). Prior to the advent of current phonomicrosurgical techniques, the procedure for RE involved vocal fold stripping in which the epithelial layer of the vocal folds was removed. However, this resulted in severe scarring, with resulting permanent dysphonia. Vocal fold stripping is not practiced currently and should never be recommended for patients with RE. It is important that any vocal fold irritants be identified and eliminated before surgery, such as gastroesophageal reflux and smoking. Voice rest after surgery is usually prescribed in order for the vocal folds to heal without scarring or web formation. Voice therapy is essential following surgery in order to prevent the polyp from reoccurring.

Leukoplakia

Leukoplakia is a clinical descriptor indicating the presence of keratin (a type of protein) on an epithelial surface (Figure 8.3) (Isenberg et al., 2008).

FIGURE 8.3 **Leukoplakia**

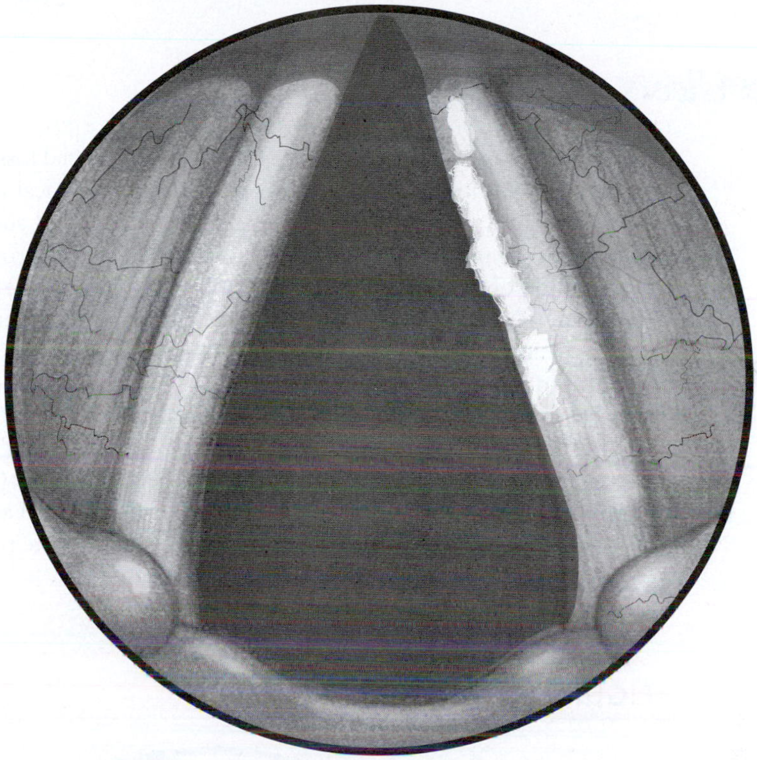

Recall that normal vocal fold epithelium is nonkeratinizing, so the presence of leukoplakia is an indication of an abnormal change in the epithelium. Approximately 50% of these lesions are benign and about 50% are premalignant with around a 6–7% chance of developing into carcinoma (Isenberg, Crozier, & Dailey, 2008). There appears to be an association between the degree of dysplasia (abnormal tissue development) and the conversion to carcinoma. The more severe is the dysplasia, the higher is the risk of malignancy (Isenberg et al., 2008). Whether or not a malignant change has occurred is determined through a biopsy.

TREATMENT

Treatment of leukoplakia can be problematic. Surgically removing the abnormal tissue can injure the vocal folds, while not treating the condition runs the risk of malignant conversion. Some voice professionals have found that antireflux treatment such as PPI therapy can be beneficial in reducing or eliminating the leukoplakia (e.g., Simpson, Archilla, Velazquez, & McGuff, 2006). Another option aside from surgery is photodynamic therapy (PDT). This is an experimental treatment currently being evaluated for a wide variety of neoplasms of the head and neck (Franco, 2007). A drug is topically administered that is retained in abnormal cells to a greater degree than in surrounding normal tissue. The drug kills the tumor cells while sparing the normal cells. Franco (2007) used this technique with patients with moderate vocal fold leukoplakia and dysplasia and reported a 78% reduction in the amount of keratosis.

Contact Ulcers and Granulomas

An **ulcer** is a lesion on a mucus surface caused by superficial loss of tissue, and usually occurs in conjunction with inflammation. Contact ulcers of the vocal folds occur when the mucosa covering the vocal processes collides repeatedly with a hard surface. Because the mucosa is thin and delicate and overlies the less flexible cartilage, it is prone to being crushed between any unyielding object (e.g., endotracheal tube, or the opposite arytenoid cartilage) and the cartilage beneath it. This causes the mucosa to break down, creating the ulcer. A granuloma is a mass of tissue consisting of inflammation, a large amount of blood cells and connective tissue, covered by squamous epithelium (Figure 8.4) (Garnett, 2001). Granulation tissue is created by fibroblasts during the wound healing process and typically grows from the base of a wound or injury. Vocal process granulomas may be the end result of inflammation caused by chronic irritation and thus represent a post-traumatic healing process (Wang et al., 2009; Yun, Lee, & Park, 2008). An ulcer can become granulated as the affected area is covered by granulation tissue (Yun et al., 2008). Ulcers and granulation occur on the posterior cartilaginous part of

FIGURE 8.4 **Granuloma**

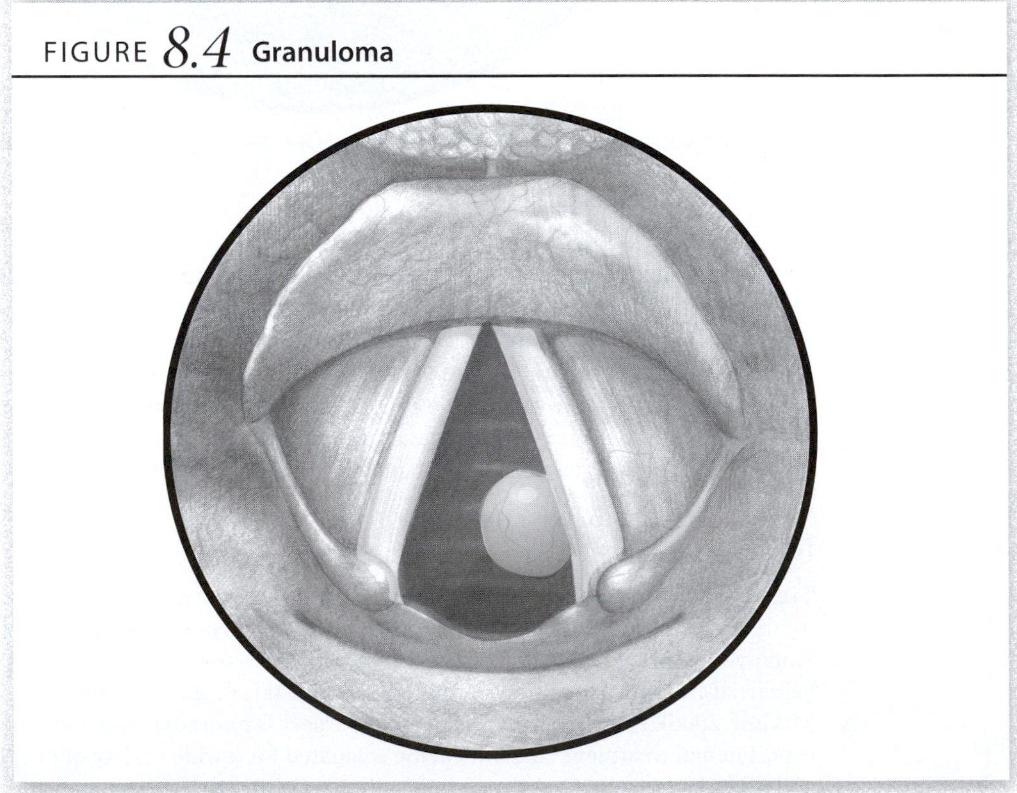

the vocal fold, where the folds attach to the vocal processes of the arytenoid cartilages. The lesion may be unilateral or bilateral. Although the lesion is located in the back portion of the glottis, the anterior sections may also look unhealthy, with thickening of the vocal fold cover (Mathieson, 2001). The tissue on the arytenoid cartilages looks swollen and inflamed. Granulomas may be pedunculated or sessile and vary in color from pale to red (Garnett, 2001). Refer to color insert photos 25 through 27.

CAUSES

For many years, the primary cause of contact ulcers and granulation was thought to be phonotrauma, characterized by the use of an extremely low pitch in conjunction with an effortful voice quality. This configuration of the glottis causes the vocal processes to collide with excessive force. Over time this can create the mucosal breakdown that results in ulceration and granulation.

Other causes of contact ulcer have become apparent over the years. One major cause is gastroesophageal reflux. The refluxate irritates and inflames the sensitive laryngeal tissues in the posterior part of the larynx. It has been found that a large proportion of patients with granuloma suffer from laryngopharyngeal reflux (e.g., Lemos, Sennes, Imamura, & Tsuji, 2005; Ylitalo, 2006). Endotracheal intubation can also cause ulceration and granulation by exerting pressure against the vocal folds, particularly in the posterior region. Individuals who need to be ventilated for long periods of time tend to be prone to contact ulcers. Indeed, laryngeal granuloma has been reported to be the most common late complication of endotracheal intubation in adults (Yun et al., 2008). Other factors that have been implicated in the formation of ulcers and granuloma include smoking, allergies, infections, postnasal drip, and chronic throat clearing (Garnett, 2001). Psychosocial elements may also contribute to contact ulcer formation, such as aggressive personality, introversion, depression, and emotional tension. One should keep in mind that all these conditions (phonotrauma, acid reflux, personality factors, etc.) can coexist in the same patient, so it is important to treat all factors that may be contributing to the ulcer and/or granuloma.

SYMPTOMS

The most common laryngeal symptoms in patients with contact ulcers and/or granuloma are reported to be throat clearing, hoarseness, restricted pitch range, vocal fatigue, sore throat, globus pharyngeus, chronic cough, hyperemia and edema of the arytenoid region, excessive tissue in the interarytenoid area, subglottic edema, and dyspnea (Garnett, 2001; Lemos et al., 2005; Ylitalo, 2006; Yun et al., 2008). In addition, unlike other benign lesions such as nodules and polyps, contact ulcers are painful. The pain may occur as a burning sensation in the larynx, or as a shooting pain in the ear. The pain may be particularly acute when the individual coughs, swallows, or clears his or her throat (Garnett, 2001; Mathieson, 2001). Even if the patient does not show symptoms, the ulcer and/or granuloma should be treated to prevent possible complications, including airway obstruction, vocal fold fixation, and posterior laryngeal stenosis (Garnett, 2001).

EVALUATION AND TREATMENT

Correct diagnosis of the cause or causes of contact ulcer is essential, so that the appropriate treatment plan can be developed. Tests for acid reflux must be done, as well as laryngoscopic visualization of the larynx. On laryngeal examination, the arytenoid cartilages often look bulky and inflamed (Mathieson, 2001). Laryngoscopy may reveal either epithelial ulceration or a reddish or grayish mass (Devaney, Rinaldo, & Ferlito, 2005). As with other phonotraumatic lesions a thorough voice evaluation by the speech-language pathologist is critical, in order to assess the type and amount of vocally damaging behaviors.

Voice Therapy. Voice therapy is typically recommended for individuals with contact ulcers. Treatment usually focuses on the causes of the problem. A program of vocal hygiene and vocal education is essential to reduce or eliminate phonotraumatic behaviors. Treatment is also directed at any underlying conditions such as acid reflux, allergies, and postnasal drip. It has been reported that most patients whose underlying cause of ulcer is phonotrauma respond well to voice therapy in conjunction with medical management, and most patients whose underlying cause is reflux respond well to medical management (Garnett, 2001).

Surgery. When nonsurgical means are not effective, or when the airway is compromised, or malignancy is suspected, surgery using microlaryngeal instruments to excise the granuloma may be indicated. However, there are some problems with surgical management. First, there is a high recurrence rate after surgery, around 37–50% (Garnett, 2001). The high postsurgical recurrence rate has been associated with a lack of voice treatment before and after the surgery, lack of antireflux treatment, and continuing phonotrauma. Second, the surgery may cause the granuloma to migrate along the edge of the wound (Garnett, 2001). When surgery is the appropriate treatment, a steroid may be injected into the interarytenoid and immediate cricoarytenoid regions just before the surgical removal of the granulation tissue. Injecting a steroid directly at the site of the lesion improves its effects by concentrating the dosage directly on the laryngeal mucosa. Other treatments include inhaled corticoids and Botox injection. Reportedly, inhaled corticoids can be effective in resolving granulomas, although resolution may take as long as 6–8 months (Lemos et al., 2005). Botox injection is aimed at preventing forceful closure of the arytenoids and has been used successfully when granulomas are resistant to behavioral treatment (e.g., Emami, Morrison, Rammage, & Bosch, 1999; Nasri, Sercarz, Mcalpin, & Berke, 1995; Orloff & Goldman, 1999).

Even when surgery is necessary, behavioral voice treatment is beneficial to prevent recurrence of the problem (Devaney et al., 2005).

Vascular Lesions of the Vocal Folds

The microcirculation in the vocal folds is designed to allow an uninterrupted and continuous flow of blood even during the high collision forces of vibration. Blood vessels in the superficial lamina propria (SLP) run in a longitudinal direction with many connections (anastomoses) between the arterial and venous capillaries. This arrangement facilitates the blood flow. There is no direct communication between the blood capillaries in the SLP and the thyrovocalis muscle, allowing the cover to move freely over the vocal ligament and muscle (Zeitels et al., 2006). The subepithelial blood vessels are able to accommodate to changes in the length and viscoelastic tension of the vocal folds without affecting the blood supply (Zeitels et al., 2006). However, high effort vocal fold vibration can cause the blood vessels to dilate or rupture, resulting in hemorrhage, varices, or ectasias. Vocal fold hemorrhage is a condition of diffuse subepithelial bleeding (see color insert photos 28, 29, and 30) (Gokcan & Dursun, 2009). A **varix** is a prominent dilated vein on the surface of the vocal fold; **ectasias** are characterized by a proliferation of blood vessels that looks like a neoplasm (Gokcan & Dursun, 2009; Schweinfurth & Ossoff, 2008).

Varices and ectasias are more likely to rupture and bleed into the vocal folds than are normal blood vessels (Zeitels et al., 2006). Constant trauma may further weaken the blood vessel walls. Repeated trauma may also result in the formation and proliferation of new blood vessels. Resulting hemorrhage and edema can lead to scarring and stiffness, or to the formation of a hemorrhagic polyp or cyst (Neely & Rosen, 2000; Neuenschwander & Dollar, 2005; Schweinfurth & Ossoff, 2008; Zeitels et al., 2006).

CAUSES

Vascular lesions of the vocal folds are strongly associated with vocal fold trauma, particularly in female vocalists. Postma et al. (1998) reported that 3.1% of their dysphonic patients had vocal fold vascular lesions. Of these patients, approximately three-quarters were female, and the vast majority were occupational voice users including singers and teachers.

SYMPTOMS

The clinical manifestations of varices and ectasias are variable, ranging from no symptoms to severe dysphonia. The dysphonia may have a sudden onset following an episode of vocal trauma, or may manifest as vocal fatigue or a loss of vocal range (Gokcan & Dursun, 2009; Neely & Rosen, 2000; Schweinfurth & Ossoff, 2008). Patients with recurrent hemorrhage may report an ongoing history of episodes of hoarseness (Schweinfurth & Ossoff, 2008). The bleeding may result in **ecchymosis** (a purplish patch caused by leaking out of blood into the skin) and **hemosiderosis** (an accumulation of **hemosiderin**—yellow or brown protein) in the affected vocal fold. In women the appearance of the lesion may depend on the stage of the menstrual cycle.

In addition to phonotrauma and vocal strain, there are several risk factors for vocal fold hemorrhage. One is aspirin, which has anticoagulant properties (Neely & Rosen, 2000; Neuenschwander & Dollar, 2005). Other risk factors include anatomic abnormalities and hormonal changes during different phases of a woman's cycle or with oral contraceptive use.

EVALUATION AND TREATMENT

Videostroboscopy usually identifies the vascular lesion in conjunction with vocal fold stiffness and loss of mucosal wave and amplitude (Neuenschwander & Dollar, 2005). As with all voice disorders, a thorough exploration of the patient's vocal usage and medical and lifestyle factors must be undertaken to identify potential causes of the problem.

Voice Therapy. In most cases hemorrhages resolve spontaneously or with conservative behavioral management. Conservative management typically includes 7 days of complete voice rest, followed by a variable period of reduced voice usage (e.g., Gokcan & Dursun, 2009; Neuenschwander & Dollar, 2005). Aspirin and other anticoagulants such as Coumadin should be avoided if at all possible, and women should stop hormone therapy and/or contraceptive pills. The patient should be encouraged to keep well hydrated, and a mucolytic agent such as guaifenesin may be prescribed to thin vocal fold secretions. Any underlying condition such as reflux disease, cough, or respiratory infection should be controlled (Neuenschwander & Dollar, 2005). Gokcan and Dursun (2009) described a systematic treatment protocol for their patients with vascular lesions. All patients were placed on strict voice rest for 7 days, and if necessary, for relative voice rest for an additional 3–6 weeks. Vocal hygiene was stressed, including increased water intake and avoidance of caffeine, alcohol, and smoking. Singers were advised to work with vocal coaches to develop better singing technique. If LPR was evident, PPI treatment was provided. The authors reported that behavioral therapy was completely successful in approximately one-third of patients.

Surgery. Surgery may be necessary in cases of recurrent hemorrhage, enlargement of the lesion, development of a mass, or a degree of dysphonia that is not acceptable to the patient (Gokcan & Dursun, 2009; Neely & Rosen, 2000; Schweinfurth & Ossoff, 2008). The surgery involves laser ablation, electrocautery, or removal of enlarged blood vessels with cold instrument dissection. Voice rest and voice therapy are strongly indicated following surgery (e.g., Hochman, Sataloff, Hillman, & Zeitels, 1999; Zeitels et al., 2006).

Vocal Fatigue

Vocal fatigue involves a physiological decline in the force of muscle contraction via central and peripheral factors. Vocal fatigue does not involve specific lesions or structural changes of the larynx and/or vocal folds, but is associated with factors related to excessive voice use, poor vocal technique, and emotional and/or physical stress (Milbrath & Solomon, 2003). The condition may occur as an independent entity, or as a component of other voice disorders (Solomon, 2008). The essential characteristic of vocal fatigue is a subjective perception of progressive increase in phonatory effort with increasing difficulty in producing and sustaining a stable voice quality (McCabe & Titze, 2002; Rantala, Vilkman, & Bloigu, 2002; Welham & Maclagan, 2003). As the vocal muscles fatigue the increased effort to produce voice may be perceived by the speaker as tightness in the throat or upper body, dry throat, odynophonia (pain upon phonation), and an overall sensation of increased muscular effort with little vocal output (McCabe & Titze, 2002). Other symptoms of vocal fatigue include hoarseness, reductions in dynamic range and pitch range, and reduced respiratory support for phonation (Welham & Maclagan, 2003). Eventually the severity of the symptoms may reach a point where the individual finds it too difficult or painful to continue talking. However, individuals have different levels of susceptibility to vocal fatigue, and there is considerable variability in the extent to which prolonged strenuous vocal activity causes adverse effects on laryngeal function (e.g., Mann et al., 1999).

CENTRAL FATIGUE

Central fatigue involves a reduction of neural stimulation to muscles by the central nervous system. This is thought to be a protective strategy to avoid muscle damage. The reduction in neuromuscular stimulation results in a reduction of the muscle's ability to sustain tension under repeated stimulation. There is a corresponding decline in the muscle's ability to contract and yield a stable output. As this occurs and the muscle fatigues, increasing numbers of muscle fibers must be recruited to maintain a specific muscular force (Boucher & Ayad, 2010). With continuing effort, the recruitment of additional fibers can extend to adjacent muscles, resulting in a general stiffening of laryngeal structures (Boucher, 2008). Thus a vicious cycle is created whereby increased phonatory effort results in greater stiffness of the vocal mechanism, which can lead to tissue changes such as edema, nodules, polyps, varices, or ectasias.

PERIPHERAL FATIGUE

Peripheral fatigue occurs due to changes in muscle and tissue chemistry and composition. During any type of vigorous exercise, chemical compounds that provide energy to the muscles become depleted, resulting in insufficient energy supplies to meet the needs for contraction (Westerblad & Allen, 2002). In addition to muscle changes, laryngeal tissue fatigue is caused by temporary changes or damage to the epithelium and lamina propria (Hunter & Titze, 2009; Milbrath & Solomon, 2003; Welham & Maclagan, 2003). Phonotrauma can cause epithelial cells to die and collagen and elastin fibers to separate from the extracellular matrix at the basement membrane (Hunter & Titze, 2009).

RECOVERY

Recovery from fatigue occurs relatively quickly in muscles, whereas damage to the epithelium and basement membrane zone (BMZ) takes considerably longer to resolve. When the BMZ is injured it is repaired by fibroblasts, a process that involves removing and reusing old protein debris to make new protein fibers (Titze, 1999). The repair process can take as long as 72 hours to complete. The process of destruction and repair during recovery from fatigue takes place continually, even during normal phonation. When the individual uses his or her voice on a protracted daily basis, the healing mechanism is in a state of continual repair (Hunter & Titze, 2009). With moderate vocal fatigue, the voice typically recovers overnight or over a period of reduced vocal usage (Hunter & Titze, 2009). However, longer recovery times may be needed with greater degrees of injury (Chang & Karnell, 2004). Further, permanent injury may result if the individual does not allow enough recovery time after strenuous phonatory activity (Titze, 1999).

FATIGUE AND PHONATION THRESHOLD PRESSURE

Vocal fatigue and the accompanying increase in perceived phonatory effort (PPE) have been linked to increased phonation threshold pressure (PTP). Experimental studies have shown that PTP increases and glottal closure patterns change with induced vocal fatigue. For example, Solomon, Glaze, Arnold, and van Mersbergen (2003) had vocally normal men read loudly for two hours and reported increased PTP, particularly at high fundamental frequencies. Videostroboscopy performed before and after the loud reading demonstrated changes in vocal fold physiology including anterior glottal gaps and a spindle-shaped glottis. Videostroboscopic data obtained from patients complaining of vocal fatigue corroborate the changes to glottal shape during phonation (e.g., Eustace, Stemple, & Lee, 1996).

A relationship exists between PTP, vocal fold hydration levels, vocal fatigue, and vocal recovery. Chang and Karnell (2004) used a vocally demanding task (2 hours of loud reading at 3 different pitches) and measured PTP and PPE. On average, PTP recovered within 1 hour, and PPE recovered within 1 day. However, there was considerable individual variability in recovery time.

Vocal folds that are well hydrated require less PTP to be set into vibration. The viscosity of the vocal fold mucosa is influenced by increasing or decreasing systemic and/or superficial hydration (Sivasankar, Erickson, Schneider, & Howes, 2008). The greater the vocal fold viscosity, the greater is the amount of PTP required, and vice versa. Solomon and DiMattia (2000) manipulated hydration levels and fatigue in vocally healthy speakers and reported that even under the most hydrated condition, PTP increased after loud reading. However, PTP returned to baseline levels after only 15 minutes of vocal silence. This relationship was also demonstrated in the speakers' perception of effort. All participants rated effort for speaking to be higher after prolonged loud reading and to be lower after the brief period of vocal rest. Sivasankar et al. (2008) had speakers with and without vocal fatigue breathe orally and nasally in different ambient humidity conditions. Fifteen minutes of oral breathing at low humidity significantly increased PTP in both groups, but to a greater extent in the speakers with vocal fatigue. Nasal breathing showed a decrease of PTP in all healthy speakers and more than half of the speakers with vocal fatigue. The authors noted that mouth breathing increases the viscosity of surface fluid and reduces mucocillary clearance. Inhalation of dry air also increases the adhesiveness of mucus and can cause accumulation of mucus on the airway surface. Sivasankar et al. (2008) suggested that dehydration may be especially detrimental to individuals with vocal fatigue even when they are not speaking.

Occupational Voice Users

People who use their voices occupationally, such as teachers, singers, salespeople, lawyers, preachers, aerobics instructors, and so on, are particularly prone to vocal fatigue and benign mucosal lesions of the vocal folds. The discussion that follows focuses on teachers, but many of the principles apply to all occupational and professional voice users.

It is estimated that teachers comprise approximately 5.09% of the United States workforce (U.S. Department of Labor, Bureau of Labor Statistics, 2006). This translates to over three million primary and secondary school teachers in the United States (Thibeault, Merrill, Roy, Gray, & Smith, 2004). Prevalence rates for voice disorders in teachers range from 20–50% (Lowell et al., 2008). Voice problems in teachers are not unique to the United States, but have been reported around the world, including Spain (Preciado-Lopez, Perez-Fernandez, Calzada-Uriondo, & Preciado Ruiz, 2007), Australia (Russell, Oates, & Greenwood, 1998), Finland (Sala, Laine, Simberg, Pentti, & Suonpaa, 2001), Brazil (De Medeiros, Barreto, & Assuncao, 2007), Sweden (Fritzell, 1996), Hong Kong (Yiu, 2002), Taiwan (Chen, Chiang, Chung, Hsiao, & Hsiao, 2010), and England (Comins, 1992). A large body of research from countries around the world as well as in the United States has focused on teachers' vocal problems. The findings of this research can be categorized into five related areas, including occupational risk factors for teachers, most commonly reported symptoms, student teachers, vocational and societal effects of teachers' voice problems, and prevention/treatment strategies for teachers.

OCCUPATIONAL RISK FACTORS

The very nature of the teaching process poses vocal risks. Factors contributing to the risk include phonation time, background noise, environmental pollutants, teaching level, and gender (Table 8.3).

Phonation Time. The most important factor contributing to vocal risk is the amount of talking required on a daily basis. Phonation time is a way of quantifying voice use and is measured as phonation per hour. Teachers have been found to have considerably higher phonation times than other professionals. Teachers' phonation times have been reported as approximately 17–20%, compared to nurses and speech pathologists whose phonation times were 5.3% and 6.9%, respectively (Masuda, Ikeda, Manako, & Komiyama, 1993; Sodersten,

TABLE *8.3* **Occupational Risk Factors for Teachers**

Phonation Time	
Teachers	17–20%
Nurses	5.3%
Speech pathologists	6.9%
Background Noise	
Recommended	50–55 dBA
Classrooms	50–90 dBA (range)
	65–76 dBA (average)
Environmental Pollutants	
Chalk	
Chemicals	
Teaching Level	
Kindergarten—highest incidence of voice disorders	
Elementary/primary—lower incidence of voice disorders	
Gender	
Males	14.3% reporting voice problems
Females	22.5% reporting voice problems

Sources: Information from Bovo et al. (2007); Marcelino et al. (2005); Masuda et al. (1993); Russell et al. (1998); Sodersten et al. (2002); Thibeault et al. (2004); Van Houtte, in press, doi:10.1016/j.voice.2010.04.008.

Granqvist, Hammarberg, & Szabo, 2002). Exacerbating the problem is that teachers have few opportunities for resting their voice.

Background Noise. Teachers often must speak above high levels of noise in the classroom. The recommended noise level in environments where speech communication is important is 50–55 dBA (Bovo et al., 2007). Noise levels in day care centers and in primary and secondary classrooms have been reported to range from 50–90 dBA, with an average ranging from 65–76 dBA (Bovo et al., 2007; Sodersten et al., 2002; Thibeault et al., 2004). The background noise in classrooms comes from multiple sources including heating, ventilation, and air conditioning noise; transmitted noise from outside the building; transmitted noise from other classrooms; and noise from the children in the classroom (Thibeault et al., 2004). In order to make themselves heard and to keep the students' attention, teachers must increase their vocal intensity levels for extended periods of time. Increased fundamental frequency levels have been reported in conjunction with the increased intensity (e.g., Rantala et al., 2002; Sodersten et al., 2002). Sodersten et al. (2002) reported that female teachers in their study spoke at a level of 85.4 dB during the working day, which was on average 9.1 dB higher than during baseline. In addition, vocal fundamental frequency increased from 202 Hz during baseline to 247 Hz during work. High intensity and high frequency phonation results in a high level of vocal fold collision forces (Bovo et al., 2007). The elevated vocal loudness has been shown to increase by a factor of 4 the probability of developing a voice disorder (Chen et al., 2010).

Environmental Pollutants. Environmental pollutants such as chalk may be implicated in some teachers' voice dysfunction. The main component of chalk is calcium carbonate (Marcelino & Oliveira, 2005). Particles of this substance can cause coughing and can injure the mucosa of the vocal folds (Marcelino & Oliveira, 2005). Further, the dust in the vocal tract can reduce the secretions of the salivary and mucous glands, creating a vicious cycle in which breathing dry air results in dryness and irritation of the mucosa (Marcelino & Oliveira, 2005). Science teachers may be exposed to additional pollutants. In a survey of teachers, Thibeault et al. (2004) found that the percentage of chemical science teachers experiencing a voice disorder increased with the number of chemicals to which they were exposed. Many chemicals to which these teachers are exposed are listed by the Committee on Chemical Safety as corrosive, carcinogenic, and/or highly toxic, and the relationship between inhalation of fumes and tissue injury of the aerodigestive tract is well documented (Thibeault et al., 2004).

Teaching Level. There is some evidence that teaching level (i.e., kindergarten, primary, secondary) affects vocal usage. Bovo et al. (2007) reported that the maximum incidence of voice disorders is reported by kindergarten teachers, with increasingly reduced incidence for elementary and primary school teachers.

Gender. Gender may also play a role in the development of teachers' voice problems. The incidence of vocal disorders is reported to be considerably higher in female teachers compared to their male peers (Bovo et al., 2007; Russell et al., 1998; van Houtte, Claeys, Wuyts, & Van Lierde, 2010). The gender difference may be due to the lower amounts of HA in female vocal folds, as well as to the higher frequency of vocal fold vibration resulting in higher collision forces during phonation (Lauri, Alku, Vilkman, & Sihvo, 1997).

SYMPTOMS

A wide range of vocal symptoms has been reported in teachers with voice disorders (Table 8.4).

Benign lesions including nodules, sulcus vocalis, and cysts are also common (e.g., Chen et al., 2010; Nguyen, Kenny, Tran, & Livesey, 2008; Tavares & Martins, 2007; van Houtte et al., 2010). Vocal fatigue and increased phonatory effort are core complaints of teachers with voice problems (De Medeiros et al., 2007; Lowell et al., 2008; Preciado-Lopez et al., 2007; Solomon et al., 2003; Welham & Maclagan, 2003). Kooijman, Thomas, Graamans, and De Jong (2007) surveyed 6,000 teachers, of whom more than half reported voice complaints during their professional career. Interestingly, the authors found that teachers in the latter portions of their career had fewer voice complaints than those in the beginning years. They suggested that teachers may develop coping strategies to deal with the amount of talking required as well as with the stresses involved in their work. The results indicate that special attention should be paid to teachers in the beginning of their career, and more attention should be focused on preventive programs in teacher education. De Medeiros et al. (2007) found that 17% of the teachers surveyed in their study reported voice problems at work in the last 2 weeks before the interview. Further, during those two weeks 3% were absent from work and 7% sought medical help or saw a speech therapist due to voice problems. Fifteen percent reported daily or frequent voice symptoms during the past 15 days. During their teaching career 30% of teachers reported

TABLE 8.4 Vocal and Physical Symptoms Reported in Teachers with Voice Disorders

Vocal Symptoms	Physical Symptoms
Hoarseness	Sore throat
Strain	Increased throat mucus
Edema	Neck and chest discomfort
Erythema	
Breathiness	
Difficulty projecting voice	
Low pitch	
Limited pitch and loudness range	
Loss of voice	
Vocal fatigue	
Increased phonatory effort	

Sources: Information from Chen et al. (2010); De Medeiros et al. (2007); Lowell et al. (2008); Nguyen et al. (2008); Preciado-Lopez et al. (2007); Solomon et al. (2003); Tavares & Martins, (2007); van Houtte et al. (2010); Welham & Maclagan (2003).

having had leave from work due to voice disorders. Only one-third of the teachers reported no voice symptoms during the past 15 days.

STUDENT TEACHERS

Student teachers are also subject to high vocal demands, and as a group have been found to be at risk for voice disorders. Many students demonstrate similar voice complaints to practicing teachers, including dryness in the throat, throat tightness, and vocal fatigue, as well as throat discomfort or pain, hoarseness, and reduced pitch (Sapir, Keidat, & Mathers-Schmidt, 1993). Thomas, Kooijman, Donders, Cremers, and De Jong (2007) found an incidence of 17.2% of voice complaints among student teachers, compared to 9.7% for other students. Student teachers have reported significantly more vocal symptoms than non–student teachers, including throat clearing/coughing, fatigue, hoarseness, pain or lump in the throat, and difficulty in being heard (Timmermans, De Bodt, Wuyts, & Van de Heyning, 2005). These findings indicate the need for more voice training to cope with the high vocal demands of their profession. While research in this area is sparse, there is some evidence to suggest that training during the student years can be effective in preventing the onset of voice disorders in teachers. Ilomaki, Maki, and Laukkanen (2005) surveyed teachers in Finland to determine the amount of voice education received during their teacher training. About two-thirds received no vocal education, a small percentage received short-term education, and approximately 20% of the teachers had received longer term voice education. The authors reported that the incidence of symptoms such as strain, hoarseness, and vocal fatigue was lowest among those with longer term training. An additional advantage of vocal education is that students and practicing teachers may seek treatment earlier and thus prevent a more severe voice problem from developing later on.

VOCATIONAL AND SOCIAL EFFECTS

It is clear that teaching poses a high risk for voice disorders, particularly among women. Voice dysfunction interferes with job satisfaction, job performance, and job attendance. Around 18.3% of teachers have been reported to miss at least one day of work per year due to a voice disorder (Thibeault et al., 2004). Teachers may become confused and frustrated due to the discrepancy between their perception of the severity of the voice disability and the public view of vocal fatigue as a minor and inevitable consequence of teaching (McCabe & Titze, 2002). Teachers with voice disorders have reported reduced job satisfaction levels, reduced communicative ability, chronic stress or frustration, reduced social interaction, and increased emotional distress (Chen et al., 2010; Sapir et al., 1993). The presence of a voice disorder can threaten, shorten, or even end a teacher's career (van Houtte et al., 2010). It is not uncommon for individuals in this situation to retire early or to change professions. This can have negative financial consequences for the individual, resulting in even more frustration.

Economic loss resulting from vocal problems and limitations on occupational performance affects not only individual teachers, but society as a whole. Based on factors including the number of teachers in the United States, days of work lost due to voice difficulties, the cost of substitute teachers to cover those days, and treatment costs, Verdolini and Ramig (2001) estimated that the overall cost to the United States is around $2 billion annually. This amount, according to the authors, does not include other monetary costs related to pharmaceutical treatment, worker's compensation, and change/loss of job. Thus, preventing and treating voice disorders in teachers has both personal and societal benefits.

PREVENTION AND TREATMENT

From the previous discussion it is clear that prevention and treatment of voice disorders in teachers, student teachers, and all occupational voice users is of utmost importance. While prevention programs for teachers reported in the literature are sparse, a few have been described. Bovo et al. (2007) examined data from 30 teachers who participated in a 12-hour vocal care course and 30 teachers who did not. The vocal care course included lectures and "hands-on" group sessions. The lectures focused on anatomy and physiology of phonation, causes and predisposing factors of vocal pathology, warning symptoms of vocal fatigue, vocal hygiene, classroom acoustics, and amplification systems. The group sessions focused on efficient breathing, muscle relaxation, and manual circumlaryngeal therapy; relaxed voicing with elimination of hard glottal attack; resonant voice therapy; and exercises for developing greater oral opening. Participants also kept a chart of phonotraumatic behaviors. After 3 months, 85% of teachers who took the course reported that they practiced good vocal hygiene, and 90% had adopted strategies for reducing vocal demand in the classroom. Other programs for teachers with voice problems have described positive results from treatment strategies such as resonant voice therapy (Chen et al., 2007), chanting (McCabe & Titze, 2002), vocal hygiene, and vocal exercises (Gillivan-Murphy, Drinnan, O'Dwyer, Ridha, & Carding, 2006).

chapter SUMMARY

NODULES ARE BENIGN GROWTHS THAT develop on the epithelium of the vocal folds as a consequence of vocal hyperfunction and resulting inflammation of the folds. The high collision forces generated during high effort vocal fold vibration disrupt the epithelium and basement membrane zone. Personality factors have been associated with the likelihood of developing nodules, particularly in young women and in prepubertal boys. Symptoms range from mild to severe and include hoarseness, breathiness, lowered pitch, straining, and vocal fatigue. Treatment for nodules focuses on vocal education, improved vocal usage, and direct therapy approaches to reduce muscle tension and hyperfunction. Surgery is only occasionally recommended to remove recalcitrant nodules.

Polyps are benign growths on the vocal fold mucosa that may result from laryngeal hyperfunction as well as from other causes such as chronic infections of the upper airway, allergies, smoking, and gastroesophageal reflux. Reinke's edema is a condition of polypoid degeneration that affects the entire vocal fold. Polyps are characterized histologically by disruption of the basement membrane zone, epithelial thickening, capillary proliferation, and inflammation, suggesting that the polyp may represent an interruption or stoppage of the wound healing process in the acute inflammatory stage. Dysphonia is characterized by hoarseness, breathiness, low pitch, and possible stridor and dyspnea on exertion. Frequent throat clearing and globus sensation have also been reported. Voice therapy approaches include vocal hygiene and direct techniques to improve vocal production. Surgery may be required to remove RE and large or persistent polyps.

Leukoplakia is a clinical descriptor indicating the presence of keratin on an epithelial surface. Leukoplakia may be benign or premalignant. Treatment may be behavioral such as treating underlying GERD, or surgical.

Contact ulcers of the vocal folds occur when the mucosa covering the vocal processes collides repeatedly with a hard surface resulting in superficial loss of tissue and inflammation. Vocal process granulomas may be the end result of inflammation caused by chronic irritation, and thus represent a post-traumatic healing process. Causes include phonotrauma, gastroesophageal reflux, smoking, allergies, infections, postnasal drip, chronic throat clearing, and endotracheal intubation. Symptoms include throat clearing, hoarseness, restricted pitch range, vocal fatigue, sore throat, globus pharyngeus, chronic cough, hyperemia and edema of the arytenoid region, excessive tissue in the interarytenoid area, subglottic edema, and dyspnea. Voice therapy focuses on vocal hygiene and vocal education to reduce or eliminate phonotraumatic behaviors. Underlying conditions such as acid reflux, allergies, and postnasal drip are also addressed. Surgery is recommended when nonsurgical means are not effective, or when the airway is compromised or malignancy is suspected.

High effort vocal fold vibration can cause the blood vessels in the vocal folds to dilate or rupture, resulting in hemorrhage, varices, or ectasias. Symptoms may be minimal or severe. Treatment is typically seven days of complete voice rest, followed by a variable period of reduced voice usage; aspirin and other anticoagulants, as well as hormone therapy and/or contraceptive pills should be avoided. Surgery may be necessary in cases of recurrent hemorrhage, enlargement of the lesion, development of a mass, or a degree of dysphonia that is not acceptable to the patient.

Vocal fatigue involves a physiological decline in the force of muscle contraction via central and peripheral factors. This is perceived subjectively as a progressive increase in phonatory effort with increasing difficulty in producing and sustaining a stable voice quality. The increased effort to produce voice may be perceived by the speaker as tightness in the throat or upper body, dry throat, odynophonia, and an overall sensation of increased muscular effort with little vocal output. Other symptoms of vocal fatigue include hoarseness, reductions in dynamic range and pitch range, and reduced respiratory support for phonation. Vocal fatigue is associated with excessive voice use, poor vocal technique, and emotional and/or physical stress, and it is particularly prevalent in people who use their voices occupationally, such as teachers, singers, salespeople, lawyers, preachers, and aerobics instructors. Teaching poses specific occupational risks due to high vocal demands, including increased phonation time, high levels of background noise, environmental pollutants, teaching level, and gender. Student teachers are also at risk for voice disorders. Prevention and treatment of voice disorders in teachers, student teachers, and all occupational voice users is of utmost importance.

review QUESTIONS

1. Describe the relationship between age, personality, and the development of vocal nodules.
2. Compare nodules and polyps in terms of etiology, histology, symptomatology, and treatment.
3. Differentiate between polyps and Reinke's edema, and explain why vocal fold stripping should not be used to treat Reinke's edema.
4. Identify the composition of leukoplakia and describe why it can be difficult to treat.
5. How is the process of ulceration and granulation related to wound healing in the vocal folds?
6. Describe similarities and differences between vocal fold varices, ectasias, and hemorrhage.
7. Define vocal fatigue and then explain the central and peripheral factors that contribute to this condition.
8. List and describe the factors that have been found to contribute to vocal fatigue and the development of benign lesions in teachers.

PREPARING FOR THE PRAXIS

CASE STUDY 8.1: Vocal Nodules

Directions: Please read the case study and answer the five questions that follow. The answers can be found at the bottom of the page.

Chauncey W. Barrington Jr is an 8-year-old male. He spends much of his time yelling at the maid, the cook, the chauffeur, and his mother. The rest of the time he talks incessantly to his friends on his gold-plated cell phone. Recently his mother became alarmed when his voice started to sound very hoarse, breathy, and low pitched. She took him to a laryngologist who diagnosed bilateral vocal nodules. The physician suggested that rather than having the nodules removed surgically, Chauncey should try voice therapy.

1. Chauncey's vocal habits likely resulted in
   a. irritation and inflammation of the vocal folds
   b. disruption of the basement membrane zone of the vocal folds
   c. increased levels of fibronectin within the lamina propria
   d. high collision forces between the vocal folds
   e. all of the above
2. Other professionals who should be included on a team include a
   a. pulmonologist
   b. neurologist
   c. physical therapist
   d. classroom teacher
   e. all of the above
3. The perceptual symptoms of hoarseness, breathiness, and low pitch result from
   a. tight approximation of the vocal folds during phonation
   b. incomplete vocal fold closure during phonation in conjunction with the increased vocal fold mass
   c. stretched and tense vocal folds due to excessive cricothyroid muscle contraction
   d. medial compression of the false vocal folds in conjunction with the true vocal folds
   e. differences between the vertical levels of the left and right vocal folds
4. Which of the following (if any) would NOT be an appropriate treatment approach?
   a. program of vocal hygiene and vocal education
   b. invite Chauncey's parents to participate in some therapy sessions so they learn strategies to facilitate less damaging vocal fold behaviors
   c. use a child-friendly acoustic analysis program as a form of visual biofeedback
   d. recommend surgery as it is unlikely that Chauncey will be able to modify his vocal behavior
   e. provide Chauncey with alternative strategies for communicating with people in his household
5. Differences between nodules and polyps include
   a. locations of lesions
   b. causes of lesions
   c. fibronectin levels
   d. blood supply
   e. all of the above

Answers for Case Study 8.1: 1. (e); 2. (d); 3. (b); 4. (d); 5. (e)

CASE STUDY 8.2: Vocal Fatigue

Directions: Please read the case study and answer the five questions that follow. The answers can be found at the bottom of the page.

Lauren Matthews, a 23-year-old female, comes to see you because she is having trouble talking. Her voice is important in her job—she is an elementary school teacher. She loves the children, but complains that she has a hard time making them listen to her, and by the end of the day she struggles to speak. She says that she has seen a laryngologist who found that her larynx was normal. However, her voice sounds tight and strained, with intermittent hoarseness, and you notice visible tension in the neck and facial areas.

1. Lauren's sensation of struggling to speak is best evaluated objectively through
   a. acoustic analysis of jitter, shimmer, and harmonics-to-noise ratio
   b. electroglottography
   c. pulmonary function testing
   d. phonation threshold pressure
   e. none of the above
2. Factors that may contribute to Lauren's vocal difficulties include
   a. poor classroom acoustics
   b. possible sensitivity to chalk
   c. shouting to make herself heard above noise
   d. possible lifestyle factors such as excessive talking, poor diet, etc.
   e. all of the above
3. Which of the following would be the most appropriate evaluation and treatment approach for Lauren?
   a. direct laryngoscopy under general anesthesia to determine the possibility of malignant growth on the vocal folds
   b. a trial of Botox injection
   c. recommendation to give up teaching and get a job that involves less vocal usage
   d. program of vocal hygiene and vocal education
   e. all of the above
4. Which of the following statements (if any) is NOT true of vocal fatigue?
   a. results from both central and peripheral factors
   b. is associated with degree of vocal recovery
   c. may be associated with other benign lesions of the vocal folds
   d. is common in occupational voice users
   e. all of the above statements are true
5. Which of the following statements (if any) is NOT true of phonation time?
   a. is a way of quantifying voice use measured as phonation per hour
   b. is the most important factor contributing to vocal risk
   c. is higher in teachers than in other professionals
   d. is directly proportional to phonation threshold pressure
   e. all of the above statements are true

Answers for Case Study 8.2: 1. (d); 2. (e); 3. (d); 4. (e); 5. (d)

Chapter 9
Movement Disorders

LEARNING OBJECTIVES

1. Become familiar with the Darley, Aronson, and Brown (1969) classification system of dysarthrias.
2. Describe types of vocal fold paresis and paralysis resulting from damage to the vagus nerve and appropriate treatment protocols for each type.
3. Identify the primary symptoms of and treatments for myasthenia gravis.
4. Compare and contrast spastic and ataxic dysarthria in terms of etiology, symptoms, and treatment options.
5. Explain how loss of dopamine results in the typical symptoms associated with Parkinson's disease.
6. Describe behavioral and medical/surgical options for the treatment of Parkinson's disease and voice-related symptoms.
7. Distinguish between the extrapyramidal symptoms of chorea and dystonia.
8. Understand spasmodic dysphonia as a focal dystonia.
9. Identify similarities and differences between the mixed dysarthrias of amyotrophic lateral sclerosis and multiple sclerosis.

Movement disorders are associated with problems in vocal fold function that may manifest in hyper- or hypoadduction, problems in pitch and/or loudness control, and problems in breathing and/or swallowing. Most causes of movement disorders are neurological, such as strokes, degenerative diseases, infectious diseases, and traumatic brain injury, although some movement disorders may also be caused by or have an associated psychological and/or physiological component. Neurological voice disorders comprise a subset of dysarthria. *Dysarthria* is a collective term that refers to neurologically based speech production disorders in which the primary problem is weakness, paralysis, or incoordination of any or all of the muscles of respiration, phonation, articulation, and resonance. Dysarthrias were classified by Darley, Aronson, and Brown (1969) on the basis of the primary site of the brain damage, the resulting type of movement disorder, and the perceptual symptoms of the disorder. Their classification scheme is widely used and includes six categories of motor speech disorders: flaccid, spastic, ataxic, hypokinetic, hyperkinetic, and mixed (Table 9.1). This chapter is organized according to the Darley et al. classification.

TABLE 9.1 Classification System for Dysarthrias

Type of Dysarthria	Site of Brain Damage	Primary Voice Symptoms
Flaccid	Lower motor neuron	Breathy, weak
Spastic	Upper motor neuron	Low pitch, strain-strangle
Ataxic	Cerebellum	Prosodic abnormality, scanning speech
Hypokinetic	Basal ganglia	Monotone, weak
Hyperkinetic	Basal ganglia	Chorea: Prosodic abnormality Dystonia: Effortful, strain-strangle
Mixed	Various	Depends on affected areas

Source: Information from Darley, Aronson, & Brown (1969).

Flaccid Dysarthria

Flaccid dysarthria results from damage to the **lower motor neuron (LMN)** of the brain. The LMN includes the spinal and cranial nerves, as well as the myoneural junction between the nerve ending and the muscle fibers that it innervates. Examples of disorders resulting in flaccid dysarthria are vocal fold paresis, vocal fold paralysis, and myasthenia gravis.

VOCAL FOLD PARESIS

Paresis refers to a slight or partial paralysis resulting in partial loss of muscle strength and movement. The intrinsic laryngeal muscles may be paretic if either the recurrent laryngeal nerve (RLN) or superior laryngeal nerve (SLN) is involved. Although the vocal folds are able to move, their ability to adduct, abduct, or regulate their tension is reduced, particularly when the patient performs repetitive phonatory tasks (Heman-Ackah & Batory, 2003; Heman-Ackah & Barr, 2006). The condition may be unilateral or bilateral. The degree of loss of mobility usually depends on the severity of the injury and can range from mild to severe.

Causes. Causes of paresis can include inflammation, endotracheal intubation, trauma, a mass pushing on the nerve, as well as medical conditions such as autoimmune disorders and diabetes (Mortensen & Woo, 2008). Bilateral vocal fold paresis may also be related to progressive neurological diseases such as multiple systems atrophy (Blumin & Berke, 2002). It is fairly common for an upper respiratory infection to precede the onset of symptoms, suggesting a viral cause of the problem (Rubin et al., 2005). Onset of the dysphonia may be gradual, sudden, or episodic (Simpson et al., 2009).

Symptoms. Symptoms can include breathiness, hoarseness, vocal fatigue, loss of volume, loss of projection, diplophonia, and decreased pitch range in the upper registers (Mortensen & Woo, 2008; Rubin et al., 2005; Simpson et al., 2009). Symptoms may become more pronounced with increased vocal usage. Patients with more severe paresis may present with airway obstruction or swallowing problems (Rubin et al., 2005). Videostroboscopic findings are typically extremely subtle, but may include decreased vocal fold tone, glottic gap and bowing, decreased range of motion, incomplete abduction, and asymmetric mucosal wave (Heman-Ackah & Barr, 2006). The affected vocal fold may be reduced in size due to atrophy. Because the affected muscle or muscles do retain some function but are weaker than the unaffected muscles, there may be asymmetrical muscle forces that act on the vocal folds. The distribution of muscular tension along the length of the vocal fold is unequal, resulting in different closing forces during vibration (Mortensen & Woo, 2008). Furthermore, the normally functioning muscles may compensate for the relative weakness of the affected muscles, and the compensation can result in hyperfunction and vocal fatigue (Heman-Ackah & Barr, 2006; Rubin et al., 2005).

Diagnosis and Evaluation. Diagnosing vocal fold paresis may be difficult because the signs of vocal fold hypomobility are very subtle and can be masked by the patient's compensatory vocal behaviors. The speaker's efforts to produce adequate phonation can result in hyperfunctional glottal and supraglottal compression. Thus, the patient may be incorrectly diagnosed with a muscle tension dysphonia. Further, patients tend to complain of vague symptoms that are not readily apparent on examination (Heman-Ackah & Batory, 2003).

Because of these issues, laryngeal EMG (LEMG) is the best method of diagnosing vocal fold paresis. LEMG studies of vocal fold paresis show reduced nerve activity in affected nerves (e.g., Heman-Ackah & Barr, 2006; Nierengarten, 2009). The degree of reduction can be quantified in terms of percentage to determine the severity of the paresis. Thus, 1–29% decrease in nerve activity is considered mild, 30–59% is considered to be moderate, and 60% or greater is considered to be severe (Rubin et al., 2005).

Additional tests may be necessary to confirm the diagnosis and determine the cause of the vocal fold paresis. These include a CT scan of the patient's skull base to the chest in order to rule out the presence of masses that may be impinging on the RLN; laboratory tests for diabetes, thyroid disease, and other infectious and immune disorders; and tests to determine whether the hypomobility may be due to non-nerve-related causes such as injury to the cricoarytenoid and/or cricothyroid joints, or stiffness of the joints resulting from arthritis.

A comprehensive case history is important in determining the effect of the vocal dysfunction on the individual's quality of life. Acoustic and aerodynamic tests can help to quantify the degree of disruption to the vocal signal.

Treatment. A patient may choose to leave the condition untreated if his or her voice is functional and does not interfere with vocal needs. When treatment is necessary, it may be behavioral and/or surgical. Voice therapy is critical to reduce excessive hyperfunction that may exacerbate the dysphonia. Techniques to reduce tension include yawn-sigh, general relaxation, laryngeal massage, resonant voice therapy, accent method, and other holistic approaches.

To improve glottal closure the patient may elect to undergo either **injection augmentation** or medialization thyroplasty. Studies have shown that these techniques are effective for vocal fold paresis. For example, Hertegard et al. (2004) compared the long-term effects of Hylaform and Zyplast in a series of patients with glottal insufficiency resulting from vocal fold paresis. Both of these treatments were demonstrated to be effective, with improvements in glottal closure and increased maximum phonation time. While a normal voice was not achieved for the majority of the individuals, most rated their voices as significantly improved.

VOCAL FOLD PARALYSIS

Vocal fold paralysis (VFP) is the most common vocal disorder associated with flaccid dysarthria and accounts for 10% of all laryngeal problems (Andrews, 1995). It may occur at any time over a person's lifespan. The paralysis may affect one or both vocal folds (unilateral or bilateral), and the vocal fold(s) may be paralyzed in an adducted, paramedian, or abducted position.

Unilateral Vocal Fold Paralysis. Unilateral paralysis (see color insert photos 31 and 32) is considerably more common than is bilateral vocal fold paralysis. Unilateral paralysis results from damage to the vagus nerve and its laryngeal branches (recurrent laryngeal nerve [RLN] and superior laryngeal nerve [SLN]).

Causes. The causes of unilateral vocal fold paralysis (UVFP) are numerous, including viral infections, stroke, progressive neurological diseases (e.g., multiple sclerosis), head trauma, infectious diseases, cancer that invades the vagus nerve, and thyroid surgery (Table 9.2). The cause of the paralysis may be unknown, in which case the disorder is called *idiopathic vocal fold paralysis*. In some cases paralysis that seems to be idiopathic may actually have underlying viral cause related to conditions such as herpes simplex, varicella zoster (shingles), Epstein-Barr syndrome, influenza, and upper respiratory infections (Dworkin & Treadway, 2009). Many patients who present with idiopathic UVFP have been shown to have preexisting central nervous system conditions such as recurrent cranial neuropathies, transient ischemic attack, postpolio syndrome, blacking out/numbness/blurred vision, and laryngeal spasms (Urquhart & St. Louis, 2005). In infants, UVFP may result from birth trauma, or may be secondary to congenital heart problems, surgery, or other medical procedures (Andrews, 1995).

Surgery in the area close to the RLN is a major cause of UVFP, particularly thyroid and thoracic/cardiac surgeries. Because the RLN courses close to the thyroid glands, it can be injured during thyroid surgery by being stretched, pulled, compressed, or cut. The nerve can

TABLE 9.2 Causes of Unilateral Vocal Fold Paralysis

Viral infections
Stroke
Progressive neurological diseases
Head trauma
Infectious diseases
Pulmonary, thyroid, esophageal cancer
Thyroid surgery
Thoracic/cardiac surgery
Anterior cervical spine surgery
Birth trauma
Cardiac problems

also be damaged by thermal or electrical energy generated during surgery (Rosen & Simpson, 2008; Witt, 2005). Vocal fold paralysis has also been reported following anterior cervical spine surgery (Merati, Shemirani, Smith, & Toohill, 2006). Nonlaryngeal pulmonary, thyroid, and esophageal malignancies are another major cause of UVFP because these cancers can spread and invade the RLN (Rosen & Simpson, 2008; Witt, 2005). Because the left RLN is considerably longer than the right, it is more susceptible to injury. Therefore, the left vocal fold is more commonly affected in UVFP than the right (e.g., Merati et al., 2006).

Symptoms. Several factors contribute to the specific symptoms exhibited by patients with UVFP, including the position of the paralyzed fold and the location of the nerve damage (Table 9.3). The fold can be immobilized in the adducted, paramedian, or abducted position. The position of the paralyzed fold can change over time, due to factors such as muscle atrophy, joint fibrosis, and the degree of reinnervation and synkinesis that occurs (Azadarmaki, Mirza, & Soliman, 2010; Rosen & Simpson, 2008). **Synkinesis** refers to an involuntary movement that occurs in conjunction with a voluntary movement, and results when a damaged nerve regenerates and reinnervates an incorrect muscle. When both adductor and abductor muscles are randomly innervated, the antagonistic muscular contraction can result in immobility or hypomobility of the affected fold (Azadarmaki et al., 2010). In addition, the positioning of the arytenoid cartilage on the affected side tends to shift to a more forward and medial position. This occurs due to activity of undamaged intrinsic laryngeal muscles (e.g., the interarytenoid muscle, which has bilateral innervation), passive action of ligaments within the larynx, and possible restriction of joint movement due to inflammation and fibrosis (Rontal & Rontal, 2003). The result is a bowed and shortened vocal fold that is at a lower vertical level than the healthy fold (Hong & Jung, 2001). The paralyzed vocal fold also loses tone, resulting in bowing at the midline.

The location of the nerve damage is another factor that affects the resulting voice. Proper vocal function and resonance depend on an intact nerve supply from the superior laryngeal, recurrent laryngeal, and pharyngeal branches of the vagus nerve. Injury to the vagus nerve at a level superior to the branching results in a loss of innervation to the pharyngeal, superior laryngeal, and recurrent laryngeal nerves. Thus, all muscles innervated by these nerves will be paralyzed, including the soft palate and all the intrinsic laryngeal muscles. The individual's voice is likely to be hypernasal, breathy, weak, and limited in pitch range. If only the pharyngeal branch is damaged, the patient may be mildly hypernasal, but phonation is not impacted. With damage to only the superior laryngeal nerve, the patient likely will demonstrate some restriction in pitch range, but vocal fold abduction and adduction are unaffected. When the recurrent laryngeal nerve is the only one affected, abduction and adduction are disordered, but pitch control is relatively intact.

TABLE 9.3 Factors That Influence the Position of the Paralyzed Vocal Fold

Reinnervation/synkinesis
Muscle atrophy
Joint fibrosis
Position of arytenoid cartilage

Symptoms can include problems in vocal production, breathing, and airway protection for swallowing and coughing (Table 9.4). If the fold is paralyzed close to the midline, the patient's voice may be slightly breathy, with decreased loudness, difficulty in projecting voice, vocal fatigue, and increased phonatory effort (Leydon, Bielamowicz, & Stager, 2005). Diplophonia may be present. Symptoms of airway obstruction such as stridor and dyspnea when speaking may occur (Woo & Carroll, 2009). The dyspnea is not usually due to true airway obstruction, but typically occurs when the individual uses increased supraglottic constriction as a compensatory strategy (Azadarmaki et al., 2010). With the fold paralyzed further from the midline the breathiness and weakness will be more pronounced. Coughing may be ineffective, and the patient may complain of increased throat mucus (Woo & Carroll, 2009). The airway is not affected, so pulmonary symptoms will not be present. However, swallowing may be problematic as the vocal folds are unable to approximate completely to close the glottis.

Diagnosis and Evaluation. A comprehensive assessment of the patient's vocal function should include videostrobolaryngoscopy, acoustic and aerodynamic measures of voice, and perceptual evaluation of his or her vocal quality. The impact of the disorder is assessed using an appropriate quality of life outcomes instrument such as the VHI (Table 9.5). Videostroboscopy allows the examiner to observe detailed mechanics of vibratory function including the mucosal wave, vibratory amplitude, periodicity, and symmetry of vibration (Baylor et al., 2006). A useful way of assessing the degree of paralysis is to have the individual alternately produce the /i/ vowel and sniff (the "/i/-sniff" maneuver), which causes the vocal folds to alternately adduct and abduct to their maximum extent possible (Rosen & Simpson, 2008). Flexible endoscopy is helpful in evaluating various phonatory and nonphonatory laryngeal maneuvers such as

TABLE 9.4 Position of Paralyzed Vocal Fold and Effects on Voice, Airway, and Swallowing

Median Position		
Voice	**Airway**	**Swallowing**
Slight breathiness	Mild stridor	Not affected
Slightly decreased loudness	Mild dyspnea	
Diplophonia		
Difficulty projecting voice		
Increased phonatory effort		
Vocal fatigue		
Paramedian/Abducted Position		
Voice	**Airway**	**Swallowing**
Severe breathiness/aphonia	Ineffective cough	Dysphagia
Moderate/severely decreased loudness		

TABLE 9.5 **Comprehensive Evaluation of Vocal Fold Paralysis**

Evaluation	Parameters Measured
Videostroboscopy	Glottal closure
	Mucosal wave
	Vibratory symmetry, periodicity, amplitude
Flexible nasoendoscopy	/i/-sniff maneuver
	Whistle, cough, sustained vowels, connected speech
	Supraglottal constriction
FEES	Swallowing
CT scan/x-ray	Detect masses impinging on the RLN
Laryngeal EMG	Synkinesis, nerve function
Acoustic	F0, intensity, jitter, shimmer, HNR
Aerodynamic	Air volume, flow, pressure
	MPT, s/z ratio
EGG	Phases of vibration
Perceptual	Breathiness, roughness, strain, pitch, loudness
QOL	VHI
	V-RQOL

whistle, cough, swallow, sustained vowels at high and low F0 and intensity, and connected speech (Woo & Carroll, 2009). Nasoendoscopy also allows assessment of supraglottic constriction (Woo & Carroll, 2009). As appropriate, patients may also undergo CT scans and chest x-rays to detect possible masses that may be impinging on the RLN (Dworkin et al., 2006). Laryngeal EMG is helpful is assessing presence and degree of synkinesis and is the strongest prognostic test of nerve function (Azadarmaki et al., 2010; Woo & Carroll, 2009).

Because patients with vocal fold paralysis often have weakness in vocal fold valving, their ability to cough is decreased, leaving them susceptible to aspiration pneumonia (Dworkin et al., 2006). In these cases it is important to evaluate the individual's swallowing abilities by means of modified barium swallow and Fiberoptic Endoscopic Evaluation of Swallowing (FEES) or Fiberoptic Endoscopic Evaluation of Swallowing with Sensory Testing (FEESST).

Treatment. Treatment for UVFP may be behavioral, surgical, or a combination of both. It is not unusual for the paralysis to resolve spontaneously within 6 months to a year of onset. Because of this possibility, surgery is usually not performed immediately following onset of paralysis. Many surgeons require the patient to wait 9 months to a year, unless he or she has serious problems with swallowing and aspiration. In such a case surgery may be appropriate at an earlier time. Surgery is very seldom indicated for young children, who tend to improve naturally by means of compensatory strategies, even if the affected vocal fold does not regain movement (Smith & Sauder, 2009).

Voice Therapy. Behavioral therapy is the first option for unilateral paralysis (Bergamini et al., 2010). An important goal of therapy is to prevent the individual from developing maladaptive compensatory behaviors in an effort to increase loudness, or to reduce such behaviors if they are already present. Patients can learn to lessen the muscle tension dysphonia that often accompanies their attempts to compensate for the problem. Therapy focuses on reducing vocal effort, increasing vocal efficiency, and improving voice quality (Smith & Sauder, 2009). The most common techniques are those that focus on teaching the patient good vocal hygiene, including education regarding the anatomy and physiology of voice production, modification of voice use, improved communication strategies, changing the environment to facilitate less abusive vocal usage, and suggesting assistive devices such as voice amplifiers (Baylor, Yorkston, Eadie, Strand, & Duffy, 2006; Rosen, 2002; Woo & Carroll, 2009). Approaches such as resonant voice therapy, accent therapy, and other techniques that facilitate easy onset of phonation and improved breath control can be helpful.

A few recent studies have evaluated the effectiveness of behavioral voice therapy in speakers with UVFP. Schindler et al. (2008) focused therapy on improving glottal closure while avoiding undesirable compensatory behaviors. Techniques included training the patient to produce better breath support for speech, as well as utilizing humming and resonant voice to achieve forward focus with no tension in the oral and pharyngeal musculature. Laryngeal strength and agility were targeted by vocal exercises such as sustaining vowels and gliding from the patient's highest to lowest note or vice versa. Following therapy, videolaryngoscopy demonstrated improvements in glottal closure related to compensation of the healthy vocal fold, as well as changes in the position of the paralyzed fold. Reportedly, the severity of the dysphonia lessened following behavioral intervention, confirmed by improvements in jitter, shimmer, and HNR. Patients also indicated improvements in their quality of life as shown on the VHI.

Khidr (2003) used the accent technique with 3 individuals with unilateral vocal fold paralysis, and reported post-therapy improvements in voice quality, aerodynamic values, vibratory patterns, and patients' VHI scores.

Surgery. Surgery is indicated for treatment of UVFP when swallowing is compromised, when the patient is severely breathy, or when voice therapy has not been successful (Dworkin et al., 2006; Woo & Carroll, 2009). Even when surgery is recommended, the speech-language pathologist should be actively involved in helping to determine the patient's optimal vocal quality and in facilitating his or her most effective use of the vocal mechanism. The two most commonly used surgical approaches are injection laryngoplasty and medialization thyroplasty. Laryngeal reinnervation techniques are used to a lesser degree (Blumin & Merati, 2008).

Injection augmentation has been combined with other procedures in order to maximize glottal closure and facilitate a stronger and clearer voice quality in individuals with UVFP. For example, Rontal and Rontal (2003) used Gelfoam to augment the paralyzed vocal fold in conjunction with Botox injection to block residual and synkinetic muscle activity. They also manipulated the cricoarytenoid joint in order to eliminate any stiffness or fibrosis. The authors reported both an immediate improvement of the patient's voice as well as a long-term repositioning that held the vocal fold and arytenoid in an appropriate position. Videostroboscopy showed that the arytenoid returned to an improved position on the cricoid cartilage, allowing the vocal folds to adduct at the same vertical level. Patient satisfaction with vocal quality was high on the V-RQOL. Moreover, the researchers reported that long-term follow-up (up to 4 years) of these patients demonstrated that the vocal folds maintained their functional position very near the midline. Dworkin et al. (2006) compared short-term and long-term outcomes in patients who had augmentation injection with Cymetra compared to those who underwent medialization thyroplasty. Videostroboscopy demonstrated excellent medialization for both groups. However, the effects of the medialization thyroplasty lasted longer than the injection.

Both injection laryngoplasty and medialization thyroplasty have been shown to be safe and effective, with good outcomes. However, in cases where the results of medialization thyroplasty are not satisfactory, or when complications such as airway difficulties, infection, throat discomfort, or dysphagia occur, a revision procedure may be performed. This may entail either another open procedure to reposition, replace or remove the implanted material, or an injection laryngoplasty to augment the vocal fold if a glottal gap still remains (Andrews et al., 2008; Umeno, Chitose, Sato, & Nakashima, 2008).

While not as common as medialization thyroplasty or injection laryngoplasty, laryngeal reinnervation (LR) procedures have some important advantages. The surgical technique itself is relatively simple and does not involve implants or injections that may affect the vibratory wave or that may extrude or migrate (Smith et al., 2008). One of the major advantages of LR is that it prevents atrophy of the paralyzed vocal fold and provides vocal fold tone, bulk, tension, and position stability (Baylor et al., 2006; Blumin & Merati, 2008; Lorenz et al., 2008). There are reports that LR results in improved pitch and loudness control compared to thyroplasty (Smith et al., 2008). Another advantage is that other medialization procedures can be used in conjunction with laryngeal reinnervation. For example, the procedure can be combined with vocal fold injection with Gelfoam to temporarily medialize the vocal fold while awaiting physiological reinnervation (Lorenz et al., 2008). LR has also been performed with simultaneous arytenoid adduction (e.g., Blumin & Merati, 2008).

Outcomes Studies. Baylor et al. (2006) reviewed 92 studies that reported outcomes of injection, thyroplasty, and voice therapy treatments. Across the studies outcomes were documented utilizing videostroboscopy, acoustic measures, aerodynamic measures, respiratory-phonatory measures, perceptual voice quality, and psychosocial measures. Fifty percent of the studies used videostroboscopy, and of these, 20% showed statistically significant changes in terms of glottal closure and/or mucosal wave. Fifty-five percent of the studies used acoustic measures, including jitter, shimmer, HNR, and F0. More than half of the studies that employed jitter or HNR demonstrated statistically significant positive changes. Around one-third of the studies (35%) reported on amount of airflow as the outcome, and almost two-thirds (61%) of these documented statistically significant improvements. More than half the studies (55%) employed respiratory-phonatory measures including MPT and the s/z ratio. Fifty-three percent of studies using MPT and 63% of studies using the s/z ratio reported significant improvements in these measures. Change in voice quality was the most prevalent outcome measurement, with 70 studies (76%) including perceptual voice quality measures. Measures included formal and informal rating scales as well as anecdotal reports. Almost half (47%) of studies that used the GRBAS scale showed statistically significant change in perceptual ratings of patients' voices following treatment. Baylor et al. (2006) noted that the VHI was the most common quality of life measure, and all studies using VHI demonstrated statistically significant improvements in patients' quality of life after treatment. Only a few papers focused on the role of voice therapy in managing UVFP. Baylor et al. (2006) pointed out that while many authors commented that voice therapy was part of routine clinical protocols, there was very little evidence that voice therapy for UVFP has been studied in a controlled fashion.

Bilateral Vocal Fold Paralysis. When both vocal folds are paralyzed, not only is voice production severely impacted, but respiration and/or swallowing can also be problematic. When both folds are paralyzed in the adducted position (abductor paralysis), immediate surgical attention is necessary to establish an adequate airway. Bilateral paralysis of the vocal folds in an abducted position (**adductor paralysis**) results in aphonia as well as in swallowing problems such as aspiration of liquids and foods. In severe cases of bilateral paralysis patients may need to use an alternative source of nutrition such as a nasogastric or gastronomy tube to prevent aspiration (Stemple et al., 2000). Bilateral vocal fold paralysis (BVFP) can occur in individuals of all ages, including infants. Refer to color insert photos 33 and 34.

Causes. The most common cause of bilateral paralysis in adults is thyroid surgery (Olthoff et al., 2005; Witt, 2005), although some investigators have suggested that nonlaryngeal malignancies such as pulmonary tumors are becoming increasingly common as an etiology (Feehery et al., 2003; Hillel et al., 1999). While thyroid surgery is still the leading cause of bilateral vocal fold paralysis, the number of cases has decreased due to careful identification of the RLN as well as improved surgical techniques (Bosley, Rosen, Simpson, McMullin, & Gartner-Schmidt, 2005; Feehery et al., 2003). Other causes include blunt trauma to the neck and neurological conditions such as Parkinson's disease, multiple systems atrophy, multiple sclerosis, amyotrophic lateral sclerosis, and Guillain-Barr syndrome (Feehery et al., 2003; Hillel et al., 1999; Li et al., 2008). The condition may also be idiopathic.

In infants, the primary causes of bilateral vocal fold paralysis are neurologic defects, upper motor neuron disorders, brain stem lesions, genetic syndromes, and birth trauma (Lewis, Carron, & Vedanarayanan, 2010; Tarin, Martinez, & Shapiro, 2005). Birth trauma accounts for 20% of congenital cases, because the use of forceps or complicated delivery can damage the RLN (Tarin et al., 2005). Cardiothoracic or esophageal surgeries can also cause injury to the RLN (Tarin et al., 2005). In some cases the condition is idiopathic (Aubry et al., 2010).

Symptoms. The most common symptoms of BVFP are dyspnea, stridor, voice impairment, and dysphagia (Aubry et al., 2010; Feehery et al., 2003). In adults, symptoms of abductor vocal fold paralysis are related to airway obstruction and respiratory difficulties, but phonation is relatively intact. Adductor paralysis is associated with severe phonatory weakness and breathiness, and possibly aphonia. Swallowing difficulties are also likely. In infants, symptoms include high-pitched inspiratory stridor and respiratory distress, weak cry, cough, cyanosis, difficulty feeding, and aspiration (Tarin et al., 2005). Obstructive sleep apnea caused by bilateral vocal fold paralysis has occasionally been reported (Aziz & Ejnell, 2003).

Evaluation and Treatment. BVFP is evaluated in a similar manner as UVFP (Table 9.5). In infants, evaluation often includes a brain MRI, as well as sleep apnea studies, neurological assessment and imaging studies, tests for GERD, and swallowing studies (Smith & Sauder, 2009).

The most important goals of treatment are to establish a patent airway and safe swallowing, while maintaining or developing as functional a voice as possible (Lagier et al., 2009). For patients with abductor paralysis, a tracheotomy or emergency intubation may be necessary (Bosley et al., 2005). Other surgical procedures for abductor paralysis are designed to enlarge the airway and include total arytenoidectomy, medial arytenoidectomy, and transverse cordotomy (see Chapter 5). Good results (i.e., patent airway and functional voice) have been reported using these procedures (e.g., Ossoff et al., 1984).

Botox injection has shown good results in improving airway function in bilateral abductor paralysis. El-Hakim (2008) injected Botox in the cricothyroid muscle, sternothyroid muscle, and sternohyoid muscle in children with bilateral vocal fold immobility. Reportedly, after injection, most of the children in the study showed less stridor and significantly fewer cyanotic spells. The majority of the children had a complete return of laryngeal mobility bilaterally, and

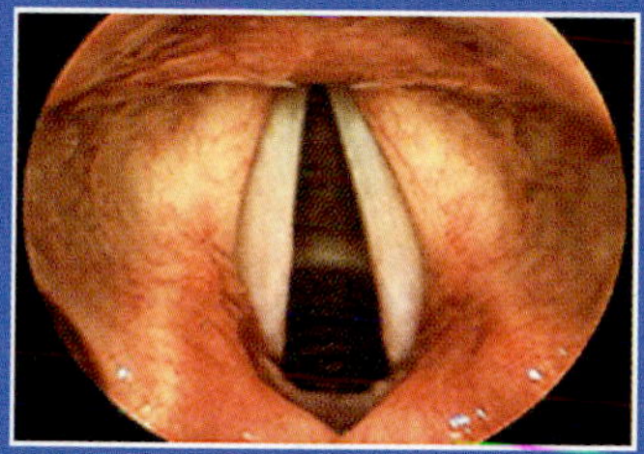

1 Normal Vocal Folds

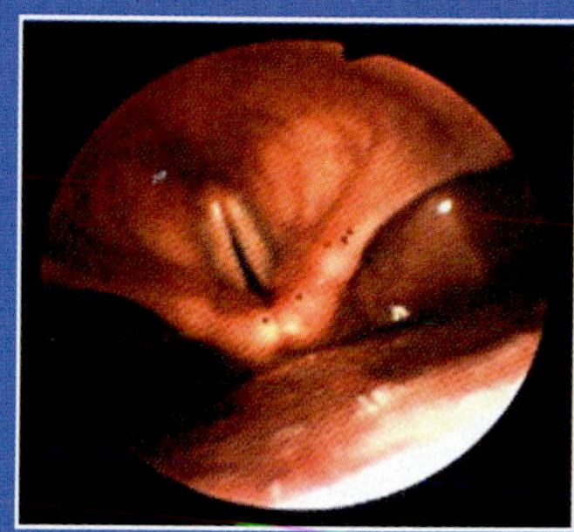

2 Aging

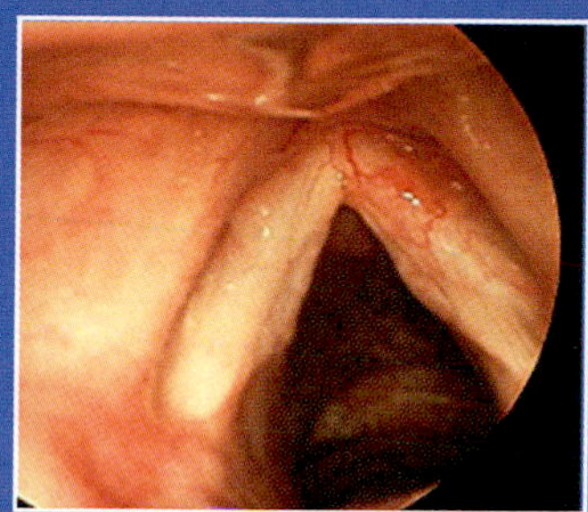

3 Scar 1

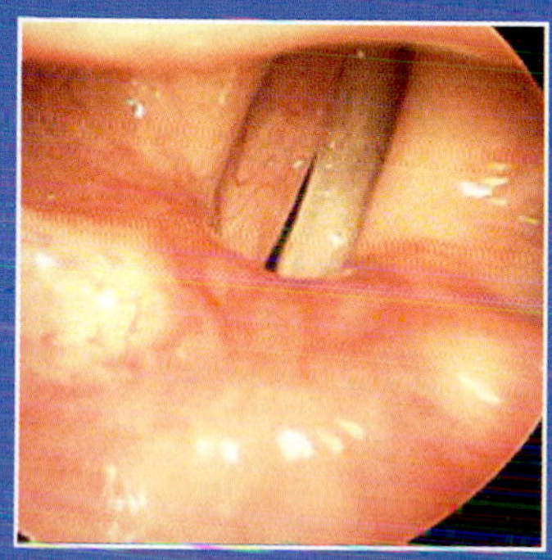

4 Scar 2

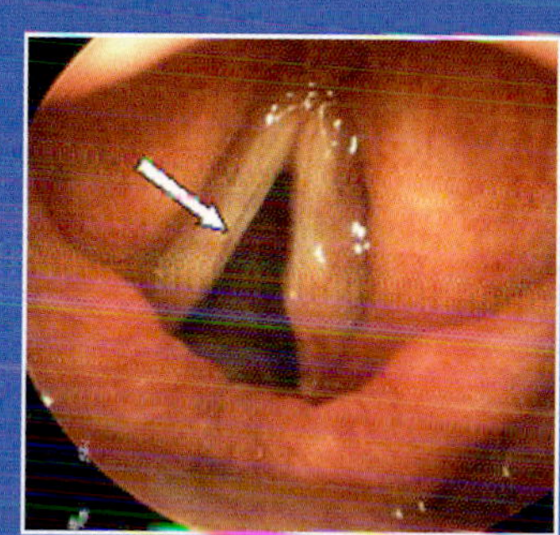

5 Sulcus

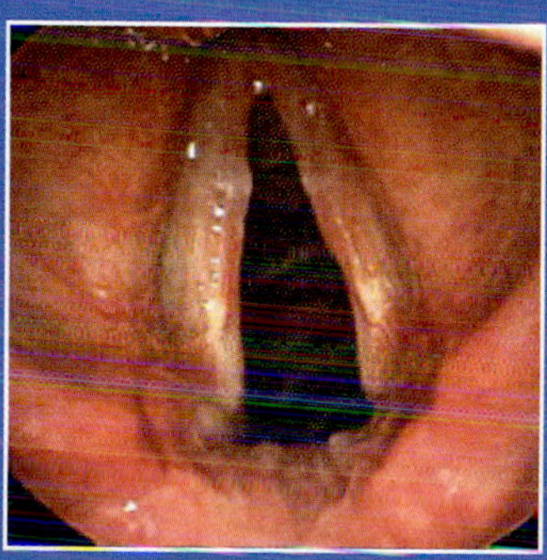

6 Laryngitis 1

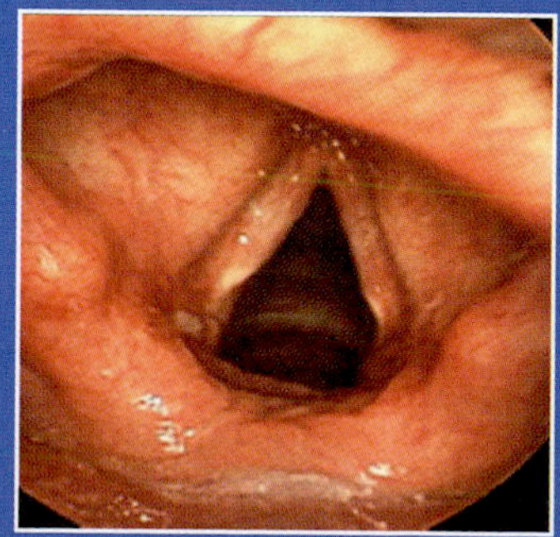

7 Laryngitis 2

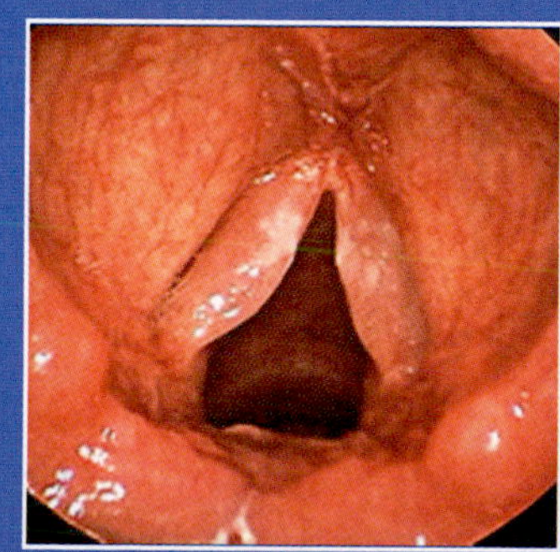

8 Reflux 1

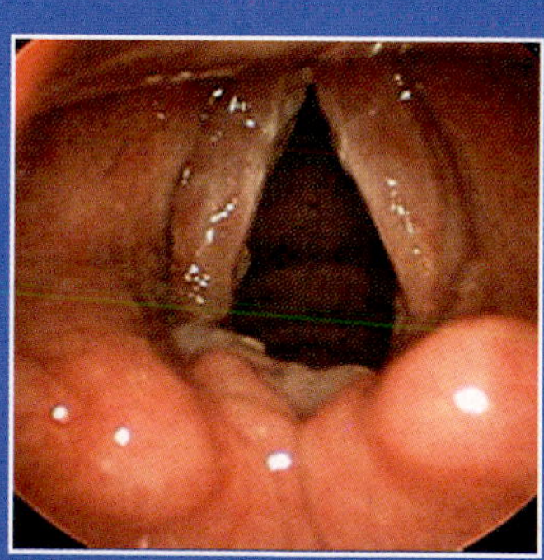

9 Reflux 2

All photos courtesy of Lucian Sulica , MD—www.voicemedicine.com

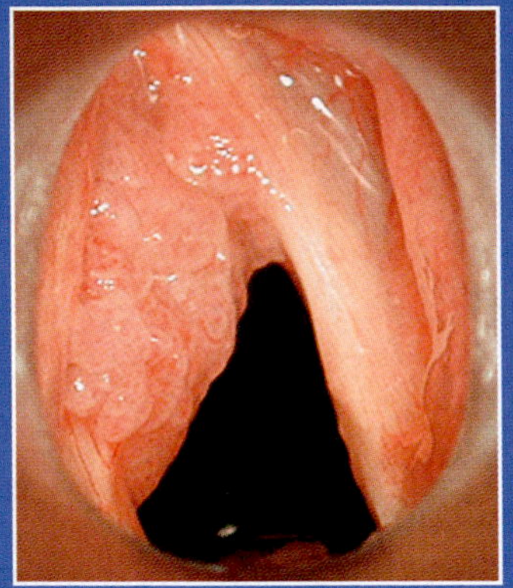
10 Papilloma 1

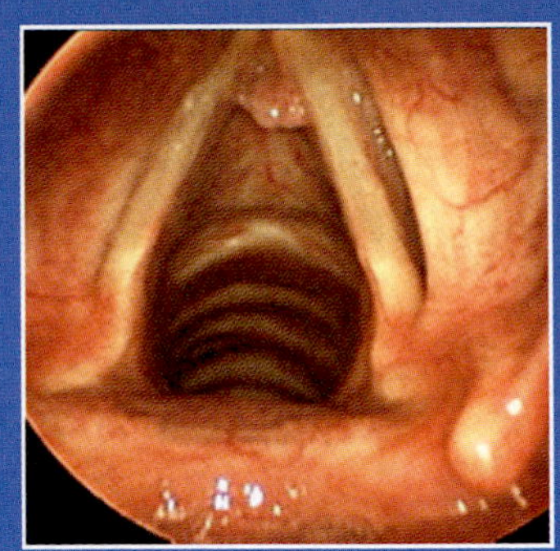
11 Papilloma 2

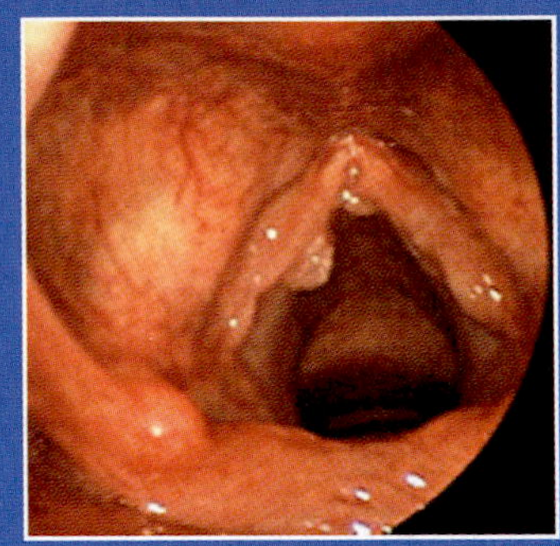
12 Papilloma 3

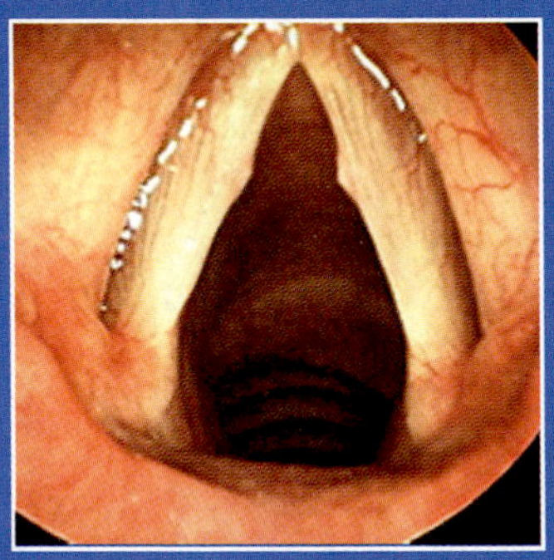
13 Nodules 1

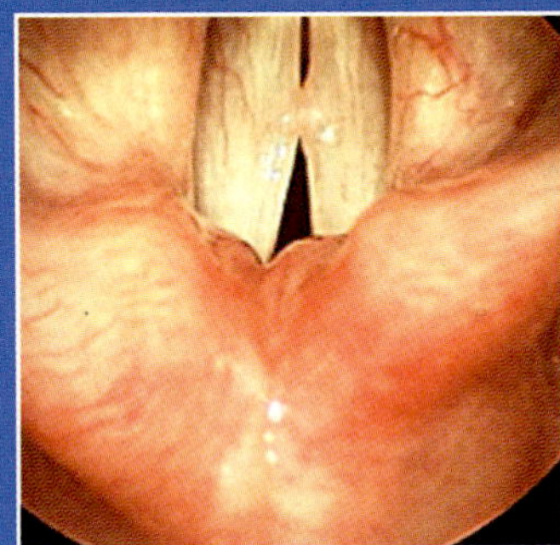
14 Nodules 2

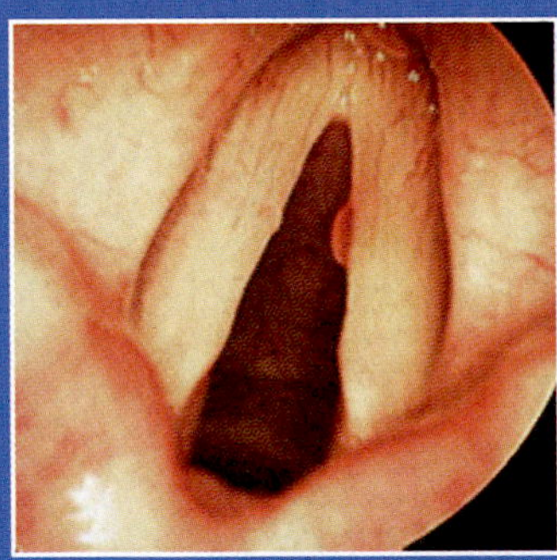
15 Polyp 1

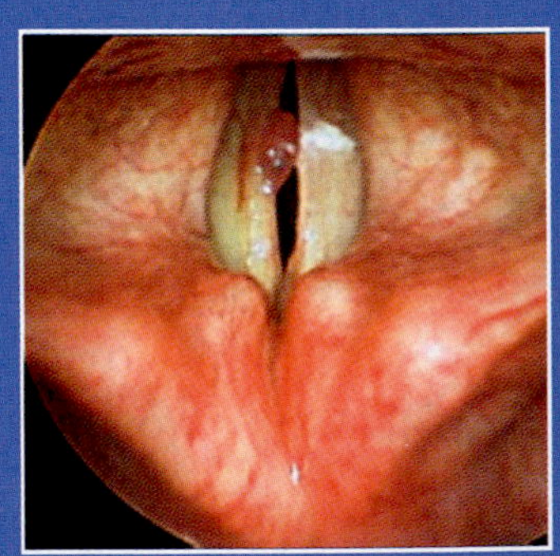
16 Polyp 2

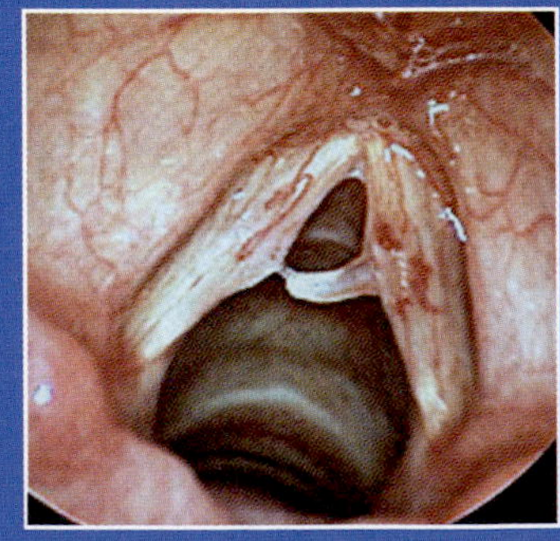
17 Polyp 3

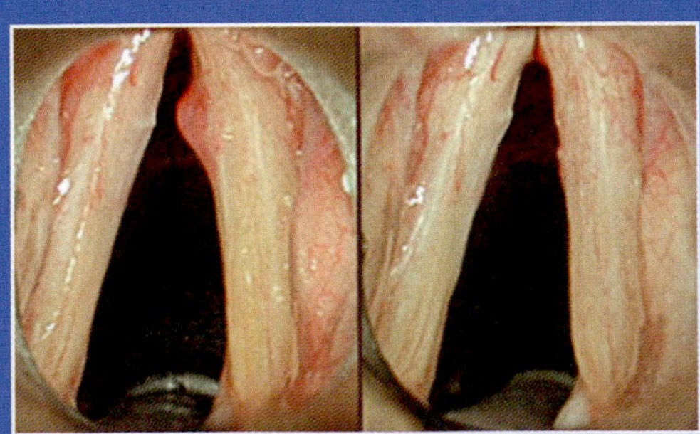
18 Polyp 4

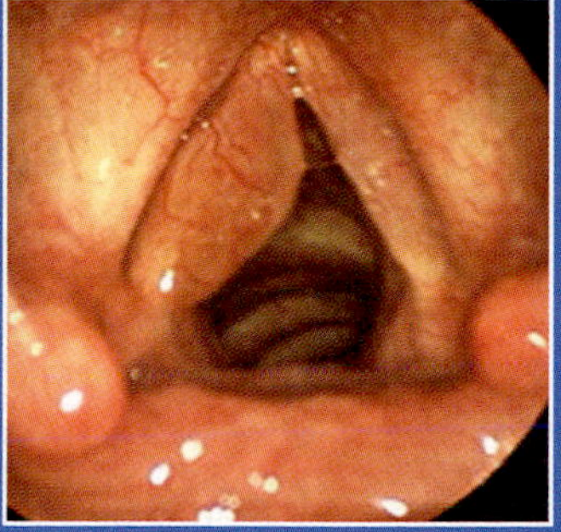
19 Reinke's Edema 1

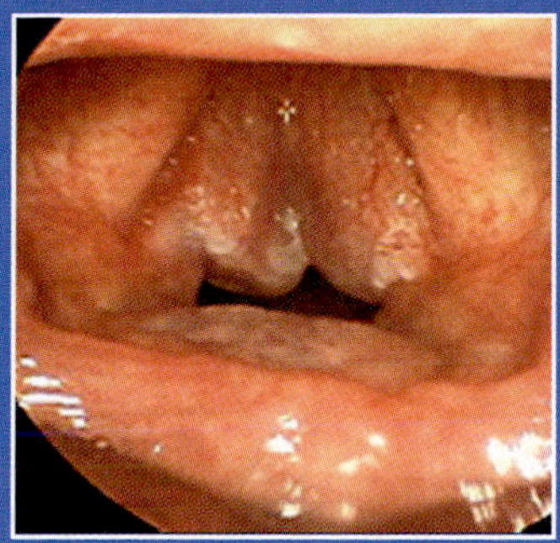
20 Reinke's Edema 2

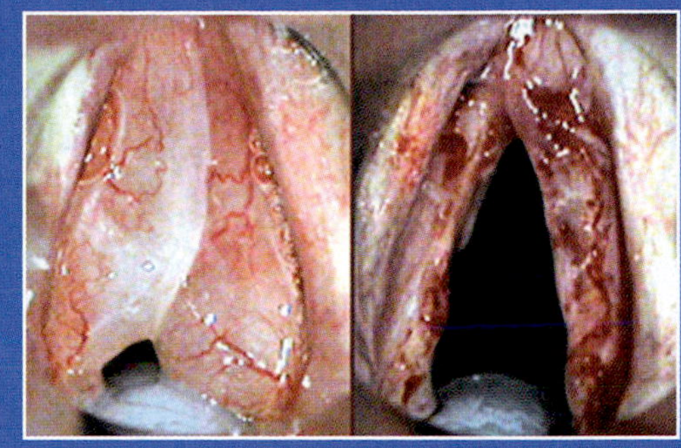
21 Reinke's Edema 3

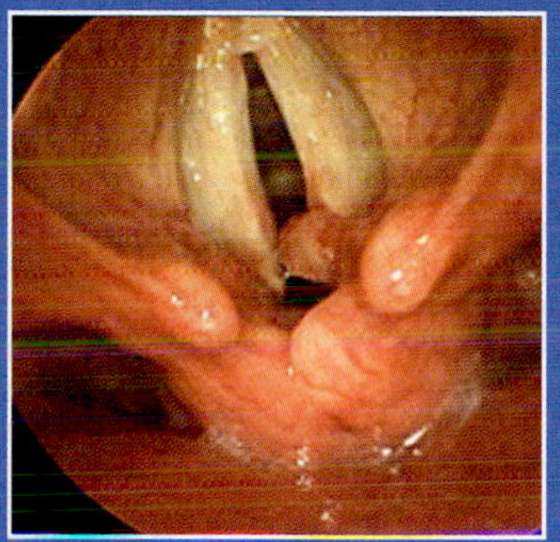
22 Granuloma 1

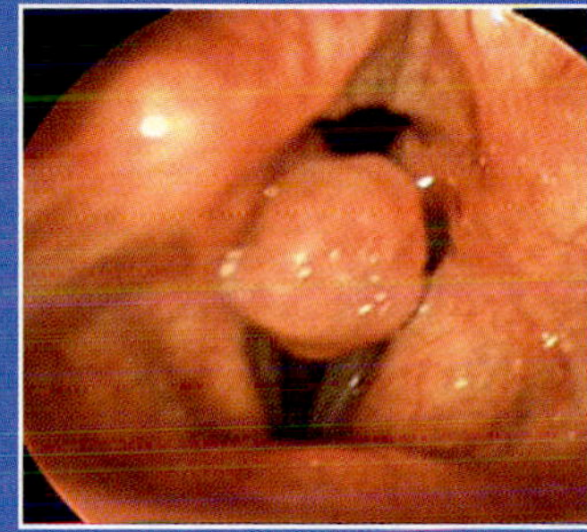
23 Granuloma 2

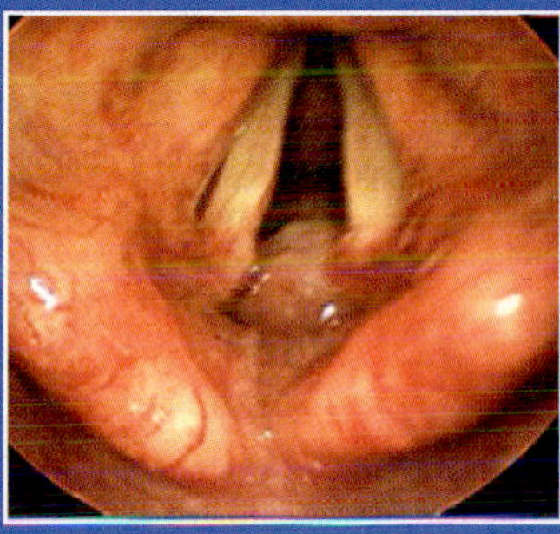
24 Granuloma 3

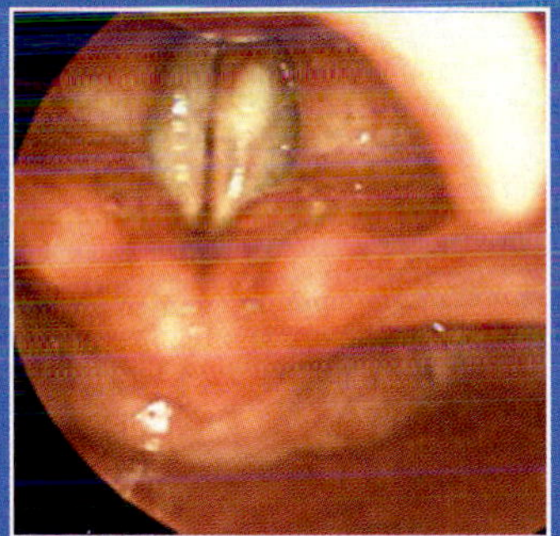
25 Cyst 1

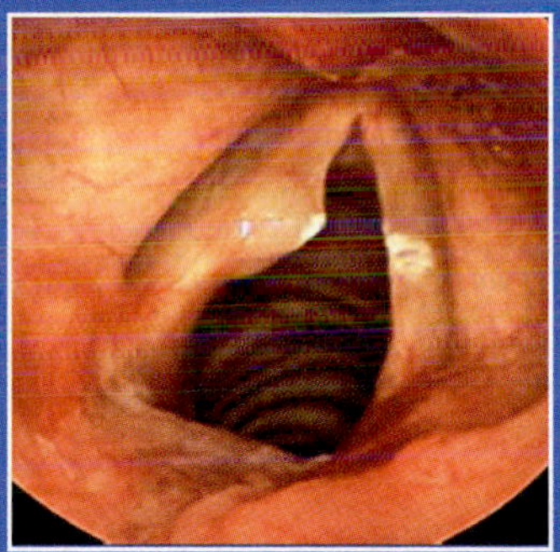
26 Cyst 2

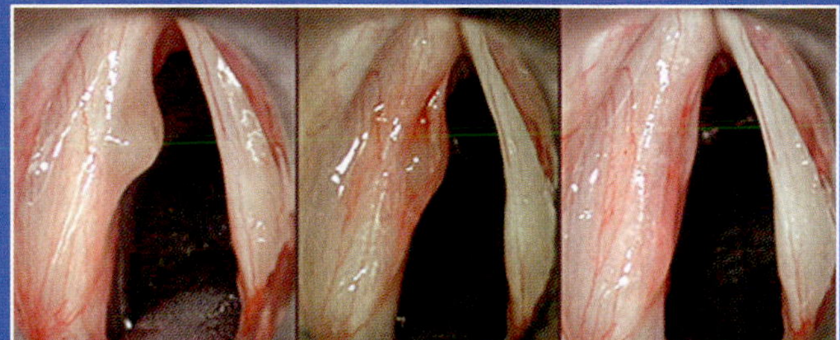
27 Cyst 3

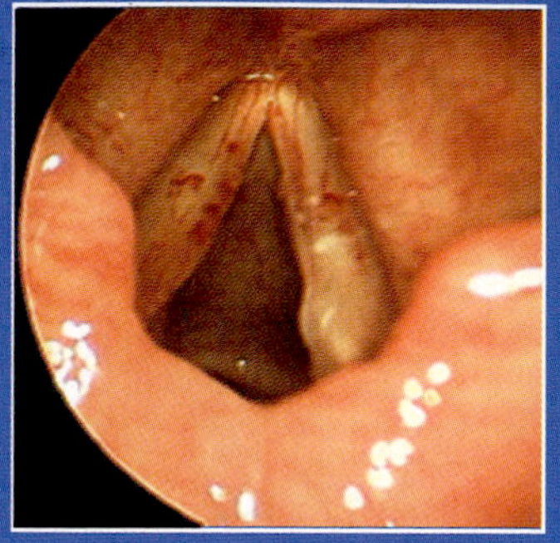
28 Hemorrhage 1

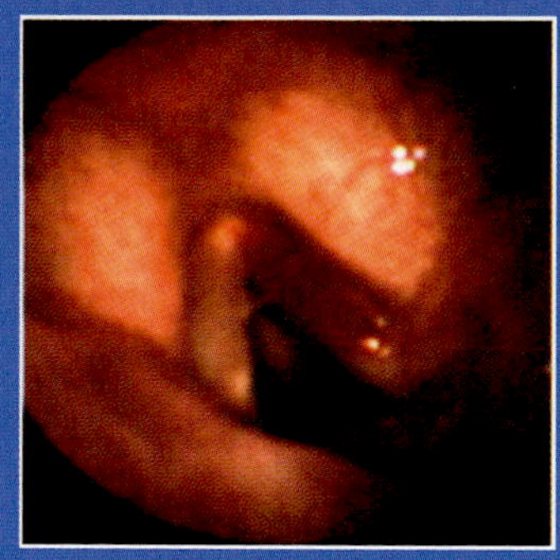
29 Hemorrhage 2

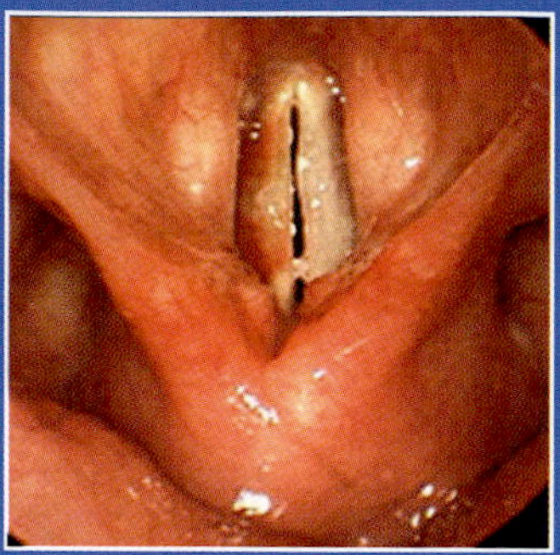
30 Hemorrhage 3

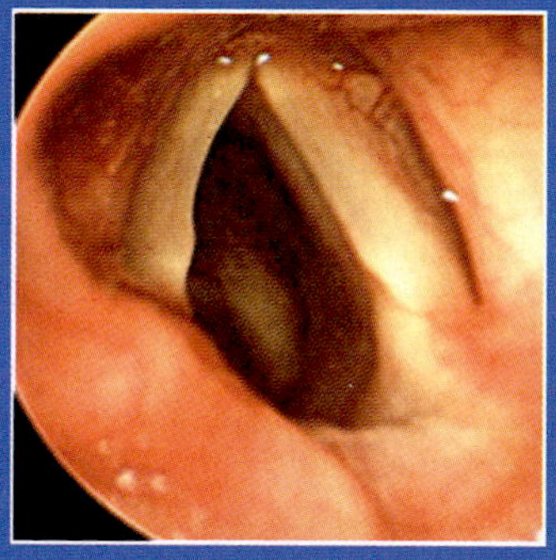
31 Unilateral Paralysis 1

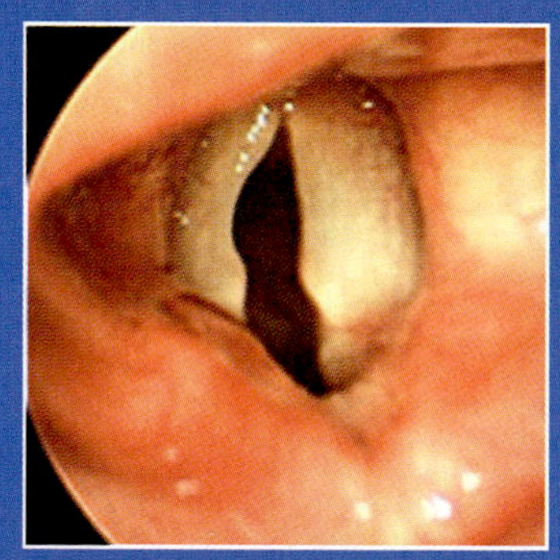
32 Unilateral Paralysis 2

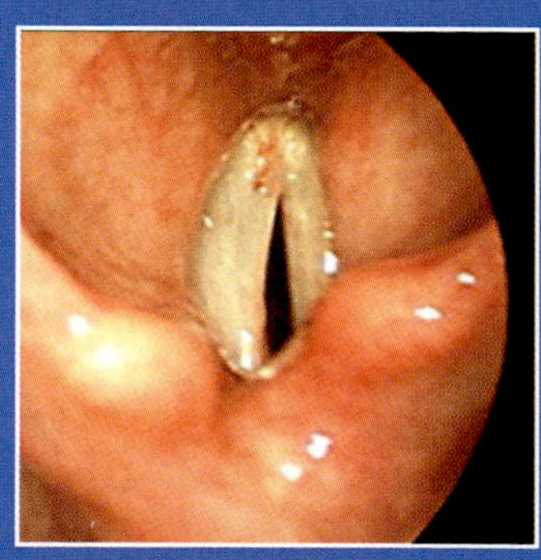
33 Bilateral Paralysis 1

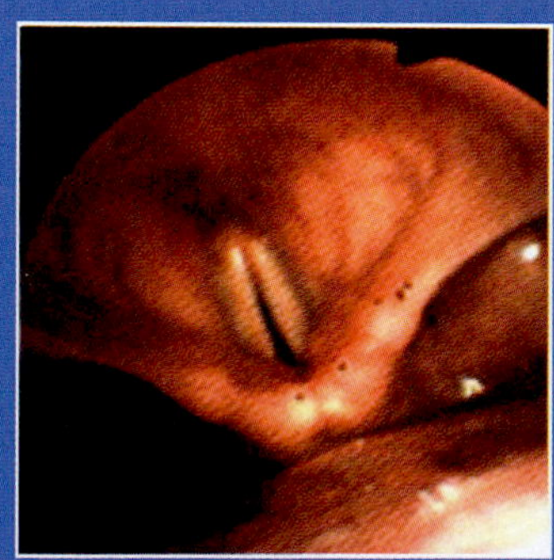
34 Bilateral Paralysis 2

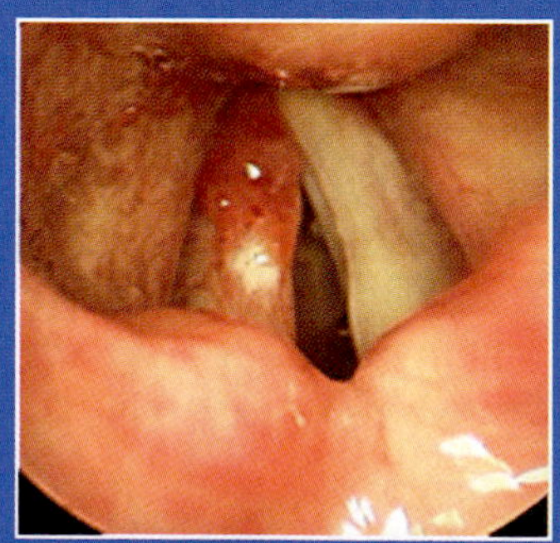
35 Cancer 1

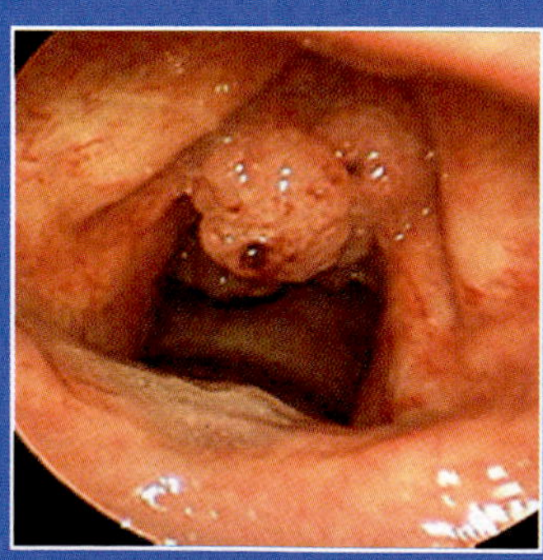
36 Cancer 2

one child showed unilateral return of vocal function. Filho and Rosen (2004) injected Botox into the thyroarytenoid and **lateral cricoarytenoid** muscles with the aim of improving vocal fold abduction, enlarging the glottis, and reducing the tension in the laryngeal adductors, and they reported satisfactory results. The advantage of Botox treatment is that it is reversible, not overly invasive, and safe. The disadvantage of this approach is the necessity for repeated injections.

Another surgical approach for bilateral abductor paralysis is electrical pacing. This method involves applying electrical stimulation to the paralyzed posterior cricoarytenoid muscle, which causes it to contract and open the airway (Hillel et al., 1999). Very few of these surgeries have been performed due to the demanding requirements for stimulating denervated muscle, which requires high current pulses to cause a full contraction (Hillel et al., 1999). Therefore the electrode delivering the current must be implanted near or in the muscle, but in such a way that it will not injure the muscle. Hillel et al. reported that results of the few surgeries have been promising. Further refinements of this procedure are under development.

MYASTHENIA GRAVIS

Myasthenia gravis (MG) is another example of a nervous system disorder that results in flaccid dysarthria. The outstanding characteristic of this disease is that the individual's movements in the affected structure(s) become progressively weaker with repetition in an extremely short period of time, i.e., seconds or minutes. Thus, if the person's larynx is involved, he or she may start out phonating relatively normally, but within a minute or less, the voice becomes progressively weaker, breathier, and more hypernasal. There are often other symptoms typical of flaccid muscle movement, such as difficulty chewing and swallowing, a weak and ineffective cough, and dulled facial expression resulting from difficulty contracting the facial muscles (Juel & Massey, 2007; Turner, 2007). **Ptosis** (drooping) of the eyelid is very common as the eye muscles are usually affected.

Causes. MG is an acquired autoimmune disorder of neuromuscular transmission in which antibodies destroy the acetylcholine receptors (AChR) at the myoneural junction between the nerve and muscle fiber (Ashraf, Taley, Veerendrakumar, & Rao, 2006; Kanemaru et al., 2007; Rieder, Conley, & Rowe, 2004; Turner, 2007; Xu, Han, Hou, Hu, & Wang, 2009). In normal neuromuscular function, **acetylcholine** (ACh) declines with repeated activity (Rieder et al., 2004). In MG, the combination of normal ACh decline with decreased efficiency in neuromuscular transmission causes fewer muscle fibers to be activated with each successive nerve impulse, resulting in rapid muscular fatigue (Kanemaru et al., 2007; Mao et al., 2001; Rieder et al., 2004). There is also a form of the disease related to pharmacological agents such as penicillamine, calcium channel blockers, quinine, and curare (Turner, 2007). These drugs can create changes in the patient's immune system, allowing for the formation of anti-AChR antibodies (antibodies that attack the acetylcholine receptors). There have also been reports of MG following a viral or bacterial infection and occurring in conjunction with herpes simplex. Rarely, infants born to mothers with MG have a transient form of the disease (Shah, 2009). There is a 10–15% incidence in children of mothers with MG, and symptoms generally resolve by age 2 months (Rieder et al., 2004). There is also a congenital form of the disorder that is not related to maternal disease and which is thought to be genetic in nature (Rieder et al., 2004; Turner, 2007).

MG is a rare disease with a prevalence rate of 20 per 100,000 individuals (Juel & Massey, 2007). MG is more common in young and middle-aged women, but does also occur in men.

Age and gender play a role in the incidence of MG, with female incidence peaking in the third decade of life, and male incidence peaking in the fifth to seventh decade (Shah, 2009; Turner, 2007; Xu et al., 2009). However, in the fifth decade new cases are evenly distributed between males and females (Juel & Massey, 2007). Rarely, MG occurs in children (Ashraf et al., 2006).

Symptoms. Muscles innervated by the cranial nerves seem to be particularly prone to MG (Chang, Lee, & Kuo, 2004). The most common initial signs of the disease are weaknesses of the eye muscles, resulting in ptosis (drooping eyelid) and **diplopia** (double vision) (Xu et al., 2009). Jaw-closing muscles are often affected, while jaw-opening muscles may maintain normal strength. The head and neck muscles tend to be involved at the early stages of the disease; in fact, the structures that are important for speech and swallowing are often the first to be affected. Speech and swallowing difficulties have been reported as early symptoms in up to 27% of cases (Mao et al., 2001). Dysphonia and dysphagia are the most common otolaryngological manifestations of MG (Kanemaru et al., 2007). Dysphonia may be the first symptom of the disease (e.g., Chang et al., 2004). Even if not the presenting symptom, dysphonia has been reported to develop at some time during the course of disease in 60% of cases (Mao et al., 2001). Sometimes the disorder is localized to the larynx, in which case it is called *myasthenia laryngis*. However, MG can progress to affect other structures.

When present, dysphonia is characterized by hypernasality, breathiness, difficulty sustaining pitch, vocal fatigue, intermittent aphonia, and stridor. In some cases, the signs and symptoms mimic unilateral vocal fold paresis or paralysis (Hartl et al., 2007). In such cases it is important to look for clues such as a personal or family history of autoimmune disease and fluctuating symptoms in order to distinguish between the two conditions (Hartl, Leboulleux, Klap, & Schlumberger, 2007). The symptoms of the disease are not consistent throughout the day, but fluctuate depending on factors such as the individual's level of stress and exertion, temperature, medications, infections, surgery, and hormonal changes that occur with pregnancy and the menstrual cycle (Turner, 2007). Symptoms are typically worse later in the day (Juel & Massey, 2007). Dysphagia and nasal regurgitation are not uncommon.

Diagnosis and Evaluation. Diagnosis of MG is based on the patterns of fatigue and recovery of affected muscles. When the larynx is involved, the patient undergoes a "stress test" to fatigue the muscles, such as counting from 1 to 100. An **anticholinesterase** agent (i.e., an agent that prevents the breakdown of acetylcholine) is injected while the patient is phonating. If the drug improves the function within a very short period of time, MG is suspected. Tensilon is one such anticholinesterase, and this kind of diagnostic measure is called the *Tensilon test*, but other drugs, such as neostigmine (Prostigmin) and pyridostigmine (Mestinon), are used for the same diagnostic and treatment purposes. The Tensilon test is highly sensitive and has been found to be positive in 95% of patients with generalized MG (Mao et al., 2001). Other tests are utilized to assess neuromuscular function more directly (Table 9.6).

The **repetitive stimulation test (RST)** involves repetitive electrical stimulation of a motor nerve at a rate of 2–3 times per second. Patients with MG show a decrease in successive nerve impulses, and the test is considered positive if a 10% or greater decrease occurs (Liu, Xia, Men, Wu, & Huang, 2007; Mao et al., 2001). The disadvantage of RST is its lack of sensitivity. A false-negative rate as high as 50% has been reported (Mao et al., 2001). Another type of test is single fiber electromyography (SFEMG). This is a form of EMG in which electrical activity is recorded from individual muscle fibers. The variation in action potentials between two parallel muscle fibers (called jitter) is determined and has found to be increased in up to 95% of patients with generalized MG (Liu et al., 2007; Mao et al., 2001; Woodson, 2008). In addition to

TABLE 9.6 **Diagnostic Tests Used for Myasthenia Gravis**

Test	Expected Result
Tensilon	Muscle/structure recovers rapidly
Repetitive stimulation test	Decline in successive nerve impulses
Single fiber electromyography	Increase in muscle fiber jitter
Blood test	Detectable presence of anti-AChR antibodies
Chest CT scan	Possible thymoma

these tests, blood testing can also be performed to check for anti-AChR antibodies. Antibodies against AChR are detectable in the serum of up to 90% of patients with generalized MG (Liu et al., 2007; Mao et al., 2001; Woodson, 2008). However, these antibodies are not as commonly seen in patients with primarily laryngeal or pharyngeal involvement (Woodson, 2008).

The patient should also undergo a chest CT scan to check for a possible tumor on the thymus gland (**thymoma**). The thymus gland is responsible in early life for the development and maturation of cells involved in immune functioning (Miller & Kline, 2007). After puberty the gland shrinks. Approximately 70% of individuals with MG have an enlarged (**hyperplasic**) thymus, and around 10–20% have a (usually benign) thymoma (Saito et al., 2005; Woodson, 2008). MG has also been found to be associated with other **autoimmune diseases**, particularly those associated with thyroid disease, and patients should undergo thyroid function testing if appropriate (Juel & Massey, 2007).

Vocal Function. Several investigators have used laryngoscopic and acoustic measures to evaluate vocal function in patients with MG. Vocal difficulties include hoarseness, vocal fatigue, difficulties with pitch, and difficulty with volume or projection. Asymmetries in mucosal wave phase and amplitude are frequent. A consistent finding is incomplete glottic closure and decreased glottal efficiency, often resulting in a compensatory muscle tension dysphonia (Liu et al., 2007; Mao et al., 2001). Mao et al. (2001) also reported decreased values for speaking fundamental frequency, maximum phonational frequency range, and maximum phonation time.

Treatment. While medical management is the primary treatment for MG, voice therapy may be a useful adjunct. Implementing a vocal hygiene program may help the individual to avoid tension-inducing compensatory phonatory behaviors. Patients should also be counseled to rest their voices frequently and to explore environmental modifications such as the use of a portable amplification system. The use of an appropriate AAC system may be beneficial during periods of voice rest or severe unintelligibility (Coppens, 2007). For patients with severe hypernasality, a palatal lift may be helpful.

Medical Management. The choice of treatment for MG depends on the severity of the disease, as well as the patient's age and general condition. The most popular treatment is the administration of long-acting **cholinesterase inhibitors**, such as Mestinon and Prostigmin. These agents prevent acetylcholine from being reabsorbed by the presynaptic neuron too soon, so the neurotransmitter is available in the myoneural junction for a longer period of time. Mestinon and Prostigmin have similar properties, but their times of onset of effects and duration of effectiveness differ. Mestinon has an onset of 20 minutes and duration of 50–60 minutes, and Prostigmin has an onset of 30 minutes and a prolonged duration that peaks at 2 hours (Liu et al., 2007). Most patients are reported to respond well to this type of medication (Woodson, 2008). However, to date there are no controlled clinical trials of these medications (Juel & Massey, 2007).

Removal of the thymus gland (**thymectomy**) is also recommended for most patients, because of the strong correlation between thymus function and MG. Thymectomy has been reported to cause remission or improvement of symptoms even in patients without evidence of thymomas (Mao et al., 2001). Other treatments include corticosteroids such as prednisone, which often provide patients with relief of symptoms. Immunosuppressant drugs such as azathioprine and cyclosporine may also be helpful in symptom relief. A procedure called **plasmaphoresis** (plasma exchange), is used when a patient's symptoms suddenly become markedly worse, or when the patient has not responded to the other types of treatment. In this procedure the individual's plasma is filtered and the antibodies that are causing the problem are removed (Mao et al., 2001). This treatment is short-term, with improvements lasting only a few weeks (Juel & Massey, 2007).

A treatment that has become more widespread recently is intravenous immunoglobulin. **Immunoglobulins** are antibodies produced by the immune system. In this procedure antibodies from thousands of blood donors are used to flood the body, providing temporary relief of symptoms (Scheinfeld & Goodwin, 2010). The procedure is used where a patient is experiencing worsening weakness, or may be useful as an adjunct to other treatments (e.g., Arsura, Brunner, & Grob, 1988; Gajdos, Chevret, Clair, Tranchant, & Chastang, 1997; Zinman, Ng, & Bril, 2007).

Spastic Dysarthria

Spastic dysarthria results from damage to the corticobulbar tracts of the upper motor neuron. The nerve supply from the corticobulbar pathway to the cranial nerves is mostly bilateral, with innervation from the cortical motor areas of both the left and right hemispheres. Thus, if only one side of the corticobulbar tract is affected, the vagus nerve still receives innervation from the other side. Speech is affected when the damage to the corticobulbar tract is bilateral, with few effects on the speech subsystems from unilateral damage (Duffy, 2005). There are many causes of bilateral corticobulbar damage including multiple strokes, traumatic brain injury, tumors, infection, and diseases such as progressive supranuclear palsy, multiple sclerosis, and amyotrophic lateral sclerosis (e.g., Skodda, Visser, & Schlegel, 2010; Solomon, McKee, & Garcia-Berry, 2001).

SYMPTOMS

Damage to the corticobulbar tract causes weakness and spasticity that have the effect of slowing the movement of the affected structure(s) and reducing the range and force of motion (Duffy, 2005). Individuals with spastic dysarthria demonstrate a wide range of involvement of the speech musculature, including tongue, lips, jaw, velum, larynx, and respiratory muscles. In terms of laryngeal function the range of motion of the vocal folds is limited by their weakness and spasticity. The resulting vocal symptoms are typically a very low-pitched voice with a strong strained-strangled component and reductions in intonational variability (Skodda et al., 2010). In addition, the false folds may adduct, resulting in a harsh voice quality (Andrews, 1995). Hypernasality is common because of lack of coordination of the velum with the other articulators. Speech breathing patterns tend to be uncoordinated and uncontrolled. The patient may have difficulty in coordinating breathing and phonation, resulting in very short phrases of one or two words. Dysphagia is common (Duffy, 2005; Mathieson, 2001). A very characteristic symptom is uncontrollable laughter or crying that is either unrelated or vastly out of proportion to the individual's actual emotional status (Miller, 2006).

TREATMENT

Treatment is usually pharmacological, with the aim of reducing the spasticity. Muscle relaxants such as Valium may be helpful, and **antispasmodics** such as Dantrium and Lioresal (Baclofen) are often prescribed. However, because these medications work through the spinal cord, they are not effective in relieving the laryngeal symptoms (McHenry, Whatman, & Pou, 2002).

Very few descriptions of behavioral voice techniques for this disorder are available. Relaxation procedures have been suggested such as full-body relaxation stretches for the head and neck, and use of the yawn-sigh technique to facilitate easy onset of phonation (Dworkin, 1991). McHenry et al. (2002) used the confidential voice approach to establish easy onset of phonation in one patient with spastic dysarthria. The patient was able to reduce her loudness level, but she still demonstrated a strained vocal quality and was not able to generalize the soft voice outside therapy. The authors then investigated the effects of Botox injection in an attempt to relieve the patient's vocal symptoms. They reported that volume of airflow during speech increased after injection, and the patient went through a long period of hypofunction. Perceptual ratings improved after injection in terms of pleasantness of voice and more relaxed vocal quality.

Ataxic Dysarthria

Ataxic dysarthria results from damage to the cerebellum and/or its sensory and motor nerve pathways (Ackermann & Hertrich, 2000). The cerebellum functions to coordinate complex movement in terms of speed, direction, timing, range, and force and is also involved in the regulation of muscle tone (Deem & Miller, 2000; Mathieson, 2001). Damage results in a breakdown in the timing, accuracy, and coordination of the movements necessary for speech production (Cornwell, Murdoch, Ward, & Kellie, 2003). Because the cerebellum also regulates muscle tone, there is often a hypotonic component as well. Damage may occur from stroke, tumors, cerebral palsy, infectious diseases, and progressive neurological conditions such as multiple sclerosis. Genetic syndromes with ataxia as one of the characteristics are not uncommon and include Fragile-X syndrome, Friedreich's ataxia, familial episodic cerebellar ataxia, and a variety of spinocerebellar ataxias (a group of hereditary degenerative diseases). There is also an acute childhood version that can occur following a viral infection.

SYMPTOMS

Speech- and voice-related symptoms of ataxia are related to the breakdown of motor organization as well as to the associated hypotonia (Schalling, Hammarberg, & Hartelius, 2007). Physiological studies have documented errors of direction and range of movements, impaired ability to increase muscular forces in order to produce rapid movements, and reduced or exaggerated range of movements involving the respiratory, phonatory, or articulatory systems (Sapir et al., 2003). The individual's speech is often abnormally slow, and all syllables are stressed equally, a condition called **scanning speech**. This occurs because the speaker loses the ability to rapidly coordinate the muscular adjustments needed to regulate the subtle pitch and loudness changes that contribute to the rhythm and stress of the language. To stress a word or syllable the pitch is raised slightly, volume is increased, and the syllable is briefly extended in duration. Without the ability to make these fine distinctions, the prosody and rhythm of the language are lost. Acoustic analysis has shown that healthy speakers vary prosodic patterns in a systematic fashion, whereas speakers with ataxia do not differentiate between accented and unaccented syllables (Casper, Raphael, Harris, & Geibel, 2007). In addition, the associated hypotonia may contribute to reduced pitch and loudness variation, and hoarseness and tremor may be evident (Ackermann & Hertrich, 2000; Cornwell et al., 2003). Harsh voice, pitch breaks, vocal instability, strained-strangled quality, and glottal fry have also been reported (e.g., Schalling et al., 2007).

TREATMENT

Treatment of cerebellar ataxia relies primarily on surgical or pharmacological intervention for the underlying cause (e.g., surgical excision of cerebellar tumor) or for associated symptoms (e.g., medication for tremor). Few accounts of voice treatment are available. However, one such report is provided by Sapir and colleagues (2003), who used the Lee Silverman Voice Treatment to treat the vocal symptoms of a patient with ataxic dysarthria. The patient's voice was weak, although there were occasional increases in intensity. Pitch was low, with decreased and inappropriate prosody. The patient also demonstrated intermittent increases or decreases in breathiness or hoarseness, and perceptually sounded vocally unstable. After treatment, perceptual ratings indicated improved intonation and articulatory precision as well as improved speech intelligibility. Other behavioral strategies focus on enhancing the patient's respiratory control, improving rate of speech to increase intelligibility, and teaching the patient to increase duration of speech segments to signal stress patterns (Duffy, 2005). Acoustic instrumentation that provides visual biofeedback may be helpful in monitoring and modifying speech rate and prosodic parameters.

Hypokinetic Dysarthria

Hypokinesia refers to movements that are abnormally reduced in amplitude. Hypokinetic dysarthria is associated with Parkinson's disease (PD). PD is a neurological syndrome that results from the loss of **dopamine**, a neurotransmitter manufactured in the substantia nigra of the basal ganglia. In patients with PD, at least 80% of the cells that produce dopamine have died or been damaged (Henkel, 1998). The disease can result from degenerative, vascular, or inflammatory changes in the basal ganglia and related neural networks. It can also result from neuroleptics (drugs used to treat certain psychiatric illnesses) and can occur following encephalitis. Most cases of Parkinson's disease, however, are idiopathic. Approximately 1.5 million people in the United States suffer from PD, with more than 40,000 new cases being diagnosed each year (Schulz & Grant, 2000). The disease is most common in individuals in the middle years (50 and over), but it can also occur in younger adults. Both men and women can be affected.

SYMPTOMS

Loss of dopamine results in muscular rigidity, tremor, **bradykinesia** (slowness in initiating and executing movements), and postural instability (Harel et al., 2004; Skodda et al., 2010). The tremor arises from the imbalance between the diminished levels of dopamine and resulting excess of acetylcholine. Tremor usually occurs when the affected structure is at rest. When the tremor affects the patient's hands, there is often a characteristic rolling movement of the fingers, called a "pill-rolling" movement. The muscular rigidity typically results in a blank look on the individual's face, resulting from the inability to move the facial muscles. This is termed a **masked facies**.

In terms of phonation, the rigidity and resistance to movement of the vocal folds make it difficult to achieve normal vibration (Sachin et al., 2008). Perceptually, speech is characterized by reduced intensity, monopitch, and varying degrees of harshness and breathiness (e.g., Holmes, Oates, Phyland, & Hughes, 2000; Plowman-Prine et al., 2009; Skodda et al., 2009, 2010). Vocal symptoms can be the first obvious sign of the neurological problem, or can develop later as the disease progresses.

Videolaryngoscopy has revealed a high occurrence of bowed vocal folds and incomplete glottic closure (e.g., Blumin, Poolinsky, & Atkins, 2004; Schulz & Grant, 2000). Acoustic analysis has demonstrated reduced F0 variability, difficulty in modulating F0 and intensity, reductions in maximum F0 range, higher jitter and shimmer levels, and shorter maximum phonation times (e.g., Cheang & Pell, 2007; Harel et al., 2004; Holmes et al., 2000; Plowman-Prine et al., 2009). The acoustic decrease in F0 variability has been reported to be evident years before the onset of clinically significant symptoms (Harel et al., 2004; Skodda et al., 2009).

In addition to motor symptoms, sensory symptoms are often present in PD and include numbness, tingling, pain and achiness, and coldness or burning sensations (Fox, Morrison, Ramig, & Sapir, 2002). Both sensory and auditory forms of feedback are important for laryngeal control of pitch and loudness, and deficits in somatosensory function can significantly affect phonatory control (Hammer et al., 2010; Larson, Altman, Liu, & Hain, 2008). Fox et al. (2002) proposed that individuals with PD experience difficulty in generating and monitoring the right amount of effort to produce adequate loudness due to two factors: the reduced amplitude of neural input to the muscles of the speech mechanism, and the associated deficit in sensory processing. This combination of factors results in decreases in subglottal air pressure and peak flow, decreased laryngeal resistance, decreased air expended per syllable, and decreased voice intensity (Hammer et al., 2010).

STAGING OF PD

Because PD is a progressive disease, it is helpful for professionals involved in clinical decision making to have guidelines in terms of the various stages of the disease. The most common staging systems are the **Hoehn and Yahr Staging of Parkinson's Disease (H&Y)** and the **Unified Parkinson Disease Rating Scale (UPDRS).** The H&Y was originally developed in 1957 and consists of five levels ranging from mild symptoms in Stage 1 to complete debilitation in Stage 5. The scale was revised in 2004 to include additional stages (Table 9.7).

The Unified Parkinson Disease Rating Scale (UPDRS) is a more comprehensive classification system that categorizes the assortment of problems in PD in terms of three scales: Mentation, Behavior, and Mood (MBM), which assesses cognition and personality; Activities of Daily Living (ADL), which rates everyday living ability; and Motor, which assesses movement, including tremor and posture. The MBM scale includes categories such as intellectual

TABLE 9.7 Hoehn and Yahr Staging of Parkinson's Disease: Original and Modified Scales

Original Scale	
Stage 1	Unilateral signs and symptoms
Stage 2	Bilateral signs and symptoms
Stage 3	Moderately severe generalized dysfunction with significant slowing of body movements
Stage 4	Severe symptoms with limited walking; patient not able to live independently
Stage 5	Cannot stand or walk; patient requires constant nursing care
Modified Scale	
Stage 0	No signs of disease
Stage 1	Unilateral symptoms only
Stage 1.5	Unilateral and axial involvement
Stage 2	Bilateral symptoms, no impairment of balance
Stage 2.5	Mild bilateral disease with recovery on pull test
Stage 3	Balance impairment, mild to moderate disease, physically independent
Stage 4	Severe disability, but still able to walk or stand unassisted
Stage 5	Needing a wheelchair or bedridden unless assisted

Sources: Information from Goetz et al. (2004); Hoehn & Yahr (1967).

impairment, thought disorder, and depression. ADL includes speech intelligibility, swallowing, handwriting, walking, and hygiene. The Motor scale focuses on speech production, facial expression, resting tremor, action tremor, rigidity, and posture. All categories are ranked on a 5-point scale from 0 to 4, with 0 indicating no problem and 4 indicating a severe problem. Table 9.8 presents the speech-related categories of the scale.

TREATMENT

Clinical management for PD is designed to improve the motor symptoms of the disorder by pharmacologic or surgical means, and the speech and voice components by means of voice therapy.

Pharmacologic Treatment. The primary treatment of PD is pharmacological, and many different drugs have been developed to treat the symptoms of the disease (Table 9.9).

The most commonly used drug is **levodopa (L-dopa).** Levodopa is converted into dopamine in the brain by means of "converter" cells, thus replacing the dopamine that is lacking in the basal ganglia. This reduces the primary problems of rigidity and tremor. However, levodopa can have severe side effects such as involuntary tics (dyskinesia) and nausea.

TABLE 9.8 **Speech- and Swallowing-Related Categories of the Unified Parkinson Disease Rating Scale (UPDRS)**

Activities of Daily Living
Speech
0—normal
1—mildly affected, no difficulty being understood
2—moderately affected, may be asked to repeat
3—severely affected, frequently asked to repeat
4—unintelligible most of the time
Swallowing
0—normal
1—rare choking
2—occasional choking
3—requires soft food
4—requires NG tube or G-tube
Motor Exam
Speech
0—normal
1—slight loss of expression, diction, volume
2—monotone, slurred but understandable, moderately impaired
3—marked impairment, difficult to understand
4—unintelligible
Facial Expression
0—normal
1—slight hypomimia, could be poker face
2—slight but definite abnormal diminution in expression
3—moderate hypomimia, lips parted some of the time
4—masked or fixed face, lips parted 1/4 inch or more with complete loss of expression

Therefore, the drug is often taken in combination with other drugs (e.g., carbidopa) to reduce the side effects and to enhance treatment effectiveness. Sinemet, a drug that combines L-dopa with carbidopa, is the primary medication for treating PD (Schulz & Grant, 2000). Sinemet is highly effective, but a disadvantage is that doses usually have to be increased over time. Additionally, an "on-off" pattern can occur in which the drug does not work for unpredictable periods of time (Goberman, Coelho, & Robb, 2002; Henkel, 1998; Schulz & Grant, 2000). Patients typically experience a consistent reduction of symptoms for 2–5 years, an interval

TABLE 9.9 Pharmacologic Agents Used in the Treatment of Parkinson's Disease

Agent	Action
Levodopa	Converted to dopamine in the brain by means of converter cells
Anticholinergics	Block the action of acetylcholine
Dopamine agonists	Enhance dopamine receptor sites in the brain
COMT inhibitors	Slow the breakdown of levodopa
MAOIs	Prevent the breakdown of dopamine and enhance release of dopamine from nerve cells

that Goberman et al. (2002) called the "levodopa honeymoon period." Thereafter side effects and the "on-off" pattern start to occur in around 50% of patients (Goberman et al., 2002). The reduction of symptoms during the "on" period begins to decrease and become shorter in duration, and symptoms reappear during the "off" period. These "on-off" swings gradually become more rapid and violent, increasing the patient's need for higher doses of the drug (Schulz & Grant, 2000).

While L-dopa is generally effective for the motor aspects of PD, effects on speech and voice are equivocal. Some researchers have reported improvements in voice quality, speech breathing, pitch variability, and loudness (e.g., De Letter et al., 2005, 2007; Goberman et al., 2002). Others have failed to demonstrate any speech-related improvements associated with the drug (e.g., Plowman-Prine et al., 2009; Skodda et al., 2010).

Other pharmacological treatments used to relieve disabling tremor include anticholinergics, dopamine agonists, COMT inhibitors, and monoamine inhibitors. Anticholinergic drugs block the action of acetylcholine (Schulz & Grant, 2000). Two common anticholinergics are Artane and Cogentin. While they can be effective in reducing limb tremor, these drugs have not been found to improve speech (Schulz & Grant, 2000). Dopamine agonists act directly on dopamine receptors in the brain. One of the problems with levodopa is that the cells that convert the levodopa into dopamine die off, so dosages must continually be increased. Dopamine agonists, on the other hand, act directly on the dopamine receptor sites, and therefore do not need the converter cells to exert their benefit. It has been found that low doses of dopamine agonists in conjunction with levodopa work for longer periods of time and have less severe side effects. Examples of dopamine agonists include Bromocriptine, Pergolide, and Lisuride. **COMT** stands for **catechol-O-methyltransferase**. This is an enzyme that breaks down levodopa before it can be converted to dopamine. COMT inhibitors prolong the availability of a dose of levodopa by inhibiting the action of the enzyme and slowing the breakdown of the levodopa. These drugs, taken in conjunction with levodopa, may help to reduce on-off fluctuations and dyskinesias and prolong the duration of symptom relief (Henkel, 1998). Examples include Tasmar, Comtan, and many others. Stalevo is a newer combination tablet that combines carbidopa/levodopa with a COMT inhibitor. The carbidopa reduces the side effects of levodopa, while the COMT inhibitor extends the time levodopa is active in the brain. **Monoamine oxidase inhibitors (MAOIs)** are also used for symptom relief in PD. These drugs prolong the effects of dopamine in the brain by preventing its breakdown. They also may prevent the removal of dopamine between nerve endings and enhance release of dopamine from nerve cells. Rasagiline and Selegiline are selective monoamine oxidase (MAO-B) inhibitors. These drugs can be effective in advanced stages of the disease in reducing motor fluctuations, increasing the effective time of the levodopa, and decreasing the amount of levodopa needed to control symptoms.

Surgical Treatments. Pharmacologic therapy is reasonably effective for a majority of individuals with PD. However, drugs have potentially severe side effects including nausea, hypotension, confusion, dementia, hallucinations, and delusions (Schulz, Greer, & Friedman, 2000). Further, these medications may not be effective for some individuals. There has, therefore, been much interest in the use of surgical techniques to treat the rigidity, bradykinesia, and tremors that are characteristic of PD. Techniques that have been used include pallidotomy, thalamotomy, deep brain stimulation, and fetal cell transplantation. Pallidotomy and thalamotomy both involve destruction of specific brain areas within the basal ganglia and thalamus, and have been shown to markedly reduce tremors, rigidity, and bradykinesia. Deep brain stimulation (DBS) involves insertion of implant wires into a brain area such as the thalamus and implantation of a pulse generator in the patient's chest. When activated by the patient, the device transmits electrical impulses to the brain, which has the effect of blocking the tremors (Deem & Miller, 2000; Henkel, 1998). This technique has been shown to be effective in reducing tremor (D'Alatri et al., 2008; Schulz & Grant, 2000). It also has the advantage of decreased risk of permanent neurological damage due to a smaller lesion than those in pallidotomy and thalamotomy (Solomon et al., 2000). Other advantages include its reversibility and adjustability for optimizing benefits by varying stimulation parameters, the possibility of bilateral implantation with a single procedure, and the small risk of cognitive damage (Solomon et al., 2000). It can also reduce the need for medication, even in the long term (D'Alatri et al., 2008). **Fetal cell transplantation** aims to increase the production of dopamine by implanting fetal cells directly into the basal ganglia. Research on a small number of patients has shown that while the procedure has beneficial effects on the motor system in general, the effects on voice production are not pronounced (e.g., Schulz & Grant, 2000).

While these surgical techniques have demonstrated effectiveness in reducing the motor aspects of PD, reported effects on voice and speech are conflicting. Schulz et al. (2000) reported positive changes in phonatory/articulatory measures such as greater intensity, more syllables per second, and longer maximum vowel durations. Putzer, Barry, and Moringlane (2008) reported that some of the patients who had undergone DBS demonstrated improvement of glottal closure while others demonstrated increased adductory weakness. Other researchers have reported either no or limited effects on speech and voice, or deterioration of speech and voice parameters (e.g., D'Alatri et al., 2008; Farrell, Theodoros, Ward, Hall, & Silbum, 2005; Narayana et al., 2009; Solomon et al., 2000). Because speech and voice problems in PD typically do not respond to pharmacologic or surgical treatment, researchers have speculated that other neurotransmitters such as serotonin may be more important than dopamine in voice and speech function (Biary, Pimental, & Langenberg, 1988; Sandyk, 1997).

Voice Therapy. In addition to pharmacological and/or surgical management for the motor difficulties, voice therapy has been found to be extremely beneficial in managing the vocal problems associated with PD. One of the most distressing vocal characteristics for individuals with PD is the severely reduced loudness level of their speech. The weak and monotone voice has been shown to have negative communicative and social consequences. Individuals with

PD report feeling that they have lost control in communicating, are less confident, and find it difficult to get their message across (Miller, Noble, Jones, Allcock, & Burn, 2008). The resulting frustration, feelings of inadequacy, and sense of loss of independence may lead to withdrawal and social isolation (Miller et al., 2008). The voice quality may also negatively influence listeners' perceptions of the speaker's personality. Speakers with PD were rated by listeners who were unaware of their condition as sounding significantly less happy, friendly, interested, and involved, as compared to healthy speakers (Jaywant & Pell, 2010). The social withdrawal and negative stereotypes may contribute to the high incidence of anxiety and depression reported in patients with PD (e.g., Manor, Balas, Giladi, Mootanah, & Cohen, 2008).

Over the past 20 years, Ramig and her colleagues have developed and evaluated a systematic protocol to help patients achieve and maintain a louder voice (e.g., Dromey, Ramig, & Johnson, 1995; El-Sharkawi et al., 2002; Fox et al., 2002; Ramig, Countryman, Thompson, & Horii, 1995; Ramig, Sapir, & Fox, 2001; Sapir et al., 2001, 2003). Called the Lee Silverman Voice Treatment (LSVT), this program is designed to help patients to use a higher level of effort to overcome the rigidity and hypokinesia of the laryngeal system and to make this new level habitual. The LSVT program takes into account important principles of exercise physiology, skill acquisition, and motor learning. The principles include targeted training, high effort, multiple repetitions, intensive sessions, exercises that are simple to understand and perform, and focus on sensory and proprioceptive awareness (Fox et al., 2002; Russell, Ciucci, Connor, & Schallert, 2010). One of the essential features of the LSVT program is training patients to recalibrate their perception of normal loudness (Spielman, Ramig, Mahler, Halpern, & Gavin, 2007). It is common for speakers with PD to perceive that their voice is loud enough or too loud, despite listeners' perceptions that the voice is abnormally weak and soft. The concept of calibration is extremely important, because the sensory mismatch between the patient's subjectively perceived vocal effort and the actual vocal output may hinder the individual from generalizing the new behavior to everyday situations and maintaining the necessary loudness levels over time (Fox et al., 2002). LSVT teaches the individual to recognize how much effort to use in order to produce a consistently louder voice, as well as to accept and internalize the increased level (Fox et al., 2002; Schulz & Grant, 2000).

The program includes 4 hourly sessions per week and lasts for one month. Patients perform vocal loudness exercises such as maximum duration of sustained vowel phonation, maximum F0 range, and maximum functional speech loudness drills. External cues are provided, such as the instruction to "think loud." Individuals practice multiple repetitions of stimuli using the higher effort level, and attention is focused on enhancing sensory awareness of the increased effort (Spielman et al., 2007). The intensive practice and repetition during therapy sessions, in conjunction with required homework, can decrease the patient's perception of effort required to perform the task and help to make the new loudness level more automatic (Spielman et al., 2007). LSVT is well suited to patients with PD who may have slowed or impaired cognitive processing because the goals and procedures are simple to understand and carry out.

Outcomes studies have shown LSVT to be highly effective in helping patients to generate and maintain higher levels of vocal volume and increased intelligibility. Many studies have demonstrated vocal benefits of the program including consistent use of increased loudness levels, increased duration of sustained vowel phonation, increases in maximum range of F0, increased F0 variability during speech, and reductions in speech rate (Fox et al., 2002). Lasting improvements have been documented by videostroboscopy as well as by LEMG increases in thyroarytenoid muscle activity post-treatment (Russell et al., 2010).

Several modifications to the LSVT program have been reported. For example, the program has been modified to be provided over 8 weeks rather than 4 weeks, with two rather than four 1-hour sessions per week. Results have been positive, with similar increases in vocal SPL following treatment as the 4-week model (Spielman et al., 2007).The LSVT has also been used successfully as a home-based remotely delivered service. Many patients with PD have difficulties in accessing clinical care, and telepractice has enormous potential for reaching large numbers of patients due to increasing access to the Internet and improved telecommunications systems (Little, McSharry, Hunter, Spielman, & Ramig, 2009). Constantinescu et al. (2010) reported on such a program with one client with PD. One computer was located at the speech-language pathology site, and the other at the client's home. The system was able to provide videoconferencing, present reading material, manipulate the Web cameras with a robot arm, obtain acoustic measures, and capture high-quality video. The clinician presented the LSVT in the traditional format, which included sessions for 1 hour per day, 4 days per week, for 4 weeks. The real-time videoconferencing feature allowed for giving instructions to the participant; assisting with shaping correct voice productions and calibrations; monitoring the individual's loudness level, pitch level, and vocal quality; and maintaining good rapport with the client. The authors reported substantial treatment gains for loudness tasks, and the client reported high degrees of motivation for and satisfaction with the clinical service. In another telepractice approach, Howell, Tripoliti, and Pring (2009) used remotely delivered LSVT with 3 patients with PD. Of the 16 sessions (4 per week), one session each week was delivered face to face in participants' homes in order to build a personal relationship, to measure SPL during treatment, to review weekly homework sheets, and to deliver tailored materials for carryover from short phrases to longer utterances. During Web cam sessions recordings were made using HotRecorder, which allows recording of conversations during Skype calls and which can also play and/or save recorded files. The authors reported that the patients achieved gains in loudness levels (dB SPL) comparable to those from face-to-face sessions, and these outcomes were maintained at a 2-month follow-up. However, the authors cautioned that the benefits of telepractice may not apply to individuals with cognitive deficits who may have difficulties engaging with a clinician via a monitor and small screen image, as well as difficulty following directions and managing desktop operations. Tindall, Huebner, Stemple, and Kleinert (2008) used a videophone to provide standard LSVT in the home setting to patients with PD. They collected acoustic data face-to-face in the clinic setting. Following treatment patients compared costs of the videophone and traditional face-to-face delivery options, and completed the Telemedicine Satisfaction Questionnaire. Gains were made in vocal intensity demonstrated by statistically significant increases in dB levels. The cost analysis demonstrated savings in both money and time over the course of the program. Participants reported moderate to very strong satisfaction with the videophone program.

While most therapy for patients with PD is provided on an individual basis, group therapy may be an effective means of improving voice and communication skills. Manor, Posen, Amir, Dori, and Giladi (2005) described a group intervention model facilitated jointly by a speech pathologist and social worker. The program focused on teaching core skills of increased vocal loudness using the LSVT approach. Participants practiced these skills in the context of turn-taking in conversation, engaging in an argument, communicating with more than one person, asking and answering different people's questions, and talking in front of a group of people. The authors reported improvement in objective measures of F0 range and amplitude range, as well as in patient perceptions of speech clarity and voice loudness. Many patients reported that increasing their loudness in a group setting felt more natural than doing it in isolation.

Hyperkinetic Dysarthria

Hyperkinetic dysarthria is characterized by random, involuntary, uncontrollable movements that interfere with normal motor function. Hyperkinetic movements can be choreic or dystonic. Choreic movements are quick and jerky; dystonic movements are slower and more sustained. The movements may occur in the limbs and /or the muscles of the face, jaw, tongue, and larynx. Hyperkinetic dysarthria results from damage to the basal ganglia and/or its connections to other brain regions. Hyperkinetic dysarthrias can result from numerous causes including degenerative neurological diseases, stroke, trauma, inflammation, and metabolic diseases (Duffy, 2005).

CHOREA

The most common disease resulting in **chorea** is Huntington's disease (HD). This is a genetic disease caused by a problem with a gene protein called huntingtin on chromosome 4 (Harper, 2005). The disease is autosomal dominant with full penetrance, so that if one parent is affected, each of the offspring has a 50% probability of inheriting the disease. Typically, the disease manifests itself later in life, between ages 35 to 50 years. By this time it is likely that the person has had children, who in turn have a 50% probability of inheriting the disease. Occasionally, the disease manifests itself earlier in life. Young children who develop the disease usually do not survive until adulthood. HD is a rare disease, with a prevalence of 4–7 affected individuals per 100,000 in the United States, and affects an equal proportion of men and women (Hartelius, Carlstedt, Ytterberg, Lillvik, & Laakso, 2003). The disease is progressive and results in death 15–25 years after initial diagnosis. Rigidity and spasticity tend to emerge later in the progression of the disease, and coexist with the chorea (Rosenblatt, Ranen, Nance, & Paulsen, 1999).

Symptoms. Huntington's disease is characterized by a set of clinical features that includes psychiatric, cognitive, and motor disturbances. Symptoms include chorea, clumsiness, slurred speech, depression, anxiety, irritability, apathy, impulsivity, memory loss, and attention deficits (Rosenblatt et al., 1999). Severe dysphagia is common as the disease progresses, with difficulty coordinating swallowing and respiration (Kagel & Leopold, 1992). At the late stages of the disease death often occurs from aspiration or asphyxiation (Hunt & Walker, 1989; Leopold & Kagel, 1985).

Voice and speech are commonly affected when laryngeal and articulatory muscles are involved, and vocal difficulties may be early symptoms of the disease. Vocal impairment has been reported in 80% of patients studied (Garcia et al., 2009). Vocal quality may be harsh or strained-strangled, with excessive loudness variations, prosodic disruptions due to erratic and unpredictable fluctuations in pitch and loudness, breathiness, prolonged silent intervals, inappropriate silences, and excess and equal stress. Sudden hyperadductory and hyperabductory vocal fold movements and unpredictable inhalations and exhalations result in unpredictable voice breaks and stoppages (Garcia et al., 2009; Hartelius et al., 2003). Hartelius et al. (2003) reported that even patients with recent onset and mild disease showed marked vocal changes including harshness, intermittent breathiness, glottal fry, and hoarseness.

Articulation may also be disrupted by random and uncontrollable movements of the tongue, lips, jaw, and velum. The individual may make facial grimaces, as well as sucking and lip-smacking movements (Rosenfield, 1991). Voice and speech problems appear early in the disease and progressively worsen. The individual typically becomes unintelligible and may become completely nonverbal at later stages.

Treatment. In the past several years the genetic marker for HD has been identified, and it is now possible for individuals who are affected or at risk to be tested for the defective gene. However, although research is underway, there is currently no specific treatment for the disease, and no cure. Treatment is targeted to particular symptoms, such as drugs to treat the motor disturbances, antidepressants to treat the depression, antipsychotics, and mood stabilizers (Bonelli, Wenning, & Kapfhammer, 2004; Rosenblatt et al., 1999). As with Parkinson's disease, surgical techniques such as fetal tissue transplantation, pallidotomy, and thalamotomy may be attempted to alleviate the motor symptoms.

Voice Therapy. Although there is no specific treatment for HD, the speech-language pathologist can play an important role in educating caregivers, family, and friends in how to communicate effectively with the patient. People in the patient's environment should be encouraged to allow him or her enough time to communicate in specific situations. The individual may benefit from interacting in a quiet and nondistracting environment. Communication may be enhanced by simplifying conversation, by asking the individual yes/no questions, and by providing a few choices rather than requiring open-ended responses (Table 9.10).

The clinician can also help the patient to maximize communication by teaching him or her to slow the rate of speech. If appropriate, the speech professional may consider alternative means of communication for the individual. However, it is important for the speech-language pathologist to keep in mind the significant cognitive impairments associated with Huntington's disease and the limitations on direct therapeutic interventions this may impose. Swallowing therapy is important before the onset of dysphagia, in order to accustom the patient to strategies such as eating slowly, sitting in an upright position, taking small bites, and clearing the mouth of food after each bite (Rosenblatt et al., 1999). Eventually the patient may require an alternative nutrition source such as a gastronomy tube.

DYSTONIA

The primary features of dystonia are involuntary and uncontrollable movements. The movements in dystonia are more sustained than those in chorea. Simultaneous contraction of agonist and antagonist pairs of muscles cause prolonged twisting movements and abnormal

TABLE 9.10 Strategies for Caregivers to Enhance Communication in Huntington's Disease Patients

Allow the person enough time to answer questions.
Offer cues and prompts to get the person started.
Give choices. For example, rather than asking "What do you want for dinner?," ask "Do you want hamburgers or meatloaf?"
Break the task or instructions down into small steps.
If the person is confused, speak more simply and use visual cues.
Ask the person to repeat unintelligible phrases or spell the words.
Alphabet boards, yes-no cards, or other communication devices may be helpful.

Source: Information from Rosenblatt et al. (1999).

postures of the affected structure(s) (Berardelli et al., 1998). The movements build up to a peak and gradually subside. The dystonia may be generalized to the entire body, may affect several structures, or may be limited to one particular structure. These latter are known as **focal dystonias** and are typically induced by a specific type of task or activity involving the affected muscles. Focal dystonias include blepharospasm (involuntary contractions of the eye muscles resulting in uncontrolled squinting and/or eye closing), oromandibular dystonia (OMD, involving spasms of the tongue, mouth, jaw, and pharyngeal muscles), spasmodic torticollis (spasms of the cervical neck muscles), **Meige's syndrome** (combination of blepharospasm and OMD), and spasmodic dysphonia (involuntary contractions of the intrinsic laryngeal muscles). Dystonia can be isolated, with no other neurological problems, or it can occur in conjunction with other problems such as tremor (Berardelli et al., 1998). The most common type of focal dystonia that a speech-language pathologist is likely to encounter is laryngeal dystonia, usually called spasmodic dysphonia.

SPASMODIC DYSPHONIA

Spasmodic dysphonia (SD) is a descriptive term that refers to a voice disorder characterized by spasms of either the adductor and/or abductor intrinsic laryngeal muscles. Spasms are induced by voluntary phonatory activity. Thus, when the person tries to talk normally the problem manifests itself, but when he or she uses the laryngeal apparatus reflexively, such as for coughing, the muscle function is normal. Vocal function is also within normal range for phonatory activities such as singing, speaking at a higher than normal pitch, and whispering. While this disorder is rare, affecting an estimated 30,000–50,000 people in North America (Duffy & Yorkston, 2003), SD is the third most prevalent form of dystonia (estimated at 1 per 100,000) after cervical dystonia and blepharospasm (Ludlow et al., 2008). About 10% of affected individuals have a family history of dystonia with onset in the forties (Ludlow et al., 2008). SD is typically gradual in onset and begins to manifest itself in the third or fourth decade of life. The disorder is more prevalent in women than men (Blitzer, 2010; Hogikyan, Wodchis, Spak, & Kileny, 2001; Watts, Nye, & Whurr, 2006). SD can be extremely disruptive to the affected individual's quality of life. Duffy and Yorkston (2003) noted that job performance is affected in 77–93% of patients, with a substantial proportion of untreated people (26–37%) needing to change jobs or be reclassified within their work setting.

Cause. The cause of this disorder used to be considered psychogenic. In the past, individuals with spasmodic dysphonia were shunted from therapist to therapist, often trying such methods as psychiatry, hypnosis, acupuncture, and others, to try to find some relief from this debilitating problem. However, research conducted over the past three decades has demonstrated that most cases of SD are neurogenic in nature and are most likely due to a focal dystonia. Currently, SD is thought to be a central motor processing disorder of the basal ganglia and its connections that results in task-specific, action-induced involuntary spasms of the muscles of the larynx (Holden, Vokes, Taylor, Till, & Crumley, 2007). Recent brain imaging studies have implicated a sensory component in addition to the motor abnormalities in SD. Reportedly, patients with SD who underwent PET scans had reduced brain activation in sensory as well as motor regions during symptomatic intervals (Ali et al., 2006; Ludlow et al., 2008). Thus, the symptoms of SD may result from a failure of cortical areas to effectively process sensory information and make it available to motor regions to regulate laryngeal movements (Ali et al., 2006).

In an effort to pinpoint the location of the brain dysfunction in SD, Simonyan et al., (2008) used diffusion tensor imaging (DTI) as well as post mortem examination to detect changes in the microstructure of nerve pathways in the brain. DTI is a form of magnetic resonance imaging (MRI) that is extremely sensitive to subtle pathology in the brain and can visualize damage to nerve fibers that connect brain areas (Le Bihan et al., 2001). Simonyan et al. (2008) reported that conventional MRI of patients with SD was normal, but DTI imaging showed changes in the corticobulbar and corticospinal tracts as well as in the brain regions directly or indirectly contributing to these tracts in patients with SD. To corroborate this finding, the authors conducted a postmortem study of the brain of one patient with SD who died of unrelated causes. They reported abnormalities in specific brain regions related to the corticobulbar tract. Interestingly, the authors found no differences between patients with SD and normally speaking controls in the areas of the brain involved with voluntary control of emotional vocal expression. This finding may help to explain why speakers with SD are able to laugh, cry, and sing normally, but undergo laryngeal spasms during purposeful phonation.

SD has been associated with a combination of genetic and environmental factors. These include a personal history of blepharospasm and tremor; a history of mumps or other viral infections such as measles, meningitis or upper respiratory infections; and a family history of voice disorders, meningitis, tremor, tics, cancer, and compulsive behaviors (Tanner et al., 2009). Many individuals with SD also have a history of intense occupation and avocational voice use (Tanner et al., 2009).

Types of SD. Three categories of SD have been identified based on laryngeal symptoms: adductor, abductor, and mixed. Any of these types may or may not be accompanied by tremor. The primary form of the disorder may occasionally change over time, i.e., from adductor to abductor (Blitzer, 2010).

Adductor SD. Adductor SD (ADSD) is characterized by laryngospasms of the adductor muscles. Ninety percent of cases fall into this category (Ludlow et al., 2008). Depending on the severity of the disorder the supraglottic structures and the pharyngeal muscles may hyperadduct in addition to the true vocal folds. The spasms result in a voice quality that is strained-strangled, with an effortful, jerky tone that sounds as if the person is struggling to push out his or her voice. Sudden voice arrests are common and can result in speech that sounds stuttered. In severe cases the individual may grimace with the effort. The increased effort needed to produce voice may be felt by the patient in his or her articulators, in a sensation of being strangled, a burning sensation in the throat, or tightness across the chest and abdomen when speaking (Stewart, 1997). Some patients may strain so intensely to produce voice that they produce grunts, groans, and squeaks along with the voice. In around 20–25% of cases the disorder coexists with a tremor (Blitzer, Brin, & Stewart, 1998; Kendall & Leonard, 2009; Tanner et al., 2009), giving the voice a quavery, tremulous quality in addition to the other symptoms.

Onset of the disorder is typically in adulthood and is usually gradual, becoming progressively worse over some years. Often (but not always) patients report first noticing symptoms either coinciding with or immediately after a viral infection or some kind of unusual emotional stress. Symptoms usually worsen with stress, illness, or fatigue (Ludlow & Connor, 1987).

Abductor SD. The abductor form of the disorder (ABSD) is much rarer. In this condition, the involuntary spasms of the abductor muscles cause the glottis to open inappropriately during phonation, particularly during voiced sounds (e.g., Schlotthauer, Torres, & Jackson-Menaldi, 2010). The individual's speech has a breathy, jerky quality, but without the severe strained-strangled feature of the adductor type. The overall flow of speech is disrupted by intermittent periods of aphonia. Voiceless consonants are inappropriately prolonged, and the transitions from voiceless to voiced sounds are difficult. This results in an effortful whisper being produced or brief periods of silence between sounds. In some cases the person's speech has a more sustained, whispery quality (Edgar, Sapienza, Bidus, & Ludlow, 2001; Woodson, Hochstetler, & Murry, 2006). It has been suggested that ABSD may be a "negative dystonia" in which activation of adductor muscle activity at the onset of phonation is delayed or inadequate (Bielamowicz, Stager, Badillo, & Godlewski, 2002). This might explain the persistent breathiness. As with adductor SD, a vocal tremor may be present. Acoustic findings in ABSD include abnormal fundamental frequency fluctuations, abnormally long voice onset time for voiceless consonants, increased aperiodicity, and abnormally long word and sentence duration.

Mixed SD. The mixed form of SD is uncommon, but when it does occur the individual presents signs and symptoms of both forms of the disorder.

Tremor. All types of SD may be accompanied by vocal tremor. Vocal tremor is characterized by periodic fluctuations in the voice frequency or intensity at a rate between 3 and 12 Hz (Barkmeier, Case, & Ludlow, 2001). Tremor of the laryngeal structures is usually at 5 Hz and may be isolated to speech, but also may occur during quiet breathing. Other patterns associated with vocal tremor include reduced magnitude of the tremor during softer or high-pitched voice production. Tremor intensity increases during louder voice production. Laryngeal examination may show a rhythmic medial displacement of the arytenoid cartilages involving the body of the cartilage, consistent with contraction of the interarytenoid muscles (Kendall & Leonard, 2009).

Diagnosis and Evaluation. Diagnosing SD is not straightforward, as there is no specific test to confirm the presence of the disorder. Rather, other conditions must be eliminated, and the diagnosis of SD is based on perceptual, acoustic, behavioral, and physiological evidence.

Because of overlap in symptoms it is important to distinguish between SD and other types of voice disorders, particularly muscular tension dysphonia (Rees, Blalock, Kemp, Halum, & Koufman, 2007; Roy et al., 2007; Schlotthauer et al., 2010). Individuals with SD often attempt to control or prevent their symptoms by increasing laryngeal muscle tension (Barkmeier et al., 2001). This can result in an accompanying muscle tension dysphonia (MTD) along with the SD, which may even obscure the underlying symptoms of the SD (Schlotthauer et al., 2010). In addition, both ADSD and MTD may be associated with excessive supraglottic contraction (Rees et al., 2007). Distinguishing between ADSD and MTD is crucial as treatment approaches for each disorder are distinctly different (Lundy, Roy, Xue, Casiano, & Jassir, 2004; Sapienza et al., 2000). While MTD responds well to voice therapy as a primary measure, ADSD is typically treated with periodic Botox injection (Rees et al., 2007; Sapienza, Walton, & Murry, 2000), with voice therapy as an important adjunct.

Flexible nasoendoscopic assessment during speech can yield important diagnostic clues, as the abnormal vocal fold movements are triggered by speech and tend to be within normal range during other types of vocal activities. Laryngeal assessment should include continuous and stroboscopic light with different phonatory and nonphonatory tasks (Schlotthauer et al., 2010). Videoendoscopy may also demonstrate the presence of a posterior or anterior glottal gap during sustained phonation. Laryngoscopic features suggestive of SD include excessive phonatory activation of intrinsic laryngeal muscles, extrinsic muscle hyperfunction, possible tremor with phonation and at rest, and presence of spasmodic movements during respiration (Cannito & Woodson, 2000). Both glottic and supraglottic compression and intermittent spasms may be observed on prolonged vowels and during sentences (Sapienza et al., 2000). In abductor SD the arytenoids can be seen to pull open inappropriately during phonation.

Perceptual evaluation of voice is an important part of the diagnostic process (Chhetri et al., 2008). Evaluation should assess the patient's overall severity of dysphonia, as well as presence and degree of roughness, breathiness, strained-strangled quality, abrupt voice initiation, voice arrest, aphonia, tremor, expiratory effort, related movements, and grimaces. The examiner should note the presence of normal or near-normal-sounding whispered speech, improved voice quality for nonspeech vocalizations and phonation at high pitch levels, and reported worsening of dysphonia with increased stress (Cannito & Woodson, 2000).

Reported acoustic findings in ADSD include a high incidence of phonatory breaks, abrupt frequency shifts, aperiodic segments, irregular widely spaced vertical striations, well-defined formants, and some high-frequency spectral noise (Rees et al., 2007; Sapienza et al., 2000).

Several assessment protocols have been developed that attempt to distinguish between spasmodic dysphonia types, vocal tremor, and MTD. Barkmeier et al. (2001) developed a perceptual speech symptom assessment protocol for patients with ADSD, ABSD, and vocal tremor (Table 9.11).

The protocol takes into account the number of occurrences of specific symptoms such as adductor voice breaks, abductor breathy breaks, and tremor. The material is designed to elicit symptoms characteristic of each type of disorder, providing a profile that can help determine which disorder the patient has. Individuals with higher scores for adductor breaks than abductor breaks and fewer occurrences of tremor would be classified as having ADSD. Individuals with breathy breaks and little tremor are classified as ABSD. Speakers demonstrating a consistent voice quality abnormality but few adductor or abductor breaks and few occurrences of tremor may be classified as having MTD.

Ludlow et al. (2008) recommended a three-tiered approach to the diagnosis of SD. The recommendation is based on findings from a multidisciplinary working group that included scientists and clinicians in the fields of otolaryngology, neurology, speech pathology, genetics, and neuroscience (Tables 9.12 and 9.13). The approach includes screening questions to suggest possible SD, a speech examination to identify probable SD, and nasolaryngoscopy for definitive diagnosis. A way to distinguish between SD and MTD is also included.

To determine probable SD patients are asked to repeat sentences in their normal voice and in a whisper. One or more voice breaks during speaking and fewer during whispering are required for probable SD, and the number of breaks in 10 sentences provides a measure of severity. Shouting "No" or "Not now" in a loud voice should be symptom free. To differentiate between ADSD, ABSD, and MTD the patient repeats sentences from the abductor and adductor lists, indicating which type is more effortful. Patients with MTD typically demonstrate equal difficulty with both lists. Ratings of a choked strained voice should be made on a visual analogue scale with "normal" on the left and "constantly severely strained" on the right to identify MTD without breaks. Prolonged vowels for 5 seconds at a normal pitch can identify voice tremor, which usually reduces at high pitches.

In addition to laryngoscopic and perceptual measures of SD, the speaker's own perceptions of vocal effort must be taken into consideration. This is particularly important because while listeners only have access to the sound of the individual's voice to help in assessing features such as vocal effort and strain, the speakers themselves use kinesthetic and tactile cues that are interpreted in terms of vocal effort. Eadie et al. (2007) compared self-evaluations of speakers with SD to evaluations by naïve and experienced listeners and found no differences for perceptual ratings of overall strain and vocal effort across groups. Speakers with SD also completed the VHI. Individuals with SD demonstrated a correlation between their perceived vocal effort and the VHI. However, listener judgments were only weakly related to the speaker's VHI. This suggests that a patient's rating of his or her own voice handicap is not related to the listeners' perception of voice quality.

TABLE *9.11* **Speech Symptom Assessment Protocol for ADSD, ABSD, and Vocal Tremor**

Tremor Rating Scale

0 = normal

1 = mild (or intermittent)

2 = moderate (draws attention to itself)

3 = severe (interferes with speech intelligibility

Intermittent __________ Continuous __________ Overall rating __________

	Vowel Breaks	Breathy Breaks	Tremor
The puppy bit the tape			
We mow our lawn all year			
The dog dug a new bone			
Did he go to the right or to the left			
When he comes home we'll feed him			
Total			

Predominant Symptom Type (circle one)

ADSD

ABSD

AD tremor

AB tremor

ADSD/ABSD + tremor

Other

ADSD/ABSD + other

WNL

Source: From "Identification of Symptoms for Spasmodic Dysphonia and Vocal Tremor: A Comparison of Expert and Nonexpert Judges," by J. M. Barkmeier, J. L. Case, and C. L. Ludlow, 2001, *Journal of Communication Disorders, 34*, pp. 30–33. Copyright 2001 by Elsevier. Reprinted with permission.

Treatment. Treatment for SD has undergone great changes over the past few decades. SD is typically highly resistant to traditional behavioral voice therapy, although mild cases sometimes do respond to techniques for lessening the force of vocal fold closure, such as yawn-sigh and gentle onset. Treatment aimed at alleviating the voice problem via psychological techniques has become less popular, as the cause of the disorder has been reclassified as neurological rather than psychological. Counseling techniques and/or psychological referrals are appropriate, however, if the person does have serious issues and concerns, and to help the patient deal with the effects of the disorder on his or her life.

Currently, surgical techniques are the most prevalent form of clinical management. In the late 1970s, a surgical technique called recurrent laryngeal nerve resection (RLN section) was introduced. This procedure aims to decrease the force of vocal fold vibration by

TABLE 9.12 Screening Questions for Spasmodic Dysphonia

Screening Questions	Required for SD	Not Expected
Does it take a lot of work for you to talk?	Yes	No
Is it sometimes easier and sometimes more difficult to talk?	Yes	Sometimes entirely normal without treatment
How long has it been difficult for you to talk?	3 months or more	Less than 3 months
Can you do any of the following normally:	Some should be normal	Affected
shout		Can't shout
cry		Not normal
laugh		Not normal
whisper		Affected same as speech
sing		Affected more than speech
yawn		Not normal

Source: From "Research Priorities in Spasmodic Dysphonia," by C. L. Ludlow, C. H. Adler, G. S. Berke, S. A. Bielamowicz, A. Blitzer, S. B. Bressman, M. Hallett, H. A. Jinnah, U. Juergens, S. B. Martin, J. S. Perlmutter, C. Sapienza, A. Singleton, C. M. Tanner, and G. E. Woodson, 2008, *Otolaryngology-Head and Neck Surgery, 139,* pp. 498–500. Copyright 2008 by Elsevier. Reprinted with permission.

TABLE 9.13 Speech Exam Findings Expected for Probable SD

Task	Required for Probable SD	MTD
Repeat adductor sentences (glottal stops & vowels)	ADSD: breaks on vowels (1 or more on 3 sentences)	Equal symptoms on vowels & voiceless consonants
Repeat abductor sentences	ABSD: prolonged voiceless consonants; 1 or more breaks per 3 sentences	Equal symptoms (p, t, k, s, h, f)
Shout	Normal	Affected same as speech
Prolonged vowel	Strained choked voice	Consistent
	Less at higher pitch	No tremor, same as speech
	May have tremor; less affected than speech	
Counting 1–10	Breaks on vowels or prolonged voiceless consonants	No voice breaks

Source: From "Research Priorities in Spasmodic Dysphonia," by C. L. Ludlow, C. H. Adler, G. S. Berke, S. A. Bielamowicz, A. Blitzer, S. B. Bressman, M. Hallett, H. A. Jinnah, U. Juergens, S. B. Martin, J. S. Perlmutter, C. Sapienza, A. Singleton, C. M. Tanner, and G. E. Woodson, 2008, *Otolaryngology-Head and Neck Surgery, 139,* pp. 500–501. Copyright 2008 by Elsevier. Reprinted with permission.

severing the recurrent laryngeal nerve, thus inducing a unilateral vocal fold paralysis or paresis. However, over several years, follow-up studies of the effectiveness of this technique showed that while the patient's voice was much improved after surgery, long-term results were poor, with many patients' voices becoming as bad as or worse than they had been before surgery.

Botox Injection. Botox injection is the current treatment of choice in the United States among physicians who treat adductor spasmodic dysphonia (Chang et al., 2009). For ADSD, injection is into the thyroarytenoid muscle; in the case of abductor SD the posterior cricoarytenoid muscle is injected. The needle is passed through the cricothyroid membrane, which has been locally anesthetized. EMG is used to monitor the muscle activity and to make sure that the needle has been properly placed. The Botox causes the nerve terminal to atrophy over a period of 1–2 weeks, with clinical effects occurring within 24–48 hours (Holden et al., 2007). After Botox injection the laryngospasms are reduced or eliminated, and the individual is able to speak with less effort. Improvement typically lasts for 2–5 months, until new nerve terminals sprout and the muscle returns to its pre-injection state (Holden et al., 2007).

Dosage Considerations for ADSD. Two factors are important in terms of dosage of Botox for the most effective treatment results: amount of toxin and unilateral versus bilateral injection. The optimal treatment goal is 3–4 months of usable voice that fulfils the vocal needs of the individual and with acceptable side effects limited to 2 weeks (Bielamowicz et al., 2002; Birkent et al., 2009; Cannito & Woodson, 2000). Side effects typically include breathiness, cough, and mild dysphagia, which are more pronounced with bilateral injection (e.g., Blitzer, 2010; Elmiyeh et al., 2010; Paniello, Edgar, & Perlmutter, 2009). Dosages are adjusted for each patient based on the degree and duration of voice improvement and duration and severity of side effects. Injections are usually repeated every 3–6 months. It has been reported that the length of time of voice improvement often increases with sequential injections, or that the amount of Botox necessary to maintain a stable duration of treatment effects decreases over time (Birkent et al., 2009; Cannito & Woodson, 2000). These effects may occur due to permanent and irreversible changes that occur to the muscles at the injection site, such as muscle atrophy and fibrosis, scarring, and changes in distribution of laryngeal muscle fiber types (Birkent et al., 2009; Inagi, Ford, Bless, & Heisey, 1996). Damrose, Goldman, Groessl, and Orloff (2004) suggested that although the increasing duration of vocal improvement may reflect a cumulative benefit of repeated injections, it may also be explained in part by patients returning more frequently for repeat injections before their symptoms worsened significantly.

Botox may be injected unilaterally or bilaterally. Some researchers have reported more effective results with unilateral injections (e.g., Bielamowicz et al., 2002; Elmiyeh et al., 2010). Others have found better results with bilateral injection (e.g., Blitzer, 2010). In order to maximize treatment benefit and minimize side effects, dosage schemes and patterns should be tailored to individual patients in terms of amount of toxin, unilateral or bilateral injection, and injection schedule (Blitzer, 2010; Kendall & Leonard, 2009).

Dosage Considerations for ABSD. The use of Botox for ABSD involves different considerations than those for ADSD. First, airway safety is of primary importance. Because the posterior cricoarytenoid muscle is the sole laryngeal abductor, care must be taken to balance the degree of muscle weakness needed to eliminate the spasms with the patient's ventilatory requirements. The patient should be able to open the glottis widely enough so that there is no stridor or dyspnea during rest or light to moderate activity. Second, because ABSD also involves weakness of the thyroarytenoid muscle, individuals may continue to demonstrate glottal insufficiency and breathiness even after injection (Cannito & Woodson, 2000). Third, the spasms in ABSD are typically asymmetric, with one posterior cricoarytenoid muscle demonstrating larger amplitude spasms than the other. Therefore unilateral injections may not be enough to control the patient's symptoms, because smaller spasms continue in the uninjected muscle (Cannito & Woodson, 2000). Bilateral injections are often preferred, with the more affected muscle receiving a greater dose of the toxin than the less affected muscle (e.g., Stong, DelGaudio, Hapner, & Johns, 2005; Woodson et al., 2006). Some clinics begin with a unilateral injection into the more spasmodic PCA muscle and delay injecting the opposite side for some weeks, depending on the degree of improvement of the patient's symptoms and occurrence of any airway difficulties. The fourth consideration is that Botox injection is reportedly less effective for ABSD than it is for ADSD (e.g., Blitzer et al., 1998; Woodson et al., 2006). There are several reasons for this difference, including difficulty in localizing the PCA for injection, limitations due to airway safety issues, and the concurrent adductor muscle weakness. Despite these considerations and limitations, Botox has been reported to be effective in relieving abductor spasms (Woodson et al., 2006).

Advantages of Botox injection for either form of spasmodic dysphonia include a less invasive procedure compared to surgery, no permanent damage to nerve or laryngeal structures, wide availability, and the opportunity to adjust dosages (Sanuki, Yumoto, Minoda, & Kodama, 2010). Disadvantages include the need for repeated injections over the individual's lifespan, the unpredictable relationship between dosage and response, risk of resistance to treatment, cost, inconvenience, and adverse side effects (Hussain & Shakeel, 2010; Sanuki et al., 2010).

Outcome Measures and Quality of Life After Botox Injection. Botox injection is endorsed by the American Academy of Otolaryngology-Head and Neck Surgery as the primary treatment for laryngeal dystonia (Birkent et al., 2009). There is no doubt that Botox injection is safe, well tolerated by most patients, and highly effective, particularly for ADSD. Many patients have been receiving injections for 20 years or more. A few individuals may develop a resistance to Botox, while others may become increasingly sensitive to the drug (Birkent et al., 2009; Park, Simpson, Anderson, & Sataloff, 2003).

Outcomes studies have utilized a variety of measures to validate treatment effectiveness including clinician/listener perception of voice quality, patient perception of voice quality, acoustic and aerodynamic measures, laryngeal imaging, EEG, EMG, and quality of life instruments (Braden et al., 2010). Several systematic reviews of treatment literature confirm the effectiveness of Botox injection for SD, although there is significant variation across patients, measurements, and treatment conditions (Boutsen, Cannito, Taylor, & Bender, 2002; Watts et al., 2006). Results from acoustic, perceptual, aerodynamic, laryngeal, neurophysiological, and psychosocial outcomes showed improvement ranging from 74–91% (Whurr, Nye, & Lorch, 1998).

Studies pre- and post-Botox injection show less impairment, fewer limitations in activity and participation, and large improvements in quality of life (Duffy & Yorkston, 2004; Hogikyan et al., 2001; Rubin, Wodchis, Spak, Killeny, & Hogikyan, 2004). Studies have consistently found a weak relationship between dysphonia severity as rated by a clinician and patient-perceived quality of life (e.g., Braden et al., 2010). Quality of life depends not only on the severity of the voice impairment but also on environmental factors, personal factors, coping mechanisms, communication partners, and the individual's vocal habits and needs. Many speakers with SD report a substantial degree of voice-related handicap (Kapstein, Hughes, Scharloo, Hondebrink, & Langeveld, 2010). Baylor, Yorkston, Eadie, and Maronian (2007) employed in-depth interviews with speakers with SD to explore the psychosocial consequences of SD and Botox injection. They reported that consequences of SD could be grouped in three categories: the experience of physical symptoms such as voice quality, effort, and unpredictability of the voice; internal personal experiences such as affective responses, changes in the patient's self-view, and personal coping; and consequences associated with the external or social environment such as obstacles in the physical environment, other people's reactions, and altered participation in social roles. In terms of Botox injection, three major themes emerged. The first dealt with experiences with Botox changing over time. This theme included the individual acknowledging that something was wrong with his or her voice, finding a way to the answer, making the decision to get Botox, and learning how Botox affected them. Participants reported that the decision to get Botox was difficult, largely due to fears of injecting poison into the body and of getting an injection in the throat. Despite these fears, however, participants were motivated to get the treatment due to occupational voice demands and frustration over how SD was impacting their lives. Issues related to the injections included adjusting to the cycle of symptoms and side effects and dealing with the reemergence of symptoms as the toxin wore off. Other concerns included the long-term use of Botox and moving to a location where Botox is not available. All participants reported improved voice quality with Botox, improved dependability of voice, and relief from physical effort and fatigue. An important factor was the relief of not having to worry about their voices. Importantly, the Botox treatments allowed patients to return to valued activities and to resume participation in social and community life.

Other Surgical Procedures. Aside from Botox injection, several surgical procedures have recently been described, including thyroplasty type II and thyroarytenoid myectomy. Thyroplasty type II involves incising the thyroid cartilage at the midline with the patient under local anesthetic. The edges of the thyroid cartilage are pulled apart to various distances while the patient phonates (Sanuki et al., 2010). Increasing the distance between the thyroid edges has the effect of preventing the vocal folds from approximating too tightly. When the optimum voice quality is determined at which the patient can phonate easily but without any breathiness or weakness, titanium bridges are inserted above and below the anterior commissure to maintain the separation (Isshiki & Sanuki, 2010). Patients are required to rest their voices for up to 7 days. The advantages of this procedure are that it maintains an intact nerve and muscle system in the larynx, provides a stable, long-term improvement of voice function, avoids risk of scarring or damage to the vocal folds, and is reversible and readjustable (Isshiki & Sanuki, 2010). **Thyroarytenoid myectomy/myotomy** involves resecting the thyroarytenoid muscle either with microinstruments or laser. This creates a permanent muscular weakness that prevents the vocal folds from hyperadducting during laryngospasms. The procedure has been reported to yield complete relief of the ADSD symptoms, with improvements in voice quality, fluency, and sustainability (Hussain & Shakeel, 2010). However, following surgery patients may experience glottic insufficiency, breathiness, and hoarseness for up to 6 months (Nakamura et al., 2008). Nakamura et al. (2008) stress the importance of voice therapy in conjunction with surgery to facilitate easy onset of phonation and decrease laryngeal tension.

Voice Therapy. Behavioral voice therapy has been shown to be a valuable adjunct to Botox treatment and can prolong the effective interval between Botox injections. Voice therapy is recommended by many physicians who treat adductor SD in the United States (e.g., Chang et al., 2009). As part of the therapeutic process, the speech-language pathologist can provide information for the patient regarding the injection procedure, discuss the individual's vocal expectations postinjection, and counsel him or her about the side effects of breathiness and mild dysphagia. It is important for the patient to learn principles of good voice usage and to eliminate vocally traumatic behaviors. Voice therapy is also designed to decrease the amount of respiratory effort used to power voice production, thus decreasing hyperfunctional vocal fold closure. A technique that has been utilized with some success is inverse phonation. Cannito and Woodson (2000) noted that spasms are less likely to occur during this mode of phonation, likely because it is a profoundly different motor task than normal phonation. The authors reported that some patients are able to use inverse phonation as the primary means of communication, while others are able to generalize the glottic relaxation achieved by this technique to speech produced on exhalation. Other approaches include the use of a whisper voice, continuous airflow, establishing easy voice onset, using /h/ onset, and speaking with an overall higher pitch. Cannito and Woodson (2008) described their therapy for abductor SD in which the patient is taught to use a "continuous voicing" technique. This involves maintaining phonation during normally unvoiced consonants and maintaining weak vocal fold vibration between syllables. According to the authors, this helps to avoid the sudden onsets and offsets of voicing that provoke many of the spasms in abductor SD.

ESSENTIAL TREMOR

Essential tremor (ET) is considered by some voice researchers and clinicians to be a hyperkinetic dysarthria (e.g., Rammage et al., 2001), although no specific site of brain damage has been identified. It can occur in conjunction with other dystonias, including SD. The tremor may be isolated to the laryngeal muscles or may be evident in other articulators such as the lips, jaw, tongue and soft palate, as well as in the head and hands. When the larynx is involved the condition is sometimes called *essential tremor of the voice (ETV)* and occurs in 10–20% of individuals with ET (Jenkins et al., 2006). The rate of the tremor is around 4–8 Hz (Jenkins, Adams, Dykstra, & Jog, 2006; Mathieson, 2001; Stemple et al., 2000; Rammage et al., 2001). If the tremor is familial, as occurs in approximately 50% of cases (Jenkins et al., 2006), then it is inherited as an autosomal dominant gene. However, in many cases there is no obvious cause of the disorder (Newman & Ramadan, 1998). The disease usually manifests itself in the middle to later years of life. The onset may be gradual or sudden (Andrews, 1995). This is not a progressive disorder, but the tremor is worsened by stress, fatigue, and excitement (Dromey, Warrick, & Irish, 2002). The tremor tends to be more conspicuous when the person is using the affected structure for some kind of purposeful activity. When the laryngeal muscles are affected the vocal characteristics include rhythmic alterations of pitch and loudness that give the voice a quavery quality, as well as voice arrests. Often it is possible to see the person's larynx moving vertically in concert with the voice arrests. Because voice arrests are common in SD as well, SD and essential tremor are sometimes confused and misdiagnosed. ET should also be differentiated from tremors associated with other disorders such as Parkinson's disease and cerebellar disease. Laryngeal EMG has demonstrated that the thyroarytenoid muscle is affected in most cases of ET, although other intrinsic and extrinsic laryngeal muscles and muscles of the soft palate may also be involved (Dromey et al., 2002; Woodson, 2008).

Treatment. Treatment is typically pharmacological or surgical. Drug treatments include beta blockers such as propranolol, or anticonvulsants such as primidone (Jenkins et al., 2006; Woodson, 2008). These medications can reduce the amplitude of the tremors, but the problem is difficult to eliminate entirely (Deem & Miller, 2000). Side effects include vertigo, nausea, sedation, unsteadiness, bradycardia, fatigue, nausea, diarrhea, rash, impotence, and depression (Jenkins et al., 2006). A broad spectrum antiepileptic medication called topiramate has recently been found to be effective in the treatment of ET of the upper limbs. However, side effects such as impaired memory or concentration, fatigue, paresthesias, stomach upset, weight loss, impaired balance, and dysarthria can be problematic (Jenkins et al., 2006).

When the tremor is severe and resistant to medications, surgery may be considered. Surgical techniques are similar to those used to alleviate the tremors in Parkinson's disease, such as thalamotomy or deep brain stimulation (e.g., Sataloff, Heuer, Munz, Yoon, & Spiegel, 2002).

Botox injection into the thyroarytenoid muscle is another option that has been used in an attempt to reduce or eliminate the tremor. This can be helpful when the tremor involves primarily the vocal folds themselves. Success rates of 50–65% have been reported on the basis of a variety of perceptual and acoustic measures (Dromey et al., 2002). However, Botox injection may result in unacceptable breathiness in individuals who have vocal fold atrophy as well as ET, a not uncommon finding (Woodson, 2008).These patients may benefit from behavioral voice therapy such as vocal function exercises that can help to reduce the effort of phonation by strengthening the laryngeal muscles and decreasing glottal insufficiency. Injection augmentation can also be useful in improving glottic closure and reducing the effortfulness of phonation. This can in turn reduce the amplitude of the tremor.

Mixed Dysarthrias

Discussion so far has focused on dysarthrias primarily associated with a specific brain area. However, damage to the brain can be more widespread, affecting several regions that are involved in voice production. The resulting problems are characterized by different combinations and degrees of dysarthrias, such as flaccid-spastic or spastic-cerebellar. Two of the most common disorders that result in mixed dysarthrias are amyotrophic lateral sclerosis and multiple sclerosis.

AMYOTROPHIC LATERAL SCLEROSIS

Amyotrophic lateral sclerosis (ALS), also known as Lou Gehrig's disease, is a progressive neurological disease that strikes the lower and upper motor neurons (LMN and UMN). Nerves degenerate with resulting scarring and hardening of the nerve tissue. LMN damage results in muscle weakness, atrophy, and fasciculations. Signs of UMN damage include spasticity and abnormal reflexes (Chen & Garrett, 2005).

The disease usually affects individuals in the 40- to 70-year age range, although it can affect much younger individuals as well. There are around 30,000 cases in the United States, with 5,000 new cases diagnosed each year (www.alsa.org). The average time that it takes from diagnosis to death is around three years (Deem & Miller, 2000), with 20% of patients surviving beyond 5 years, and 10% living more than 10 years with the disease (Chen & Garrett, 2005). There are a few well-known cases of individuals who contracted ALS in their young adulthood and who have lived for 30 or more years with the disease, such as the renowned British physicist Stephen Hawking.

The cause of the disease is not known conclusively, but research is focusing on several potential candidates, such as genetic, viral, autoimmune, and neurotoxic agents (Walling, 1999). Only around 10% of cases are genetic, with an autosomal dominant pattern (Vance et al., 2009). Theories attempting to explain causes of nongenetic cases are being explored. One such theory focuses on the role of the neurotransmitter glutamate. Too much of this neurotransmitter is toxic to nerve cells, and researchers in the 1990s found that ALS patients had excessive amounts of glutamate in their nervous systems (Bristol & Rothstein, 1996; Rothstein, Martin, & Kuncl, 1992). This finding led to the development of a drug called Riluzole, which inhibits the release of glutamate from neurons. The drug has been shown to be fairly successful with some patients in increasing survival rates (e.g., Lacomblez, Bensimon, Leigh, & Meininger, 1996).

Symptoms. Because the disease affects both lower and upper motor neurons, symptoms of both flaccid and spastic dysarthria occur. The disease affects all the speech subsystems including respiration, phonation, articulation, and resonance. Swallowing is also affected. Phonatory symptoms of flaccid dysarthria include breathiness and weakness, while symptoms of spastic dysarthria include low pitch and a very tense and harsh voice quality. The patient may also demonstrate tremor, unusual pitch patterns, limited pitch range, hypernasality, abnormally slow rate of speech, and a hyperactive gag reflex (Andrews, 1995). The patient's voice often has a wet, gurgly, hoarse quality as the individual is not able to swallow properly and clear the buildup of secretions. Weakness and spasticity in the respiratory muscles also contribute to the patient's speech production difficulties, and the uncontrollable laughter and crying associated with spastic dysarthria may be present.

Impaired articulation, dysphonia, hypernasality, and dysphagia are considered to be bulbar (LMN) symptoms of ALS. Most patients present initially with UMN symptoms of weakness and spasticity, but around 14–40% are initially seen with LMN symptoms (Chen & Garrett, 2005; Hadjikoutis & Wiles, 2001; Paiva et al., 2001; Seneviratne & Ross, 2008). Laryngoscopic signs of dysphonia in ALS include incomplete vocal fold closure, vocal fold bowing, supraglottic hyperfunction, decreased abduction, and mucus pooling (Chen & Garrett, 2005). Bulbar symptoms early in the disease tend to yield a poor prognosis for survival because of compromised respiration.

Diagnosis and Evaluation. There is no specific test for ALS, and diagnosis relies on ruling out other diseases that could explain the signs and symptoms. This is done on the basis of laboratory tests, muscle and/or nerve biopsy, analysis of cerebrospinal fluid by means of a spinal tap, magnetic resonance imaging (MRI), electromyography (EMG), and nerve conduction velocity tests (www.alsa.org). Diagnosis of ALS can be made with three levels of certainty, depending on the presence and spread of UMN and LMN signs: definite, probable, or possible. The Revised El Escorial Criteria is a classification system used to determine definite, probable, or possible status (Brooks, Miller, & Swash, 2000). This system is based on the spread of physical signs over time in areas of the central nervous system including the brainstem, cervical spinal cord, thoracic spinal cord, and lumbosacral spinal cord (Table 9.14). Physical signs include those related to LMN involvement such as weakness, wasting, and fasciculation and those related to UMN degeneration such as spasticity and increased reflexes.

Evaluation of voice and speech production has demonstrated that acoustic aspects of the voice signal are affected even when the individual has no perceptible voice symptoms. Numerous researchers have reported higher levels of jitter and shimmer and decreased HNR in patients either with or without overt bulbar symptoms and with perceptually normal voices (e.g., Kent et al., 1991, 1992; Ramig, Scherer, Titze, & Ringel, 1988; Ramig, Scherer, Klasner, Titze, & Horii, 1990; Robert, Pouget, Giovanni, Azulay, & Triglia, 1999; Silbergleit, Johnson, & Jacobson, 1997; Strand, Buder, Yorkston, & Ramig, 1994; Watts & Vanryckeghem, 2001).

Treatment. There is no cure for ALS, and typically a combination of medications is used to control the signs and symptoms of the disorder, as well as physical aids such as walkers,

TABLE 9.14 **Revised El Escorial Criteria for ALS**

Diagnostic Category	Criteria
Definite ALS	UMN & LMN signs in 3 regions
Definite familial ALS	UMN & LMN signs in 1 region plus DNA evidence of familial ALS
Probable ALS	UMN & LMN signs in 2 regions
Probable ALS lab supported	UMN & LMN signs in 1 region or UMN signs in > 1 region plus EMG evidence of LMN signs in > 2 limbs
Possible ALS	UMN & LMN signs in 1 region

Source: Information from Brooks et al. (2000).

wheelchairs, and braces. Only one drug, Riluzole, is currently on the market for ALS. While the drug does not stop the progression of the disease, studies have shown that survival rates have increased for some patients taking the drug, particularly those with bulbar onset of the disease (Chen & Garrett, 2005; Walling, 1999). Other medications are used for different symptoms, such as Baclofen, Valium, and Dantrium to relieve spasticity; anti-inflammatory agents to relieve pain from muscle cramping; medications to reduce excess saliva production; and antidepressants to treat anxiety and depression. Botox injection and medialization thyroplasty may be helpful to alleviate troubling vocal symptoms such as excessive vocal folds spasms or vocal fold paresis/paralysis.

Voice Therapy. In the later stages of the disease, the individual may become aphonic, but he or she may be able to use augmentative communication devices such as a communication board or some type of computerized system. Swallowing is typically a problem and requires appropriate treatment (Walling, 1999). Like other disorders that are far-reaching in their effects, treatment of the individual with ALS is best done in an interdisciplinary setting, so that all areas of concern can be addressed. The speech-language pathologist plays a particularly important role in providing education about the disease and communication options to the patient and his or her caregivers.

MULTIPLE SCLEROSIS

Multiple sclerosis (MS) is thought to be an autoimmune disorder in which antibodies attack the myelin coating surrounding nerve axons, resulting in inflammation and scarring. The nerve axons themselves may be damaged or destroyed. The problem can occur anywhere within the central nervous system, including the cerebrum, spinal cord, cerebellum, brainstem, and spinal pathways (Andrews, 1995; Deem & Miller, 2000; Feijo et al., 2004; Mathieson, 2001). The progression of the disease is highly variable, both between and within individuals. Onset of the disease is typically between ages 20 to 40 years, with an average age of 30. The disease affects more than 400,000 people in North America, with a prevalence ranging from 2–150 per 100,000 (Rosati, 2001).

The National Multiple Sclerosis Society defined four different forms of the disease. Each is characterized by a different pattern of acute flare-ups of symptoms (called *relapses* or *exacerbations*) and remissions (Lublin & Reingold, 1996). The most common form, affecting 85–90% of patients, is called **relapsing-remitting MS,** in which periods of remission are interspersed with relapses. The patient may go for weeks or months without symptoms, and then suffer a relapse lasting for months or even years. Without treatment at an early stage of the disease, 50% of patients with this form will progress to a more severe form, called **secondary progressive MS.** Secondary progressive MS is also characterized by relapses and remissions, but the relapses start to predominate, and the remissions become less frequent over time. Twenty to thirty percent of sufferers have this form of the disease. The third type, **primary progressive MS,** affects 10–15% of individuals with the disease. In this form of the disease there is a gradual but steady loss of function over a period of years, with no remissions in between. Finally, the **progressive-relapsing** form of the disease is characterized by steady worsening from the onset, in conjunction with acute relapses. Only around 5% of MS patients have this form of the disease (www.nationalmssociety.org).

Symptoms. MS is characterized by muscular weakness and spasticity due to damage to the corticospinal pathways, as well as ataxia resulting from cerebellar involvement (Deem & Miller, 2000). However, because the demyelinization and inflammation can occur anywhere within the nervous system, individual symptoms and the course and progression of the disease vary greatly. Early symptoms often include impaired vision. As the disease progresses, the individual may develop other symptoms such as an intention tremor, dysarthria, and swallowing problems. Speech and swallowing disorders are common, affecting around 50–70% of patients with MS (Feijo et al., 2004; Woodson, 2008). When speech and voice are affected, the resulting symptoms are characteristic of ataxic and/or spastic involvement, including reduced pitch and loudness ranges, vocal instability, changes in prosody, harsh or breathy voice quality, and vocal fatigue (Deem & Miller, 2000; Dogan et al., 2007; Sapir et al., 2001). The individual may also demonstrate abnormal pitch and loudness control, hypernasality, impaired breath support, and the scanning speech that is characteristic of ataxic dysarthria (Feijo et al., 2004; Merson & Rolnick, 1998). Videolaryngostroboscopy has demonstrated incomplete glottic closure patterns including posterior chink and spindle-shaped glottis (Dogan et al., 2007).

Diagnosis and Treatment. Diagnosis of MS is based on tests of nervous system structure and function. MRI is useful in visualizing the specific defects in the white matter and can also help to differentiate between old and new lesions. A lumbar puncture or spinal tap is done to extract cerebrospinal fluid and test it for the presence of inflammation. Tests of evoked potentials are used to measure how rapidly nerve impulses are conducted in the body. A slowing of nerve conduction rates suggests a problem in impulse transmission. In order for a diagnosis of MS to be made, signs of disease must be present in different areas of the nervous system, and there must be signs of at least two separate relapses.

There is currently no cure for the disease, but drugs are available that reduce the duration of relapses and that can slow the progression of the disability. Current forms of therapy are designed to change the response of the immune system (www.neurologychannel.com/multiplesclerosis/symptoms.shtml). For example, corticosteroids can shorten the duration of the relapses. High doses of beta interferon may decrease the demyelinating activity by regulating the abnormal immune response and reducing the inflammation. This can reduce the frequency of relapses as well as physical disability in the relapsing-remitting form of the disease (www.neurologychannel.com/multiplesclerosis/symptoms.shtml). Some examples of commercially available interferons are Avonex, Betaseron, Rebif, and Copaxone. Other types of drugs are also becoming available. For example, taking a form of bovine myelin by mouth may stimulate remission of the disease (National MS Society, www.nationalmssociety.org). Amino acids such as glatiramer acetate can also reduce the frequency of relapses and the resulting physical disability (www.neurologychannel.com/multiplesclerosis/symptoms.shtml). Certain chemotherapeutic drugs are used to treat progressive forms of the disease, as well as in cases of remitting-relapsing MS which is getting worse. Antispasmodic drugs such as Baclofen and Zaniflex can help to alleviate spastic muscles, as can Botox injection. Shaking and tremors may be controlled with the use of propranolol and other similar drugs. Deep brain stimulation is another option, although the effects on phonation may be to increase the spastic hyperfunctional aspect of phonation (e.g., Putzer, Barry, & Moringlane, 2007). Fatigue is often a problem, and medications such as amantadine can work well. Antidepressants may be used to treat concurrent depression.

Behavioral voice treatment that focuses on respiration training and pushing exercises may be helpful in improving the individual's vocal fold closure and increasing loudness. Implementation of the LSVT has been reported to significantly improve loudness and maximum phonation time in patients with MS, and the improvement was maintained 6 months after treatment (Sapir et al., 2001).

chapter SUMMARY

FLACCID DYSARTHRIA RESULTS FROM damage to the lower motor neuron (LMN) of the brain. Examples of disorders resulting in flaccid dysphonia are vocal fold paresis, vocal fold paralysis, and myasthenia gravis. Causes of paresis can include inflammation, endotracheal intubation, trauma, a mass pushing on the nerve, as well as medical conditions such as autoimmune disorders and diabetes. Symptoms can include breathiness, hoarseness, vocal fatigue, loss of volume, loss of projection, diplophonia, and decreased pitch range in the upper registers. Laryngeal EMG is the best method of diagnosing vocal fold paresis. Injection augmentation or medialization thyroplasty can improve glottal closure. Voice therapy is critical to reduce excessive hyperfunction that may exacerbate the dysphonia.

Vocal fold paralysis is the most common disorder associated with flaccid dysphonia. The paralysis may affect one or both vocal folds (unilateral or bilateral), and the vocal fold(s) may be paralyzed in an adducted, paramedian, or abducted position. Causes include viral infections, stroke, progressive neurological diseases, head trauma, infectious diseases, cancer that invades the vagus nerve, and thyroid surgery. The cause of the paralysis may be unknown, in which case the disorder is called idiopathic vocal fold paralysis. Symptoms can include problems in vocal production, breathing, and airway protection for swallowing and coughing. Behavioral therapy is the first option for unilateral paralysis with the goal of preventing or reducing maladaptive compensatory behaviors. The two most commonly used surgical approaches are injection laryngoplasty and medialization thyroplasty. Laryngeal reinnervation techniques are used to a lesser degree. Surgical procedures for abductor paralysis are designed to enlarge the airway and include total arytenoidectomy, medial arytenoidectomy, transverse cordotomy, and Botox injection.

Myasthenia gravis is characterized by rapidly progressing weakness of movement in an extremely short period of time, i.e., seconds or minutes. MG is an acquired autoimmune disorder of neuromuscular transmission in which antibodies destroy the acetylcholine receptors at the myoneural junction between the nerve and muscle fiber. The structures that are important for speech and swallowing are often the first to be affected, and dysphonia and dysphagia are the most common otolaryngological manifestations of the disease. Dysphonia is characterized by hypernasality, breathiness, difficulty sustaining pitch, vocal fatigue, intermittent aphonia, and stridor. The Tensilon test and other tests of nerve function are used to diagnose the disorder. The disease is managed by medical/surgical treatment including long-acting cholinesterase inhibitors, which prevent acetylcholine from being reabsorbed by the presynaptic neuron too soon, and removal of the thymus gland.

Spastic dysarthria results from damage to the corticobulbar tracts of the upper motor neuron with resulting weakness and spasticity of the tongue, lips, jaw, velum, laryngeal, and respiratory muscles. Vocal symptoms are typically a very low-pitched harsh voice with a strong strained-strangled component, reductions in intonational variability, and hypernasality. Uncontrollable laughter or crying occurs that is either unrelated or vastly out of proportion to the individual's actual emotional status. Treatment is usually pharmacological, with the aim of reducing the spasticity.

Ataxic dysarthria results from damage to the cerebellum and/or its sensory and motor nerve pathways. Damage results in a breakdown in the timing, accuracy, and coordination of the movements necessary for speech production. Causes include stroke, tumors, cerebral palsy, infectious diseases, progressive neurological conditions, genetic syndromes, and viral infection. Speech is often abnormally slow, and all syllables are stressed equally. Treatment is primarily surgical or pharmacological intervention for the underlying cause (e.g., surgical excision of cerebellar tumor) or for associated symptoms (e.g., medication for tremor).

Hypokinetic dysarthria is associated with Parkinson's disease (PD). PD is a neurological syndrome that results from the loss of dopamine, a neurotransmitter manufactured in the substantia nigra of the basal ganglia. PD can result from degenerative, vascular, or inflammatory changes in the basal ganglia and related neural networks. It can also result from neuroleptics, following encephalitis or be idiopathic. Symptoms are muscular rigidity, tremor, bradykinesia, and postural instability. Sensory symptoms include numbness, tingling, pain and achiness, and coldness or burning sensations. Speech is characterized by reduced intensity, monopitch, and varying degrees of harshness and breathiness. The primary treatment of PD is pharmacological, and many different drugs have been developed to treat the symptoms of the disease, including levodopa, levodopa plus carbidopa, anticholinergics, dopamine agonists, COMT inhibitors, and monoamine inhibitors. Surgical techniques to alleviate motor symptoms include pallidotomy, thalamotomy, deep brain stimulation, and fetal cell transplantation. Voice therapy is extremely beneficial in managing the vocal problems associated with PD. The Lee Silverman Voice Treatment has been shown to be effective in helping patients to use a higher level of effort to overcome the rigidity and hypokinesia of the laryngeal system, and to make this new level habitual.

Hyperkinetic dysarthria is characterized by random, involuntary, uncontrollable movements that interfere with normal motor function. Hyperkinetic movements can be choreic or dystonic. Huntington's disease is associated with chorea and is characterized by a set of clinical features that includes psychiatric, cognitive, and motor disturbances. Symptoms include clumsiness, slurred speech, depression, dysphagia, anxiety, irritability, apathy, impulsivity, memory loss, and attention deficits. Vocal quality may be harsh or strained-strangled, with excessive loudness variations, prosodic disruptions due to erratic and unpredictable fluctuations in pitch and loudness, breathiness, prolonged silent intervals, inappropriate silences, excess and equal stress, and unpredictable voice breaks and stoppages. Treatment is targeted to particular symptoms, such as drugs or surgery to treat the motor disturbances, antidepressants to treat the depression, antipsychotics, and mood stabilizers. Surgical techniques such as fetal tissue transplantation, pallidotomy, and thalamotomy may be attempted to alleviate the motor symptoms. The speech-language pathologist can play an important role in educating caregivers, family, and friends in how to communicate effectively with the patient.

Spasmodic dysphonia (SD) is a descriptive term that refers to a voice disorder characterized by spasms of either the adductor and/or abductor intrinsic laryngeal muscles. SD is a focal dystonia in which spasms are induced by voluntary phonatory activity. Adductor spasms result in a voice quality that is strained-strangled, with an effortful, jerky tone, and sudden voice arrests. The increased effort may result in a sensation of being strangled, a burning sensation in the throat, or tightness across the chest and abdomen when speaking. In abductor SD involuntary spasms of the abductor muscles cause the glottis to open inappropriately during phonation, particularly during voiced sounds. This results in a voice that has a breathy and jerky quality, but without the severe strained-strangled feature of the adductor type. Voiceless consonants are inappropriately prolonged, and the transitions from voiceless to voiced sounds are difficult resulting in an effortful whisper or brief periods of silence between sounds. Both types of SD may be accompanied by vocal tremor. Diagnosis is based on perceptual, acoustic, behavioral and physiological evidence, and ruling out other conditions. Botox injection is the current treatment of choice. For adductor SD injection is into the thyroarytenoid muscle; in the case of abductor SD the posterior cricoarytenoid muscle is injected. Behavioral voice therapy has been shown to be a valuable adjunct to Botox treatment and can prolong the effective interval between Botox injections.

Essential tremor is considered to be a hyperkinetic dysarthria although no specific site of brain damage has been identified. It can occur in conjunction with other dystonias, including SD. The tremor may be isolated to the laryngeal muscles, or may be evident in other articulators such as the lips, jaw, tongue and soft palate, as well as in the head and hands. When the laryngeal muscles are affected the vocal characteristics include voice arrests as well as rhythmic alterations of pitch and loudness that give the voice a quavery quality. Treatment is typically pharmacological or surgical.

Mixed dysarthrias occur when damage to the brain is more widespread, affecting several regions that are involved in voice production. Two of the most common disorders that result in mixed dysarthrias are amyotrophic lateral sclerosis (ALS) and multiple sclerosis (MS). ALS affects both lower and upper motor neurons, resulting in symptoms of both flaccid and spastic dysarthria. Phonatory symptoms of flaccid dysarthria include breathiness and weakness, while symptoms of spastic dysarthria include low pitch and a very tense and harsh quality. Tremor, unusual pitch patterns, limited pitch range, hypernasality, abnormally slow rate of speech, and a hyperactive gag reflex may also occur. A combination of medications is used to control the signs and symptoms of the disorder, as well as physical aids such as walkers, wheelchairs, and braces. The speech-language pathologist plays a particularly important role in providing education about the disease and communication options to the patient and his or her caregivers, as well as by helping the patient to maintain his or her most effective communication and swallowing for as long as possible.

Multiple sclerosis (MS) is an autoimmune disorder in which antibodies attack the myelin coating surrounding nerve axons, resulting in inflammation and scarring. The problem can occur anywhere within the central nervous system, including the cerebrum, spinal cord, cerebellum, brainstem, and spinal pathways. Progression of the disease is highly variable. When speech and voice are affected, the resulting symptoms are characteristic of ataxic and/

or spastic involvement, including reduced pitch and loudness ranges, vocal instability, changes in prosody, harsh or breathy voice quality, vocal fatigue, abnormal pitch and loudness control, hypernasality, impaired breath support, and scanning speech. Pharmacological treatment helps to reduce the duration of relapses and can slow the progression of the disability. Behavioral voice treatment that focuses on respiration training and pushing exercises may be helpful in improving the individual's vocal fold closure and increasing loudness.

review QUESTIONS

1. Describe the Darley, Aronson, and Brown (1969) classification system of the dysarthrias, including site of damage, type of dysarthria, and perceptual features.
2. Explain how different locations of damage to the vagus nerve result in different vocal signs and symptoms in unilateral and bilateral vocal fold paralysis.
3. Compare and contrast behavioral and surgical treatment approaches used for patients with unilateral or bilateral vocal fold paralysis.
4. What are the differences between spastic and ataxic dysarthria in terms of etiology, symptomatology, and intervention?
5. Identify the basic neuropathology in Parkinson's disease, and describe treatments for the motoric aspects of the disorder.
6. Describe the Lee Silverman Voice Treatment, and explain why it is effective for many individuals with Parkinson's disease.
7. Distinguish between choreic and dystonic movements in hyperkinetic dysarthria.
8. Why is it difficult to diagnose and evaluate spasmodic dysphonia and to distinguish it from muscle tension dysphonia?
9. Compare the effectiveness of Botox injection for adductor and abductor spasmodic dysphonia.
10. Amyotrophic lateral sclerosis and multiple sclerosis are both mixed dysarthrias. Describe and explain similarities and differences in the signs and symptoms of each disorder.

PREPARING FOR THE PRAXIS

CASE STUDY 9.1: Vocal Fold Paralysis

Directions: Please read the case study and answer the five questions that follow. The answers can be found at the bottom of the page.

Jennifer Abel, a 47-year-old female, underwent thyroid surgery a month ago. Upon recovery from the anesthetic, she asked a nurse for a glass of water. She was horrified to find that her voice was extremely weak and breathy.

After a month, when her voice remained weak and breathy, she consulted a laryngologist, who diagnosed right unilateral vocal fold paralysis and referred her to a voice disorders specialist.

1. The most likely explanation for the paralysis is
   a. endotracheal intubation during surgery
   b. damage to the recurrent laryngeal nerve during surgery
   c. preexisting vocal nodule
   d. side effect of the anesthesia
   e. none of the above
2. Vocal weakness and breathiness result from
   a. flaccid dysarthria
   b. spastic dysarthria
   c. hyperkinetic dysarthria
   d. ataxic dysarthria
   e. all of the above
3. Acoustically, one would predict
   a. jitter, shimmer, and harmonics-to-noise ratio within normal limits
   b. decreased values of jitter and shimmer and increased values of harmonics-to-noise ratio
   c. increased values of jitter and shimmer and decreased values of harmonics-to-noise ratio
   d. no relationship between jitter, shimmer, harmonics-to-noise ratios, and perceptual levels of weakness and breathiness in the voice
   e. none of the above
4. Aside from the speech-language pathologist and otolaryngologist, the most appropriate professional to include on a team would be a
   a. pulmonologist
   b. endocrinologist
   c. physical therapist
   d. nutritionist
   e. neurologist
5. The best way to treat Ms. Abel is to
   a. explain the advantages of medialization thyroplasty and injection laryngoplasty and recommend that she undergo either one of these procedures immediately
   b. recommend against medialization surgery because of the possibility of further damage to the nerve
   c. discuss the possibility of recovery of vocal fold function and recommend a trial of voice therapy for several months
   d. recommend further evaluation with laryngeal EMG before beginning any behavioral and/or medical treatment
   e. none of the above

Answers for Case Study 9.1: 1. (b); 2. (a); 3. (c); 4. (e); 5. (c)

CASE STUDY 9.2: Hypokinetic Dysarthria

Directions: Please read the case study and answer the five questions that follow. The answers can be found at the bottom of the page.

Rose Mason is a 66-year-old female. She comes to you complaining that her voice is weak in volume and that she sounds monotonous and can't vary her pitch very much. In addition, she can say only 4–5 words per breath before running out of air. At the ends of sentences her voice is so weak and soft she can hardly be heard. Her rate of speech is extremely fast, and often the sounds are indistinct and slurred. Her facial expression does not seem to change at all, no matter what she says, and she also exhibits a pill-rolling tremor in her right hand.

1. Based on her symptoms, Ms. Mason probably has
   a. spasmodic dysphonia
   b. Huntington's disease
   c. myasthenia gravis
   d. Parkinson's disease
   e. essential tremor
2. Which is NOT a characteristic of Parkinson's disease?
   a. bradykinesia
   b. muscle rigidity
   c. strained/strangled voice quality
   d. tremors
   e. masked facies
3. Which would be the most appropriate treatment approach for the vocal symptoms exhibited by Ms. Mason?
   a. Botox injection
   b. Lee Silverman Voice Treatment
   c. deep brain stimulation
   d. yawn-sigh approach
   e. all of the above
4. Which of the following neurotransmitters is reduced in Parkinson's disease?
   a. dopamine
   b. acetylcholine
   c. serotonin
   d. glutamate
   e. none of the above
5. Huntington's disease is a disorder that
   a. can only be identified after age 50
   b. is autosomal dominant with full penetrance
   c. is curable in certain cases
   d. is characterized vocally by low intensity, weakness, and breathiness
   e. is a form of dystonia

Answers for Case Study 9.2: 1. (d); 2. (c); 3. (b); 4. (a); 5. (b)

CASE STUDY 9.3: Spasmodic Dysphonia

Directions: Please read the case study and answer the five questions that follow. The answers can be found at the bottom of the page.

Alice Whittier, a 56-year-old woman, comes to your voice clinic complaining of extreme effort in vocalizing. She reports that this problem started to occur about three years ago, and since then it has gradually worsened. You note that her voice sounds strangled, almost as if it is being squeezed out forcefully through very tightly closed vocal folds. After ruling out other causes, you conclude that she has spasmodic dysphonia.

1. Spasmodic dysphonia is considered to be a type of
   a. hypokinetic dysarthria
   b. focal dystonia
   c. vagal nerve dysfunction
   d. cerebellar problem
   e. psychogenic problem
2. Which of the following laryngeal findings (if any) is NOT suggestive of spasmodic dysphonia?
   a. excessive phonatory activation of intrinsic laryngeal muscles
   b. glottic and supraglottic compression and intermittent spasms during phonation
   c. phonatory breaks, abrupt frequency shifts during phonation
   d. consistent and continuous voice quality abnormality
   e. All of the above findings suggest spasmodic dysphonia.
3. It is important to differentiate between spasmodic dysphonia and muscle tension dysphonia because
   a. correct labeling of the disorder helps the patient to accept the diagnosis
   b. giving a name to the disorder facilitates patient trust
   c. treatment strategies for spasmodic dysphonia and muscle tension dysphonia are very different
   d. the term *spasmodic dysphonia* is more intimidating than the term *muscle tension dysphonia*
   e. none of the above
4. Alice received Botox injection, and the following data for pre- and postevaluation measures are compared. Which of the following is most strongly indicated by the data?
   a. Alice's voice has improved.
   b. Alice's voice has deteriorated.
   c. jitter is worse, but the other measures are better.
   d. Alice's voice is still abnormal.
   e. none of the above

Pitch	185 Hz	187 Hz
Phonation duration	10 sec.	15 sec.
Jitter	1.2%	.68%
Average airflow during connected speech	67 ml/sec.	150 ml/sec.

5. Behavioral voice therapy techniques to help Alice maximize the benefits of Botox injection include
   a. providing information about the injection procedure
   b. helping Alice to develop realistic vocal expectations post injection
   c. counseling Alice about the side effects of breathiness and mild dysphagia
   d. implementing a program of vocal hygiene and vocal education
   e. all of the above

Answers for Case Study 9.3: 1. (b); 2. (d); 3. (c); 4. (a); 5. (e)

Chapter 10
Voice Disorders Related to Self and Identity

LEARNING OBJECTIVES

1. Appreciate the link between voice, self-concept, identity, and personality.
2. Identify symptoms and features related to disorders of self and identity.
3. Understand the relationship between stress and vocal function.
4. Describe muscle tension dysphonia in terms of etiology, symptomatology, and treatment approaches.
5. Discuss the relationship between conversion disorders and psychological factors.
6. Identify similarities and differences between conversion aphonia/dysphonia and functional dysphonia.
7. Describe the basis of mutational falsetto and treatment techniques appropriate for this disorder.
8. Gain familiarity with the terminology used in gender identity disorders.
9. Describe behavioral and surgical treatments for voice feminization in male-to-female transsexual patients.

One's voice, self-concept, identity, and personality are inextricably intertwined, and the voice is remarkably sensitive to emotional and psychological moods and states of mind. Not only are self-concept and identity strongly tied to an individual's vocal self-perception, but a person's voice can have an emotional impact on his or her listeners (Bliss-Moreau, Owren, & Barrett, 2010). Vocal characteristics such as quality and pitch provide listeners with information about the speaker's emotional status, social status, feelings, moods, attitude to the communication partner(s), subject matter, and the situation (Gobl & Chasaide, 2003; Gregory, Green, Carrothers, Dagan, & Webster, 2001). For example, high pitch levels and increased use of pitch inflections have been associated with strong emotions such as joy, anxiety, or fear, while low pitch levels and decreased use of pitch inflections are associated with sadness or calmness (Rodero, 2010). Specific aspects of voice have also been linked to certain mental illnesses. For example, patients with clinical depression have been reported to use decreased levels of pitch inflections (Alpert, Pouget, & Silva, 2001; Mundt, Snyder, Cannizzaro, Chappie, & Geralts, 2007).

Voice disorders that are linked to psychological, personality, identity, and gender issues have been called by various names, such as nonorganic dysphonia, psychogenic dysphonia, conversion disorder, muscle tension dysphonia, and functional dysphonia. What one clinician or researcher calls functional dysphonia, another calls muscle tension dysphonia, nonorganic dysphonia, or psychogenic dysphonia. The lack of clarity in terminology has resulted in confusion regarding specific clinical entities. In order to avoid confusion, in this chapter the phrase *voice disorder related to self and identity* will be used generically, and the terms *functional dysphonia, muscle tension dysphonia,* and *conversion disorder* will be used to denote specific voice disorders. The chapter begins with a discussion of the symptoms of disorders related to self and identity, followed by a description of psychiatric caseness. The effects of stress on the body and the relationship between stress and vocal function are described. Consideration then turns to specific disorders of muscle tension dysphonia, conversion disorder, functional dysphonia, and mutational falsetto. Finally the chapter explores vocal issues related to transgender voice.

Symptoms and Features of Voice Disorders Related to Self and Identity

A characteristic of most voice disorders related to personality and identity issues is that the larynx is structurally normal, and there is no detectable organic or neurologic basis for the problem. Vocal function, however, is impaired in terms of quality or capacity (Seifert & Kollbrunner, 2005). Vocal symptoms of these types of disorders are extremely varied and can include any one or a combination of features such as breathiness, hoarseness, harshness, strain, and pitch and loudness problems. Dysphonia can range from slight to severe, or in extreme cases to complete aphonia. While there are many different symptoms and characteristics of voice problems related to self and identity, there are also certain commonalities (Table 10.1). First, the symptoms are inconsistent with the clinical examination,

TABLE *10.1* Features of Dysphonias Related to Self and Identity

Symptoms are inconsistent with the clinical examination
Vocal folds may behave normally
Voice may be worse than vocal fold appearance suggests
Larynx may be positioned high in the neck
Palpation of the extrinsic muscles is painful
Presentation of symptoms is not consistent
Patient's voice varies depending on context, subject matter, or mood
History and presentation of symptoms are not consistent with any known conditions
History of related stressful events or prolonged stress

and the vocal folds may either behave normally, or the patient's voice may be much worse than the vocal fold appearance would suggest (Rubin & Greenberg, 2002). The larynx may be positioned high in the individual's neck, and palpation of the extrinsic muscles may be painful. Second, the presentation of symptoms is not consistent, and the patient's voice may vary depending on the context, subject matter, and mood. Third, it is often the case that the history and presentation of symptoms are not consistent with any known condition. Finally, there is typically a history of related stressful events or prolonged stress (Mathieson, 2001). It is important to keep in mind, however, that certain neurological problems can result in similar features. For example, a patient with spasmodic dysphonia is likely to be able to laugh or cough normally, and the voice problem only presents itself on voluntary phonation for speech. There are also numerous clinical accounts and case studies of patients with coexisting neurological and personality-related voice problems, and differentiating the two components may or may not be possible. Underlying problems such as GERD may also complicate the diagnostic picture.

Psychiatric Caseness in Patients with Voice Disorders

Caseness refers to the presence of clinically significant psychological distress that is indicative of an active psychiatric disorder (Mirza, Ruiz, Baum, & Staab, 2003). Mirza et al. (2003) investigated the presence of psychiatric caseness in patients with vocal fold paralysis, spasmodic dysphonia, and functional dysphonia. The prevalence of major psychiatric disorders varied among groups, with those with vocal fold paralysis demonstrating the highest percentage (63.6%). Evidence of major psychiatric disorders was demonstrated by 29.4% of individuals with functional dysphonia and 7.1 % of those with spasmodic dysphonia. Individuals with functional dysphonia were prone to interpersonal sensitivity, estrangement, and mistrust. Patients with vocal fold paralysis had high rates of major depression mixed with anxiety, and the more severe was the dysphonia, the higher were the levels of these problems. Willinger, Volki-Kernstock, and Aschauer (2005) and Willinger and Aschauer (2005) evaluated 61 patients with functional dysphonia. Of this group, 33% were reported to have mood disorders, including depression; 20% had anxiety disorders, including panic disorder, social phobia, post-traumatic stress disorder, and generalized anxiety disorder; and 4% had adjustment disorders.

Stress

Stress has been described as the set of emotional, cognitive, and physiological reactions to psychological demands and challenges, and is influenced by an individual's coping ability (Demmink-Geertman & Dejonckere, 2002). Stress arises from many external and internal factors (Table 10.2) and may be neutral, positive, or negative (Panzarino, n.d.). Internal factors play an important role in an individual's ability to respond to and deal with the external stress-inducing factors (Panzarino, n.d).

Stress is a highly subjective sensation, and individuals deal with stress in very different ways. People have more or less tolerance for stress, influenced by such factors as degree of social and emotional support from friends and family, sense of being in control of the situation, and overall attitude and outlook on life. Individuals have different coping

TABLE 10.2 **Internal and External Factors Related to Stress**

External Factors	Internal Factors
Interpersonal relationships	Health status
Divorce	Nutritional status
Moving	Fitness level
Death in the family	Emotional well-being
Difficulties at work or school	Coping strategies
Financial problems	Pessimistic outlook on life
Hectic schedule	Perfectionism

strategies, defined as the person's cognitive and behavioral efforts to manage stress by reducing the imbalances between the demands of the stressors and the capacities of the individual (Epstein et al., 2009).

There are many signs and symptoms of stress, including cognitive, emotional, physical, and behavioral (Table 10.3).

Whether stress is internally or externally generated, the body responds to stress by activating the autonomic nervous system, limbic system, and thalamus (Demmink-Geertman & Dejonckere, 2002). The nervous system response (called the *stress response*) prepares the body to react to the stress by increasing adrenaline. Increased adrenaline results in increases in heart rate, breathing rate, and blood pressure. The stress response is designed to enhance the individual's ability to respond quickly and effectively to dangerous situations. However, over a longer period of time continuing and chronic stress can cause problems such as high blood pressure, increases in heart rate, decreases of vocal tract secretions, suppression of the immune system, GERD, pain syndromes, chronic fatigue, anxiety, and depression (e.g., Carleton, Peluso, Collimore, & Asmundson, 2011; Pruett, 2003; Schmidt et al., 2010; Schubert et al., 2009). Severe or prolonged stress is also associated with increased muscle tension, particularly in the head and neck area (Caputo-Rosen & Sataloff, 1998). These stress responses can affect vocal function. For instance, increases in acid production can result in acid reflux disease, which itself is a common cause of vocal problems. Increased tension in the head and neck region may affect the intrinsic and extrinsic laryngeal muscles (Case, 2002) resulting in vocal fold hyperadduction and a strained, tense voice. In addition, when the larynx and vocal folds are extremely tense and constricted, the entire larynx may be elevated in the neck, resulting in an abnormally high pitch. The vocal symptoms experienced by the individual may themselves act as an additional stressor, thus increasing the level of musculoskeletal tension and further interfering with vocal production. The disturbance in vocal function can be particularly devastating for professional voice users. Patients with severe or life-threatening conditions such as cancer or degenerative neurological diseases are subject to highly stressful situations and must cope with fear, anxiety about the future, pain, loss of income, loss of control, and expenses related to treatment, in addition to the difficulties arising from the voice problem. Family roles and relationships may be changed, adding yet another source of stress. Complex relationships exist between an individual's day-to-day emotions and states of mind, long-term emotional status,

TABLE 10.3 Signs and Symptoms of Stress

Cognitive
Memory problems
Inability to concentrate
Constant worrying
Emotional
Moodiness
Irritability
Agitation
Depression
Physical
Aches and pains
Nausea
Dizziness
Chest pain
Hyperventilation
Changes in saliva flow
Changes in gastric acid production
Changes in skin temperature
Behavioral
Changes in eating habits
Changes in sleeping habits

physical correlates of emotional stress, way of coping with stress and anxiety, and the way in which these factors affect the voice. Usually these factors are interwoven and result from a mixture of physiological and psychological features occurring in a social context (Caputo-Rosen & Sataloff, 1998; Rammage et al., 2001). Such factors can be the cause of a voice problem, play a role in maintaining an existing voice problem, or result from a voice problem. All these psychological, social, and emotional issues are critically important to address during the diagnostic and treatment process for an individual with a stress-related voice disorder.

Muscle Tension Dysphonia

Muscle tension dysphonia (MTD) is a clinical diagnosis in which several etiological factors may play a role (Van Houtte, Van Lierde, & Claeys, 2011). The term describes dysphonia that results from hypercontraction of the intrinsic and extrinsic laryngeal muscles as well as muscles in other areas such as the face, jaw, tongue, neck, and shoulders (Lee & Son, 2005; Mathieson et al., 2009; Nguyen & Kenny, 2008; Roy, Nissen, Dromey, & Sapir, 2009; Van Houtte et al., 2011). The tension is noticeable in the patient's neck, jaw, shoulders, and throat, and the individual often reports pain in these areas, as well as excessive vocal effort and vocal fatigue (Stemple et al., 2000). Often, the patient's larynx is elevated in the neck due to increased tension of the extrinsic laryngeal muscles (Van Houtte et al., 2011). The condition may be exacerbated by inappropriate posture, which influences the muscular patterns and tension of the head and neck (Rubin, Blake, & Mathieson, 2007).

Muscle tension dysphonia may be primary or secondary. Primary MTD results from many interacting factors, including psychological and/or personality factors that induce tension, psychosocial issues, poor vocal technique, and excessively high occupational and/or social voice usage (Altman, Atkinson, & Lazarus, 2005; Dietrich, Verdolini, Abbott, Gartner-Schmidt, & Rosen, 2008; Dromey et al., 2008; Mathieson et al., 2009; Nguyen & Kenny, 2008). Stress, GERD, and seasonal allergies may also play a part (Altman et al., 2005; Nguyen & Kenny, 2008; Van Houtte et al., 2011). Stress in patients with MTD has been reported to be linked to daily anxieties rather than to psychiatric problems (Dietrich et al., 2008). Secondary MTD is associated with vocal tension, which results from compensation for underlying glottal insufficiency (Dromey et al., 2008; Nguyen, Kenny, Tran, & Livesey, 2008). Glottal insufficiency can be caused by benign or malignant vocal tumors, vocal fold bowing, or vocal fold paralysis. The abnormal vocal fold vibratory patterns develop as the patient exerts excessive muscular force to compensate for the insufficiency (Belafsky et al., 2002; Dworkin, Meleca, Simipson, & Garfield, 2000).

MTD is seen most often in young and middle-aged individuals (Nguyen et al., 2008), but it has also been reported in children ranging from around 4 years to 12 years of age (Lee & Son, 2005).

SYMPTOMS

Symptoms of MTD range from mild to severe, with vocal qualities including breathiness, hoarseness, strain, effortful phonation, vocal fatigue, pitch breaks, voice arrests, and reduction in vocal range (Belafsky et al., 2002; Dworkin et al., 2000; Lee & Son, 2005; Nguyen & Kenny, 2008; Nguyen et al., 2008). Pain on phonation has also been noted (Altman et al., 2005). Other features that have been reported include hard glottal attacks, poor breath support, and obvious cervical neck tension (Altman et al., 2005; Andrade et al., 1999). The symptoms tend to worsen with increased voice use (Ford & Bless, 1996). Patients with MTD may also complain of vocal tract discomfort including burning, tightness, dryness, aching, tickling, soreness, and globus sensation (Mathieson et al., 2007). Mathieson et al. (2009) suggested that the sensations of dryness, tickling, irritability, burning, and soreness may be associated with inflammatory changes or tissue damage in the laryngeal and/or pharyngeal mucosa. The aching, tightness, and globus sensation may arise from the musculoskeletal tension.

Certain laryngoscopic patterns have been associated with MTD, in particular anterior-posterior compression of the true vocal folds and medial compression of the false vocal folds (e.g., Behrman, Dahl, Abramson, & Schutte, 2003; Koufman & Blalock, 1988; Nguyen et al., 2008; Nguyen & Kenny, 2008a, 2008b; Stager, Bielamowicz, Regnell, Gupta, & Barkmeier, 2000). Medial compression (MC) of the false vocal folds occurs during phonation. In some cases the true vocal folds may also be adducted, while in others the true vocal folds remain open (Rammage et al., 2001). The resulting voice is low-pitched and hoarse, and pitch range is often decreased as well. Medial compression of the false vocal folds is usually due primarily to poor vocal technique. In anterior-posterior compression of the true vocal folds (AC) the front and back portions of the vocal folds are squeezed toward each other, with the arytenoid cartilages pulled forward toward the base of the epiglottis. This may occur due to excessive contraction of the thyrohyoid muscles, which pull the hyoid bone close to the thyroid cartilage, thus decreasing or even closing the thyrohyoid space (Angsuwarangsee & Morrison, 2002). The pattern of anterior-posterior compression is typically seen in conjunction with an extremely low-pitched speaking voice, with extreme effort levels and rapid vocal fatigue. In addition, the finding of poor breath support is very common (Blalock, 1992), which increases the degree of muscle tension needed to produce the desired pitch and volume of the voice (Koufman & Blalock, 1988). Other laryngoscopic findings may include signs of GERD and/or chronic laryngitis, polyps, nodules, cysts, vocal fold bowing, scar, hemorrhage, granuloma, and vocal fold paralysis (Altman et al., 2005).

DIAGNOSIS AND EVALUATION

A comprehensive evaluation is important to diagnose MTD and to differentiate it from other disorders such as spasmodic dysphonia (Table 10.4). In addition to an in-depth case history, perceptual assessment, and acoustic analysis of the patient's voice, videolaryngoscopy is used to detect any underlying laryngeal pathology that may contribute to glottal insufficiency. The presence and degree of medial compression of the false vocal folds and/or anterior-posterior compression of the true vocal folds is determined. AC and MC are often used as hallmarks to identify MTD (Behrman et al., 2003). However, these patterns are also common in speakers without MTD (Behrman et al., 2003; Stager et al., 2001) and may not, therefore, be diagnostically useful. In addition to videolaryngoscopy, the clinician can use manual circumlaryngeal assessment to determine regions of tension and/or pain. The clinician applies pressure over the major horns of the hyoid bone, the superior horns of the thyroid cartilage, and into the suprahyoid muscles (Ford & Bless, 1996). MTD is suspected when the pressure causes discomfort or pain for the patient. The discomfort tends to be unilateral, but may radiate to one or both ears. The clinician also attempts to move the individual's larynx gently from side to side and notes the ease with which it moves. Difficulty in the lateral motion indicates generalized tension in the suprahyoid muscles. In addition, the clinician can feel the thyrohyoid space between the posterior borders of the hyoid bone to the thyroid notch. A restricted thyrohyoid space suggests that the excessive muscular tension is causing the larynx to be carried abnormally high in the neck. During the manual examination, there are methods of manipulating the larynx that may improve the patient's voice, indicating that muscle tension may be the primary factor in the dysphonia. For instance, while the patient phonates, the clinician can exert gentle downward pressure on the larynx, or compress the larynx by putting pressure on the hyoid bone, or both. By briefly interrupting the excessive tension and stabilizing the larynx, these movements may result in an improved voice, indicating that MTD is likely to be the cause of the problem (Ford & Bless, 1996). As well as being diagnostic, these types of applications of manual pressure can be used as part of treatment.

Morrison (1997) proposed a three-tier assessment of patients with MTD, which includes obtaining visual, auditory, and tactile information. Visually, it is important to note the patient's movement and postural patterns, shoulder and neck motion and alignment, extrinsic muscle tension, laryngeal movements on phonation, breathing patterns, and jaw movements. These movements often tend to be restricted and tense in individuals with MTD. Auditory information is based on the patient's vocal symptoms including strain, vocal steadiness, pitch levels, resonance, and vocal fatigue. The clinician should also note how the patient's voice changes

TABLE 10.4 **Comprehensive Evaluation Protocol for Muscular Tension Dysphonia**

Laryngoscopic
Underlying vocal fold pathology
Medial compression of false vocal folds
Anterior/posterior compression of true vocal folds
Auditory/Perceptual/Acoustic
Consistent voice quality
Limited adductor/abductor breaks
Limited occurrences of tremor
Strain
Breathiness
Vocal steadiness
Pitch level
Resonance
Vocal fatigue
Hard glottal attack
Visual
Movement/postural patterns
Shoulder/neck motion and alignment
Extrinsic laryngeal muscle tension
Laryngeal movements on phonation
Breathing patterns
Jaw movements
Tactile
Palpable laryngeal tension during voicing
Palpable laryngeal tension during nonphonatory tasks

when he or she hums, and with movements of the tongue, jaw or head. In addition, the individual's voice may change depending on the topic of conversation, or with strong emotion, and this is an important diagnostic indicator of MTD. Tactile information is obtained by palpating the larynx both at rest and during voicing. Tension and abnormal contraction of the larynx may be present in some patients only during voicing, with the larynx returning to normal during rest (Morrison, 1997). Other patients may keep the muscles tightly contracted during both phonatory and nonphonatory activities. Extrinsic muscle tension around the larynx may be graded on a scale of 0–3, with 0 indicating normal tension and 3 indicating a severe increase in palpable muscle tension (Angsuwarangsee & Morrison, 2002).

Because MTD and spasmodic dysphonia share many perceptual features, it is important to differentiate between the two conditions. Unlike the intermittently strained/strangled quality of speakers with spasmodic dysphonia, individuals with MTD typically demonstrate a consistent voice quality abnormality but few adductor or abductor breaks, and few occurrences of tremor. Acoustic analysis can be helpful in supplementing the clinician's subjective perception of these features.

VOICE THERAPY

Because stress and excessive muscular tension are strongly related to MTD, treatment typically focuses on relaxation of the head and neck muscles. A general progressive relaxation approach may help the patient to identify specific sites in the body where excessive muscular tension occurs. The individual learns to identify the feeling of the state of tension and contrast it with that of relaxation. He or she then learns to consciously and systematically control the bodily tension. More direct techniques of reducing laryngeal tension may also be valuable. Laryngeal massage is helpful because a tense muscle is overly contracted and shortened, and massaging the muscle helps to lengthen and relax it (Verdolini, 1998). Studies examining the effectiveness of laryngeal massage techniques have reported good results. Based on the assumption that the larynx is held in a lower position after massage, theoretically all the vocal tract formant frequencies should be lowered. Significant lowering of formant frequencies and perceptual improvement of voice quality pre- and post-therapy has been reported for both children and adults with MTD following laryngeal massage (e.g., Dromey et al., 2008; Lee & Son, 2005; Roy & Ferguson, 2001).

Some treatment techniques for MTD are more holistic in their focus. Andersson and Schalen (1998) developed an intervention protocol focusing on direct and indirect vocal exercises, communicative exercises, and interactive therapeutic discourses. Vocal exercises included relaxation, deep diaphragmatic breathing, and coordination of respiration and phonation. Communicative exercises involved teaching the patient the link between emotional, vocal, and bodily expression. Interactive therapeutic discourse focused on helping the patient to identify and develop strategies (e.g., assertiveness training) for coping with conflicts in his or her life. The authors asserted that this three-pronged therapeutic model was successful in most cases, with a high proportion of patients regaining a normal voice after only one to five sessions. A similar holistic approach was described by Rubin and Greenberg (2002). Their approach is a team effort that involves the speech-language pathologist, voice teacher, physical therapist, and psychologist. The patient is helped to overcome the feeling of helplessness as well as the belief that the problem is somehow his or her fault. Rubin and Greenberg's approach takes into account the physical elements of the problem, the musculoskeletal issues, and other possible underlying problems such as gastric reflux that could contribute to the voice difficulty. Cognitive behavioral therapy has been used successfully for MTD. Cognitive behavioral therapy is based on the assumption that predisposing and precipitating factors such as personality traits, childhood adversity, and stressful life events precipitate an initial period of physical symptoms. Symptoms are maintained by the interaction of physical, cognitive, behavioral, social, and cultural factors (Daniilidou, Carding, Wilson, Drinnan, & Deary, 2007; Sudhir, Chandra, Shivashankar, & Yamini, 2009). The therapeutic strategy involves helping the patient to identify and clarify his or her assumptions. In the case of children, the MTD may be related to developmental problems, life situation, social context, and/or tension within the family structure (Nienkerke-Springer, McAllister, & Sundberg, 2005). Family therapy has been reported to have positive effects on children's dysphonia, with improvements in hyperfunction, hoarseness, and mean F0 (Nienkerke-Springer et al., 2005).

Conversion Disorders

Conversion disorders are categorized in the *Diagnostic and Statistical Manual of Mental Disorders,* 4th edition (DSM-IV, American Psychiatric Association, 1994) as somatoform disorders. A **somatoform disorder** is one in which symptoms suggest a physical etiology such as a medical condition, disease, or injury. However, no physical cause is evident, and the condition is actually an expression of psychological conflict (Duffy, 2008; Verdolini, Rosen, & Branski, 2006; Willinger et al., 2005). The affected individual is not malingering and can be seriously impacted by the symptoms in all areas of his or her life.

CHARACTERISTICS OF CONVERSION DISORDERS

Certain features are characteristic of conversion disorders (Table 10.5). First, the problem exists despite the apparently normal structure and function of the neuromuscular system. Second, the individual is not consciously producing the symptoms, and the symptoms cannot be explained by malingering, substance use, or any other external factor (Verdolini et al., 2006). Third, the problem is caused by anxiety, stress, and/or conflict, and the disorder has symbolic significance for that conflict. Thus, a person whose conflict has to do with some aspect of communication may present with conversion aphonia or dysphonia. Fourth, the disorder may enable the person to avoid facing the situation directly, and/or it extricates him or her from the situation (primary or secondary gain). Fifth, some patients may show a surprising indifference to the symptoms (called ***la belle indifference***). Sixth, in a true conversion disorder, the symptoms conform to the patient's knowledge about and idea of the disability. In terms of voice, most people are not aware that the vocal folds are used for vegetative purposes such as coughing and laughing, so someone with a true conversion aphonia will likely cough and laugh normally.

TABLE 10.5 **Characteristics of Conversion Disorders**

Normal structure and function of the neuromuscular system
Symptoms cannot be explained by any external factors
Problem is caused by anxiety, stress, and/or conflict
Disorder has symbolic significance for the conflict
Disorder may provide primary or secondary gain
Patient may be indifferent to the symptoms (*la belle indifference*)
Symptoms conform to the patient's knowledge of the disability

In terms of personality factors, individuals with conversion disorders tend to suffer acute or chronic stress, suppressed anger, immaturity and dependency, a history of frequent minor health problems, and mild-to-moderate depression (Caputo-Rosen & Sataloff, 1998; Duffy, 2008; Seifert & Kollbrunner, 2005). Patients report feeling tense and overburdened, cannot admit to weaknesses, and attach great importance to social conventions (Seifert & Kollbrunner, 2005). Conversion disorders are more prevalent in women, particularly those who feel overburdened with responsibilities and unable to control their environment (House & Andrews, 1987). The individual may also be reluctant to express negative emotions in general (Baker, 2003). Some patients, particularly women, may present as tense, anxious, and upset, often crying or being close to tears as they describe their situations (Mathieson, 2001). Men in highly stressful situations such as war are also prone to conversion disorders. Conversion disorder may coexist with depression, and a proportion of sufferers have a history of sexual abuse, incest, and/or drug abuse. However, the condition may occur in psychologically stable people who are in unusually stressful situations (Duffy, 2008).

Onset of the conversion aphonia or dysphonia may either be sudden or the patient may experience recurring episodes. The onset may be linked to acute stress/trauma, but may occur months or years following the precipitating stressor(s) (Duffy, 2008). Many patients associate the onset with some kind of illness or infection (Duffy, 2008). Many also report some kind of chronic health problems related to the respiratory tract (e.g., asthma, bronchitis, frequent upper respiratory infections), and/or digestive tract (Andersson & Schalen, 1998; Baker, 1998).

It has been suggested that some cases of conversion aphonia or dysphonia may represent a form of posttraumatic stress syndrome. In this case traumatic events that have not been fully processed by the individual are suppressed from conscious memory but give rise to vocal symptoms (Baker, 2003).

DIAGNOSIS AND EVALUATION

The diagnosis of conversion disorder may be complicated, because it is not unusual for neurological and psychological disorders to occur together, a condition called **somatic compliance**. In addition, conversion symptoms have a tendency to develop in an organ that is already affected by organic disease, for example, conversion aphonia in those with preexisting vocal fold weakness (Duffy, 2008). In addition, sometimes what may seem to be a conversion disorder turns out to be the first signs of a neurological disease (Caputo-Rosen & Sataloff, 1998). Thus, a comprehensive evaluation is important in order to rule out any possible organic or neurologic causes of the problem. This involves a thorough laryngeal examination. The vocal folds in a conversion disorder are capable of movement, and the patient is typically able to cough, laugh, and perform other reflexive laryngeal behaviors. However, during volitional phonation, the vocal folds either do not move at all, resulting in aphonia, or do not move adequately, resulting in dysphonia. The vocal folds may abduct rather than adduct, or they may only partially adduct during vibration (Deem & Miller, 2000). Sometimes the patient presents with a falsetto voice and may also demonstrate pitch breaks (Baker, 1998). Typically, the larynx is kept in a state of excessive tension. Patients with conversion aphonia typically communicate by whispering (Seifert & Kollbrunner, 2005).

A comprehensive interview and case history is carried out to establish a link between the voice problem and psychological issues the patient is currently experiencing or has in the past experienced. Gentle probing and exploration of the patient's emotional and psychological functioning in relevant areas of his or her life is called for. Should the clinician uncover psychoemotional difficulties that do not fall within his or her professional purview, or if the patient's emotional issues warrant more in-depth investigation, referral to a mental health specialist may be appropriate.

VOICE THERAPY

Treatment focuses on both restoring normal vocalization and exploring the psychological issues that underlie or contributed to the voice problem.

Circumlaryngeal massage may be helpful in releasing the muscular tension. Another strategy is based on the fact that most patients are able to vocalize reflexively for nonphonatory purposes such as coughing, laughing, crying, gargling, throat clearing, grunting, and so on. The clinician can make use of these vocalizations by helping the patient to shape them into voluntary phonation. For example, the patient is instructed to cough gently or to clear the throat, and to deliberately extend the vocalization. Once he or she is able to achieve this easily, the reflexive vocalization is faded while the voluntary vocalization is maintained. As the individual gains control of vocalization, phonation is shaped into vowels, syllables, words, phrases, and longer utterances. When working directly with the voice, it is important to keep in mind that the person's vocal quality may go through many stages before normal quality is achieved, and that some of the stages may actually sound perceptually worse than the previous dysphonia (Baker, 1998).

Counseling techniques are important to help the patient uncover and deal with the conflict in more open and productive ways. As the patient talks about concerns and conflicts in his or her life, it is not uncommon that the voice spontaneously reverts to a more normal quality. While there are anecdotal reports in the literature describing the success of indirect and direct voice therapy techniques, there are no controlled research studies that document treatment effectiveness for conversion aphonia/dysphonia.

Functional Dysphonia

Functional dysphonia (FD) has been defined as a voice disorder in the absence of any organic or neurogenic cause (Daniilidou et al., 2007). FD is classified by the DSM-IV as a somatoform disorder, subclassified as a conversion disorder with motor symptom or deficit. The disorder appears to be strongly related to internal and external stressors and to personality characteristics (Table 10.6). Individuals with FD have been reported to demonstrate higher scores than controls in terms of specific anxiety symptoms related to health concerns and somatic complaints; to be cautious, careful, tense, fearful, apprehensive, nervous, timid, doubtful, discouraged, and passive; to feel insecure, victimized, resentful, and pessimistic; and to experience life as stressful and disturbing (Roy, Bless, & Helsey, 2000; Willinger et al., 2005; Willinger & Aschauer, 2005). Speakers with FD have described themselves as introverted, reserved, reflective, and serious; more afraid of illness, more conscious of health, more fearful of physical injury and of medical treatment, as treating themselves with more care, and as having expectations that other people will provide solutions for their needs and desires (Deary, Wilson, Carding, & Mackenzie, 2003; Seifert & Kollbrunner, 2006; Willinger et al., 2005; Willinger & Aschauer, 2005). Additional features that have been reported include helplessness, inability to manage their life situation, difficulty in asserting themselves, social anxiety, nonassertiveness, a tendency to exhibit self-restraint, anxiety concerning everyday

TABLE 10.6 Personality Features Reported in the Literature for People with Functional Dysphonia

Anxiety regarding health	Cautious	Careful
Tense	Fearful	Apprehensive
Nervous	Timid	Doubtful
Discouraged	Passive	Insecure
Victimized	Resentful	Pessimistic
Introverted	Reserved	Reflective
Serious	Helpless	Social anxiety
Inability to manage life situations	Nonassertiveness	Difficulty in emotional expression

Sources: Information from Andersson & Schalen (1998); Deary et al. (2003); Roy et al. (2000); Seifert & Kollbrunner (2005); Seifert & Kollbrunner (2006); van Mersbergen et al. (2008); Willinger et al. (2005); Willinger & Aschauer (2005).

lifestyle, and difficulty in the verbal expression of emotion (Andersson & Schalen, 1998; Seifert & Kollbrunner, 2005; van Mersbergen, Patrick, & Glaze, 2008). Individuals with these personality characteristics may be sensitive to certain conditioned environmental stimuli, and exposure to that stimulus produces a high level of nonspecific autonomic arousal. The person may become overly sensitive to normal pharyngeal and laryngeal sensations and react by increasing laryngeal muscle tension (Duffy, 2008; Mirza et al., 2003).

EVALUATION AND TREATMENT

Vocal symptoms tend to be nonspecific and include varying degrees of breathiness, hoarseness, and roughness (e.g., Awan & Roy, 2005). As with conversion aphonia/dysphonia, a comprehensive evaluation is integral in establishing a diagnosis of FD.

Individuals with FD respond well to voice therapy focusing on direct treatment techniques such as vocal and breathing exercises; indirect techniques such as education, vocal hygiene, and nondirective counseling; as well as cognitive behavioral therapy (Daniilidou et al., 2007). Daniilidou et al. (2007) compared regular voice therapy in patients with FD whose voices were rough, breathy, and/or strained with voice therapy plus cognitive behavioral therapy. Outcome measures included the GRBAS Voice Symptom Scale, a measure of anxiety and depression, and a general health questionnaire. The voice outcome measures showed significant improvement in both treatment groups, but levels of general health and well-being improved significantly more in the CBT group.

Mutational Falsetto

Mutational falsetto, also called *puberphonia* or *mutational dysphonia*, occurs primarily in postadolescent males. As described in Chapter 2, the boy's larynx and vocal folds show a dramatic growth spurt during puberty. This results in the longer, more massive vocal folds of the adult male. F0 decreases by approximately 100 Hz, and the pitch is correspondingly lowered. Occasionally, despite normal laryngeal growth, a male's pitch level does not lower. The lack of lowering of the high pitch of childhood to the low pitch of adulthood is often due to psychological reasons, such as resistance to the responsibilities of adulthood, embarrassment at the pitch changes and voice arrests that often occur during the change, or desire to identify with a female role model (Remacle, Matar, Verduyckt, & Lawson, 2010). The abnormal pitch may also be the result of the boy's attempt to stabilize the unsteady pitch and quality of the changing vocal mechanism. Deafness is another cause of mutational falsetto due to the loss of auditory feedback to regulate pitch (Chernobelsky, 2002).

Whatever the cause, maintaining the high F0 requires a great deal of laryngeal muscular force and tension. Recall that the cricothyroid muscles exert considerable longitudinal tension on the vocal folds in falsetto register, and the folds do not close completely during vibration. Thus, the voice is not only abnormally high pitched, but also breathy and weak. The individual's larynx may be hypertonic, and the cartilaginous glottis may be closed too tightly, so that only the membranous portion of the vocal folds is able to vibrate (Rammage et al., 2001). This would also contribute to the excessively high pitch, because the effective vibrational length of the vocal folds is decreased. In addition, the entire larynx may be elevated due to excessive contraction of the suprahyoid muscles. Inappropriate vocal tract resonance may also be a factor in the abnormal vocal quality, as the individual may carry his tongue in an abnormally high position (Stemple et al., 2000). Other potential vocal features include hoarseness, pitch breaks, lack of pitch variability, muscle tension, vocal fatigue, and inability to project the voice (Remacle et al., 2010).

EVALUATION

Flexible and/or rigid laryngoscopy is important to document that the laryngeal mechanism is structurally intact with normal vocal fold mobility. Acoustic and perceptual measures help to determine the overall severity of the problem as well as to quantify the extent of F0 deviation. Other causes of the patient's high pitch such as endocrine problems, hearing loss, or neurological problems should be ruled out and/or addressed. The existence of psychological factors should be determined during the case history interview.

TREATMENT

With structural or other physical causes ruled out, behavioral voice therapy is the treatment of choice for mutational falsetto, although surgical techniques may be useful for severe or recalcitrant cases.

Voice Therapy. Laryngeal massage may be effective in producing a lower pitch by relaxing the extrinsic and intrinsic laryngeal muscles and decreasing the excessive hypercontraction. Another technique for eliciting a more normal pitch level is having the individual cough or laugh. These vegetative vocalizations are likely to occur at a more normal pitch level and can then be shaped into meaningful utterances. Manual compression of the larynx is another simple yet effective strategy in which the thyroid cartilage is compressed and pushed gently downward to prevent the larynx from pulling upward and increasing tension on the vocal folds. The patient is encouraged to focus on the sound and feel of the lower pitch produced by this manipulation. The digital pressure is faded as he becomes more adept at producing the lower pitch consistently. Visual feedback can be very helpful in facilitating the desired pitch. Chernobelsky (2002) used electroglottography with deaf adolescents who exhibited an abnormally high pitch with an average F0 of 436 Hz. Using the technique of voiced coughing to lower the F0 into the modal register, the boys were able to compare the electroglottographic waveforms produced in modal versus falsetto registers. Posttherapy, the average F0 of these boys lowered to 184 Hz.

Several researchers have reported successful outcomes of behavioral voice therapy with long-term maintenance of the lower pitch (e.g., Dagli, Acar, Stone, Dursun, & Eryilmaz, 2008; Lim et al., 2007). Lim et al. (2007) treated 15 patients with mutational falsetto using manual compression of the larynx. The authors conducted acoustic and aerodynamic tests before and after treatment. Reportedly, before treatment the voices of all patients were abnormally high pitched, weak, and breathy, and no patient could phonate at low pitches. Laryngeal examinations showed normal development of the larynx in the majority of cases, although many boys demonstrated a narrow thyrohyoid space, elevation of the larynx, and severe contraction of the suprahyoid muscles during phonation. Vocal fold mobility was normal in all cases. F0 was 193.41 Hz for /a/ and 198.85 Hz for connected speech. Following therapy F0 for /a/ decreased to 113.49 Hz and for connected speech to 115.62 Hz. Jitter and shimmer levels also decreased, reflecting increased vocal stability.

Counseling or psychotherapy may be helpful for some individuals who are able to lower their F0 with voice therapy, but who are strongly resistant to voice change (Remacle et al., 2010).

Surgery. For those cases that are unresponsive to voice therapy due to excessive muscular contraction of suprahyoid and/or cricothyroid muscles, Botox injection has been proposed (e.g., Lim et al., 2007; Woodson & Murry, 1994). Woodson and Murry (1994) described a case study of a 47-year-old man with an above-average F0 and thin voice quality for whom voice therapy was unsuccessful. The researchers injected Botox into the cricothyroid muscles, with a resulting drop in F0 to a normal level (around 100 Hz). Woodson and Murry (1994) proposed that Botox injection in conjunction with voice therapy should be attempted prior to considering surgical alteration such as Type III thyroplasty for individuals who do not respond to voice therapy alone. Type III thyroplasty, also called *relaxation thyroplasty*, is designed to manipulate the thyroid cartilage in a way that shortens the vocal folds and reduces vocal fold tension (Remacle et al., 2010). Using this procedure Remacle et al (2010) reported a decrease in F0 from an average of 187 Hz to 104 Hz postsurgery and a substantial improvement on the VHI for patients with mutational falsetto.

Transgender Voice

The term **transsexual** was coined in the 1960s and defined in various versions of the DSM as a condition in which an individual wishes to manifest the primary and secondary sex characteristics of the non-natal sex and live as a member of that sex, and who modifies his or her body with hormones and surgery to achieve that end (Denny, 2004). In the mid-1990s the diagnostic category Transsexualism was replaced with the more general category Gender Identity Disorder (DSM-IV-TR, 1994) and specifies four criteria for diagnosis (Table 10.7). In this version the term *transsexual* was subsumed under the more inclusive term *transgender*. The term **transgender** describes all persons whose identities, behavior, or dress vary from traditional gender norms, including transsexuals, transgenderists,

TABLE 10.7 DSM-IV-TR Diagnostic Criteria for Gender Identity Disorder

A. Strong and persistent cross-gender identification (not merely a desire for any perceived cultural advantages of being the other sex). In children, the disturbance is manifested by four (or more) of the following:
   1. Repeatedly stated desire to be, or insistence that he or she is, the other sex
   2. In boys, preference for cross-dressing or simulating female attire; in girls, insistence on wearing only stereotypical masculine clothing
   3. Strong and persistent preferences for cross-sex roles in make-believe play or persistent fantasies of being the other sex
   4. Intense desire to participate in the stereotypical games and pastimes of the other sex
   5. Strong preference for playmates of the other sex

B. Persistent discomfort with his or her sex or sense of inappropriateness in the gender role of that sex.

C. The disturbance is not concurrent with a physical intersex condition.

D. The disturbance causes clinically significant distress or impairment in social, occupational, or other important areas of functioning.

cross-dressers, and drag queens (Denny, 2004). The transgender model views transsexualism and other forms of gender variance as natural forms of human variability rather than as a mental disorder (Denny, 2004). Some clinicians and researchers have argued that gender incongruence should not automatically mandate a psychiatric diagnosis, but rather a medical one (e.g., Allison, 2010). Terms have been proposed to describe variations in gender without categorizing them in terms of a disorder. These include *gender dysphoria, gender discordance, gender dissonance, gender discomfort,* or *gender incongruence* (Allison, 2010; Cohen-Kettenis & Pfafflin, 2010).

As currently used, the term *transsexual* refers to individuals whose gender identity is fundamentally in conflict with their biological sex, and who unambiguously identify with the non-natal gender (Denny, 2004). The individual feels strong discomfort with the biological identity and the corresponding roles, expectations, and attitudes that society expects in accordance with traditional male and female genders. It is not uncommon for the person to live for years in accordance with the societal rules for the natal gender (Thornton, 2008). Indeed, the male-to-female transsexual (MFT) seeking the services of a speech-language pathologist is likely to be middle-aged, married or previously married, and the father of one or more children (Gelfer, 1999; Thornton, 2008). It is likewise not unusual for transsexual individuals to have (or have had) traditionally male-oriented occupations (Gelfer, 1999). Many have served in the military or have worked in law enforcement, construction, or some other stereotypically masculine field. The individual's masculine lifestyle may represent his attempt to suppress the gender dysphoria (Brown & Rounsley, 1996). Eventually the person may seek help and may decide to undergo surgical procedures for changing gender identity. The process of changing one's gender is a long and challenging one. The process may take years and involves stages of counseling and psychotherapy, living as a person of the target gender, enduring the surgery itself, and becoming accepted as a person of the desired gender. The treatment of the transsexual client has been described as a process of phases that one travels through to get to the other gender side (Gold, 1999).

SEX REASSIGNMENT SURGERY

Despite nonsurgical lifestyle options now open to transgendered people, transsexuals tend to view sex reassignment surgery (SRS) as the treatment of choice (Denny, 2004). It has been estimated that around 1 in 30,000 adult males and 1 in 100,000 adult females elect to undergo sex reassignment surgery (Levy, 2000). Surgery for changing one's natal gender is not something that is done lightly, and most physicians and psychiatrists require a person to live for 1–2 years as a member of the target gender before undergoing the surgery (Verdolini et al., 2006). Internationally adopted guidelines contain built-in time restraints and safeguards for the potential transsexual patient. The first version of this document was published in 1979. Originally called the Harry Benjamin Guidelines for Standards of Care, the name was changed in 2001 to the Harry Benjamin International Gender Dysphoria Association's Standards of Care for Gender Identity Disorders, 6th Version (February 2001). In 2009 the Harry Benjamin International Gender Dysphoria Association (HBIGDA) was renamed the World Professional Association for Transgender Health (Cohen-Kettenis & Pfafflin, 2010).

The Standards of Care is an extensive document that covers introductory concepts describing the purpose and standards of care; epidemiological considerations such as the natural history of gender identity disorder and cultural differences in gender identity variance throughout the world; diagnostic terminology and ICD-10 classification of gender identity disorders; responsibilities of the mental health professional; assessment and treatment of children and adolescents; psychotherapy with adults; requirements for and effects of hormone therapy for adults; the real-life experience; different forms of surgery including sex reassignment surgery, breast surgery, and other cosmetic surgeries (e.g., reduction thyroid chondroplasty); and post-transition follow-up. The entire document may be accessed at www.wpath.org/publications_standards.cfm.

Most individuals who complete sex reassignment surgery are male-to-female transsexuals. Often, the surgery is extremely successful in terms of visual appearance, with the help of appropriate hormone treatment, breast augmentation, electrolysis, and facial plastic surgery. However, the so-called "trans woman" is often left with a voice that is perceived as masculine, at odds with her new appearance. The person's pitch levels, intonational patterns, voice quality, and overall communicative characteristics often remain in the masculine domain. Mainstream culture does tend to penalize people whose voices do not match their gender, body type, and build. This is troublesome to many patients who have undergone the surgery. Reportedly, 93% of participants at a transgender conference rated voice as at least somewhat important in the transition process, and around 25% rated voice and nonverbal communication as playing the most important role in the individual's success in "passing" as a female (Johnson, 2008).

Many trans women turn to speech-language therapists for help in achieving a more feminine voice. Clinicians working with this population are faced with some unique challenges. A clinician may be reluctant to work with a transgender client for moral, ethical, and/or religious reasons, yet ASHA's Principles of Ethics state that all clients must be treated with respect. Clinicians need to be aware of their own biases and perspectives and take care that these do not negatively impact the therapeutic process. Speech-language pathologists must ensure that they are familiar with the guidelines for treatment of all transgendered clients and are cognizant of appropriate gender terminology. Table 10.8 provides terminology currently used in the transgender community.

TABLE 10.8 **Terminology Related to Sexual Orientation and Gender Identity Disorder**

Term	Definition
Gender identity disorder	Diagnostic category referring to individuals with a strong and persistent cross-gender identification
Queer	Umbrella term that includes gender identities and sexual orientations and applies to anyone who does not identify as straight/gender normative
Sexual orientation (SO)	External, sexual attraction to others; spectrum from straight to bisexual to gay (Queer SO)
Gender identity (GI)	Internal, perception of self; spectrum from male to androgynous to female (Queer GI)
Cisgender	Gender identity consistent with the gender one is identified as at birth
Transgender	Gender identity not consistent with the gender one is identified as at birth; used as an umbrella term for all queer GIs; describes persons in gender transition
Transsexual	An individual who desires to live full-time in the opposite gender; describes a person whose external genital anatomy has been changed to resemble that of the opposite sex
Cross-dresser (transvestite)	Individual who identifies on the gender spectrum but who does not wish to fully transition and presents as the opposite gender less than half time
Transition	The process one goes through to live as the opposite gender
Gender community	Cultural group where gender roles are not strictly defined by anatomical physical attributes
Passing	Ability of a TG or TS individual to be perceived by others as belonging to the target gender group

Sources: Information from Johnson (2008); King et al. (1999).

EVALUATION

As with any voice disorder a comprehensive evaluation is essential. In the case of a transgendered individual, the case history becomes even more important because of unique concerns involving privacy issues, terminology, evolving treatment goals, and unusual social circumstances (King, Lindstedt, & Jensen, 1999). Table 10.9 presents questions pertaining specifically to transgender/transsexual clients that should be incorporated in the overall case history interview.

In order to establish professional credibility, trust, and rapport with the client, the speech-language pathologist must demonstrate a high level of pragmatic appropriateness during the initial interview, ongoing evaluation, and the entire therapeutic process. When dealing

TABLE 10.9 Case History Questions Pertaining to Transgender and/or Transsexual Clients

Gender Role Information

Which name do you prefer to be called?

Is this the name to be used for contact outside the clinic?

What stage are you in the gender reassignment process?

How often do you present yourself as male? (estimate percentage of time)

How often do you present yourself as female? (estimate percentage of time)

Are you undergoing hormone treatment?

Are you under the care of a mental health specialist?

Do you plan to transition to full-time immersion in the female role?

If so, when?

What kind of woman do you wish to be?

How supportive are your friends, colleagues, and family?

Voice Information

How would you rate your present female voice? (poor, fair, good, excellent)

How do others react to your female voice?

How much of a strain is it to use your female voice (not at all, somewhat, very)

What strategies do you use to change from your male to female voice?

How important is a feminine voice to you? (not at all, somewhat, very)

What are your goals for voice therapy?

Sources: Information from Brown et al. (2000); Dacakis (2006); Gelfer (1999); Johnson (2008); King et al. (1999); Moran et al. (2008).

with individuals with sexual orientation or gender identity issues, it is critical to use appropriate current terminology and the individual's preferred form of address in order to win the person's confidence and trust. The evaluator should ask the client which name he/she prefers to be called and whether this is also the name to be used for contact outside the clinic (Dacakis, 2006; Gelfer, 1999; Johnson, 2008). For an individual who is transitioning from full-time male role to full-time female role the client will likely use both the male and female versions of his/her name (Dacakis, 2006). It is important for the clinician to respect and use the preferred name and the appropriate personal pronouns, according to the client's wishes.

During the interview process the evaluator should elicit information from the client regarding where the individual is in the gender reassignment process, whether he/she is undergoing hormone treatment, and whether he/she is under the care of a psychiatrist or other mental health professional (Gelfer, 1999). The individual should be questioned regarding the degree of support he/she is receiving or is likely to receive from family, friends, and colleagues (Gelfer, 1999; King et al., 1999). The level of support in the client's everyday environment can impact the degree to which he/she is able to apply techniques learned in the clinic to functional situations in his/her life. Information should be obtained about when the client must pass with the new voice (Johnson, 2008), what percentage of time he/she is currently living as a woman, and when he/she plans to make the transition to full-time immersion in the female role. It is likely that as the individual transitions from a more masculine role to a more feminine role, the communication situations in his/her environment will change, signaling the need for ongoing communication assessment and evaluation (Dacakis, 2006; King et al., 1999).

Identifying the client's goals for voice treatment is important to maximize the potential for a successful treatment outcome. A client may have unrealistic expectations about what her feminine voice will sound like (Gelfer, 1999). This could jeopardize the therapeutic process and negatively impact the person's perception of therapeutic success. The client's perspective regarding what kind of woman she wishes to be is another important issue, as many of the verbal and nonverbal behaviors suggested in the literature for transsexual clients reflect a female stereotype, which is rejected by many modern women but forms the target for some clients (Moran, Hague, & Roper, 2008).

In addition to specific items related to transgender issues the client's medical history should be explored. Particular attention should be paid to conditions that may affect the voice, such as a history of GERD, any neurological problems, cardiac problems, hearing difficulties, respiratory issues, and seasonal or other allergies. It is important to note whether the individual has undergone any nongender or gender-related surgeries, and whether he/she was intubated for the procedure. Any prescribed or over-the-counter medications should be noted, as these can affect voice production. Attention should also focus on the client's use of tobacco, alcohol, and recreational drugs.

As with all individuals who present for voice therapy, the speech-language pathologist should determine the client's level of daily vocal usage, vocal technique, vocal needs, and vocal habits. Vocally traumatic behaviors should be identified. It is also important to note whether and how the person has attempted to change the voice during the transition process. An individual may have tried to raise pitch by using excessive laryngeal tension, thereby creating the conditions for a possible MTD (Brown, Perry, Cheesman, & Pring, 2000). Quality of life questionnaires such as the VHI are an important means of gaining insight into the impact of the client's voice on his/her everyday life.

In addition to the extensive case history, the client should undergo laryngeal examination by an otolaryngologist to rule out any laryngeal abnormalities of structure or function. Acoustic analysis is also a critical part of the assessment process. It is important to determine the client's habitual speaking frequency level in the male role (Mordaunt, 2006), as well as maximum phonational frequency range, intensity levels, and intonational patterns. An acoustic analysis program is helpful in documenting the person's habitual average fundamental frequency in sustained phonation, reading, and spontaneous speech.

TREATMENT

Treatment for individuals wishing to develop a more feminine communication style is multifaceted and may include voice therapy, surgery, counseling, articulation therapy, assistance with nonverbal communication patterns, and focus on physical appearance. The goal of treatment is to emphasize and highlight the markers of female speech. Markers include a higher pitch, greater intonational range and pitch variability, increased vocal expression, rising intonation on statements, breathier voice quality, feminine patterns of phrasing, as well as nonverbal visual markers such as increased eye contact, increased hand/arm gestures, and increased use of touch (Parker, 2008). A good starting point for gender-specific communication work is for the client to spend time observing people who are of the chosen gender, age, culture, and social class in familiar contexts (Thornton, 2008). However, before any gender-specific work begins, any existing dysphonia and vocally traumatic behaviors must be treated (Thornton, 2008), and any medical conditions such as GERD or allergies should be addressed.

Voice Therapy. Behavioral voice therapy plays a critical part in helping the trans speaker develop a perceptually more feminine voice and more feminine communication patterns. Therapy focuses not only on raising pitch but on feminizing the client's vocal quality and resonance, intonational patterns, articulatory patterns, and nonverbal gestures. Vocal hygiene is also emphasized as the individual learns to generate and maintain the target pitch without laryngeal strain or vocal hyperfunction (Table 10.10).

Pitch. F0 is the most salient cue to gender identification for trans speakers as well as for biological men and women (Gelfer & Mikos, 2005). Therefore, raising the individual's pitch has typically been targeted as the most important goal of treatment. Research has established

TABLE 10.10 **Feminizing Strategies for Trans Speakers**

F0 and Pitch
Determine target F0 level
Establish a starting F0 slightly above the male habitual pitch
Raise F0 levels in small increments while maintaining good voice quality and appropriate intonation
Begin each F0 level with isolated vowels and progress to longer utterances
Practice using each new F0 level in different phonetic contexts and with varying intonational patterns
Use more upward pitch inflections and fewer downward pitch inflections
Voice Quality
Eliminate glottal fry and hard glottal attacks
Avoid falsetto register
Use a slightly breathy quality
Use a resonant forward focus
Articulation
Use more anterior tongue placements and lip spreading to raise formant frequencies
Use light and more precise articulatory contacts
Paralinguistic and Nonverbal
Use feminine nonverbal patterns such as increased eye contact and use of gestures
Increase use of tags at the end of utterances

a cutoff F0 of around 150–173 Hz, below which speakers are perceived as male and above which speakers are perceived as female (e.g., Brown, Perry, Cheesman, & Pring, 2000; Gelfer & Schofield, 2000; Wolfe, Ratusnik, Smith, & Northrop, 1990). The range between approximately 145–165 Hz forms a gender-ambiguous F0 zone in which the speaker's gender is not identifiable (Mordaunt, 2006; Thornton, 2008). This zone forms the initial target for pitch raising exercises.

The goal of intervention is to achieve a mean F0 level as close as possible to that of adult female speakers, which typically ranges between 180–230 Hz. An important first step in raising the client's pitch level is determining an appropriate target that takes into account the speaker's ability to vary pitch for inflectional purposes. Pitch raising protocols typically establish a starting F0 by having the client produce easy productions of vowels or nasal consonant/vowel combinations such as /a/, /ma/, or "um-hmm" at a frequency slightly above the speaker's typical male level (e.g., Gelfer, 1999; Mordaunt, 2006). The client is provided a model of a light, clear vocal quality. Most protocols use acoustic instrumentation for visual feedback and audio recordings for auditory feedback. When the client becomes able to habituate and maintain the slightly higher level with good voice quality, the target is raised again. Mordaunt (2006) recommended raising the level in increments of 10 Hz, while ensuring that the speaker maintains an acceptable voice quality, is able to use the higher level in different situations and with varying loudness levels, and can use the upward intonational patterns that give the speech a more feminine quality. The final desired pitch level must allow the speaker to easily access the upper pitch ranges for intonational purposes. As the client continues to progress to higher pitch levels, practice at each level typically begins with isolated vowels, extending utterances as the individual becomes more adept at using the new pitch. The new pitch level should be practiced in different phonetic contexts, using varying levels of meaningfulness (e.g., reciting the days of the week versus talking about an important issue), reading, and answering questions. At the sentence level, the speaker is encouraged to express different emotions such as happiness, sorrow, and annoyance, so that he/she can experiment with the feminine voice (Gelfer, 1999).

Vocal Quality. Good vocal quality is emphasized both before the pitch work begins and throughout the treatment process. The individual is taught to eliminate any instances of harshness, hoarseness, glottal fry, and hard glottal attacks and encouraged to use a slightly lower intensity and breathy quality to increase the perception of vocal femininity (Gorham-Rowan & Morris, 2006; Holmberg et al., 2009; Mordaunt, 2006). Practicing and habituating a "confidential voice" may create the desired slightly breathy voice quality. Resonant voice therapy can also be helpful in achieving this goal. The speaker is taught to produce sound with a forward focus and away from the laryngeal area, and to feel the oral vibrations produced during speech primarily in the mask of the face. This facilitates the voice resonating fully throughout the vocal tract and increasing vocal power, clarity, and flexibility without any effort or tension (e.g., Hirsch, 2006).

Individuals should avoid certain vocal acts that are more commonly used by males, such as throat clearing, low-pitched vocalized pauses, and coughing (Deem & Miller, 2000). Also to be avoided is the use of falsetto, which has a thin, reedy quality that does not sound natural or pleasant. Speakers wishing to be perceived as female may use this register in the mistaken belief that the very high pitch will be helpful.

Vocal Tract Formant Frequencies. Raising vowel formant frequencies has been a target in some intervention approaches. There are differences in formant frequency related to the size and configuration of the vocal tract in males and females. The male vocal tract is longer than the female, and the male pharynx is proportionally larger than the female (Rammage et al., 2001). The male vocal tract resonates more strongly to lower frequencies while the female vocal tract resonates to higher frequencies. These formant frequency differences also contribute to the perception of a person's voice as male or female (Gelfer & Schofield, 2000; Rammage et al., 2001). The first formant frequency (F1) is related to tongue height and the second formant frequency (F2) is associated with anterior/posterior tongue placement. The third formant frequency (F3) is correlated to degree of lip spreading (Carew, Dacakis, & Oates, 2007). Teaching the speaker to articulate with the tongue in a more forward position raises F2 frequency and may facilitate the perception of a "thinner" and more feminine voice (Gorham-Rowan & Morris, 2006; Thornton, 2008). Teaching the client to talk with lips slightly spread can raise F3 (Carew et al., 2007). Carew et al. (2007) reported that the combination of increased forward tongue carriage and increased use of lip spreading not only increased formant values, but in addition had the effect of raising F0 by up to 30 Hz. Perceptual ratings of femininity of voice following treatment increased for 70% of participants, and participant self-ratings of both satisfaction and femininity of voice were significantly higher after treatment (Carew et al., 2007).

Intonation. Pitch range and variability are aspects of intonation that are strong markers of gender identity. Female speakers typically use a wider range of F0s and a more varied pattern of pitch inflections, while male speakers tend to use a more restricted F0 range and fewer inflectional patterns (Ferrand & Bloom, 1996). Studies have demonstrated that trans speakers' voices identified as female are characterized by more pitch inflections both upward and downward, less extensive downward shifts, a greater proportion of upward shifts, and fewer level intonation patterns (e.g., Gelfer & Schofield, 2000; Wolfe et al., 1990). Women's intonational patterns differ from men's not only in range, but in phrase endings. Women tend to use more rising inflections at the end of utterances, often giving their speech a somewhat tentative sound. In fact, a speaker who uses a lower pitch, but a more feminine intonational pattern and style will sound more feminine than one who uses a higher pitch but fewer feminine patterns.

Outcomes of Voice Therapy. Many studies have demonstrated that voice therapy can be effective in helping the trans speaker achieve a more feminine sounding voice. Soderpalm, Larsson, and Almquist, (2004) evaluated a group of speakers before and after therapy. The therapy approach included vocal hygiene and pitch raising exercises, improving the clarity of articulation, and encouraging more anterior articulation. The authors reported that fewer than half the patients produced an F0 above 155 Hz at the close of therapy, but some patients reached this level at follow-up. They suggested that one of the benefits of voice therapy may be the improved vocal technique that prevents fatigue and sore throat. Mayer and Gelfer (2008) studied the effects of voice therapy in shifting listener perceptions of gender in trans speakers from male to female, and the acoustic parameters accompanying that change. Each client received 16 sessions of group voice treatment. Intervention focused on raising pitch to an individually determined level using a light, breathy quality and good breath support, improving articulatory precision, and increasing intonational variability. A group of listeners rated pre- and post-therapy voices as male or female, as well as rating the voices on a scale of pleasantness, masculinity, and femininity. Acoustic measures included speaking fundamental frequency (SFF), upper and lower limits of SFF, and F1, F2, and F3. Samples were analyzed prior to therapy, immediately following 8 weeks of therapy, and 15 months after termination of therapy. The results showed that prior to therapy only 2% of voices were rated as female, while 51% of post-therapy voices were rated as female. Gains in SFF made in therapy were maintained more than a year after therapy, although not at the level attained immediately after treatment (pretest SFF 119 Hz, post-test 178 Hz, long-term 138 Hz).

There is relatively strong consensus among experts as to recommended approaches to voice therapy (Oates, 2006). Studies indicate that voice therapy can be beneficial, although there is very little guidance as to prognostic indicators or predictors of successful intervention (Oates, 2006). However, some reports provide anecdotal suggestions as to who may benefit most from voice therapy. The trans client who is living full time in the female role will have a strong need to develop a voice consistent with her gender and will likely be more motivated to practice and comply with therapy regimes (Gelfer, 1999; Gold, 1999). Speakers who are prone to vocally traumatic behaviors or suffer from allergies or untreated GERD are likely to be less successful.

Surgical Treatments. Surgical treatments are available to raise F0 as well as to feminize laryngeal appearance. Pitch-raising surgery aims to raise the fundamental frequency by increasing vocal fold tension, decreasing vocal fold mass, or modifying vocal fold consistency (Remacle, Matar, Morsomme, Verduyckt, & Lawson, 2011). A thorough assessment of the individual's suitability for surgery is important and should be carried out by a multidisciplinary team including the consultant psychiatrist, speech-language pathologist, and otolaryngologist (Parker, 2008).

Cricothyroid Approximation. **Cricothyroid approximation (CTA)** is the most commonly used procedure to increase F0 (Remacle et al., 2011). In this technique the cricoid cartilage is tilted backward and the thyroid cartilage is tilted forward. The vocal folds are thus elongated and stretched, resulting in a higher F0 and perceptually higher pitch. By means of computed tomography Pickuth et al. (2000) calculated that F0 increased approximately 18 Hz for every millimeter of approximation of cricothyroid distance. The surgery can be performed either under general or local anesthetic. Local anesthesia has the benefit of patient participation in determining the optimal pitch level. Many researchers have reported F0 increases resulting from CTA ranging from 16 to 131 Hz (e.g., Brown et al., 2000; Debruyne, De Jong, & Oosterlinck, 1995; De Jong & Norbart, 1996; Kanagalingam et al., 2005; Kocak et al., 2009; Neuman, Welzel, & Berghaus, 2002).

The advantages of CTA include the lower degree of effort for the patient to keep up the high F0 and the rise of the lowest pitch level (Soderpalm et al., 2004). However, complications have been reported including decreased vocal range, decreased dynamic range and loudness, and worsened vocal quality (e.g., Neumann & Welzel, 2004; Spiegel, 2006).

Anterior Commissure Surgeries. Several surgical techniques have been described that modify the vocal folds at the anterior commissure. This has the effect of shortening the vocal folds and reducing the vibrating portion in order to raise the F0. Laser-assisted anterior commissure placation is designed to create a web between the anterior edges of the vocal folds. The mucosal lining of the anterior quarter of the folds is vaporized with a CO_2 laser, and the denuded folds are sutured together (Rammage et al., 2001). A similar technique, called *endoscopic vocal fold shortening*, was described by Gross (1999). Gross (1999) presented results demonstrating not only an average increase of 9.2 semitones in pitch, but also a reduction in range in the lower frequencies. **Glottoplasty** is another technique that involves suturing the deepithelialized anterior portion of the vocal folds at the anterior commissure in a V-shape. Using this procedure, Remacle et al. (2011) reported a significant increase in F0 from a median of 150 Hz presurgery to 194 Hz postsurgery. Kocak et al. (2009) used laser reduction glottoplasty in patients who were not satisfied with CTA results. This technique reduces the bulk of the thyrovocalis muscle and vocal ligament, thus shifting the vocal mass toward the female size range. Glottoplasty following CTA was reported to increase F0 from the postsurgical CTA mean of approximately 158 Hz to the postsurgical glottoplasty mean of approximately 203 Hz. Postsurgery voice quality was dysphonic, but improved substantially at the one-year follow up. However, only 4 of the 6 patients were completely satisfied with their voice outcome, while two were only partially satisfied.

Although these procedures can be effective in increasing F0, other features such as voice quality, frequency range, and intensity levels may deteriorate (e.g., Kocak et al., 2009; Neumann & Welzel, 2004; Parker, 2008; Remacle et al., 2011).

Surgical techniques can be an important means of increasing the femininity of the individual's voice, because even when behavioral voice therapy is effective, uncontrolled vegetative vocalizations (e.g., laughing, coughing, yawning) may still occur in the male register (Gross, 1999). Even with the relatively substantial increases in F0, however, research indicates that the surgery does not necessarily result in the perception of a wholly feminine voice. Neuman et al. (2002) had a panel of judges rate the femaleness of trans speakers who had undergone CTA compared with biological males and biological females. Listeners rated the postoperative voices as more female than the biological males, but less female than those of the biological females. Further, patient expectations may be extremely high, so that although the F0 increases, it does not conform to the individual's perception of a wholly female voice (Remacle et al, 2011). Table 10.11 displays average F0 levels reported in the literature before and after pitch-raising treatment.

TABLE 10.11 Average Fundamental Frequencies (F0) Reported in the Literature for Male-to-Female Transsexual Speakers before and after Pitch-Raising Treatment, and on Long-Term Follow-Up

Author(s)	Treatment	Pretherapy	Post-therapy	Follow-Up
Dacakis (2000)	Voice therapy	125 Hz	168 Hz	146 Hz
Carew et al. (2007)	Oral resonance therapy	119 Hz	133 Hz	
Gross (1999)	Surgery	117 Hz	201 Hz	
Mayer & Gelfer (2008)	Voice therapy	119 Hz	178 Hz	138 Hz
Brown et al. (2000)	Surgery	142 Hz	174 Hz	185 Hz
Yang et al. (2002)	Surgery	133 Hz	185 Hz	
Van Borsel et al. (2008)	Surgery	118 Hz	169 Hz	
Neumann & Welzel (2004)	Surgery plus voice therapy	117 Hz	155 Hz	162 Hz
Kocak et al. (2009)	Surgery	158 HZ (post CTA)	203 Hz (post glottoplasty)	
Remacle et al. (2011)	Surgery	150 Hz	194 Hz	

Other surgical procedures such as thyroid chondroplasty ("laryngeal shave") may be performed for cosmetic reasons. Thyroid chondroplasty is designed to feminize the appearance of the neck by removing the upper parts of the thyroid laminae (Matal, Cheesman, & Clarke, 2003; Parker, 2008).

CLIENT SATISFACTION

Outcomes studies have demonstrated that surgical and behavioral voice therapy can be effective in facilitating a more feminine voice for trans speakers. However, despite reported successes in raising pitch there is not universal satisfaction among clients with their feminine voice. There is often a discrepancy between the client's and clinician's perception of a satisfactory voice, particularly when success is defined solely or primarily in terms of perceptual ratings and acoustic measurements of the voice (Dacakis, 2000; Pasricha, Dacakis, & Oates, 2008). Yang, Palmer, Murray, Meltzer, and Cohen (2002) reported that 50% of their patients felt their voice after surgery now fitted with their self-perception, 20% felt neutral about their new voice, and 29% responded negatively. Wagner et al. (2003) noted that 11 of their patients experienced a postsurgery improvement in F0 and some expressed satisfaction. However, the measured improvement in F0 did not always correspond with patient satisfaction. McNeill, Wilson, Clark, and Deakin (2008) investigated the relationship between F0, perceived femininity of voice, and happiness with voice in transsexual individuals. Speakers also completed the VHI. Voice recordings were evaluated by speech language pathologists and naïve observers. Most participants described situations where they felt their voice let them down, including speaking on the telephone, coughing, and laughing. McNeill et al. (2008) cautioned that patients' happiness with their voice is not directly related to F0 and may not correlate with perceptions of the clinician or the lay public. Pickuth et al. (2000) reported that despite the increase in F0, not all the patients were satisfied with their current voice. Only 58% indicated they were satisfied, while 33% were dissatisfied, and 8% were neutral. Vocal pitch was rated as feminine by half the respondents, masculine by one-quarter, and neutral by the remainder. Pickuth et al. (2000) reported that when asked how well the individual's new voice fit with her current self-perception, 51% responded positively, 29% responded negatively, and 20% felt it to be neutral. Neumann and Welzel (2004) reported that approximately 85% of their patients who underwent surgery were satisfied with the results. Pasricha et al. (2008) held focused interviews with trans speakers who had undergone various types of therapy. Participants reported that voice was the feature of communication with which they were the least satisfied and was the principal feature likely to betray their biological gender. Dacakis (2000) followed up on trans speakers several years after therapy and obtained acoustic measures as well as measures of satisfaction with voice and pitch level. Reportedly, the more therapy sessions attended, the better the maintenance of F0 gains achieved in therapy. As a group, the subjects maintained a higher F0 at follow-up than at the initial evaluation although there was variability in the actual amount of F0 increase. The majority of the clients, including 3 whose mean F0 had returned to pretherapy levels, expressed a high level of satisfaction with their pitch level. This may reflect a client's ability to "pass" despite the lower pitch.

These studies highlight the fact that intervention should focus not only on the client's voice, but on other important aspects of communication including articulation, rate of speech, vocabulary, and body language. The client should learn to articulate more gently, yet with more precision than is typical of males (Thornton, 2008). Nonverbal gender markers such as maintaining eye contact and using touch and gestures more frequently should also be targeted in therapy. Female speakers tend to use more tags at the end of sentences (e.g., "It's a lovely day, isn't it?"), and this is a straightforward means of increasing the feminineness of the person's communication.

Physical appearance is another important factor to take into account. Van Borsel, De Cuypere, and den Berghe (2001) reported that the perception of a male-to-female transsexual as male or female was modified depending on both physical appearance and vocal characteristics. They suggested that vocal training to feminize the voice should be done in conjunction with appearance factors such as clothing and makeup. An individual with a less feminine-sounding voice may still be accepted as a woman if her physical appearance is convincingly female. Thus, treatment for trans speakers is best provided in a holistic context, with emphasis not only on vocal characteristics, but on the person's overall communicative style and presentation.

chapter SUMMARY

A CHARACTERISTIC OF MOST voice disorders related to personality and identity issues is that the larynx is structurally normal, and there is no detectable organic or neurologic basis for the problem. Vocal function, however, is impaired in terms of quality or capacity. While there are many different symptoms and characteristics of voice problems related to self and identity, there are also certain commonalities. Stress may play an important role in certain voice disorders.

Muscle tension dysphonia (MTD) is a disorder that results from hypercontraction of the intrinsic and extrinsic laryngeal muscles as well as muscles in other areas such as the face, jaw, tongue, neck, and shoulders. Muscle tension dysphonia may be primary or secondary. Primary MTD results from many interacting factors, including psychological and/or personality factors that induce tension, psychosocial issues, poor vocal technique, and excessively high occupational and/or social voice usage. Secondary MTD is associated with vocal tension, which results from compensation for underlying glottal insufficiency caused by benign or malignant vocal tumors, vocal fold bowing, or vocal fold paralysis. Symptoms of MTD include breathiness, hoarseness, strain, effortful phonation, vocal fatigue, pitch breaks, voice arrests, and reduction in vocal range. Vocal tract discomfort has also been reported including burning, tightness, dryness, aching, tickling, soreness, and globus sensation. Because MTD and spasmodic dysphonia share many perceptual features, it is important to differentiate between the two conditions. Stress and excessive muscular tension are strongly related to MTD, and treatment typically focuses on relaxation of the head and neck muscles. Cognitive behavioral therapy has been used successfully for MTD.

Conversion disorders are categorized as somatoform disorders in which symptoms suggest a physical etiology such as a medical condition, disease, or injury. However, no physical cause is evident, and the condition is actually an expression of psychological conflict. Individuals with conversion disorders tend to suffer acute or chronic stress, suppressed anger, immaturity and dependency, a history of frequent minor health problems, and mild-to-moderate depression. Patients report feeling tense and overburdened, cannot admit to weaknesses, and attach great importance to social conventions. A comprehensive evaluation is important in order to rule out any possible organic or neurologic causes of the problem. Treatment focuses on both restoring normal vocalization and exploring the psychological issues that underlie or contributed to the voice problem. Counseling techniques are important to help the patient uncover and deal with the conflict in more open and productive ways.

Functional dysphonia (FD) is strongly related to internal and external stressors and to personality characteristics. Individuals with FD have been reported to demonstrate higher scores than controls in terms of specific anxiety symptoms related to health concerns and somatic complaints; to be cautious, careful, tense, fearful, apprehensive, nervous, timid, doubtful, discouraged, and passive; to feel insecure, victimized, resentful, and pessimistic; and to experience life as stressful and disturbing. Vocal symptoms tend to be nonspecific and include varying degrees of breathiness, hoarseness, and roughness. Individuals with FD respond well to voice therapy focusing on direct treatment techniques such as vocal and breathing exercises, indirect techniques such as education, vocal hygiene, and nondirective counseling, as well as cognitive behavioral therapy.

Mutational falsetto, also called puberphonia or mutational dysphonia, occurs primarily in postadolescent males. Occasionally, despite normal laryngeal growth, a male's pitch level does not lower. This is often due to psychological reasons, such as resistance to the responsibilities of adulthood, embarrassment at the pitch changes and voice arrests that often occur during the change, or desire to identify with a female role model. The abnormal pitch may also be the result of the boy's attempt to stabilize the unsteady pitch and quality of the changing vocal mechanism. Other causes of the patient's high pitch such as endocrine problems, hearing loss, or neurological problems should be ruled out and/or addressed. Behavioral treatment is effective in helping the individual lower his pitch and can include laryngeal massage, shaping vegetative vocalizations, and manual compression of the larynx. Counseling or psychotherapy may be helpful for some individuals who are able to lower their F0 with voice therapy, but who are strongly resistant to voice change. Botox injection may be used in cases that are unresponsive to voice therapy due to excessive muscular contraction of suprahyoid and/or cricothyroid muscles.

The term *transgender* describes all persons whose identities, behavior, or dress vary from traditional gender norms, including transsexuals, transgenderists, cross-dressers, and drag queens. The term *transsexual* refers to individuals whose gender identity is fundamentally in conflict with their biological sex, and who unambiguously identify with the non-natal gender. Transsexuals tend to view sex reassignment surgery (SRS) as the treatment of choice. Often, the surgery is extremely successful in terms of visual appearance, but the person's voice is perceived as masculine in terms of pitch levels, intonational patterns, voice quality, and overall communicative characteristics. A comprehensive evaluation is essential. In the case of a transgendered individual, the case history becomes even more important because of unique concerns involving privacy issues, terminology, evolving treatment goals, and unusual social circumstances. Treatment for individuals wishing to develop a more feminine communication style is multifaceted and may include voice therapy to raise pitch and increase intonational variability, surgery such as cricothyroid approximation, counseling, articulation therapy, assistance with nonverbal communication patterns, and focus on physical appearance.

review QUESTIONS

1. How are self-concept, identity, and personality linked to voice production and vocal self-perception?

2. Explain the role of stress in generating and/or maintaining specific voice disorders.

3. Compare and contrast primary and secondary muscle tension dysphonia in terms of etiology, symptomatology, and treatment approaches.
4. Identify and describe similarities and differences between conversion disorders and functional dysphonia.
5. Why is behavioral voice therapy often very effective in treating mutational falsetto?
6. Explain the importance of using appropriate terminology when dealing with clients with gender identity differences.
7. Describe behavioral and surgical pitch-raising techniques, and explain why factors other than pitch are important in voice feminization.

PREPARING FOR THE PRAXIS

CASE STUDY 10.1: Mutational Falsetto

Directions: Please read the case study and answer the five questions that follow. The answers can be found at the bottom of the page.

Philip Gaynes is a 23-year-old college student. He is 6 feet, 2 inches tall, weighs 210 pounds, and is very good looking. However, when he starts talking, you are startled by the sound of his voice, which is extremely high pitched, weak in intensity, and hoarse. He reports that when he speaks on the telephone he is usually mistaken for a young female, and he is sick of it. He wants to know if there is anything he can do to change his voice.

1. Based on the above symptoms, the most likely diagnosis for Philip is
   a. mutational falsetto
   b. conversion disorder
   c. muscle tension dysphonia
   d. functional dysphonia
   e. transsexual voice problem
2. The most appropriate way of evaluating Phillip's voice is
   a. acoustic analysis of F0 and electroglottography
   b. aerodynamic analysis of air pressures and airflows
   c. pulmonary function testing
   d. high-speed digital imaging
   e. all of the above
3. The most appropriate clinical course of action is to
   a. refer Phillip to a psychiatrist to determine the possibility of an underlying personality disorder
   b. implement a program of vocal hygiene and vocal education
   c. contact Phillip's parents to find out if he had any unusual difficulties going through adolescence
   d. use natural vocalizations such as coughing to shape a lower pitch
   e. none of the above

4. An excessively high pitch such as that exhibited by Phillip may be due to
   a. longitudinal tension exerted by the cricothyroid muscles
   b. vibration of only the membranous portion of the vocal folds
   c. elevation of the larynx due to excessive contraction of the suprahyoid muscles
   d. inappropriately high tongue carriage that affects vocal tract resonance
   e. all of the above

5. An appropriate referral for Phillip would be to a
   a. psychiatrist
   b. physical therapist
   c. audiologist
   d. gastroenterologist
   e. social worker

CASE STUDY 10.2: Transsexual Voice

Directions: Please read the case study and answer the five questions that follow. The answers can be found at the bottom of the page.

Alexis Carter is a 25-year-old individual who has recently undergone gender reassignment surgery (male to female). She is happy with the surgery and her new lifestyle as a woman, and she is taking the recommended hormones. Her voice, however, is creating problems for her, as it still sounds like a male voice. You work at a clinic that specializes in transsexual voice, and you assure her that there are techniques and strategies that can help to make her sound more feminine.

1. The term *transgender*
   a. refers to a challenging mental illness best treated by pharmacologic means
   b. is a category in the DSM-IV that describes all persons whose identities, behavior, or dress vary from traditional gender norms
   c. should be used exclusively to refer to individuals whose gender identity is fundamentally in conflict with their biological sex, and who unambiguously identify with the non-natal gender
   d. is a synonym for gender dysphoria, gender discordance, gender dissonance, gender discomfort, or gender incongruence
   e. all of the above

2. The fact that Alexis recently underwent sex reassignment surgery means that
   a. she is really serious about living her life as a woman
   b. she has always dressed as a woman and held traditionally female jobs
   c. she probably lived for 1–2 years as a woman before undergoing the surgery
   d. she felt that all other options for a happy life were closed to her unless she had the surgery
   e. all of the above

Answers for Case Study 10.1: 1. (a); 2. (a); 3. (d); 4. (e); 5. (c)

3. Which of the following questions are appropriate for the speech professional to ask Alexis during the evaluation?
   a. Which name do you prefer to be called?
   b. Is this the name to be used for contact outside the clinic?
   c. What stage are you in the gender reassignment process?
   d. What kind of woman do you wish to be?
   e. all of the above
4. Which of the following treatment goals (if any) is NOT appropriate for Alexis?
   a. pushing technique to facilitate a strong falsetto voice
   b. developing a higher pitch
   c. increasing intonational variability
   d. developing a slightly breathy voice quality
   e. All of the above are appropriate treatment goals.
5. The range of F0s between around 145–165 Hz is called "gender neutral" because
   a. it is a range very seldom used by either men or women
   b. men who speak in that range sound female, and women who speak in that range sound male
   c. it is the range in which the speaker's gender is not identifiable
   d. it is the range in which different emotions such as happiness, sorrow, and annoyance are neutralized
   e. it is the range that best lends itself to a confidential voice that obscures the person's gender

---

Answers for Case Study 10.2: 1. (b); 2. (c); 3. (e); 4. (a); 5. (c)

Chapter 11
Disorders Related to Airway Problems and Respiration

LEARNING OBJECTIVES

1. Develop an understanding of the two primary symptoms of airway difficulty, dyspnea and stridor.
2. Gain familiarity with aspects of pulmonary function testing including flow-volume loop, bronchial challenge tests, and pulse oximetry.
3. Discuss laryngeal side effects of steroid inhalers for asthma.
4. Describe similarities and differences between paradoxical vocal fold motion and chronic cough in terms of etiology, symptomatology, evaluation, and treatment.

The primary purpose of respiration is ventilation. Ventilation is the process of moving air into and out of the airways and lungs in order to exchange oxygen (O_2) entering the lungs and carbon dioxide (CO_2) leaving the lungs. Ventilation depends on generating the forces necessary to move the appropriate volumes of air from the atmosphere to the alveoli within the lungs (Gildea & McCarthy, 2003). Respiratory and/or laryngeal disorders that obstruct the airway can hinder ventilation and pose a life-threatening risk to the individual. Adequate respiratory function is also essential for voice production. Difficulty with inhaling and/or exhaling air, with obtaining an adequate amount of air, or with maintaining appropriate breath support can adversely affect voice production. Reactive airway diseases such as asthma can interfere with voicing, and side effects of medications used to control such diseases can induce laryngeal irritation and inflammation. Other disorders related to respiratory function such as paradoxical vocal fold motion and chronic cough can interfere with respiratory and laryngeal function. This chapter begins with a description of two primary symptoms of airway difficulty, dyspnea and stridor. Discussion then turns to the importance of pulmonary function testing for disorders with a respiratory component. Respiratory-related disorders of asthma, paradoxical vocal fold motion, and chronic cough are explored, with a focus on clinical management.

Dyspnea

Dyspnea can be broadly defined as subjectively perceived discomfort in breathing. Dyspnea is common in respiratory-related conditions, but can also occur in healthy individuals during intense emotional states or exercise (De Peuter et al., 2004). The perceived sensation varies considerably in severity from mildly unpleasant to intolerable (American Thoracic Society, 1999; Hoit, Lansing, & Perona, 2007; Lansing, Im, Thwing, Legezda, & Banzett, 2005). The feeling of dyspnea is generated by a complex interaction between sensory receptors in the lungs, airways, thorax, blood vessels, and multiple brain areas and physical and psychological patient characteristics (De Peuter et al., 2004).

Dyspnea is not a unitary perception but is associated with different types of sensations including air hunger, work/effort, and chest tightness. **Air hunger,** also called "uncomfortable urge to breathe," "breathlessness," and "shortness of breath" (Hixon & Hoit, 2005), is perceived as the inability to obtain adequate air on inhalation. This results in a strong urge to breathe more deeply. The feeling can be alarming to the individual and may even cause a sense of impending death (Gracely, 2001). The physical basis for this sensation results from high levels of carbon dioxide (CO_2) in the blood (Gracely, 2001; Liotti et al., 2001). High levels of arterial CO_2 signal the nervous system centers that control motor activity for respiration to produce an increased motor drive (ventilatory drive) to the respiratory muscles. The increased ventilatory drive causes deeper breathing so that more oxygen (O_2) is brought into the lungs and more CO_2 exits the lungs (Gracely, 2001). Causes of air hunger include weak respiratory muscles, impairment of the nerves that regulate the respiratory muscles, decreased central nervous system drive to the muscles, and abnormal heart and lung function.

The sensation of having to work hard to breathe arises when an individual uses higher than normal respiratory muscle activity to maintain ventilation (Lansing et al., 2005). This sensation can result from fatigue, pulmonary diseases such as asthma, or neurological diseases that affect the respiratory muscles (Hixon & Hoit, 2005; Lansing et al., 2005). The feeling of chest tightness results when the airways are constricted, thus stimulating pulmonary sensory receptors. This sensation is almost exclusively associated with asthma (Gracely, 2001; Hixon & Hoit, 2005; Hoit et al., 2007). The sensation may occur in isolation, or in combination with air hunger and increased effort.

Dyspnea is not uncommon during speech, in which linguistic and ventilation requirements must be balanced. An imbalance can occur when an individual experiences air hunger and focuses his or her attention on obtaining an adequate air supply while simultaneously trying to speak (Hixon & Hoit, 2005). Individuals with a variety of diseases and conditions have been reported to experience some form of breathing discomfort during speaking. Hoit et al. (2007) presented findings from several survey studies, which collectively showed that 32% of participants with chronic obstructive pulmonary disease experienced dyspnea while speaking. Eighteen percent of participants with cervical spinal cord injury and 17% of participants with lung cancer reported speaking-related dyspnea when speaking for more than a few minutes. In order to investigate the nature of speaking-related dyspnea Hoit et al. (2007) induced hypercapnia (increased levels of CO_2) in healthy subjects participating in a speaking task. The resulting dyspnea was characterized by air hunger and physical exertion, which increased as the level of CO_2 was raised. Subjects also reported expending unusual mental effort in order to change their breathing patterns to accommodate the speech task. Reportedly, the mental effort focused on developing strategies to cope with the increased ventilatory demands, such as inhaling larger volumes of air and exhaling between words and phrases. Determining the effect of dyspnea on speech is particularly important for individuals with respiratory difficulties who are professional voice users.

EVALUATION OF DYSPNEA

There are many and varied contributing factors to dyspnea, including the patient's age, gender, psychoemotional status, duration of symptoms, fluctuations in the state of lungs and airways, and degree of airway inflammation (De Peuter et al., 2004). It is important, therefore, to take into account both objective measures of physiological pathology and subjective measures of patient perception of the problem (De Peuter et al., 2004). Dyspnea can be evaluated in terms of degree of breathlessness during physical and speech activities, the effect of the dyspnea on activities of daily living, and the resulting level of disability. Table 11.1 to Table 11.3 present several scales that are commonly used for this purpose. Table 11.1 presents a scale developed by the American Thoracic Society that defines five levels of dyspnea severity. Table 11.2 displays the commonly used Borg (1982) 14-item scale, which rates degree of perceived exertion and breathlessness. The Medical Research Council (MRC) dyspnea scale depicted in Table 11.3 is a simple and valid method of categorizing extent of disability in patients with respiratory disease (Bestall et al., 1999; Stenton, 2008).

Stridor

Stridor refers to an audible sound generated during respiration. The sound results from turbulent air flow in the airways as the air passes through a narrowed or obstructed segment (Sakakura et al., 2008). The stridor may be high or low pitched and may occur on inspiration, expiration, or both (Benson, Baredes, Schwartz, & Kumar, 2006). Inspiratory stridor, the most common type (Holinger, 1998), typically is caused by an obstruction above the glottis. The obstruction results from the collapse of soft tissues due to negative pressures generated in the airways during inspiration. The blockage may occur at laryngeal, nasal, or pharyngeal locations (Benson et al., 2006). Laryngomalacia is an example of an obstruction caused by collapse of the aryepiglottic folds during inspiration. **Expiratory stridor** most commonly is caused by an obstruction of the lower airways, i.e., trachea and bronchi, and is not typically related to changing pressures within the airway. **Biphasic stridor** that occurs during both phases of respiration is associated with glottic or subglottic anomalies (Benson et al., 2006).

TABLE *11.1* **Severity Scale of Dyspnea**

Grade	Degree	Characteristics
0	None	Only with strenuous activity
1	Slight	When hurrying on level ground or climbing a slight incline
2	Moderate	Needs to walk more slowly than others of the same age or has to stop for breath when walking at own pace on level ground
3	Severe	Stops for breath after 100 yards or after a few minutes
4	Very severe	Housebound or dyspnea when dressing or undressing

Source: Information from the American Thoracic Society.

TABLE 11.2 **Borg Scale of Perceived Exertion**

Degree of Exertion	Rating	Examples
None	6	Reading a book, watching TV
Very very light	7–8	Tying shoes
Very light	9–10	Chores like folding clothes that seem to take little effort
Fairly light	11–12	Walking through the grocery store or other activities that require some effort but not enough to speed up breathing
Somewhat hard	13–14	Brisk walking or other activities that require moderate effort and speed heart rate and breathing but don't generate breathlessness
Hard	15–16	Bicycling, swimming, or other activities that take vigorous effort and get the heart pounding and make breathing very fast
Very hard	17–18	The highest level of activity that can be sustained
Very very hard	19–20	A finishing kick in a race or other burst of activity that cannot be maintained for long

Source: Information from Borg (1982).

TABLE 11.3 **MRC Breathlessness Scale**

Grade	Degree of Breathlessness
1	Not troubled by breathlessness except on strenuous exercise
2	Short of breath when hurrying on the level or walking up a slight hill
3	Walks slower than most people on the level; stops after a mile or so; or stops after 15 minutes walking at own pace
4	Stops for breath after walking about 100 yards or after a few minutes on level ground
5	Too breathless to leave the house, or breathless when undressing

Source: Information from Stenton (2008).

CAUSES

There are numerous causes of stridor, including acute infections such as epiglottitis, a foreign body in the airway, laryngeal conditions (e.g., laryngomalacia, subglottic stenosis, tumors), neurological problems, pulmonary difficulties, and cardiovascular and digestive problems. Laryngomalacia is the most common cause of inspiratory stridor (Leung & Cho, 1999; Murphy

& Ren, 2009; Sakakura et al., 2008; Zoumalan, Maddalozzo, & Holinger, 2007). Subglottic stenosis is a common cause of biphasic stridor (Murphy & Ren, 2009). Other laryngeal abnormalities that can lead to stridor include webs, cysts, subglottic hemangiomas, vocal fold paralysis, papilloma, and laryngotracheoesophageal clefts (Holzki, Laschat, & Stratmann, 1998; Leung & Cho, 1999; Murphy & Ren, 2009; Rudman, Elmaraghy, Shiels, & Wiet, 2003; Sakakura et al., 2008; Zoumalan et al., 2007). There is also a strong association between stridor and GERD/LPR, particularly in infants (Nielson, Heldt, & Tooley, 1990). This may be due to acid stimulation of sensory receptors in the infant's esophagus and/or larynx, which can result in laryngospasm and airway obstruction (Orenstein, Orenstein, & Whittington, 1983). A close connection has also been established between GERD and/or LPR and several laryngeal and respiratory disorders that induce stridor, such as recurrent croup, subglottic stenosis, chronic cough, laryngeal irritation and inflammation, and obstructive apnea (Giannoni, Sulck, Friedman, & Duncan, 1998).

Stridor can be acute or chronic, congenital or acquired. Acute stridor is typically viral in etiology, while chronic stridor results from more long-term conditions. Stridor may appear at birth, within 4–6 weeks after birth (Murphy & Ren, 2009), or later during infancy or childhood (Holinger, 1998). Stridor may appear several weeks after the infant is born as the baby gains strength and the velocity of the airflow through the airways increases, creating turbulent flow (Murphy & Ren, 2009). When the onset of the stridor is slow or presents from birth or shortly thereafter, the etiology is usually congenital (Holinger, 1998; Zoumalan et al., 2007). Patients who present with symptoms of relatively short duration are more likely to have acquired lesions, infectious conditions, internal laryngeal trauma, bronchial foreign body, or tonsil and adenoid hypertrophy. In some cases the stridor is not severe except when the infant is stressed with feeding, crying, or is placed in certain positions.

EVALUATION

Because the causes of stridor are so varied, it is essential to obtain an accurate diagnosis of the underlying etiology in order to ensure appropriate treatment. This is particularly important because subjective perceptual evaluation of the severity of stridor has not been found to correlate either with the actual degree of obstruction or with treatment outcomes (Papsin, Abel, & Leighton, 1999). The diagnostic process should include an extensive case history, physical examination, and indirect or direct laryngoscopy plus bronchoscopy if appropriate (e.g., Sakakura et al., 2008). Airway fluoroscopy has been reported to be a useful way of dynamically evaluating the entire airway to determine the cause of the obstruction (Rudman et al., 2003). Chest x-rays may also be helpful in evaluating whether the trachea is being compressed. If GERD/LPR is suspected, 24-hour double probe pH monitoring or esophagoscopy may be called for. Information should be obtained regarding any eating or feeding difficulties, aspiration, and sleep patterns (Zoumalan et al., 2007).

Pulmonary Function Testing

Pulmonary function testing (PFT) is a term that covers a variety of tests designed to assess the amount of air an individual is able to inspire and expire, as well as how efficiently the person moves air into and out of the lungs. PFT is used to evaluate respiratory symptoms such as cough or dyspnea as well as for diagnosing respiratory diseases such as asthma (Gildea & McCarthy, 2003).

Spirometry is the most common type of testing (Gildea & McCarthy, 2003; McCarthy & Dweik, 2010). A spirometer is a device that senses air volumes and pressures that are generated by breathing into a mouthpiece. Spirometry is convenient, as it can be performed in the physician's office, as well as inpatient and outpatient settings (Gildea & McCarthy, 2003). Common spirometric measures are defined in Table 11.4.

Severity of disease is calculated by comparing a patient's measured spirometric values against norms that have been developed for age, gender, body height and size, and race. Severity is determined on a 5-point scale ranging from mild to very severe. See Table 11.5.

Spirometry is useful for evaluating signs and symptoms such as dyspnea, chest pain, cough, wheezing, diminished breath sounds, and cyanosis (Gildea & McCarthy, 2003). It is also useful in measuring the effect of disease on pulmonary function, assessing the outcome of therapeutic interventions, and describing the course of diseases affecting respiratory function (Gildea & McCarthy, 2003).

Measures of lung function provide a quantitative means of assessing obstructive and restrictive airway problems. Obstructive problems are those in which the flow of air is impeded as the individual exhales. This can result from narrowing of the airways due to bronchial

TABLE *11.4* **Spirometric Measures and Definitions**

MEASURE	DEFINITION
FVC	Amount of air that can be exhaled forcefully after a maximum inhalation
FEV_1	Amount of air that can be exhaled forcefully in one breath in 1 second
FEF	Amount of air that can be exhaled in an interval of time
FEF25%	Amount of air forcibly expelled in the first 25% of the total FVC
FEF50%	Amount of air forcibly expelled in the first 50% of the total FVC
FEF25–75%	Air flow during the middle half of the total FVC
PEFR	Maximum flow rate during FVC maneuver
MVV	Maximum amount of air that can be inhaled and exhaled in 12–15 seconds
SVC	Amount of air that can be slowly exhaled after a maximum exhalation
TLC	Total amount of air capable of being held in the lungs
FRC	Amount of air in remaining in the lungs at the end of a normal exhalation
ERV	Amount of air able to be exhaled following a normal breath out
FEV1%	Ratio of FEV1 to FVC indicating what percentage of the total FVC was exhaled during the first second of forced exhalation
FEF_{50}/FIF_{50}	Ratio between FEF at 50% of exhaled vital capacity and FIF at 50% of inhaled vital capacity

Note: FVC = forced vital capacity; FEV = forced expiratory volume; FEF = forced expiratory flow; PEFR = peak expiratory flow rate; MVV = maximum voluntary ventilation; SVC = slow vital capacity; TLC = total lung capacity; FRC = functional residual capacity; ERV = expiratory reserve volume; FIF = forced inspiratory flow; VC = vital capacity.

TABLE 11.5 Severity of Reductions in FVC and FEV1

Severity	Percentage of Predicted Value
Mild	70–79%
Moderate	60–69%
Moderately severe	50–59%
Severe	35–49%
Very severe	Less than 35%

spasms, inflammation and swelling of the mucosal lining of the airways, increased secretions within the airways, foreign object inside the airways, tumors, and destruction of lung tissue (McCarthy & Dweik, 2010). Obstructive lung diseases are characterized by a disproportionate reduction in the FEV_1 compared to the FVC (McCarthy & Dweik, 2010). The FEV_1 reflects the functioning of the large and medium-sized airways and is the most widely used parameter to measure the mechanical properties of the lungs (Gildea & McCarthy, 2003). In healthy individuals the FEV_1 accounts for the greatest part of the exhaled volume and is reduced disproportionately to the FVC in obstructive diseases (Gildea & McCarthy, 2003; McCarthy & Dweik, 2010).

Restrictive problems are those causing a decrease in lung volumes resulting from weakness or paralysis of the respiratory muscles or from diseases of the pleura or the chest wall (Kanaparthi, Lessnau, & Sharma, 2009). In restrictive disorders the FEV1, FVC, and total lung capacity are all reduced, and the FEV1/FVC ratio is normal or even elevated (Gildea & McCarthy, 2003).

Another type of spirometric test is the flow-volume loop (FVL). This is a graph that plots velocity of airflow on the Y axis and air volume on the X axis (Figure 11.1). The test is done by having the patient breathe in maximally, exhale maximally into the spirometer, and then inhale maximally from the spirometer (Bass, 1973). Expiratory airflow is shown as positive going on the graph, and inspiratory airflow is indicated by a negative going trace. The normal expiratory portion (limb) of the FVL is characterized by a rapid rise to the peak flow rate, followed by a nearly linear fall in flow as the patient exhales toward residual volume. The inspiratory limb is a relatively symmetrical curve. This is a very useful measure, because different airway diseases show characteristically different flow-volume relationships from normal. For example, fixed lesions such as tumors cause plateaus in both the inspiratory and expiratory limbs of the flow-volume loop (Lunn & Sheller, 1995). Lesions within the thoracic cavity are characterized by expiratory slowing and flattening of the expiratory limb. Lesions external to the thoracic cavity cause inspiratory slowing and a plateau on the inspiratory limb of the flow-volume loop. Problems in the large airways (e.g., trachea and bronchi) tend to reduce expiratory flow rates at all lung volumes, whereas difficulties in medium-sized airways have the effect of decreasing flow rates mainly at the midportion of the expiratory limb (Bass, 1973). Problems in the small airways reduce flow rates at low lung volumes more than at high and mid-lung volumes.

FIGURE 11.1 Examples of Normal and Disordered Flow-Volume Loops

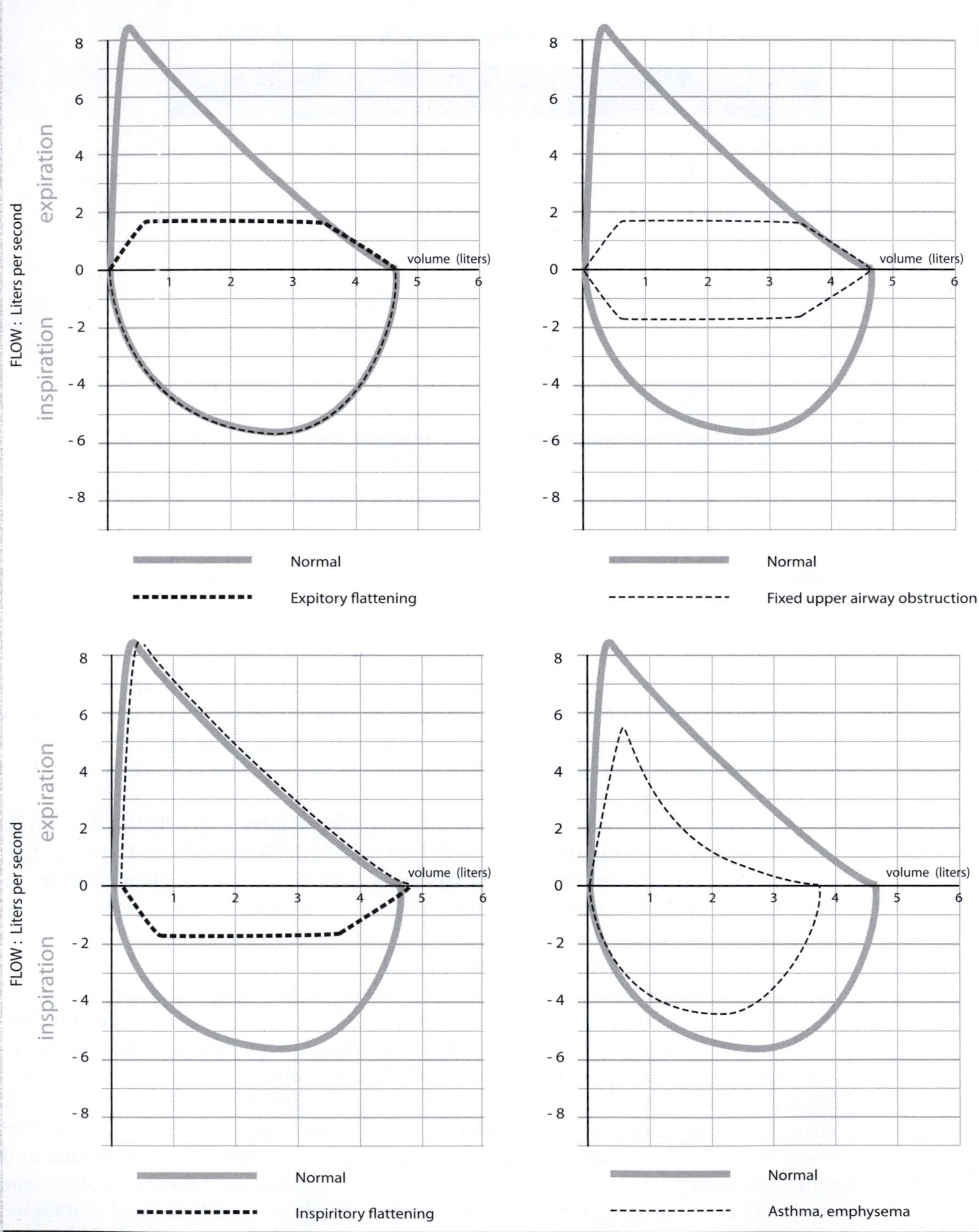

Source: From "Vocal Cord Dysfunction/Paradoxical Vocal Fold Motion," by M. Hicks, S. M. Brugman, & R. Katial, 2008, *Primary Care and Clinical Office Practice, 35,* pp. 81–103. Copyright 2008 by Elsevier. Reprinted with permission.

Bronchial challenge tests (bronchoprovocation) also make use of spirometry. In a bronchial challenge test the patient inhales a substance (methacholine, mannitol, or a histamine) that causes the airways to constrict and narrow (e.g., Chatham, Bleecker, Norman, Smith, & Mason, 1982; Spector et al., 2009; Stolz et al., 2009). A reduction of 20% in the FEV_1 with bronchial challenge is considered positive for airway hyperreactivity and/or asthma (Gildea & McCarthy, 2003).

A different type of pulmonary function test is pulse oximetry. This is a simple, noninvasive, and widely available test that uses light absorption to measure an individual's level of blood oxygenation (Pedersen, Hovhannisyan, & Moller, 2009; Schnapp & Cohen, 1990). Pulse oximetry is used to assess the severity of obstructive airway diseases and can be particularly helpful in the face of ambiguous or unusable spirometric data (Hartert, Wheeler, & Sheller, 1999).

Asthma

Asthma is a chronic inflammatory disorder of the large and small airways characterized by variable and recurring symptoms, reversible airflow obstruction, bronchial hyperresponsiveness, and underlying inflammation (Bhalla, Watson, Taylor, Jones, & Roland, 2008; National Heart, Lung and Blood Institute, 2007, www.nhlbi.nih.gov/guidelines/asthma/03_sec2_def.pdf). See Figure 11.2. The narrowing of the airways results from two factors: inflammation and swelling of the mucosal lining of the airways, and contraction of the bronchial smooth muscles (Ihre, Zetterstrom, Ihre, & Hammarberg, 2004). The airway obstruction may be reversible or partially reversible either spontaneously or with treatment.

Asthma has been shown to result from an interaction of genetic and environmental factors (Martinez, 2007), and affects 300 million people worldwide (Fanta, 2009). The prevalence of the disorder is higher in the United States than in other countries and affects ethnic groups differentially. Puerto Ricans and African Americans reportedly have the highest prevalence, and Mexicans and Koreans the lowest (Gold & Wright, 2005). The disease is highest among low-income populations. In childhood more males than females are diagnosed with asthma, but the condition is more likely to persist into adulthood in females (Osman, Hansell, Simpson, Hollowell, & Helms, 2007). The disorder is more prevalent in athletes than in the general population (Weiler, Layton, & Hunt, 1998).

While asthma is a chronic disease, it is also characterized by acute flare-ups ("attacks"). Symptoms in the chronic or steady state include nighttime coughing, dyspnea with exertion but not at rest, chronic throat-clearing and cough, and chest tightness. Depending on severity, acute attacks may be a medical emergency and are marked by dyspnea, wheezing on expiration, and chest tightness (Saunders, 2005). A type of asthma called *cough-variant asthma* has been identified in which the primary symptom is persistent cough without wheezing or dyspnea, and which responds to bronchodilation (Corrao, Braman, & Irwin, 1979; Fujimura, Ogawa, Nishizawa, & Nishi, 2003).

There are many triggers for asthma attacks, including pet hair and dander, dust, allergies, changes in the weather, viral infections, exercise, mold, pollen, chemicals, smoke, uncontrolled GERD/LPR, and stress. Speaking and singing have also been reported as triggers for asthma (e.g., Cohn, Sataloff, & Branton, 2001). Ihre et al. (2004) reported that of patients surveyed at three asthma and allergy centers, the most common factors that induced an attack were infection (67%), exercise (59%), cold air (56%), and allergy (55%).

FIGURE 11.2 **Normal versus Asthmatic Airway**

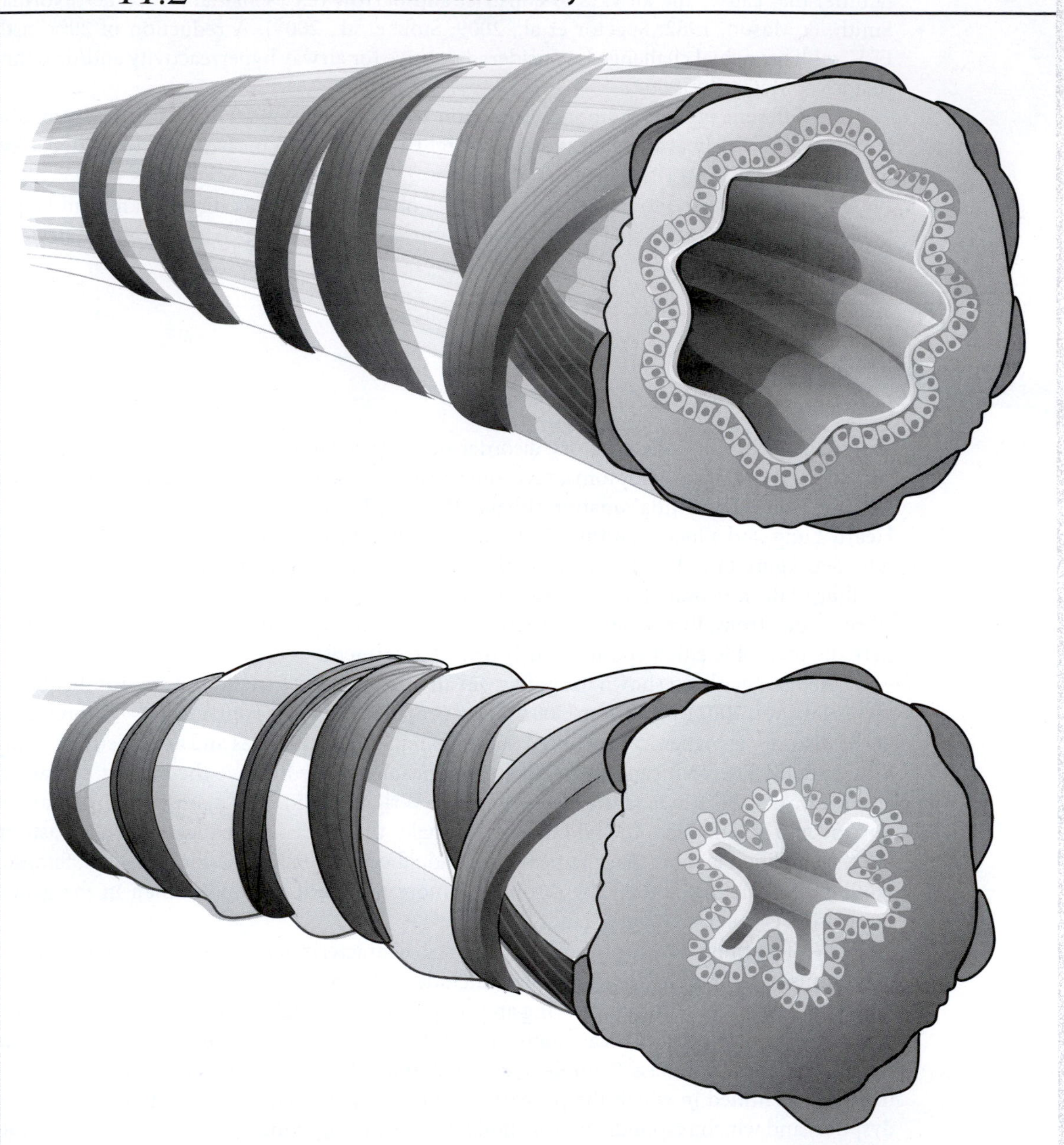

EVALUATION AND TREATMENT

Asthma is diagnosed by means of pulmonary function tests including bronchial challenge tests. Individuals with asthma are sensitive to lower doses of the challenge substance. Bronchoprovocation is a safe way to measure the degree to which an individual withstands nonspecific stimuli

TABLE *11.6* **Inhaled Corticosteroids**

Agent	Trade Name(s)
Beclomethasone	Qvar, Vanceril
Budesonide	Pulmicort, Symbicort
Ciclesonide	Alvesco
Flunisolide	Aerospan HFA, Aerobid
Fluticasone Propionate	Advair, Flovent
Mometasone Furoate	Asmanex
Triamcinolone	Azmacort

that trigger asthmatic attacks (Enright, Lebowitz, & Cockroft, 1994). A positive response to bronchodilators and/or corticosteroids is also indicative of asthma (Smith et al., 2004).

The primary treatment for asthma is inhaled corticosteroids (ICS). These are designed to reduce or eliminate the underlying inflammation of the airways and decrease the excessive mucus production associated with the disease. ICS use has been shown to be extremely effective in controlling asthma symptoms (Balter et al., 2001; Roland, Bhalla, & Earis, 2004). Many forms of ICS are available (Table 11.6). There are also medications available that combine the corticosteroid with a bronchodilator that reduces smooth muscle constriction of the airways. These medications act to improve lung function, reduce asthma symptoms and acute attacks, and decrease the rate of emergency room visits and hospital admissions.

Steroid Inhaler Laryngitis. ICS use is highly effective, well tolerated, and safe, with few serious systemic side effects (Balter et al., 2001). There are, however, numerous reports of local pharyngeal and laryngeal side effects that can significantly affect voice production. Reported incidence of pharyngeal and laryngeal side effects in patients who use ICS ranges from around 34% to 67% (e.g., Kim, Moon, Chung, & Lee, 2011; Roland et al., 2004; Stanton, Sellars, MacKenzie, McConnachie, & Bucknall, 2009; Williamson, Matusiewicz, Brown, Greening, & Crompton, 1995). Videolaryngoscopy and stroboscopy have demonstrated numerous laryngeal signs and symptoms related to ICS use (Table 11.7).

The finding of laryngeal side effects has resulted in the recognition of steroid inhaler laryngitis (SIL) as a distinct clinical entity (DelGaudio, 2002). The laryngeal changes in SIL are similar to changes seen in LPR. Before SIL was recognized as a distinct clinical entity, asthma patients with laryngeal and vocal symptoms were treated aggressively for LPR, but symptoms typically did not resolve completely (DelGaudio, 2002). Why these medications should cause laryngeal and pharyngeal side effects is not known with certainty, but may be related to several factors. One factor is that up to 80% of the inhaled dose is deposited on the mucosal surfaces of the pharynx and larynx before being swallowed (Bhalla et al., 2008; Erickson & Sivasankar, 2010; Lavy, Wood, Rubin, & Harried, 2000). The medication and/or the propellant used to project the medication into the airway may create an inflammatory response of the laryngeal and pharyngeal tissues (Bhalla et al., 2008; Lavy et al., 2000; Roland et al., 2004;

TABLE 11.7 Laryngeal Signs and Symptoms Related to Use of Inhaled Corticosteroids for Asthma

Vocal fold edema	Vocal fold atrophy
Vocal fold erythema	Hoarseness
Mucosal thickening	Throat clearing
Mucosal atrophy	Cough
Leukoplakia	Sore throat
Laryngeal candidiasis	Ventricular phonation
Posterior laryngitis	Reduced vocal fold mobility
Vocal fold hemorrhage	Mucosal wave asymmetry/aperiodicity
Vocal fold cysts	Abnormal phase closure
Sulcus vocalis	Abnormal glottic closure
Vocal fold granulation	Decreased mucosal wave amplitude
Chronic laryngitis	Supraglottic hyperactivity
Vocal fold bowing	Increased phonation threshold pressure

Sources: Information from Balter et al. (2001); DelGaudio (2002); Dogan et al. (2007); Erickson & Sivasankar (2010); Gallivan et al. (2007); Ihre et al. (2004); Kim et al. (2010); Krecicki et al. (2006); Lavy et al. (2000); Mirza, Kasper Schwartz, & Antin-Ozerkis (2004); Roland et al. (2004); Stanton et al. (2009); Williamson et al. (1995).

Williamson et al., 1995). Another factor that may contribute to laryngeal irritation is fungal infection resulting from the steroid (Stanton et al., 2009). Other consequences of steroid use can include laryngeal muscle weakness and vocal fold bowing (Roland et al., 2004). In addition to the medication effects, factors such as vocally traumatic behaviors, smoking, concurrent GERD or LPR, allergies, or rhinitis can contribute to the laryngeal symptoms. Because of the strong relationship between ICS use and laryngeal/vocal symptoms, it is important to identify possible contributors to dysphonia during the evaluation (Table 11.8).

The intensity of ICS use is related to symptom severity of the SIL. Individuals who use ICS on a regular basis have been found to have significantly more inflammation and worse vocal performance (hoarseness, vocal weakness, aphonia, sore throat, throat irritation, and cough) than occasional users and healthy controls (Bhalla et al., 2008). Further, greater dosage strength and frequency are reportedly associated with an increased incidence of symptoms and videostroboscopic findings, which improve with decreases in the dosage level (Gallivan, Gallivan, & Gallivan, et al., 2007).

SIL and the resulting laryngeal and vocal disturbances are not amenable to behavioral treatment, but the symptoms reverse when the ICS is withdrawn (Gallivan et al., 2007). Some patients respond to a different ICS or a different delivery system. Others may have such severe pharyngeal and laryngeal side effects that ICS treatment may be discontinued. Although the effects of voice treatment have not been studied, it may be worthwhile for the patient to work with a speech-language pathologist to reduce any vocally traumatic behaviors that may be contributing to the problem. Other conditions such as GERD/LPR, allergies, and so on also need to be addressed.

TABLE 11.8 Evaluation Questions for Individuals Using Inhaled Corticosteroids for Asthma or Other Respiratory Disorders

Condition for which you take steroids, e.g., asthma
How often do you take them?
Are they effective?
How long have you been on these inhalers?
Do you, or have you in the past, taken any other medicine?
Do you smoke?
How often do you get hoarse?
Is your hoarseness continuous or intermittent?
Does your hoarseness relate to inhaler use?
How soon after starting inhaled steroids did you notice hoarseness?
Do you suffer sore throats?
Do you suffer chronic cough?
Do you have to raise your voice during your everyday work?
For how many hours a day do you have to use your voice?
Have you had any other medical problems/operations in the past?

Source: From "Dysphonia Associated with Inhaled Steroids," by J. A. Lavy, G. Wood, J. S. Rubin, & M. Harried, 2000, *Journal of Voice, 14,* pp. 581–588. Copyright 2000 by The Voice Foundation. Reprinted with permission.

Paradoxical Vocal Fold Motion

Paradoxical vocal fold motion (PVFM) is a respiratory/laryngeal disorder characterized primarily by inappropriate spasmodic vocal fold adduction during the inhalation phase of breathing. PVFM has been referred to by a myriad of names (Table 11.9).

The confusion in terminology likely has arisen because the disorder itself is a confusing one, with symptoms that mimic airway diseases such as asthma (Parsons et al., 2010), and a psychological underlay in some cases. The most commonly used terms in the recent literature are *paradoxical vocal fold motion (PVFM)* and *vocal cord dysfunction (VCD).* Speech-language pathologists and otolaryngologists tend to prefer the term PVFM, while VCD is more commonly used by pulmonologists, allergists, psychiatrists, and psychologists (Christopher & Morris, 2010). In the following discussion the term paradoxical vocal fold motion (PVFM) will be used because the term accurately describes the dynamic nature of the disorder (Hicks, Brugman, & Katial, 2008).

SYMPTOMS

More females than males suffer from this disorder, with an approximate ratio of 3:1 (e.g., Doshi & Weinberger, 2006; Gurevich-Uvena et al., 2010; Husein et al., 2008; Parsons et al., 2010). The disorder is most common in adults, although children and adolescents are also

TABLE 11.9 Terms Used for Paradoxical Vocal Fold Motion

Terms
Paradoxical vocal cord movement
Paradoxical vocal fold dysfunction
Vocal cord dysfunction
Episodic laryngeal dyskinesia
Nonorganic upper airway obstruction
Irritable larynx syndrome
Episodic paroxysmal laryngospasms
Functional airway obstruction
Munchausen's stridor
Factitious asthma
Psychogenic stridor
Psychogenic wheeze

affected (Gaafar & Fasyh, 2011; Husein et al., 2008; Morris, 2006). The major symptoms of PVFM are stridor and dyspnea. Dyspnea has been reported to occur in 76–95% of patients (Morris, Perkins, & Allan, 2006). The stridor is typically heard when the patient inhales, differentiating this disorder from asthma, in which the stridor usually occurs on the exhalation. However, it is not uncommon for the exhalation phase to be affected as well, because once the laryngospasm has begun during inspiration, the hyperadduction may carry over for a brief interval into the exhalation phase (Andrianopoulos, Gallivan, & Gallivan, 2000).

Vocal symptoms are common, particularly during an attack, and can include hoarseness, strain, breathiness, and aphonia. Cough has been reported as a symptom in 25–42% of individuals with PVFM (Christopher & Morris, 2010). Videostroboscopy has demonstrated false vocal fold adduction, anterior-posterior constriction of the supraglottic larynx, decreased amplitude of vibration, and decreased mucosal wave (Yelken, Gultekin, Guven, Eyibilen, & Aladag, 2010). Laryngeal structural abnormalities may be present, such as chronic laryngitis, laryngomalacia, sulcus vocalis, nodules, and subglottic stenosis (Patel, Jorgensen, Kuhn, & Merati, 2004). Acoustic analysis has revealed significantly higher jitter and shimmer values and significantly shorter MPT than healthy controls (Yelken et al., 2010). In addition to respiratory and vocal symptoms, many other nonlaryngeal symptoms have also been reported (Table 11.10). Symptoms may or may not be precipitated or exacerbated by specific triggers (Table 11.11).

It is common for clients to report numerous visits to the emergency room or hospitalizations for their symptoms. Because of the presence of stridor and dyspnea, symptoms are often misdiagnosed as asthma or reactive airway disease. It is not uncommon for patients to undergo aggressive asthma treatment, which is usually not effective (Morris, 2006). In some cases patients have undergone invasive interventions such as intubation or tracheostomy (Newman, Mason, & Schmaling, 1995). Table 11.12 identifies similarities and differences between PVFM and asthma.

TABLE 11.10 Reported Nonvocal Symptoms of Paradoxical Vocal Fold Motion

Wheezing
Stridor
Dyspnea
Sensation of choking or suffocation
Warning signs of an impending attack such as feeling of a lump in the throat, sharp taste, sharp pain, and/or uncontrollable cough
Dizziness
Lightheadedness
Numbness or tingling of digits or around the mouth area
Chest tightness
Throat tightness
More difficulty inhaling than exhaling
Near or total loss of consciousness

Sources: Information from Buddiga (2010); Deem & Miller (2000); Hicks et al. (2008); Morris (2006); Murry et al. (2004).

TABLE 11.11 Reported Triggers for Paradoxical Vocal Fold Motion

Aromas	Postnasal drip
Perfumes	Smoke
Noxious odors	Air pollution
Soap	Exercise
Emotional stress	Depression
Cold air	Separation anxiety
Food products	Sexual abuse
Upper respiratory infections	Asthma
Eating	Intubation
Talking	Sleep
Laughing	Ammonia
Singing	Flux fumes
Coughing	Cleaning chemicals
Acid reflux	Cigarette smoke
Weather changes	Molds
Extreme temperatures	Dust

Sources: Information from Allan, Abouchahine, Harvis, & Morris (2006); Andrianopoulos et al. (2000); Buddiga (2010); Hicks et al. (2008); Murry et al. (2004); Koufman (1994); Koufman & Block (2008); Mathers-Schmidt & Brilla (2005); Morris (2006); Morrison et al. (1999); Sandage (2006).

TABLE 11.12 **Similarities and Differences between Paradoxical Vocal Fold Motion (PVFM) and Asthma**

PVFM	Asthma
Extrathoracic	Intrathoracic
Rare (never?) hypoxemia	+ hypoxemia
No hypercapnia/acidosis	+ hypercapnia/acidosis
Normal expiratory spirometry	Reduced expiratory flow
Abnormal inspiratory loop (in some)	Normal inspiratory loop
Start-stop abruptly, few symptoms between episodes	Persistent symptoms
Frequent emergency department/office visits	Frequent emergency department/ office visits
Multiple medications	Multiple medications

Source: From "Vocal Cord Dysfunction in Children," by B. E. Noyes & J. S. Kemp, 2007, *Paediatric Respiratory Reviews, 8,* pp. 155–163. Copyright 2007 by Elsevier. Reprinted with permission.

CAUSES

Similar to spasmodic dysphonia, it used to be thought that PVFM was primarily related to psychological distress, anxiety, and conflict. While some cases of PVFM may indeed have an underlying psychoemotional basis, recently it has been hypothesized that the primary cause for the laryngospasm is a hypersensitivity or hyperresponsiveness of the larynx to a wide variety of stimuli that cause the vocal folds to close as a protective reflex (Altman et al., 2002; Christopher & Morris, 2010; Hicks et al., 2008; Mirasola, Braun, Blumin, Kerschner, & Merati, 2008; Morris, 2006; Morrison, Rammage, & Emami, 1999; Vlahakis, Patel, Maragos, & Beck, 2002). Factors such as viral infection, allergic and nonallergic inflammation, LPR or GERD, and/or toxic inhalation exposures may sensitize the larynx to various irritants that inappropriately precipitate the glottic closure reflex (Christopher & Morris, 2010; Hicks et al., 2008). In addition to airway sensitivity, many other causes for PVFM have been proposed (Table 11.13).

Laryngopharyngeal reflux is reportedly the most common cause of PVFM. Patients with LPR-related PVFM usually have other clues that they have LPR (Koufman & Block, 2008). Often the attacks follow a pattern, such as occurring after a meal, after the start of exercise, or after bending over. Sometimes the attacks may wake the patient from a sound sleep. Other times the attacks may occur without any pattern or identifiable precipitant, but the patient may have symptoms and laryngeal findings of LPR.

Psychoemotional factors have been linked to PVFM including anxiety, panic disorder and hyperventilation, emotional stress, and depression (Christopher & Morris, 2010; Gavin, Wamboldt, Brugman, Roesler, & Wamboldt, 1998; Hicks et al., 2006; Koufman & Block, 2008). In some cases the PVFM may represent a conversion disorder. Husein et al. (2008) reported that 71% of patients with PVFM demonstrated symptoms of conversion disorder. The authors suggested that in these cases the abnormal laryngeal movement may serve the purpose

TABLE 11.13 Proposed Causes of PVFM

GERD/LPR
Laryngeal dystonia
Asthma
Brainstem abnormalities
Upper airway sensitivity
Viral illness
Exercise
Stress, anxiety, depression
Conversion disorder

of avoiding an unpleasant life situation or emotion, and may also provide the patients with attention and sympathy. However, of these patients, 78% also had a history of GERD, asthma, or both. Other clinicians have noted that most children with PVFM do not have psychiatric disorders, nor has there been evidence of physical, emotional, or sexual abuse (Noyes & Kemp, 2007). Thus, while a psychoemotional component may be present in some cases, such factors can coexist with physical or physiological factors, and other triggers such as reflux may also contribute to the problem. Table 11.14 lists factors suggesting an underlying psychoemotional component of PVFM.

TABLE 11.14 Factors Suggesting an Underlying Psychological Cause of Paradoxical Vocal Fold Motion

Findings resolve when the patient is distracted
Findings resolve when the patient phonates
Episode is relieved by administration of a placebo
Symptoms and findings are induced or relieved by suggestion
Episode resolves with helium, even after the gas is withdrawn
Episode is reproduced by a placebo challenge
Absence of response when the patient is blinded to exposure to a presumed agent
Findings resolve with hypnosedative administration
Episodes are absent during monitored sleep
History of sexual abuse
Respiratory complaints out of proportion to objective findings
History of psychiatric illness

Source: Information from Christopher & Morris (2010).

Neurological processes have been identified as a cause in some cases. These include respiratory-type laryngeal dystonia and brainstem abnormalities resulting from congenital causes or from stroke and head trauma (Koufman, 1994; Sandage, 2006). Treole, Trudeau, and Forrest (1999) found subtle signs of laryngeal movement disorders (e.g., phonatory instability) in patients with PVFM in between episodes of dyspnea. These signs were present even when the patients were not demonstrating any overt signs of the disorder. The authors suggested that in these cases, the vocal fold dysfunction was probably a continuous underlying dystonia, and that the episodes of airway obstruction may occur when the demands on the respiratory system exceed the capacity of the laryngeal system. Another neurologic cause of PVFM is adductor laryngeal breathing dystonia. Focal dystonias are typically triggered during a specific type of activity. In the case of adductor laryngeal breathing dystonia, the act of inhalation is the trigger to inappropriately close the vocal folds. During sleep the problem disappears. Other neurologic causes of PVFM include stroke and head injury. With these overt neurologic disorders, however, the stridor is also present during sleep (Koufman, 1994).

Other potential causes of PVFM include laryngeal irritants and exercise (Table 11.15).

LINKS BETWEEN PVFM, ASTHMA, AND GERD

Asthma has been reported to occur in a substantial number of individuals with PVFM, ranging from 33–80% (e.g., Doshi & Weinberger, 2006; Gurevich-Uvena, 2010; Koufman & Block, 2008; Morris, 2006; Newman et al., 1995; O'Connell, Sklarew, & Goodman, 1995; Parsons et al., 2010). However, it is not clear whether the asthma is a trigger of the PVFM or whether such patients have an underlying reactive airway disease that precipitates both asthma and PVFM attacks (Morris, 2006). GERD, postnasal drip, and allergies have also been reported as very common in patients with comorbid asthma and PVFM (Gurevich-Uvena, 2010; Parsons et al., 2010).

TABLE *11.15* **Irritant-Induced and Exercise-Induced PVFM**

Irritant-Induced
Absence of preceding laryngeal dysfunction or disease
Onset of symptoms after a single specific exposure or accident to a gas, smoke, fume, vapor, mist, or dust
Onset of symptoms within 24 hours after exposure
Symptoms of wheezing, stridor, dyspnea, cough, or throat tightness
Abnormal laryngoscopy either in the asymptomatic state, during symptoms, or on provocation
Exercise-Induced
Attacks triggered by competition, practice, or other strenuous activity
Symptoms occur within a few minutes of the activity
Symptoms resolve quickly
Breathing is tense and shallow
Dyspnea can contribute to struggle behavior

Sources: Information from Doshi & Weinberger (2006); Mathers-Schmidt & Brilla (2005); Perkner et al. (1998).

A combination of causes seems to be most typical of patients with PVFM. For example, Altman et al. (2000) reported that in a series of 10 patients with PVFM, 7 had psychiatric disorders (anxiety, depression, personality disorder), 8 demonstrated GERD, 6 had a prior diagnosis of asthma or a positive response to asthma treatment, and 2 subjects had neurological signs. Thus, PVFM may best be characterized as a complex disorder that can combine elements of psychoemotional, physiological, and neurological factors (Hicks et al., 2008; Sandage & Zelazny, 2004).

DIAGNOSIS AND EVALUATION

Misdiagnosis of PFVM as "refractory asthma" is common (Chiang, Goh, Tang, & Chay, 2008), and recognition of the disorder is the cornerstone for effective treatment (Mikita & Mikita, 2006). A team approach can facilitate correct diagnosis, with team members from the areas of pulmonology, otolaryngology, allergy, gastroenterology, speech-language pathology, social work or psychology, teaching, and vocal coaching. The first step is to obtain a detailed history from the individual focusing on respiratory, physical, voice and swallowing, symptomatology, and medical areas (Table 11.16).

Many people report that their symptoms have a very abrupt beginning and ending. Adults are often aware of factors that trigger the attack, such as exercise, laughing, very hot or cold air, dust, fumes, and so on (Mathers-Schmidt, 2001). Children and adolescents tend to experience the attacks during physical activity, and also during stressful times in their lives. Questions to be addressed during the evaluation should include those that focus on the client's breathing patterns, such as the location of the breathing difficulty (inhalation versus exhalation); presence of stridor when the individual is experiencing symptoms; any previously diagnosed respiratory disease including asthma or other airway obstruction; effectiveness of bronchodilators; and whether the individual reports the sensation of choking or suffocation during an attack (Sandage & Zelazny, 2004). Laryngeal symptoms are also explored, including presence of dysphonia, and laryngeal sensations such as a tight feeling in the throat. In addition, information should be elicited about bodily sensations associated with attacks, such as numbness and/or tingling in the hands or feet or around the mouth. The clinician should obtain data regarding current and previous medications and surgical history. Any changes in swallowing should be noted (Sandage & Zelazny, 2004). The clinician and client attempt to identify triggers for the attacks, including GERD, nasal symptoms such as congestion and/or postnasal drip, allergies, stress, and exercise.

The current "gold standard" for evaluation is laryngoscopy using flexible nasoendoscopy (Morris, 2006). The patient is asked to perform various tasks requiring vocal fold adduction and abduction under different circumstances such as quiet breathing, phonating, sniffing, coughing, and panting. A common vocal fold configuration that is seen as the individual inhales is adduction of the anterior two-thirds of the vocal folds with a diamond-shaped chink at the posterior portion of the glottis (Hicks et al., 2008; Morris, 2006). If present, the posterior chink may occur during both inhalation and exhalation. The false folds may also adduct (Mathers-Schmidt, 2001). However, patients whose PVFM is related to GERD may not demonstrate these laryngeal findings, and not all patients have posterior chinking (Andrianopoulos et al., 2000; Hicks et al., 2008; Koufman, 1994). Laryngeal findings may be evident even when patients are asymptomatic (Newman et al., 1995).

Laryngoscopy can also help to differentiate PVFM from a respiratory type dystonia, because patients with breathing dystonia show a different pattern of laryngoscopic findings. That is, rather than occurring spasmodically, their adductory dysfunction is continual

TABLE 11.16 Evaluation Questions for Paradoxical Vocal Fold Motion

Respiration
Have you ever been diagnosed with a respiratory disorder such as asthma?
Have you undergone pulmonary function testing?
Do you have more trouble breathing in or breathing out?
Do you make breathing-in noises (stridor) when you are having symptoms?
Do you feel breathless before or during an attack?
Do you experience upper or lower chest tightness?
Do inhaled bronchodilators prevent or abort attacks?
Physical
Do you experience throat tightness?
Does your throat feel sore or dry?
Do you have a sensation of choking or suffocation?
Do you feel light-headed or dizzy before or during an attack?
Do you experience numbness and/or tingling in your hands or feet or around your mouth with attacks?
Do you routinely experience nasal symptoms (postnasal drip, nasal congestion, runny nose, sneezing)?
Do you experience reflux symptoms?
Voice and Swallowing
Is your voice sometimes or often hoarse?
Does your voice change before or during attacks?
Do you experience swallowing difficulties before, during, or after an attack?
Symptoms
Do your symptoms come on rapidly?
How quickly do the symptoms subside?
Have you ever passed out?
Do symptoms ever occur during sleep?
Are there specific triggers for your attacks?
What do you do to resolve your symptoms?
Do you experience anxiety and/or panic before or during attacks?
Medical
Have you previously been treated for this condition?
Have you undergone any related or nonrelated surgeries?
Are you currently taking any medications?

Sources: Information from Hicks et al. (2008); Sandage & Zelazny (2004).

throughout the day, is not specific to phonation, worsens when they take a deep breath, and disappears during sleep (Koufman & Block, 2008).

One of the most critical diagnostic functions is to differentiate inspiratory stridor and dyspnea resulting from PVFM from other causes such as asthma, abductor paralysis, subglottic

TABLE 11.17 **Pulmonary Function Tests to Differentiate PVFM and Asthma**

Test	Method	PVFM	Asthma
Flow-volume loop	Plots maximum inhalation and exhalation maneuvers on a graph	Flattened inspiratory limb	Flattened expiratory limb
Pulse oximetry	Measures amount of oxygen in the blood	Normal to mildly abnormal	Abnormal
Airway reactivity testing	Pulmonary function tests completed before and after pharmacologic or other challenges	Normal response	Abnormal response

stenosis, and vocal fold fixation. Pulmonary function tests such as flow-volume loop, pulse oximetry, and airway reactivity testing are important to distinguish PVFM from asthma and other conditions (Table 11.17).

One of the distinguishing characteristics of PVFM is that spirometric values when the patient is asymptomatic are normal. This is not true of other causes of upper airway obstruction such as vocal fold paralysis or paresis, subglottic stenosis, or other fixed abnormalities of the upper airway (Doshi & Weinberger, 2006). Even when the individual with PVFM is experiencing severe respiratory symptoms, pulse oximetry is typically normal (Hicks et al., 2008; Noyes & Kemp, 2007), or may be mildly abnormal (oxygen and carbon dioxide may be slightly reduced during an acute attack). This is different from asthma, in which pulse oximetry indicates abnormal oxygen saturation levels, particularly during acute attacks. Bronchial challenge testing is usually normal in patients with PVFM (Altman et al., 2002).

Flow-volume curves tend to be different in patients with PVFM and those with asthma. Patients with PVFM often demonstrate flattening or blunting of the inspiratory limb of the loop, reflecting a reduction in the amount of inhaled air (e.g., Christopher & Morris, 2010). This is consistent with a variable extrathoracic obstruction and may be present even when the individual is asymptomatic (Buddiga, 2010; O'Hollaren, n.d.). In some cases the expiratory portion of the flow-volume loop may also be flattened (Chiang et al., 2008; Gregore, n.d.), indicating obstructive difficulty. This may occur in cases where the paradoxical vocal fold movement continues into the exhalation phase of respiration, or in patients with coexisting PVFM and asthma. Patients with asthma but without PVFM show blunting only of the expiratory limb, consistent with the exhalatory difficulty due to bronchial narrowing and inflammation. The FEF_{50}/FIF_{50} is another spirometric measure that can help in the diagnosis of PVFM. The normal ratio is less than or equal to 1, whereas it is often greater than 1 in patients with PVFM (Hicks et al., 2008). See Figure 11.3.

TREATMENT

Treatment for PVFM is aimed at relieving the patient's airway obstruction and can be divided into treatment for an acute attack and/or long-term therapy. Clinical management can include behavioral voice therapy, pharmacological therapy, respiratory procedures, or any combination of these.

FIGURE 11.3 **Flow-Volume Loops for PVFM**

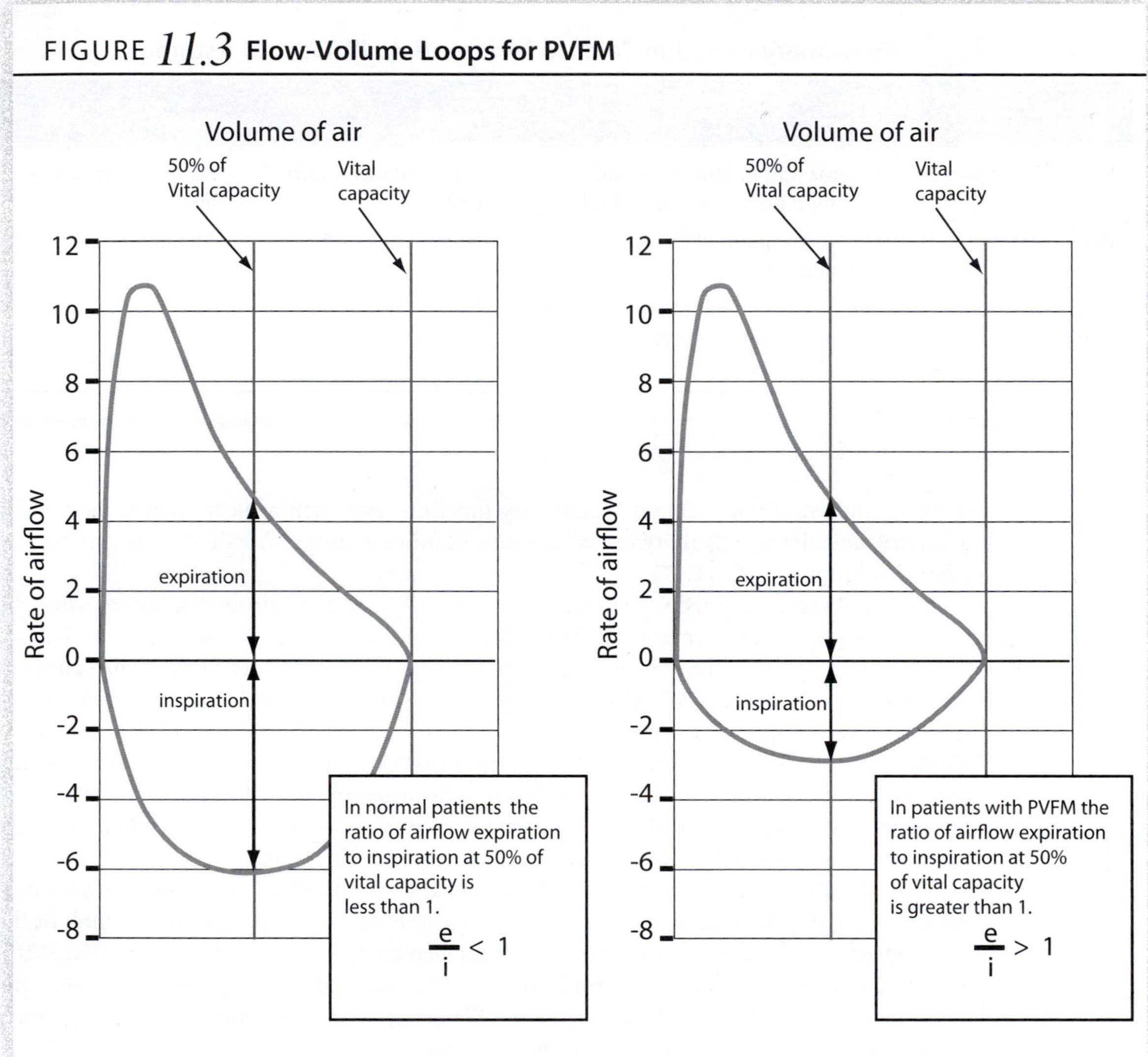

Acute Attacks. During an acute attack, the patient may be fearful and anxious. Many patients report a choking sensation that can induce a fear of dying (Vertigan, Theodoros, Gibson, & Winkworth, 2007). It is important to reassure such patients that the condition is not life-threatening and that their oxygen levels are normal. Reassurance has been reported to be effective in alleviating the symptoms in many cases (Morris, 2006). Sedating the individual may also help to reduce the symptoms. If the symptoms persist the patient may benefit from inhaling a mixture of helium and oxygen. Called *heliox*, the mixture consists of 70% helium and 30% oxygen (Deem & Miller, 2000; Mathers-Schmidt, 2001; Vlahakis et al., 2002). The less dense helium in the mixture reduces turbulent airflow and makes it easier for the individual to inhale (Christopher & Morris, 2010; Noyes & Kemp, 2007). This can reduce the patient's anxiety and prevent the attack from worsening.

The administration of continuous positive air pressure (CPAP) may be helpful in some acute cases. This procedure involves the patient wearing a nasal or facial mask, which is connected via a tube to a small instrument that delivers a steady stream of slightly pressurized air (http://ucdmc.ucdavis.edu). The high pressure overcomes obstruction in the airway and stimulates normal breathing (http://entcolumbia.org). This procedure has been reported to increase lung volume and slow the exhalation, resulting in a more widely open glottis and decreased airway obstruction (Goldman & Muers, 1991).

Pharmacological treatment may be helpful depending on the individual case. For instance, when the trigger for the attacks is GERD or other irritants, the appropriate drugs should be administered to eliminate the precipitating condition. Often an individual with PVFM feels anxiety due to the feeling of suffocation. The anxiety may in turn worsen the symptoms, and antianxiety medications may be useful in these cases. Botox injection into the vocal folds has also reportedly been successful in some patients (Vlahakis et al., 2002). As a last resort, a patient may have to be intubated or tracheotomized, if he or she does not respond to other types of therapies.

Long-Term Treatment. Because of the variety of etiologies and symptoms that characterize PVFM, a multidisciplinary approach is important. Team members should include a speech-language pathologist, pulmonologist, psychologist, and otolaryngologist (Altman et al., 2002; Lo, Ho, & Huang, 2005). Goals and methods for alleviating chronic PVFM are listed in Table 11.18.

Increasingly, speech therapy focusing on breathing management has become the primary intervention of choice for chronic PVFM (Morris, 2006). Speech therapy has been shown to be very helpful for individuals to manage the symptoms of the disorder (e.g., Jines & Drummond, 2006). Because speech-language pathologists are trained in laryngeal anatomy and physiology, they are well equipped to teach the patient how to control his or her laryngeal function for respiration. Speech therapy typically focuses on patient education, breathing techniques, raising awareness and relaxation, and vocal hygiene including reduction of coughing and throat clearing.

TABLE *11.18* Goals and Methods for Alleviating Chronic PVFM

Goal	Method
Overcome feelings of fear and helplessness	Mastery of breathing techniques
Reduce tension in intrinsic and extrinsic laryngeal muscles	Open-throat breathing, resonant voice
Divert attention away from larynx	Abdominal breathing and active exhalation
Reduce tension in neck, chest, and shoulders	Movement, stretching, progressive relaxation
Use techniques to reduce severity and frequency of attacks	Increase awareness of early warning symptoms, rehearse action plan

Source: Information from Gregore (n.d.).

Patient Education. Patient education, an essential component of intervention, is designed to increase the individual's understanding of laryngeal structure and function, the role of the larynx in the respiratory process, and the mechanics of breathing (Hicks et al., 2008). Laryngeal endoscopy is a good way to help patients visualize the vocal folds and their movements during respiration and phonation. The client watches his or her vocal fold closure during inspiration while the clinician provides an explanation of normal vocal fold functioning and compares it to the individual's paradoxical vocal fold movement (e.g., Sandage & Zelazny, 2004). The visual feedback also helps the patient to understand the rationale underlying the breathing exercises (Hicks et al., 2008). Information is provided regarding laryngeal hypersensitivity to triggers and the contribution of coughing and throat clearing to the problem (Hicks et al., 2008).

Breathing Techniques. Breathing techniques are designed to teach the patient to respond to the feeling of throat constriction with a more relaxed breathing pattern instead of the learned maladaptive response (Blager, 2006). The individual practices using abdominal rather than thoracic muscles to inhale and exhale. This involves expanding the abdominal wall on inhalation and contracting the abdominal muscles when exhaling (e.g., Altman et al., 2002; Morris, 2006). The patient simultaneously maintains his or her shoulders, neck, and jaw in a relaxed position. This respiratory pattern helps to remove the focus from the larynx.

The patient learns specific breathing patterns to use when feeling the onset of an attack in order to keep the vocal folds abducted and thus avoid the attack. For example, sniffing and panting help to open the airway (Hicks et al., 2008). The individual is taught to sniff in deeply through the nose using an abdominal inhalation without raising the shoulders. He or she then exhales for 8–10 seconds on voiceless sounds such as *s, sh*, and *f*. This has the effect of keeping the glottis open during exhalation (Gregore, n.d.; Sandage & Zelazny, 2004). Teaching the patient to breathe in and out with his or her lips pursed and an abdominal focus can be effective in facilitating a more relaxed breathing pattern and decrease anxiety and panic (Hicks et al., 2008; Mikita & Mikita, 2006). This is the basis for the technique sometimes called "relaxed throat breathing" (Table 11.19).

These types of breathing techniques have been adapted for athletes who must balance the newly learned breathing patterns with the need for extreme physical exercise. For example, Mathers-Schmidt, Brilla, Jamieson, and Parsons (n.d.) and Mathers-Schmidt and Brilla (2005) described a program of inspiratory muscle training (IMT) for athletes suffering from PVFM. Participants first learned relaxed throat breathing. Thereafter, the individuals used a custom-made inspiratory muscle-strengthening device with a mouthpiece and valve that opened when the sensor detected negative (inspiratory) pressure exceeding a threshold level. The valve remained open for exhalation. The individuals were trained to maintain an open airway against increasing levels of resistance, while using the learned respiratory patterns. The authors reported that maximum voluntary ventilation increased and patient rating of dyspnea decreased after treatment. The participants reported carryover of treatment gains to actual sports performance. Blager (2006) reported on a program of activity-based breathing techniques for athletes. This program is based on the relaxed throat breathing technique, but focuses the patient's attention on the rib cage rather than the abdomen for more rapid inhalation and exhalation. Participants are taught open mouth breathing with "gently pursed lips" and are directed to focus on the front of the mouth while breathing to avoid pulling from the larynx during competitive pressure. The patient learns the breathing pattern first at a relaxed pace and gradually integrates the new techniques into the sport.

TABLE 11.19 **Relaxed Throat Breathing Exercises and Rationales**

Exercise	Rationale
Keep your shoulders down and relaxed while breathing	Decreases upper body tension
Keep your hand on your abdomen while breathing	Facilitates conscious abdominal breath support
Breathe in quickly through your nose or mouth for approximately 1 second	Helps to open glottis
Purse your lips tightly and breathe out for 2–3 seconds	Creates pressure that helps to keep the glottis open
Practice 5–10 breaths 20 times per day during asymptomatic periods	Makes this type of breathing more automatic
Use easy throat breathing before exposure to a trigger or when you sense an attack	Can help to abort an attack

Note: These exercises can also be done with a straw.
Sources: Information from Buddiga (2010); Hicks et al. (2008).

Raising Awareness and Relaxation. It is important to help patients raise their awareness of events that trigger paradoxical attacks, in order to facilitate the use of learned strategies to avoid them. Patients are trained to use progressive relaxation techniques to develop the ability to become aware of very small changes in the body. This helps to focus attention on any physiologic sign that signals a breathing attack so that the individual can start the breathing exercises and prevent the attack (Sandage, 2006). The patient is taught to develop an awareness of throat tightness and learns to relax his or her laryngeal muscles, as well as muscles of the shoulders, neck, and chest (Sandage & Zelazny, 2004). Biofeedback can be helpful in this process (e.g., McFadden & Zawadski, 1996). Manual circumlaryngeal massage may also be beneficial in helping the patient relax the laryngeal area. By introducing breathing and relaxation techniques the patient can begin to take responsibility from the outset for eliminating the paradoxical behavior and can start to feel more in control of the problem (Sandage & Zelazny, 2004).

Vocal Hygiene. A program of vocal hygiene is essential to identify and eliminate any phonotraumatic behaviors, particularly excessive coughing and throat clearing.

Chronic Cough

Coughing is a reflex occurrence that results from a variety of stimuli. A cough is a protective mechanism designed to remove foreign substances and irritants from the airway. The cough reflex occurs when cough receptors (nerve endings) in the respiratory system are stimulated (Carney et al., 1997; Holmes & Fadden, 2004; Vertigan et al., 2006). The sensory information is sent via the vagus nerve to the brainstem, and neuromotor instructions to close the glottis are relayed to the laryngeal muscles (Altman et al., 2002). While coughing is a reflexive process mediated by the brainstem, a certain degree of cortical control is possible, allowing individuals to suppress a cough following the sensation of an urge-to-cough (Davenport, 2008; McGarvey, McKeagney, Polley, MacMahon, & Costello, 2009).

The steps of a cough include a deep inspiration, glottal closure, relaxation of the diaphragm in conjunction with increased contraction of the chest muscles, narrowing of the trachea, and finally explosive release of the built-up air pressure through the opening glottis (Altman et al., 2002; Chung & Pavord, 2008). Spontaneous cough usually occurs in a series of cough sounds called a *cough bout*, lasting a few seconds (Chung, 2006; Chung & Pavord, 2008). Stimuli that trigger the cough may be chemical, mechanical, or thermal. Chemical irritants include substances such as capsaicin (the hot ingredient in peppers), citric acid, tartaric acid, cleaning agents and nicotine, aerosols, scents, and odors. Mechanical agents include dust, constriction of the bronchi, mucus, dry crumbly foods, and foreign bodies, as well as laughing, talking, or singing (Altman et al., 2002; McGarvey et al., 2009; Gibson & Vertigan, 2009; Vertigan et al., 2007). Thermal triggers include cooking and air temperature changes (Gibson & Vertigan, 2009; McGarvey et al., 2009).

Cough may be characterized as acute or chronic. Acute cough typically results from a viral or bacterial infection and resolves within a time period of three weeks or less (Chung & Pavord, 2008). Other causes of acute cough include exacerbation of COPD, allergic rhinitis, and environmental exposure to noxious agents (Holmes & Fadden, 2004). Cough becomes chronic if it has lasted for at least eight weeks (e.g., Chung & Pavord, 2008; Holmes & Fadden, 2004; Sandage, 2006; Vertigan et al., 2006).

Chronic cough (CC) is one of the most common reasons that adults consult a physician (Altman et al., 2002). CC accounted for over 24 million visits to medical services in the United States in 1991 (Palombini et al., 1999). Sales of over-the-counter cough medications have been reported to be worth as much as $328 million in the United States (Everett, Kastelik, Thompson, & Morice, 2007). The prevalence of cough in the general population has been reported to range from 3.3% to 33% (Lorcan, McGarvey, & Elder, 2010).

CAUSES OF CHRONIC COUGH

There are numerous causes of chronic cough. The three primary causes in individuals who do not smoke are postnasal drip syndrome (also called rhinitis/rhinosinusitis and upper airway cough syndrome), asthma, and GERD/LPR (Carney et al., 1997; Dettmar et al., 2009; Everett et al., 2007; Holmes & Fadden, 2004; Lee & Woo, 2005; McGarvey et al., 2009; Palombini et al., 1999; Vernon, Leidy, Nacson, & Nelsen, 2009; Vertigan et al., 2006). See Table 11.20.

Upper airway cough syndrome, asthma, and GERD are all associated with inflammation in the upper airway. The inflammation likely increases the sensitivity of sensory nerve receptors, making the person more susceptible to stimuli that trigger the cough (Carney et al., 1997). CC may result from just one of these conditions, but it is often linked with several causes (e.g., Everett et al., 2007; Holmes & Fadden, 2004; Palombini et al., 1999).

Cough can be a side effect of angiotensin converting enzyme (ACE) inhibitors, a class of medications used to treat high blood pressure and congestive heart failure. A nonproductive cough has been reported in 5–20% of individuals taking these medications (Holmes & Fadden, 2004). Cough may also be secondary to chronic bronchitis from exposure to cigarette smoke or other irritants (Holmes & Fadden, 2004).

A form of asthma called *cough variant asthma* (CVA) accounts for between 24–35% of those referred to specialist cough clinics (Chung & Pavord, 2008). CVA is characterized by normal spirometry, but bronchial challenge testing shows airway hyperresponsiveness, and the cough

TABLE 11.20 Causes of Chronic Cough in Nonsmoking Individuals

Postnasal drip syndrome/rhinosinusitis/upper airway cough syndrome
Asthma
GERD
ACE inhibitor side effect
Chronic bronchitis
Airway hyperresponsiveness following viral infection
Psychoemotional
Paradoxical vocal fold motion
Eosinophilic bronchitis
Idiopathic

improves with bronchodilators or corticosteroids (Lorcan et al., 2010). CVA is characterized by the presence of eosinophils in the patient's airways (Gibson et al., 2002). **Eosinophils** are types of white blood cells that are components of the immune system. Normally these cells make up only 1–6% of white blood cells and should not be present in the lungs and airways (Young, Lowe, Stevens, & Heath, 2006). Researchers and clinicians have recently become aware of eosinophilic bronchitis as a cause of chronic cough (McGarvey, 2005). Eosinophilic bronchitis has also been associated with asthma, airway hyperresponsiveness, and GERD (Gibson et al., 2002).

Another cause of persistent cough may be increased airway responsiveness associated with damage to the vagus nerve following a viral infection (Altman et al., 2002; Lorcan et al., 2010). The sensitivity of the cough reflex to various forms of stimulation can fluctuate because afferent sensory nerves have a large degree of plasticity (McGarvey, 2005). Typically the cough subsides after 2–3 weeks and the reflex returns to its baseline state. Sometimes, however, the hyperreactive state persists after the initial triggering event, which can result in a chronic cough (Lorcan et al., 2010). The persistence of the cough may be a type of sensory **hyperalgesia** (increased sensitivity to pain) in which there is a reduction in sensory nerve threshold to stimulation resulting from damage to peripheral nerves or nerve endings (Ryan, Vertigan, Bone, & Gibson, 2010).

A psychoemotional basis of CC is sometimes proposed. "Psychogenic cough" has been described as a barking or honking cough that cannot be attributed to airway hyperreactivity, asthma, GERD, upper airway cough syndrome, or any other organic basis. Reportedly, the cough can be a symptom of a conversion disorder that may provide the individual with some kind of secondary gain (e.g., Gay et al., 1987; Mastrovich & Greenberger, 2002; Riegel et al., 1995). For example, a child with a persistent cough may be allowed to stay home from school. Other case reports demonstrate a strong association between the cough and depression and/or anxiety. However, the psychological distress may be a result of the debilitating cough, or a coexisting condition, rather than the cause (Carney et al., 1997; Vertigan et al., 2007). The diagnosis of psychogenic cough should only be applied after all other possible causes have been ruled out (Holmes & Fadden, 2004).

CC may be a symptom of PVFM. CC has been described to occur in as many as 56–80% of patients with PVFM (Murry et al., 2004; Ryan & Gibson, 2009). Conversely, approximately 50% of people with CC have been reported to display an abnormal pattern of vocal fold movement during respiration and following bronchial challenge testing (Milgrom, Corsello,

Freedman, Blager, & Wood, 1990; Ryan & Vertigan, 2009). Further evidence of the link between CC and PVFM is that triggers for each (e.g., talking, exercise, laughing, cold air) are similar (Vertigan et al., 2007). Both CC and PVFM are strongly associated with asthma, upper airway cough syndrome, and GERD, and they may have similar underlying mechanisms (Gibson & Vertigan, 2009; Murry & Sapienza, 2010). This suggests that the conditions may be overlapping or associated (Murry & Sapienza, 2010). Vertigan et al. (2006) suggested that CC and PVFM may fall at opposite ends of a continuum with pure cough on one end, pure PVFM at the other end, and a combination of features in the middle.

Sometimes a specific cause for the cough cannot be identified despite thorough investigation. Those cases are labeled as nonspecific or idiopathic CC (Gibson & Vertigan, 2009). When the cough persists despite appropriate treatment of specific causes, the term applied is *refractory* CC (Gibson & Vertigan, 2009). Refractory cough is reported to persist in at least 10% (Gibson & Vertigan, 2009) and as many as 46% of cases (Pavord & Chung, 2008). Individuals with either refractory or nonspecific cough reportedly are excessively sensitive to triggers that are known to activate mechanical, thermal, and chemical sensory receptors in the airway. A link has also been reported between sex hormones, viral infections, and idiopathic cough in peri- or postmenopausal women (McGarvey, 2005).

SYMPTOMS AND ASSOCIATED FINDINGS

A variety of symptoms and associated findings have been noted in patients with CC, including variations in the pattern of the cough, GERD-related symptoms, respiratory symptoms, vocal symptoms, and laryngeal findings (Table 11.21).

COMPLICATIONS OF CC

Many complications of CC have been reported, ranging in severity from mild to severely disabling (Table 11.22). Complications, which can be physical and/or psychoemotional, can seriously impact the individual's quality of life by interfering with work and social relationships (Everett et al., 2007; Gay et al., 1987).

DIAGNOSIS AND EVALUATION

Diagnosis and evaluation are optimized by a team approach including the pulmonologist, allergist, laryngologist, gastroenterologist, speech-language pathologist, psychologist, and other disciplines as appropriate. The initial evaluation typically focuses on detecting and/or ruling out underlying causes of the cough such as asthma, GERD, LPR, upper airway cough syndrome, laryngeal pathology, PVFM, ACE inhibitor therapy, and psychological issues. A thorough pulmonary assessment should be completed, including methacholine or histamine challenge to rule out asthma. Challenges are also used to induce coughing, such as capsaicin (the "hot" ingredient in red pepper) and citric acid. Capsaicin challenge is most commonly used, as the substance is well tolerated and acceptable (Chung, 2006). Usually the response is measured as the concentration of capsaicin that causes 2 or more coughs (C2) or 5 or more coughs (C5). Differences have been reported in capsaicin cough reflex in patients with CC and noncoughing volunteers (Chung, 2006). Individuals with CC have been shown to be more sensitive to capsaicin, that is, less of the substance is needed to provoke the cough (Spector, 2009).

Imaging studies (x-rays, CT scans, FEES) and endoscopic evaluations are the gold standards for identifying diseases that can contribute to CC, such as upper airway cough syndrome, GERD/LPR, chronic bronchitis, and chronic aspiration (Petty & Dailey, 2009). Endoscopic

TABLE 11.21 Symptoms and Associated Findings in Patients with Chronic Cough

Cough Patterns	Vocal Symptoms
Cough on phonation	Strain
Cough on rising	Roughness/hoarseness
Throat clearing	Breathiness
Cough with specific foods	**Laryngeal Findings**
Cough on eating	Vocal fold atrophy
Cough on lying down	Sulcus vocalis
Woken by cough	Nodules
Respiratory Symptoms	Polyps
Exertional wheeze/dyspnea	Polypoid degeneration
Breathing difficulty	Unilateral vocal fold paralysis
Symptoms of GERD	Laryngeal neoplasm
Heartburn	
Indigestion	
Choking episodes	
Globus pharyngeus	

Sources: Information from Chen (2007); Everett & Morice (2007); Vertigan et al. (2007b).

TABLE 11.22 Physical and Psychoemotional Complications of Chronic Cough

Physical	Psychoemotional
Vomiting	Embarrassment
Fatigue	Self-consciousness
Increased pressure on lumbar disks	Difficulty speaking on phone
Laryngeal trauma	Guilt
Chest pain	Social isolation
Rib fracture	Anger
Headache	Frustration
Blackouts	Feeling of being out of control
Disturbed sleep	Depression
Urinary incontinence	
Impaired vocal quality	

Sources: Information from Carney et al. (1997); Chung & Pavord (2008); Everett et al. (2007); Gibson & Vertigan (2009); McGarvey et al. (2009); Raj & Birring (2007); Vertigan et al. (2006).

assessment of the larynx should be completed on all clients to rule out laryngeal pathology that may be triggering the cough, such as contact ulcer, persistent irritation and/or inflammation, or vocal fold paralysis causing aspiration during swallowing. The individual should also be assessed for clinical signs of reflux.

The speech-language pathologist will obtain important information from the case history (Table 11.23). Questions relate to the onset of the cough, triggers for the cough, description of

TABLE *11.23* **Patient Interview Protocol for Chronic Cough**

Description of Cough	**Medical History**
Single cough	Cough preceded by illness
Repetitive cough	Hospitalizations related to cough
Normal sound	Chronic and recent illnesses and hospitalizations
Honking sound	Past and current medications
Elicits a gag reflex or vomiting	Specialists that have been consulted for cough
Follows a "tickle" or "itch" feeling	Concurrent medical conditions
Characteristics of Cough	Medical conditions of family members
Duration	Laryngological findings
Previous interventions	**Social-Emotional History**
Cough absent during sleep	Cough preceded or accompanied by a stressful event
Missed school/work	Current sources of stress, anxiety, conflict
Activities related to cough frequency	Personality characteristics
Avoidance of activities or social situations	Family, peer, teacher, work relationships
Client's reaction	School/work performance
Reaction of family, friends, peers	**Evaluation**
Triggers for Cough	Frequency (number of coughs in 10 minutes)
Perfumes	Severity
Odors	Client reaction
Changes in temperature	Presence of excessive laryngeal tension
Cooking	Voice quality, pitch, loudness
Dust	**Trial Treatment Approaches**
Fumes	Gentle abdominal inhalation
Pet dander	Lengthened exhalation with /s/
Foods	Blowing with pursed lips
Exercise	Sipping and swallowing
Talking/singing	Substituting different behavior for the cough
Laughing	Success with techniques
	Length of time cough was controlled using techniques
	Client/family reaction

Sources: Information from Gallena (2007); Murry & Sapienza (2010).

the cough, cough characteristics, medical history, and social/emotional history. The speech-language pathologist should note the frequency and severity of the cough, as well as the patient's reaction. Laryngeal palpation of the extrinsic laryngeal muscles may help to identity excessive neck tension and possible elevated laryngeal position. The clinician should also observe the individual's breathing patterns during quiet breathing and as the person speaks. A thoracic pattern of breathing characterized by shoulder lifting and chest tightening often brings on cough or shortness of breath associated with speaking (Murry & Sapienza, 2010). Finally, various therapy techniques are attempted during the evaluation to assess the patient's potential success in suppressing the cough.

QUANTIFYING COUGH

The frequency and severity of the patient's cough should be documented both objectively and subjectively. The effect of the cough on the patient's quality of life and degree of disruption to daytime and nighttime activities should also be determined (Vernon et al., 2009). Subjective measures are important to gain the patient's perspective on the severity of his or her cough. This can be done by asking the patient to self-evaluate the frequency and severity of the cough and how the cough is affecting his or her daily living and activities (Chung, 2006). The use of cough scores, cough diaries, and cough symptom questionnaires may be helpful in tracking occurrences of cough (Chung, 2006). Visual analogue scales have been developed on which the patient indicates the severity of the cough in a specific period of time (e.g., past 24 hours or past 48 hours). Various cough-related quality of life instruments are available, such as the Cough-Specific Quality of Life Questionnaire (French, Irwin, Fletcher, & Adams, 2002). This is a 28-item questionnaire that addresses the patient's physical complaints, psychosocial issues, emotional well-being, personal safety fears, and functional abilities (Table 11.24). A parent-proxy quality-of-life chronic cough-specific questionnaire (PC-QOL) (Newcombe et al., 2008) has been developed specifically for children.

Two objective ways of monitoring cough over a period of days have recently been reported. The first is a 24-hour ambulatory system that simultaneously records both the cough sound as well as EMG signals from the patient's lower respiratory muscles to measure the number of coughs (Chung, 2006). Another system is a computerized audio-timed portable recorder connected to a transmitter worn by the individual. The transmitter sends the cough sound signals to a home computer. The patient is free to move within 100 m of the computer. In addition to measuring the number of coughs in a period of time, other information including cough latency (periods between coughs), cough effort, cough intensity, and the wetness of the cough is obtained (Chung, 2006).

TREATMENT

Behavioral treatment for CC is highly recommended after all potential medical causes have been ruled out or treated. The goal of behavioral management is to suppress the cough even when the individual feels the need to cough or to clear the throat (Vertigan, Theodoros, Winkworth, & Gibson, 2008). Intervention is aimed at educating the individual about the nature of cough, reducing laryngeal irritation, training the patient to become aware of the sensations and behaviors that precipitate the cough, and teaching him or her to implement a competing and/or distracting behavior that will delay or eliminate the cough before it happens (Fulcher & Cellucci, 1997; Sandage, 2006; Vertigan et al., 2006). Vocal education focuses on the nature of cough as a reflex that can be brought under voluntary control. The patient

TABLE *11.24* **Cough-Specific Quality of Life Questionnaire**

Please indicate below how your cough bothers you. Circle the response option that best describes the degree of your agreement concerning each of the following 28 statements using the following scale: 1 = strongly disagree; 2 = disagree; 3 = agree; 4 = strongly agree

1. Family and/or close friends can't tolerate it anymore.
2. I have experienced prolonged absences from important activities such as work, school, or volunteer services.
3. I have been completely prevented from engaging in important activities such as work, school, or volunteer services.
4. I have lost my appetite.
5. I am sick to my stomach and vomit.
6. I cough and it makes me retch (dry heaves).
7. I have a fear that I might have AIDS or tuberculosis.
8. I have headaches.
9. I am concerned that I have cancer.
10. I am dizzy.
11. I wet my pants.
12. I soil my pants.
13. I sweat.
14. I am hoarse.
15. It hurts when I breathe.
16. I broke a rib.
17. I cannot sleep at night.
18. I have difficulty speaking on the phone.
19. I can no longer sing, for instance, in church.
20. I have stopped going to social activities such as movies, plays, and town meetings.
21. I have had to change my lifestyle.
22. I ache all over.
23. I am exhausted.
24. I am embarrassed.
25. I am upset by people thinking that I have something wrong with me.
26. I want to be reassured that I do not have anything seriously the matter with me.
27. I am self-conscious.
28. I am concerned that I have something seriously the matter with me.

Sources: From "Evaluation of a Cough-Specific Quality-of-Life Questionnaire," by C. T. French, R. S. Irwin, K. E. Fletcher, & T. M. Adams, 2002, *Chest, 121,* pp. 1123–1131. Copyright 2002 by the American College of Chest Physicians. Reprinted with permission.

learns that there is no physiological benefit from repeated coughing. The negative side effects from repeated coughing are explained, including laryngeal trauma, worsening of the laryngeal irritation, and perpetuation of the cycle of coughing (Gibson & Vertigan, 2009; Vertigan et al., 2008). The idea that the cough can be brought under the individual's voluntary control is emphasized, and patients are encouraged to take an active role in changing their cough behavior (Petty & Dailey, 2009; Vertigan et al., 2008). Reducing laryngeal irritation requires a program of vocal hygiene to avoid vocally traumatic behaviors and to increase vocally desirable habits. Patients should be counseled to avoid smoking or exposure to passive smoke, and to minimize consumption of substances known to have a drying effect on the larynx such as alcohol, caffeine, medicated cough lozenges, gargling, dry environment, and mouth breathing. Foods that exacerbate GERD or LPR should be avoided (Gibson & Vertigan, 2009; Sandage, 2006; Vertigan et al., 2008). Positive behaviors to be encouraged include maximizing laryngeal hydration by increasing the volume and frequency of water intake and eating "wet" snacks such as apples, melon, pears, and cucumber. Individuals should breathe through the nose rather than the mouth in order to warm and moisten inhaled air (Sandage, 2006; Vertigan et al., 2008). The humidity in the work and/or home environment should also be increased.

It is important for clients to learn to identify the triggers and the physical sensations that precede the cough (e.g., dry tickle or a strangling sensation). Once the person is aware of the triggers, he or she can use strategies to reduce their frequency (Petty & Dailey, 2009; Sandage, 2006; Vertigan et al., 2007). Monitoring the sensations that precede the cough may be more effective than monitoring the cough itself because it provides an opportunity for the patient to use the learned suppression and distraction strategies to inhibit the cough before it occurs (Petty & Dailey, 2009). Once patients are able to increase voluntary control over the cough, they learn to maintain the control while gradually increasing exposure to the triggers (Vertigan et al., 2007). Finally, clients are taught strategies to voluntarily suppress the cough. Approaches that focus on relaxation of extrinsic and intrinsic laryngeal muscles have been found to be helpful. Techniques such as yawn-sigh and easy onset can decrease laryngeal pressure receptor stimulation and thus reduce the desire to cough (Petty & Dailey, 2009). Practicing exercises that are incompatible with the cough behavior is another effective strategy. Suppression and distraction strategies are implemented by the individual when he or she feels the urge to cough (Table 11.25).

Different strategies can be taught for people who cough continuously and those who cough in bouts. Vertigan et al. (2007) suggested that people who cough continuously can be

TABLE 11.25 Suppression and Distraction Strategies for Cough Reduction

Blowing slowly through pursed lips
Taking a sip of liquid/changing the taste or temperature of the liquid
Sucking on ice chips
Effortful swallow
Nose breathing
Nasal inhalation followed by exhalation on *s, sh, f*
Silent counting to 10
Silent or whispered coughing to clear secretions
Chewing gum
Sucking nonmedicated candies

Sources: Information from Gallena (2007); Petty & Dailey (2009); Sandage (2006); Vertigan et al. (2008).

taught an exercise for suppressing the cough for gradually increasing periods of time, whereas people who cough in bouts may benefit from education about strategies to suppress the cough each time it is anticipated.

Outcomes. Speech pathology intervention for chronic cough has been shown to be effective (e.g., Molassiotis, Bryan, Caress, Bailey, & Smith, 2010). Vertigan et al. (2006) compared behavioral treatment (patient education, reduction of laryngeal irritation, increasing awareness of the sensations and behaviors that precipitate the cough, and implementation of competing/distracting behaviors) to a placebo treatment (healthy lifestyle education) for patients with CC. Patients were randomly assigned to experimental and placebo groups. Outcomes were scored in terms of breathing, cough, voice, upper airway, and limitation of activities. Participants in the experimental group had a significant reduction in all symptom scores after the intervention. Eighty-eight percent of the participants in the experimental group were rated as having a successful outcome; 80% of those in the placebo group had an unsuccessful outcome. Ryan et al. (2010) used a variety of measures including capsaicin testing, urge to cough score, and objective measures of cough frequency before and after a speech pathology program that included education, cough suppression strategies, vocal hygiene training, and psychoeducational counseling. Participants showed a significant improvement in cough-related quality of life, laryngeal function, and total symptom scores. The authors noted that improvement in cough reflex sensitivity together with decreased cough frequency was evident after the first treatment, and improved further at subsequent treatment visits. Furthermore, the improvement was sustained at the posttreatment visit. Ryan et al. (2010) concluded that the mechanism of the improvement is due to a reduction in cough reflex sensitivity facilitated by improvement in vocal hygiene leading to reduced sensory nerve stimulation. They suggested that the reduction in cough frequency subsequently reduced cough-related airway trauma. In addition, behavioral management of chronic cough has been shown to improve paradoxical vocal fold movements and extrathoracic airway hyperresponsiveness, as demonstrated by hypertonic saline challenge, capsaicin cough reflex sensitivity testing, and fiberoptic laryngoscopy before and after therapy (Ryan, Vertigan, & Gibson, 2009).

chapter SUMMARY

TWO MAJOR SYMPTOMS OF AIRWAY difficulties are dyspnea and stridor. Dyspnea is defined as subjectively perceived discomfort in breathing and is associated with different types of sensations including air hunger, work/effort, and chest tightness. Stridor refers to an audible sound generated during respiration, which results from turbulent airflow in the airways as the air passes through a narrowed or obstructed segment. The stridor may be high or low pitched and may occur on inspiration, expiration, or both. Causes of stridor include laryngeal abnormalities such as laryngomalacia, subglottic stenosis, webs, cysts, subglottic hemangiomas, vocal fold paralysis, papilloma, and laryngotracheoesophageal clefts.

Pulmonary function testing (PFT) is a term that covers a variety of tests designed to assess the amount of air an individual is able to inspire and expire, as well as how efficiently the person moves air into and out of the lungs. PFT is used to evaluate respiratory symptoms such as cough or dyspnea as well as for diagnosing respiratory diseases such as asthma.

Asthma is a chronic inflammatory disorder of the large and small airways characterized by variable and recurring symptoms, reversible airflow obstruction, bronchial hyperresponsiveness, and underlying inflammation. Symptoms include nighttime coughing, dyspnea, chronic throat-clearing, chest tightness, and wheezing on expiration. There are many triggers for asthma attacks, including pet hair and dander, dust, allergies, changes in the weather, viral infections, exercise, mold, pollen, chemicals, smoke, uncontrolled GERD/LPR, stress, speaking, and singing. The primary treatment for asthma is inhaled corticosteroids (ICS), which are designed to reduce or eliminate the underlying inflammation of the airways and decrease the excessive mucus production associated with the disease. While ICS use is highly effective, well tolerated, and safe, there are numerous reports of local pharyngeal and laryngeal side effects that can significantly affect voice production.

Paradoxical vocal fold motion (PVFM) is a respiratory/laryngeal disorder characterized primarily by inappropriate spasmodic vocal fold adduction during the inhalation phase of breathing. The primary cause for the laryngospasm is hypersensitivity or hyperresponsiveness of the larynx to a wide variety of stimuli that cause the vocal folds to close as a protective reflex. Triggers include exercise, laughing, very hot or cold air, dust, and fumes. Asthma has been reported to occur in a substantial number of individuals with PVFM. The major symptoms of PVFM are stridor and dyspnea, as well as hoarseness, strain, breathiness, cough, and aphonia. Laryngeal structural abnormalities may be present, such as chronic laryngitis, laryngomalacia, sulcus vocalis, nodules, and subglottic stenosis. One of the most critical diagnostic functions is to differentiate inspiratory stridor and dyspnea resulting from PVFM from other causes such as asthma, abductor paralysis, subglottic stenosis, and vocal fold fixation. Pulmonary function tests such as flow-volume loop, pulse oximetry, and airway reactivity testing are important to distinguish PVFM from asthma and other conditions. Speech therapy focusing on patient education and breathing management has become the primary intervention of choice for chronic PVFM.

Chronic cough is highly prevalent in the United States and other countries. The three primary causes in individuals who do not smoke are postnasal drip syndrome (also called rhinitis/rhinosinusitis and upper airway cough syndrome), asthma, and GERD/LPR. These conditions are all associated with inflammation in the upper airway. The inflammation likely increases the sensitivity of sensory nerve receptors, making the person more susceptible to stimuli that trigger the cough. Chronic cough may be a symptom of PVFM. Sometimes a specific cause for the cough cannot be identified despite thorough investigation. Those cases are labeled as nonspecific or idiopathic chronic cough. When the cough persists despite appropriate treatment of specific causes, the term applied is refractory chronic cough. Many complications of chronic cough have been reported, ranging in severity from mild to severely disabling. Complications can be physical and/or psychoemotional and can seriously impact the individual's quality of life by interfering with work and social relationships. The use of cough scores, cough diaries, and cough symptom questionnaires may be helpful in tracking occurrences of cough. Behavioral treatment for chronic cough is highly recommended after all potential medical causes have been ruled out or treated. The goal of behavioral management is to suppress the cough even when the individual feels the need to cough or to clear the throat. Intervention is aimed at educating the individual about the nature of cough, reducing laryngeal irritation, training the patient to become aware of the sensations and behaviors that precipitate the cough, and teaching him or her to implement a competing and/or distracting behavior that will delay or eliminate the cough before it happens.

review QUESTIONS

1. Distinguish between dyspnea and stridor in terms of causes, symptoms, and evaluation.
2. Define pulmonary function testing and provide examples of different measures.
3. Describe evaluation and treatment approaches for asthma, and explain the occurrence of steroid inhaler laryngitis.
4. Identify the causes of paradoxical vocal fold motion, and explain the role of airway hyperresponsiveness in many of the causes.
5. Identify similarities and differences between asthma and paradoxical vocal fold motion. Why is it so important to distinguish between them?
6. Describe a program of behavioral therapy for chronic paradoxical vocal fold motion.
7. Identify the physiology of a cough. How does the physiology relate to cough as a vocally damaging behavior?
8. Describe the causes of chronic cough, the complications that can occur from the disorder, and appropriate therapy strategies.

PREPARING FOR THE PRAXIS

CASE STUDY 11.1: Paradoxical Vocal Fold Motion

Directions: Please read the case study and answer the five questions that follow. The answers can be found at the bottom of the page.

Kimberly Stewart is a 16-year-old high school student who is very involved in soccer. She is on the varsity team and plans to obtain a soccer scholarship to university. Recently she has complained of difficulty breathing, saying, "My throat feels all closed up." She becomes very anxious during these episodes, and sometimes she feels numbness or tingling in her hands. Her parents took her to a pulmonary specialist, who ruled out asthma.

1. What was the major factor that helped the pulmonary specialist to rule out asthma in Kim's case?
   a. the occurrence of numbness and tingling in her hands
   b. the feeling of her throat being all closed up
   c. airway hyperresponsiveness
   d. stridor mainly on inhalation and normal spirometric values when Kim is asymptomatic
   e. clinical intuition
2. What other professional would you, the speech-language pathologist, refer Kim to?
   a. occupational therapist
   b. physical therapist
   c. gastroenterologist

   d. audiologist
   e. all of the above

3. What is the relationship of "triggers" to laryngeal spasms that occur in paradoxical vocal fold motion?
   a. They initiate a fear reaction.
   b. They cause the vocal folds to close as a protective reflex.
   c. They allow the person to avoid an unpleasant life situation or emotion.
   d. They differentiate between paradoxical vocal fold motion and other respiratory disorders.
   e. none of the above

4. Which of the following questions (if any) would NOT be important to ask during the evaluation?
   a. breathing difficulty during inhalation versus exhalation
   b. presence of stridor when Kim is experiencing symptoms
   c. any previously diagnosed respiratory disease
   d. effectiveness of bronchodilators
   e. all of the above are important questions

5. The most appropriate treatment approach for Kim is
   a. cognitive therapy focusing on identifying and eliminating emotional triggers for paradoxical attacks
   b. relaxed throat breathing and inspiratory muscle training
   c. recommendation to avoid physical exercise and counseling to help Kim accept this suggestion
   d. increased use of bronchodilators to eliminate paradoxical attacks
   e. all of the above

Answers for Case Study 11.1: 1 (d); 2 (c); 3 (b); 4 (e); 5 (b)

Chapter 12
Laryngeal Cancer

LEARNING OBJECTIVES

1. Understand why the prognosis for laryngeal cancer is good at early stages of the disease.
2. Become familiar with the TMN staging system for cancer.
3. Identify risk factors for laryngeal cancer.
4. Describe advantages and disadvantages of radiation therapy and chemotherapy for laryngeal cancer.
5. Compare and contrast surgical options for laryngeal cancer control including effects on voice.
6. Understand the challenges following total laryngectomy.
7. Discuss the three major methods of voice restoration following total laryngectomy, including advantages and disadvantages of each.

Head and neck cancers (HNC) are those that affect the oral cavity, salivary glands, paranasal sinuses and nasal cavities, pharynx, and larynx (National Cancer Institute, 2005). Most HNCs are squamous cell carcinomas that develop in the upper aerodigestive epithelium that lines the mouth, nose, throat, and vocal folds (Argiris, Karamouzis, Raben, & Ferris, 2009). HNCs make up around 3–5% of all cancers in the United States (National Cancer Institute, 2005).

This chapter focuses on cancer of the larynx (see color insert photos 35 and 36). The chapter begins with a discussion of survival rates and sites of disease in laryngeal cancer. The TMN staging system used to identify the specific location and extent of the tumor is presented, followed by identification of risk factors and symptoms of laryngeal cancers. Nonsurgical and surgical options for treatment are described in depth, and problems that can arise after treatment are addressed. Attention is then focused on voice therapy and voice restoration methods. The chapter ends with a discussion of quality of life following total laryngectomy.

Worldwide, approximately 182,000 new cases of laryngeal cancer are diagnosed annually, of which around 22,000 are women (Jaworowska et al., 2007). According to the American Cancer Society (2009), the number of new cases of cancer of the larynx in the United States in 2009 was 12,290. Of those, 9,920 were male, and 2,370 were female. The American Cancer Society estimated deaths from laryngeal cancer for 2009 at 3,660, with 2,900 being male and 760 female.

FIGURE 12.1 **Glottal Cancer**

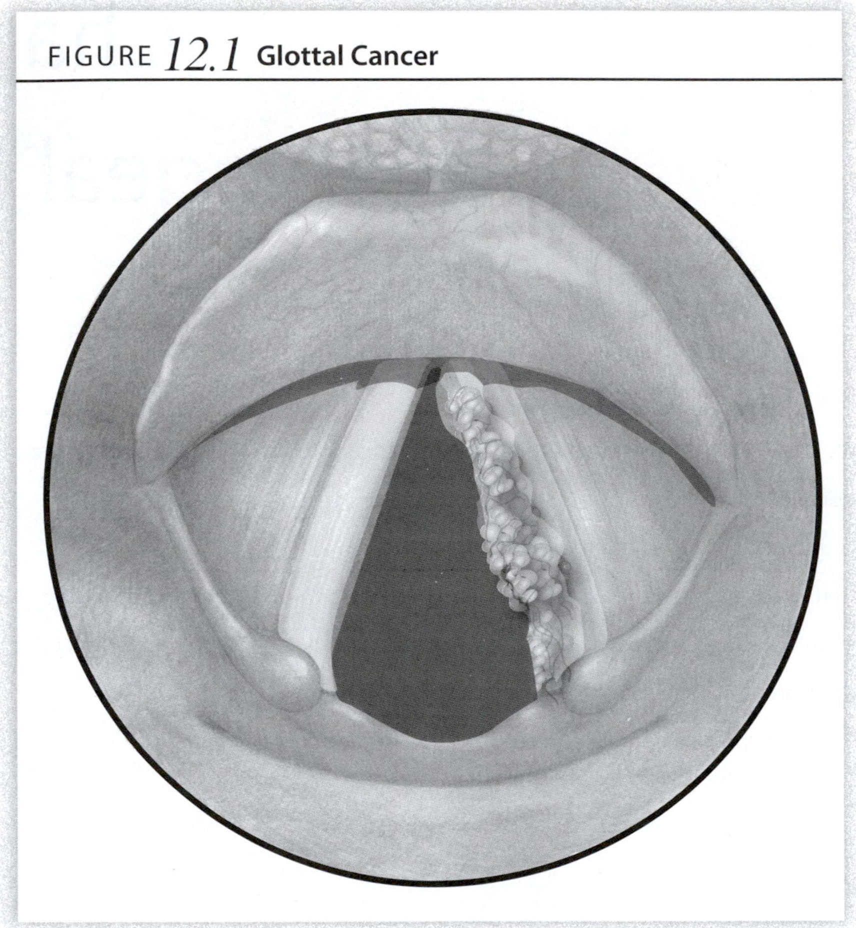

From 1975–2004 the expected five-year survival rate has been stable, averaging 67% for Caucasians and 54% for African Americans (American Cancer Society, 2009). Ethnic and demographic factors appear to play a role in the development of laryngeal cancer and survival rates for the disease. African American patients and individuals living in communities with poverty levels greater than 15% tend to be diagnosed at a younger age, present with more advanced disease, and have lower average survival rates across all age groups (Molina et al., 2008). The survival rate for laryngeal cancer depends on the site of the tumor (glottic, subglottic, or supraglottic) and how early the disease is detected and treated. In the very early stages the prognosis for glottic cancer is very good, with survival rates of 90% (Hairston & Wilson, 2006). This is because there are very few lymph nodes at the level of the glottis, so spread of the cancer is limited (Luscher, Pedersen, & Johansen, 2001; Wright, 2007). In addition, the conus elasticus, quadrangular membranes, and thyrohyoid membrane act as barriers to the spread of cancer (Wright, 2007). Glottic cancers (Figure 12.1) are often detected at an early stage because hoarseness is an early symptom that acts as a warning signal (Tamura et al., 2007). Supraglottic cancer, however, does not commonly present with hoarseness and is often only detected at a more advanced stage (Ferlito, Shaha, Lefebvre, Silver, & Rinaldo, 2002). The later the tumor is discovered the poorer the prognosis, because if left untreated eventually the cancer will spread to the lymph nodes in the patient's neck (Wright, 2007). Once the disease has invaded the lymph nodes it can spread (metastasize) to distant areas of the body. For more advanced cancers, survival is around 50% at 5 years (Hairston & Wilson, 2006).

Laryngeal cancer is more common in men than women, but in recent years, the number of women developing the disease has increased substantially, probably due to the increased rate of smoking in women (Depondt & Gehanno, 1995). Between 1970 and 1993 the incidence of cancer in males decreased by 11% while the incidence in females increased 67%; and the ratio of male to female alaryngeal speakers decreased from 10:1 to 5:1 over this same time period (Bellandese, 2009).

The most common site of disease in laryngeal cancer is the vocal folds (glottic carcinoma), making up around 55–60% of cases. Thirty-five to forty-five percent of laryngeal cancers occur supraglottally, and approximately 5% occur subglottally or overlap more than one area (American Cancer Society, 2009; Ferlito et al., 2002; Hairston & Wilson, 2006).

Laryngeal Cancer Evaluation and Staging

The presence of a cancerous tumor is determined by biopsy of removed tissue. The extent of the cancer is determined by endoscopy of the larynx and surrounding areas by means of direct laryngoscopy, bronchoscopy, esophagoscopy, and nasopharyngoscopy (Hairston & Wilson, 2006). CT scans, MRI, or PET scanning may also be used to determine the stage of the cancer (Burns, Har-El, Shapshay, Maune, & Zeitels, 2009).

The location and extent of disease is described in a system called the TNM classification developed by the American Joint Committee on Cancer (AJCC, 2002). T stands for Tumor, N stands for Nodes, and M stands for Metastasis. Each of these categories is associated with a number that indicates the degree of involvement of the affected structure. Zero indicates no involvement, and higher numbers indicate increasing involvement. Stages range from 0 to IVC. Stage 0 is the least advanced stage; Stages I and II are characterized by the increasing extent of the tumor, but at these stages there is no nodal involvement or **metastasis**. Stage III involves various combinations of tumor extent and nodal involvement, but without metastasis (e.g., T3 N0 M0, T2 N1 M0). Stages IVA, IVB and IVC also indicate increasing extent of tumor, with combinations of nodal involvement and metastasis. Staging is done separately for glottal, supraglottal, and subglottal locations. See Table 12.1.

TABLE *12.1* **TNM Staging of Laryngeal Cancer**

TNM Definition

Primary Tumor (T)

TX:	Primary tumor cannot be assessed
T0:	No evidence of primary tumor
Tis:	Carcinoma in situ

(continued)

TABLE 12.1 TNM Staging of Laryngeal Cancer (Continued)

Supraglottis	
T1:	Tumor limited to one subsite (false vocal folds, arytenoid cartilages, epiglottis, aryepiglottic folds) of supraglottis with normal vocal fold mobility
T2:	Tumor invades mucosa of more than one adjacent subsite of supraglottis or glottis or region outside the supraglottis (e.g., mucosa of base of tongue, vallecula, medial wall of pyriform sinus) without fixation of the larynx
T3:	Tumor limited to larynx with vocal fold fixation and/or invades any of the following: post-cricoid area, pre-epiglottic tissues
T4:	Tumor invades through the thyroid cartilage, and/or extends into soft tissues of the neck, thyroid, and/or esophagus
Glottis	
T1:	Tumor limited to vocal fold(s) (may involve anterior or posterior commissure) with normal mobility
T1a:	Tumor limited to one vocal fold
T1b:	Tumor involves both vocal folds
T2:	Tumor extends to supraglottis and/or subglottis, and/or with impaired vocal fold mobility
T3:	Tumor limited to the larynx with vocal fold fixation
T4:	Tumor invades through the thyroid cartilage and/or to other tissues beyond the larynx (e.g., trachea, soft tissues of neck, including thyroid gland, pharynx)
Subglottis	
T1:	Tumor limited to the subglottis
T2:	Tumor extends to vocal fold(s) with normal or impaired mobility
T3:	Tumor limited to larynx with vocal fold fixation
T4:	Tumor invades through cricoid or thyroid cartilage and/or extends to other tissues beyond the larynx (e.g., trachea, soft tissues of neck, including thyroid gland, esophagus)
Regional Lymph Nodes (N)	
NX:	Regional lymph nodes cannot be assessed
N0:	No regional lymph node metastasis
N1:	Metastasis in a single ipsilateral lymph node, 3 cm or less in greatest dimension
N2:	Metastasis in a single ipsilateral lymph node, more than 3 cm but not more than 6 cm in greatest dimension, or in multiple ipsilateral lymph nodes, none more than 6 cm in greatest dimension, or in bilateral or contralateral lymph nodes, none more than 6 cm in greatest dimension
N2a:	Metastasis in a single ipsilateral lymph node more than 3 cm but not more than 6 cm in greatest dimension
N2b:	Metastasis in multiple ipsilateral lymph nodes, none more than 6 cm in greatest dimension
N2c:	Metastasis in bilateral or contralateral lymph nodes, none more than 6 cm in greatest dimension
N3:	Metastasis in a lymph node more than 6 cm in greatest dimension

TABLE 12.1 (Continued)

Distant Metastasis (M)	
MX:	Distant metastasis cannot be assessed
M0:	No distant metastasis
M1:	Distant metastasis
Staging	
Stage 0 (Carcinoma in situ)	Abnormal cells in the lining of the larynx
Stage I	
Supraglottis:	Cancer is in one area of the supraglottis only and the folds can move normally.
Glottis:	Cancer is in one or both vocal folds and the vocal folds can move normally.
Subglottis:	Cancer is in the subglottis only.
Stage II	
Supraglottis:	Cancer is in more than one area of the supraglottis or surrounding tissues.
Glottis:	Cancer has spread to the supraglottis and/or the subglottis and/or the vocal folds do not move normally.
Subglottis:	Cancer has spread to one or both vocal folds, which may not move normally.
Stage III	
Supraglottis:	Cancer is in the larynx only and the vocal folds do not move normally, and/or cancer is in tissues adjacent to the larynx; cancer may have spread to one lymph node on the same side of the neck as the original tumor and the lymph node is smaller than 3 cm; or cancer is in one area of the supraglottis only and in one lymph node on the same side of the neck as the original tumor; the lymph node is smaller than 3 cm and the vocal folds can move normally; or cancer is in more than one area of the supraglottis or surrounding tissues and in one lymph node on the same side of the neck as the original tumor; the lymph node is smaller than 3 cm and/or the vocal folds do not move normally.
Glottis:	Cancer is in the larynx only and the vocal folds do not move normally, and/or cancer is in tissues adjacent to the larynx; cancer may have spread to one lymph node on the same side of the neck as the original tumor and the lymph node is smaller than 3 cm; or cancer is in one or both vocal folds and in one lymph node on the same side of the neck as the original tumor; the lymph node is smaller than 3 cm and the vocal folds can move normally; or cancer has spread to the supraglottis and/or the subglottis and/or the vocal folds do not move normally. The cancer has also spread to one lymph node on the same side of the neck as the original tumor and the lymph node is smaller than 3 cm.
Subglottis:	Cancer is in the larynx only and the vocal folds do not move normally; cancer may have spread to one lymph node on the same side of the neck as the original tumor and the lymph node is smaller than 3 cm; or cancer is in the subglottis only and in one lymph node on the same side of the neck as the original tumor; the lymph node is smaller than 3 cm; or cancer has spread to one or both vocal folds, which may not move normally, and to one lymph node on the same side of the neck as the original tumor; the lymph node is smaller than 3 cm.

(continued)

TABLE 12.1 **TNM Staging of Laryngeal Cancer (Continued)**

Stage IV Stage IV is divided into stage IVA, stage IVB, and stage IVC. Each substage is the same for the supraglottis, glottis, or subglottis.	
Stage IVA:	Cancer has spread through the thyroid cartilage and/or has spread to tissues beyond the larynx such as the neck, trachea, thyroid gland, or esophagus, and may have spread to one lymph node on the same side of the neck as the original tumor; the lymph node is smaller than 3 cm; or cancer has spread to one or more lymph nodes anywhere in the neck and the lymph nodes are smaller than 6 cm; cancer may have spread to tissues beyond the larynx, such as the neck, trachea, thyroid gland, or esophagus. Vocal folds may not move normally.
Stage IVB:	Cancer has spread to the space in front of the spinal column and surrounds the carotid artery, or has spread to parts of the chest and may have spread to one or more lymph nodes anywhere in the neck (the lymph nodes may be any size); or cancer has spread to a lymph node that is larger than 6 cm and may have spread as far as the space in front of the spinal column, around the carotid artery, or to parts of the chest. Vocal folds may not move normally.
Stage IVC:	Cancer has spread beyond the larynx to other parts of the body.

Source: Information from National Cancer Institute, www.cancer.gov/cancertopics/pdq/treatment/laryngeal/Patient/page2.

Risk Factors for Laryngeal Cancer

The main risk factors for developing laryngeal cancer are tobacco and alcohol consumption (e.g., De Stefani et al., 1987; Hinds, Thomas, & O'Reilly, 1979; Muscat & Wynder, 1992). Reportedly individuals who smoke more than 35 cigarettes per day have a relative risk of developing cancer that is 7 times greater than for nonsmokers. The combination of smoking and alcohol consumption increases the relative risk by 22 times (Mathieson, 2001). Heavy alcohol consumption even without smoking increases the risk of supraglottal cancer (Altieri, Garavello, Bosetti, Gallus, & La Vecchia, 2005; De Stefani et al., 1987; Hinds et al., 1979; Muscat & Wynder, 1992).

Factors other than tobacco and alcohol have also been associated with increased risk of laryngeal cancer, including HPV infection, GERD, consumption of red meat, inadequate intake of fruit and vegetables, and genetic susceptibility, particularly in women (Andrews, 1995; De Stefani et al., 1987; El-Serag, Hepworth, Lee, & Sonnenberg, 2001; Jaworowska et al., 2007; Koufman, 1991; Oreggia et al., 2001; Smith et al., 2000). On the other hand, it has been reported that a diet rich in fruit and vegetables can decrease the risk of laryngeal cancer independent of age, tobacco use, and alcohol consumption (Garavello et al., 2009).

Symptoms

Symptoms of laryngeal cancer vary depending on the location and stage of the disease. Glottic tumors result in hoarseness, breathiness, reduced loudness, increased vocal effort, and/or pain on phonation (Starmer, Tippett, & Webster, 2008). While hoarseness is most commonly associated with glottic and subglottic tumors, it can also occur with supraglottic disease, particularly if the cancer has spread to the vocal folds (Raitiola & Pukander, 2000). The greater is the extent of the tumor, the more severe is the dysphonia. The patient may also experience stridor and dyspnea if the tumor obstructs the airway. Supraglottic tumors tend to produce dysphagia (uncoordinated swallow, painful swallowing, aspiration), otalgia (pain in the ear), globus sensation, and swelling of the neck (Raitiola & Pukander, 2000; Starmer et al., 2008). Tumors in the subglottal area may result in pain and airway obstruction. Other symptoms can include persistent throat-clearing and coughing, persistent sore throat, halitosis (bad breath) and unexplained weight loss (Hairston & Wilson, 2006; Stemple et al., 2000).

Diagnosis

Cancer is diagnosed using a number of techniques. These include a physical examination by the physician to check for abnormal lumps and/or swelling of the lymph nodes in the neck, followed by flexible and/or rigid laryngeal endoscopy. Other diagnostic measures include CT scans and MRI to evaluate the extent of the tumor as well as to check for evidence of spread and/or invasion of cartilage (Holsinger, Howard, & McWhorter, 2008). As necessary, x-rays, modified barium swallow, and PET scans may be helpful.

Multidisciplinary Approach

Cancer is a disease that requires a team approach in order to provide the best possible clinical management and outcomes for the patient and his or her family. There are many options available for treatment, and often treatment includes a combination of modalities, requiring different areas of professional expertise. Table 12.2 lists the potential members of a laryngeal cancer team and a description of the primary responsibilities of each.

TABLE 12.2 Potential Members of an Interdisciplinary Laryngeal Cancer Diagnostic and Treatment Team

Team Member	Responsibilities
Head and neck surgeon	Diagnosis, organization of treatment plan; referral to other team members
Radiation oncologist	Evaluates viability of radiotherapy; optimal dosage levels and type
Medical oncologist	Administration of chemotherapy; palliative/pain care
Radiologist/nuclear medicine specialist	Performs and determines results of imaging studies; works with surgeon to plan appropriate treatment approaches
Pathologist	Examines tissue; reports on type of tumor; determines completeness of surgical excision of tumor
Internal medicine	Postoperative management of medical comorbidities such as heart disease, diabetes, and high blood pressure

(continued)

TABLE 12.2 Potential Members of an Interdisciplinary Laryngeal Cancer Diagnostic and Treatment Team (Continued)

Team Member	Responsibilities
Plastic surgeon	Performs reconstructive surgery to lessen the appearance of scarring or to improve function
Dental/maxillofacial prosthodontist	Makes prostheses for removed teeth or other oral structures
Nurse	Patient care in all phases of diagnosis and treatment; patient education regarding stoma care
Speech-language pathologist	Evaluates and provides treatment for short-term and long-term communication needs; evaluates and treats possible dysphagia; patient education
Registered dietician	Evaluates nutritional health prior to and following treatment; recommends caloric intake for optimal health and weight; counsels patient and families regarding nutritional health and well-being
Respiratory therapist	Evaluates and treats breathing and/or respiratory disorders; ventilator management; tracheostomy care
Mental health counselor	Provides counseling to patient and family regarding serious illness, potential death, end of life issues, postoperative depression, self-image, anger, role of family and/or caregivers
Physical/occupational therapist	Restores impaired movement or skills resulting from head and neck surgery, e.g., limited mobility of shoulder, neck, arms, or hands
Laryngectomized visitor	Helps to improve patient's morale and comfort with alaryngeal speech and other posttreatment issues

Source: Information from Sapienza & Ruddy (2009).

Medical Treatment

There are two primary modes of treatment for laryngeal cancer: radiation and/or chemotherapy either alone or in combination (called organ-preservation therapy), and surgery. Surgical techniques include various methods of tumor removal and resection of the whole or portions of the laryngeal structure, as well as neck dissection where indicated. Many treatments demonstrate comparable cancer control and survival rates, so choice of treatment is determined based on several factors. These include stage of cancer, potential side effects, probable functional outcomes in terms of voice and swallowing, patient needs and expectations, and quality of life considerations (Boscolo-Rizzo, Zanetti, Carpene, & Da Mosto, 2008; Chawla & Carney, 2009; Schindler et al., 2004; van der Torn, Verdonck-de-Leeuw, Kuik, & Mahieu, 2002).

RADIATION THERAPY

Radiation therapy (RT) has become quite popular in recent years as radiation treatment has become more refined, less time consuming, and less destructive of healthy tissue. RT preserves laryngeal function and is relatively cost-effective (Leeper, Parsa, Jamieson, & Heeneman,

TABLE 12.3 Potential Side Effects of Radiation Therapy

Loss of salivary and mucous glands
Xerostomia
Laryngitis sicca
Muscle atrophy
Fibrosis of soft tissues
Keratosis
Edema
Inflammation
Excess mucus accumulation
Erythema (redness)
Sore throat
Dysphagia
Loss of taste
Tooth damage
Tissue necrosis
Mucositis (mucosal injury characterized by erythema and ulcerative lesions)
Scar formation

Sources: Information from Bertino et al. (2001); Boscolo-Rizzo et al. (2008); Chawla & Carney (2009); Gultekin et al. (2010); Hairston & Wilson (2006); Leeper et al. (2002); Nakashima, Tomita, & Chitose (2005); Orlikoff & Krauss (1996); Pauloski (2008).

2002). Cure rates have been reported to be similar for radiotherapy and other approaches (Schindler et al., 2004; van der Torn et al., 2002). Cure rates of 80–90% have been reported after three years without recurrence, with fewer than 10% of patients needing a subsequent salvage laryngectomy (Mathieson, 2001). Radiotherapy may be used definitively as a single modality treatment; may be used concomitantly in conjunction with another treatment such as chemotherapy; or may be used as an adjuvant therapy following surgery to increase the potential for a successful outcome (Sapienza & Ruddy, 2009).

Side Effects. While radiation therapy preserves the larynx, it is associated with many side effects that can adversely impact both vocal and swallowing function (Table 12.3). Radiation dries out salivary and mucous glands resulting in xerostomia (dry mouth) and dehydrated laryngeal mucosa (Burns et al., 2009; Chawla & Carney, 2009; Leeper et al., 2002; Orlikoff & Kraus, 1996). Dehydrated mucosa can result in laryngitis sicca, a condition in which the vocal fold mucosa become dry and crusty. The dryness of the tissues is also associated with thick mucus accumulation and cracked epithelium within the vocal tract (Orlikoff & Kraus, 1996).

CHEMOTHERAPY

Chemotherapy may be used to treat laryngeal cancer either alone before surgery or radiation, or in conjunction with radiation therapy. Chemoradiation therapy is used as an alternative to primary laryngectomy (Fung et al., 2005). The aim is to reduce local and regional disease not only at the site of the tumor but also in more distant lymph nodes (Hairston & Wilson, 2006). An additional course of chemotherapy (adjuvant chemotherapy) may be necessary to eliminate any remaining disease after the initial treatment with radiation or chemotherapy (Hairston & Wilson, 2006). Chemotherapy may also be used to prevent or reverse the transformation of premalignant lesions (Hairston & Wilson, 2006). One such chemopreventive agent is cetuximab (Erbitux), which is a type of antibody that stops the growth of cancer cells. Radiotherapy plus cetuximab has been reported to significantly improve progression-free survival in patients with head and neck cancer (Bonner et al., 2006).

Voice and Swallowing Following Organ Preservation Treatment. While organ preservation therapy spares the larynx, the patient may be left with persisting voice and swallowing difficulties (Dworkin et al., 2003). Patients have reported symptoms such as speaking with effort, vocal fatigue, hoarseness, reduced dynamic range, reduced loudness, excessive coughing and/or throat clearing, unpredictable voice, and discomfort or pain on phonation (Hocevar-Boltezar, Zargi, & Strojan, 2009; Orlikoff & Kraus, 1996; Van Gogh et al., 2006). Videolaryngostroboscopy has shown various degrees of vocal fold edema, vocal fold atrophy, excessive supraglottic activity, tissue defects, scars, and changes in the mucosal wave following treatment (Hocevar-Boltezar et al., 2009; Krengli et al., 2004). Voice symptoms are exacerbated in patients who continue to smoke during and after treatment (Agarwal et al., 2009; Hocevar-Boltezar et al., 2009).

Individuals may also use maladaptive compensatory supraglottic behaviors to deal with their changed laryngeal status (Starmer et al., 2008). Because the vocal folds may be dehydrated they tend to be more susceptible to injury and inflammation. Throat irritation might lead to increased throat clearing and coughing that can further dry and irritate the tissues. The irradiated larynx may also be more susceptible to the effects of drying agents such as caffeine, alcohol, and antihistamines. However, despite the poorer vocal quality, it has been reported that patients with an intact larynx scored higher on voice-related quality of life measures than did laryngectomized patients (Fung et al., 2005). Many patients report a subjective improvement in voice quality after treatment, possibly resulting from loss of tumor bulk and resulting improved vibratory function of the vocal folds (e.g., Agarwal et al., 2009; Kazi et al., 2008; van Gogh et al., 2006). While vocal function does not become completely normal, improvements continue to be reported by patients and documented by acoustic measures one year after completion of radiation therapy (Kazi et al., 2008).

Patients whose vocal function is preserved but who demonstrate poor vocal quality and/or vocal effort and fatigue may benefit from voice therapy focusing on vocal hygiene, increased hydration, and more efficient vocal production. Maladaptive compensatory vocal behaviors such as glottic or supraglottic hyperfunction should be identified. Techniques to improve vocal function may be beneficial, including abdominal breath support, vocal function exercises to increase flexibility, resonant voice therapy, and circumlaryngeal massage (Starmer et al., 2008).

Swallowing dysfunction reportedly results from fibrosis, which affects movements of the oral tongue, tongue base, pharyngeal constrictors, and larynx, as well as from reduced salivary flow, xerostomia, and mucositis (Pauloski, 2008). Dysphagia may result in psychological distress and a sense of loss of the expected pleasure and satisfaction associated with eating (McQuestion, Fitch, & Howell, 2011). Swallowing disorders may persist many years after completion of radiotherapy (Pauloski, 2008).

Penetration of food or liquid into the larynx is common following chemoradiation, and swallowing problems may persist for a year following treatment (Logemann et al., 2008). If swallowing is affected, the speech-language pathologist can assist the patient in developing compensatory techniques such as chin-tuck and head rotation, or maneuvers such as supraglottic swallow.

Surgical Options for Laryngeal Cancer

Sometimes it is necessary to remove part or all of the larynx and some or all of the lymph nodes in the neck in order to eradicate the cancer. There are different types of surgical options depending on the site and extent of the tumor. A variety of partial laryngectomy procedures have been developed that are designed to remove cancerous tissue while preserving as much of the healthy structure as possible (Sewnaik, Hakkesteegt, Meeuwis, De Gier, & Kerrebijn, 2006). The goals of partial laryngectomy are to eliminate the need for a permanent tracheostomy, maintain laryngeal speech, and preserve the patient's swallow function (Robitschek, Peck, Klem, & Rassekh, 2009). The type of procedure that is chosen depends on the location and staging of the lesion, as well as other factors such as where the patient lives and his or her premorbid health status (Kempster, 2005). Procedures include resection of part or all of the affected vocal fold(s), vertical partial laryngectomy, supraglottic laryngectomy, supracricoid laryngectomy, near total laryngectomy, and total laryngectomy (Table 12.4). Because of the wide array of nonsurgical and surgical options that are available, it is important that a multidisciplinary team be involved in treatment decisions, including the head and neck surgical oncologist, radiation oncologist, medical oncologist, speech-language pathologist, as well as the patient and his or her family/caregivers (Moore, Holsinger, Diaz, & Weber, 2005).

TABLE 12.4 Partial Laryngectomy Procedures

Procedure	Indication	Structure(s) Removed
Cordectomy/resection	Single vocal fold; T1-T2; mobile folds	Portion of diseased fold plus a margin of healthy tissue
Vertical partial laryngectomy	Single side of larynx; T1-3; mobile folds; possible anterior commissure involvement	Vocal fold on affected side; possible vocal process or entire arytenoid; possible false vocal folds
Supraglottic laryngectomy	Epiglottis, false vocal folds; T1-T4	Hyoid, epiglottis, false vocal folds, aryepiglottic folds, superior portion of thyroid, possible portion of tongue base; possible arytenoid(s)
Supracricoid laryngectomy	Extensive spread beyond traditional Indications for VPL and SGL	
CHEP		True and false vocal folds; thyroid cartilage
CHP		True and false vocal folds; thyroid cartilage; epiglottis
Near total laryngectomy	Extensive spread confined to one side of the larynx	Entire vertical half of larynx plus a large portion of the healthy side

RESECTION

Resection, also called cordectomy, may be performed for a small (T1 or T2), well-defined tumor limited to the vocal fold. This surgery involves removing the diseased tissue together with a margin of healthy tissue around the tumor. The procedure can be performed either through an open approach or endoscopically. In an open approach for a glottic tumor the surgeon cuts through the anterior part of the thyroid cartilage to reach the affected fold. For a T1a glottic carcinoma the vocal ligament may be preserved (Brondbo & Benninger, 2004). More extensive T2 tumors may necessitate removal of the vocal ligament and part of the thyroarytenoid muscle (Brondbo & Benninger, 2004). The remaining tissue may either heal spontaneously, or may be reconstructed by means of a tissue flap taken from the false vocal folds (Bertino et al., 2001). The flap helps to maintain the bulk of the resected vocal fold because it maintains its blood and nerve supply (Robitschek et al., 2009).

The resection can be performed endoscopically with a laser. There is debate regarding the appropriateness of laser resection when the anterior commissure is involved. Some surgeons have proposed that laser resection is only appropriate for T1–T2 glottic and supraglottic lesions in which there is minimal to no involvement of the anterior commissure (Luscher et al., 2001; Moore et al., 2005). Other researchers have reported good results with the procedure in terms of cancer control and laryngeal function for speech and swallowing even when the anterior commissure is involved (Hartl et al., 2007; McWhorter & Hoffman, 2005).

Laser resection has several advantages. First, it is less invasive than open surgery (Holsinger et al., 2008). Second, it avoids the side effects of radiation and may preserve remaining vibratory tissue (Burns et al., 2009; Moore et al., 2005). Third, the procedure leaves open the possibility of laser re-excision or later radiation in case the cancer recurs or spreads (Burns et al., 2009; Chawla & Carney, 2009; Hartl et al., 2007; Luscher et al., 2001; Moore et al., 2005). Fourth, laser endoscopy preserves the sensory innervation of the larynx with better swallowing results (Chawla & Carney, 2009; Holsinger et al., 2008). Fifth, patients undergoing laser resection do not require a tracheotomy or feeding tube, can be discharged on the day of the surgery, and can resume normal activities immediately (Hartl et al., 2007; Moore et al., 2005; Schindler et al., 2004).

Voice and Swallowing Following Resection. The individual's voice quality after resection depends on several factors including the depth of the resection, the amount of tissue excised, whether or not the anterior commissure is preserved, and whether or not the patient uses maladaptive glottic or supraglottic compensatory behaviors (Bertino et al., 2001; Burns et al., 2009; Krengli et al., 2004; Moore et al., 2005; Schindler et al., 2004; Starmer et al., 2008). Patients may report increased vocal effort, the need to take frequent breaths, and difficulty with pitch and loudness control (Samlan & Webster, 2002). Videostroboscopic assessment may reveal glottic incompetence, decreased mucosal wave, and vocal fold stiffness (Starmer et al., 2008). When deeper layers of tissue (i.e., vocal ligament) have been excised, a band of scar tissue known as the *neocord* develops and can be used as a surrogate fold (McWhorter & Hoffman, 2005). However, the shape of the neocord is usually concave, which results in glottal insufficiency (Zeitels, 2004). Voice quality is not normal, and severe dysphonia has been observed in 70% of patients after laser surgery (Krengli et al., 2004). Despite the poor vocal quality, quality of life is not dramatically affected, with patients reporting minimal long-term handicap (e.g., Brondbo & Benninger, 2004; Cohen et al., 2006; Loughran, Calder, MacGregor, Carding, & MacKenzie, 2005).

Techniques such as injection medialization and Type I thyroplasty have been shown to improve glottic closure and improve voice quality after resection (McWhorter & Hoffman, 2005; Sittel, Friedrich, Zorowka, & Eckel, 2002; Zeitels, 2004). Behavioral voice therapy is important in helping the patient to acquire the most effective phonatory patterns and to decrease hyperfunctional behaviors (Bertino et al., 2001; Schindler et al., 2004; Zeitels, 2004). A program of vocal hygiene that focuses on improving hydration, avoiding vocally damaging behaviors, and reducing laryngeal irritants such as acid reflux or smoke can be extremely beneficial (Starmer et al., 2008). Vocal function exercises and resonant voice therapy can help to improve glottal closure, reduce supraglottal tension, and improve vocal fold flexibility (Starmer et al., 2008).

Because glottal insufficiency and the risk of aspiration may be present following resection, the patient's swallow function should be evaluated via modified barium swallow and/or FEES, and swallowing therapy techniques be used as appropriate (Pauloski, 2008; Starmer et al., 2008).

VERTICAL PARTIAL LARYNGECTOMY

Vertical partial laryngectomy (VPL) refers to a group of surgical procedures that vary in complexity and amount of tissue excised (Chawla & Carney, 2009; Wein & Weber, 2005). The procedures are all performed by vertically transecting (cutting across) the thyroid cartilage and resecting glottic tissue (Chawla & Carney, 2009; Wein & Weber, 2005). VPL is designed to treat early T1 and T2 glottic cancers and is suitable for tumors confined to one side of the larynx with mobile vocal folds (Chawla & Carney, 2009). VPL is done either as the initial procedure or as a salvage operation in cases where radiation or chemotherapy has not been successful (Robitschek et al., 2009; Yiotakis et al., 2003). High cure rates have been reported with preservation of laryngeal function (Dedivitis et al., 2008). The procedure has been used even when the anterior commissure is involved, with good control of the cancer and satisfactory laryngeal function (Davis, Hadley, & Smith, 2004).

The surgery involves removing the vocal fold on the affected side. Other structures on the affected side may be excised as well, including either the vocal process of the arytenoid cartilage or the entire cartilage, and the false vocal fold. The cricoid cartilage and epiglottis are typically left intact. A neocord forms as healing occurs, allowing the patient to produce a functional, although dysphonic voice.

Voice and Swallowing Following VPL. Reported laryngeal findings postsurgery include incomplete glottic closure, decreased and irregular mucosal wave and amplitude, abnormal arytenoid movement, supraglottal involvement in phonation, reduced maximum phonation time, high and more variable pitch, and restricted vocal intensity range (Pfuetzenreiter, Dedivitis, Queija, Bohn, & Barros, 2010; Singh et al., 2008; Starmer et al., 2008). Voice rehabilitation is important to maximize the patient's laryngeal function after all surgical procedures have been completed. Surgical medialization procedures such as injection or thyroplasty may be helpful in facilitating glottal closure following VPL (Woo, 1999). Alternatively, reconstruction of the glottic region using a flap of tissue taken from the sternohyoid muscle (Dedivitis et al., 2008; Dedivitis et al., 2010; Kempster, 2005) or from the false vocal folds (Wein & Weber, 2005) may be used to fill in the defect and allow for glottic and/or supraglottic function (Pfuetzenreiter et al., 2010). Reconstructive flap techniques have been shown to facilitate glottal and/or supraglottal vibration, with active participation of the flap during glottal vibration (Dedivitis et al., 2010). Videostroboscopy has demonstrated that structures involved in vibration include the remaining and reconstructed vocal folds, false vocal folds, and arytenoid mucosa (Dedivitis et al., 2010; Woo, 1999).

Individuals who have undergone VPL, either with or without reconstructive surgery have been reported to demonstrate poorer acoustic and perceptual results compared to normal speakers (Dedivitis et al., 2008; Singh et al., 2008). The main advantage of VPL is the avoidance of a permanent tracheostoma and preservation of swallowing (Singh et al., 2008). Patient satisfaction rates of greater than 95% have been reported following this type of procedure (Wein & Weber, 2005).

Aspiration of food and/or liquids is not typically a problem unless the arytenoid cartilage is removed, which decreases the effectiveness of airway closure (Pauloski, 2008). Reportedly, patients can tolerate oral intake the day following surgery (Pfuetzenreiter et al., 2010). Most patients regain normal swallowing with one month of surgery (Starmer et al., 2008).

SUPRAGLOTTIC LARYNGECTOMY

A supraglottic laryngectomy (SGL) may be performed when the tumor occurs on the epiglottis and false vocal folds, without any spread to more inferior structures such as the thyroid cartilage or anterior commissure (Rosen & Pou, 2000). Structures excised in this procedure depend on the extent of the tumor and may include the epiglottis, aryepiglottic folds, false vocal folds, and the superior portion of the thyroid cartilage (Hornig, Wilhoit, Sonne, & Schaefer, 2008; Remacle et al., 2009; Sasaki, Leder, Acton, & Maune, 2006). The hyoid bone may or may not be removed (Pauloski, 2008). Part of the tongue base may also be resected if the cancer has spread upward (Kempster, 2005). The epiglottis may be surgically reconstructed to prevent aspiration (Andrews, 1995). Occasionally one or both arytenoid cartilages may be removed, in which case the vocal fold is sutured to the cricoid cartilage (Hornig et al., 2008). The vocal folds themselves are left intact, thus preserving the patient's phonatory function (Chun et al., 2010; Remacle et al., 2009).

SGL can be performed through an open approach via the thyroid cartilage, or endoscopically via laser. Open procedures are more appropriate for bulky T2 lesions and selected T3/T4 lesions (Wein & Weber, 2005). Endoscopic removal is considered when the lesion is small and can be completely visualized (Burns et al., 2009; Wright, 2007). In addition, it is crucial that sufficient margins of tissue around the tumor can be excised (Chun et al., 2010; Remacle et al., 2009). The advantages of the endoscopic laser procedure include avoiding a tracheostomy, preserving phonatory function, shorter hospital stay, and shorter time for recovery of swallowing (Chun et al., 2010; Peretti et al., 2006; Remacle et al., 2009). Swallowing recovery is enhanced because the extrinsic laryngeal muscles and hyoid bone are left intact, and the superior laryngeal nerve is preserved (Remacle et al., 2009; Starmer et al., 2008).

Voice and Swallowing Following SGL. Changes to the supraglottic larynx can alter the resonant characteristics of the vocal tract resulting in a "muffled" voice quality that is difficult to project (Chun et al., 2010; Starmer et al., 2008). Patients may therefore use hyperfunctional phonatory patterns to order to produce a louder voice. Voice rehabilitation focuses on reducing hyperfunctional phonation, encouraging good vocal hygiene, and increasing vocal capacity through resonant voice therapy and vocal function exercises.

The risk of aspiration is increased following surgery because structures important in airway protection during swallowing are affected (Oeken, Hansch, Thiel, & Bootz, 2001; Pauloski, 2008; Starmer et al., 2008). Resection of the superior laryngeal nerve interferes with sensory function, which results in difficulties with bolus recognition and also weakens the glottic closure reflex (Sasaki et al., 2006). Sasaki et al. (2006) compared swallow function in patients who underwent open versus laser resection. All subjects with laser resection exhibited a glottic closure reflex both before and after surgery and demonstrated minimal aspiration of saliva. Patients who had undergone open supraglottic laryngectomy demonstrated increased aspiration and decreased glottic closure reflex. Patients are likely to need intensive swallow rehabilitation, particularly following open surgery. Individuals are taught strategies for airway protection during swallowing, such as the supraglottic and super supraglottic maneuvers. These techniques facilitate airway closure before and during the swallow (Starmer et al., 2008).

SUPRACRICOID LARYNGECTOMY

Supracricoid laryngectomy (SCL) is a partial but extensive laryngectomy used for selected T3 or T4 lesions in which the cancer has spread beyond the point where VPL or SGL would be appropriate (Ferlito et al., 2002; Lai & Weinstein, 2009). There are two versions of the surgical procedure, depending on the extent of the cancer and whether or not the epiglottis is preserved (Schindler et al., 2005). Both versions involve creating a surgical fixation (**pexy**) between remaining laryngeal structures. In a cricohyoidoepiglottopexy (CHEP) the membranous portion of the true vocal folds, false vocal folds, and the entire thyroid cartilage are resected. The larynx is then reconstructed by suturing the cricoid cartilage to the hyoid bone and the epiglottis. Following reconstruction the arytenoid cartilages adjoin each other as well as the epiglottis, changing the normal V-shape glottis to a T-shape (Lai & Weinstein, 2009). Cricohyoidopexy (CHP) is more extensive, with resection of the membranous portions of the true vocal folds, false folds, the epiglottis, and the entire thyroid cartilage. Reconstruction involves suturing the cricoid cartilage to the hyoid bone. After CHP the arytenoids adjoin each other and the tongue base, which also gives the glottis a T-shape (Lai & Weinstein, 2009).

SCL with CHEP or CHP can be used either as the initial approach or for surgical salvage after radiation (Holsinger et al., 2005; Luna-Ortiz, Pasche, Tamez-Velarde, & Villavicencio-Valencia, 2009; Marchese-Ragona, Marioni, Chiarello, Staffieri, & Pastore, 2005). Reportedly, the surgical reconstruction recreates the airway and improves swallowing to the point where even one arytenoid can be sacrificed if necessary (Holsinger et al., 2005). Because the surgery spares at least one functioning cricoarytenoid joint laryngeal phonation is possible (Dworkin et al., 2003; Eksteen, Rieger, Nesbitt, & Seikaly, 2003; Ferlito et al., 2002; Goncalves et al., 2010; Makeieff, Giovanni, & Guerrier, 2007; Schindler et al., 2005; Sewnaik et al., 2006; Webster, Samlan, Jones, Bunton, & Tufano, 2010). Vibration is produced when the functioning arytenoid cartilage makes contact against either the epiglottis or the base of the tongue (Makeieff et al., 2007; Schindler et al., 2005; Sewnaik et al., 2006). When both arytenoid cartilages are intact the arytenoids adduct and contact each other, with one arytenoid cartilage generally moving to a greater extent and overlapping the other cartilage (Makeieff et al., 2007).

Voice and Swallowing Following SCL. Voice quality after SCL with either CHEP or CHP has been reported to be breathy, hoarse, rough, and strained, with difficulties in pitch and intensity variation (Makeieff et al., 2007; Nakayama et al., 2008; Portas et al., 2009; Schindler et al., 2005; Sewnaik et al., 2006; Torrejano & Guimaraes, 2009; Webster et al., 2010). Anatomic factors such as the degree of arytenoid mobility, site of mucosal vibration, and sphincteric closure of the reconstructed glottis have been reported to be widely variable among speakers (So, Yun, Baek, Jeong, & Son, 2009). Acoustic analysis has demonstrated reductions of MPT as well as excessive noise in the signal and a variable and inconsistent F0 (e.g., Di Nicola, Fiorella, Spinelli, & Fiorella, 2006; Dworkin et al., 2003; Saito, Araki, Ogawa, & Shiotani, 2009). Despite the dysphonia, however, most speakers who have undergone SCL have been reported to show minimal handicap on the VHI. Individuals have indicated satisfaction with their voice-related quality of life, and many have been able to return to work or to other premorbid activities (e.g., Moore et al., 2005; Nakayama et al., 2008; Portas et al., 2009; Saito et al., 2009; Schindler et al., 2005; Sewnaik et al., 2006). Some speakers, however, have expressed moderate difficulty in their ability to communicate because of the need to exert physical effort in order to phonate (Dworkin et al., 2003).

Because the structures that participate in airway protection during swallowing are resected (i.e., vocal folds and epiglottis), swallowing function after surgery is affected, and patients may be at risk for aspiration (Simonelli et al., 2010; Webster et al., 2010). Swallowing therapy is therefore indicated until the patient's feeding tube can be safely removed (Dworkin et al., 2003). Usually, patients are able to return to a normal oral diet by the end of the rehabilitation period (Dworkin et al., 2003; Nakayama et al., 2008; Saito et al., 2009; Simonelli et al., 2010). However, silent aspiration has been reported as prevalent and as persisting for some patients even at 12 months postsurgery (e.g., Webster et al., 2010).

NEAR TOTAL LARYNGECTOMY

When the cancerous lesion is extensive but confined to one side of the larynx and there is no invasion of the interarytenoid space, a near total laryngectomy (NTL) may be the most appropriate surgical procedure (Kavabata, Neto, Goncalves, Alcadipani, & Menezes, 2004). This procedure is also called an extended hemilaryngectomy or subtotal laryngectomy. The entire vertical half of the cancerous larynx is removed, as well as a large portion of the healthy side. This procedure creates a shunt that connects the trachea and pharynx (Bernaldez et al., 2003; Kempster, 2005). The shunt is formed by the tracheal wall on the healthy side, a portion of the subglottic area, a small remnant of the vocal fold and arytenoid cartilage, the false vocal fold, and the aryepiglottic fold. The intrinsic laryngeal muscles and the recurrent laryngeal nerve of the healthy side must be preserved to prevent aspiration (Bernaldez et al., 2003; Globlek et al., 2004, 2005; Kempster, 2005). However, the patient still needs a permanent tracheostoma through which to breathe, because the shunt is too narrow and flaccid for respiration (Globlek et al., 2004, 2005). The advantage of this procedure is that voicing is possible without a voice prosthesis when the patient occludes the stoma and pulmonary air from the trachea is directed through the shunt into the pharynx (Ferlito et al., 2002). The upper end of the shunt appears to be the vibratory source for phonation (Kasperbauer & Thomas, 2004).

Voice and Swallowing Following Near Total Laryngectomy. Most individuals who have undergone NTL are reportedly able to produce a functional, although dysphonic, voice (e.g., Bernaldez et al., 2003; Hanamitsu, Kataoka, Takeuchi, & Kitajima, 1999; Kavabata et al., 2004; Pearson, DeSanto, Olsen, & Salassa, 1998). It is necessary to occlude the stoma in order to produce voice, and patients may do this either manually or with a tracheostoma valve (Kasperbauer & Thomas, 2004). Aspiration may be a problem if the shunt is too large, and persistent moderate or severe aspiration may necessitate revision or closure of the shunt (Kasperbauer & Thomas, 2004).

TOTAL LARYNGECTOMY

When the cancer is extremely extensive or when other methods of treatment have failed, a total laryngectomy (TL) (Figure 12.2) may be required. Reportedly, 25–37% of individuals who have undergone chemotherapy and/or radiation require a subsequent total laryngectomy (called a salvage total laryngectomy) to control the cancer (Graville, Palmer, Wax, & Andersen, 2009). In a total laryngectomy the entire laryngeal framework is removed including the hyoid bone, and often the upper tracheal rings as well. The trachea is bent forward and sutured to a permanent tracheostoma created in the patient's neck (Figure 12.3).

FIGURE 12.2 **Total Laryngectomy**

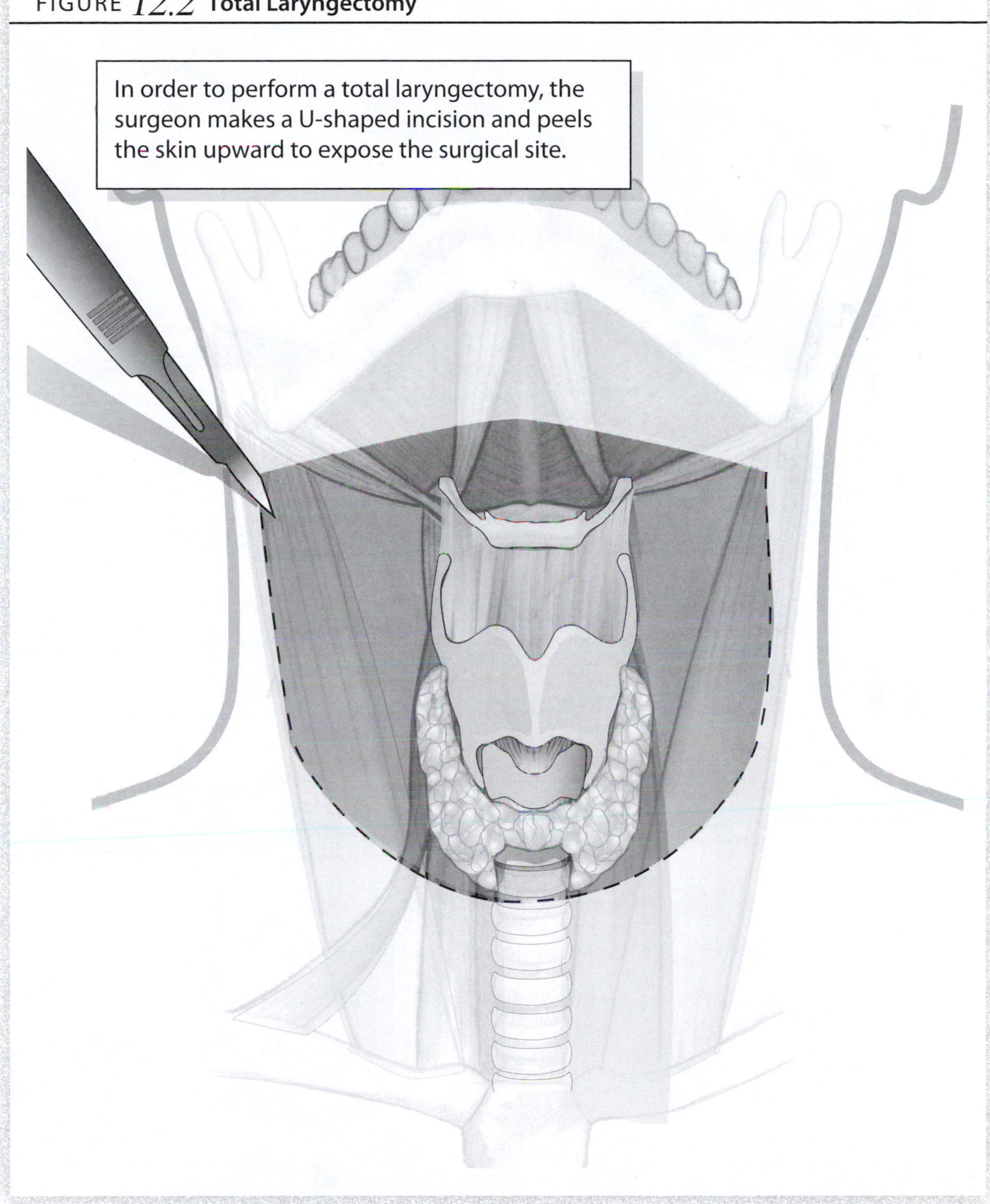

FIGURE 12.3 Trachea Sutured to Stoma

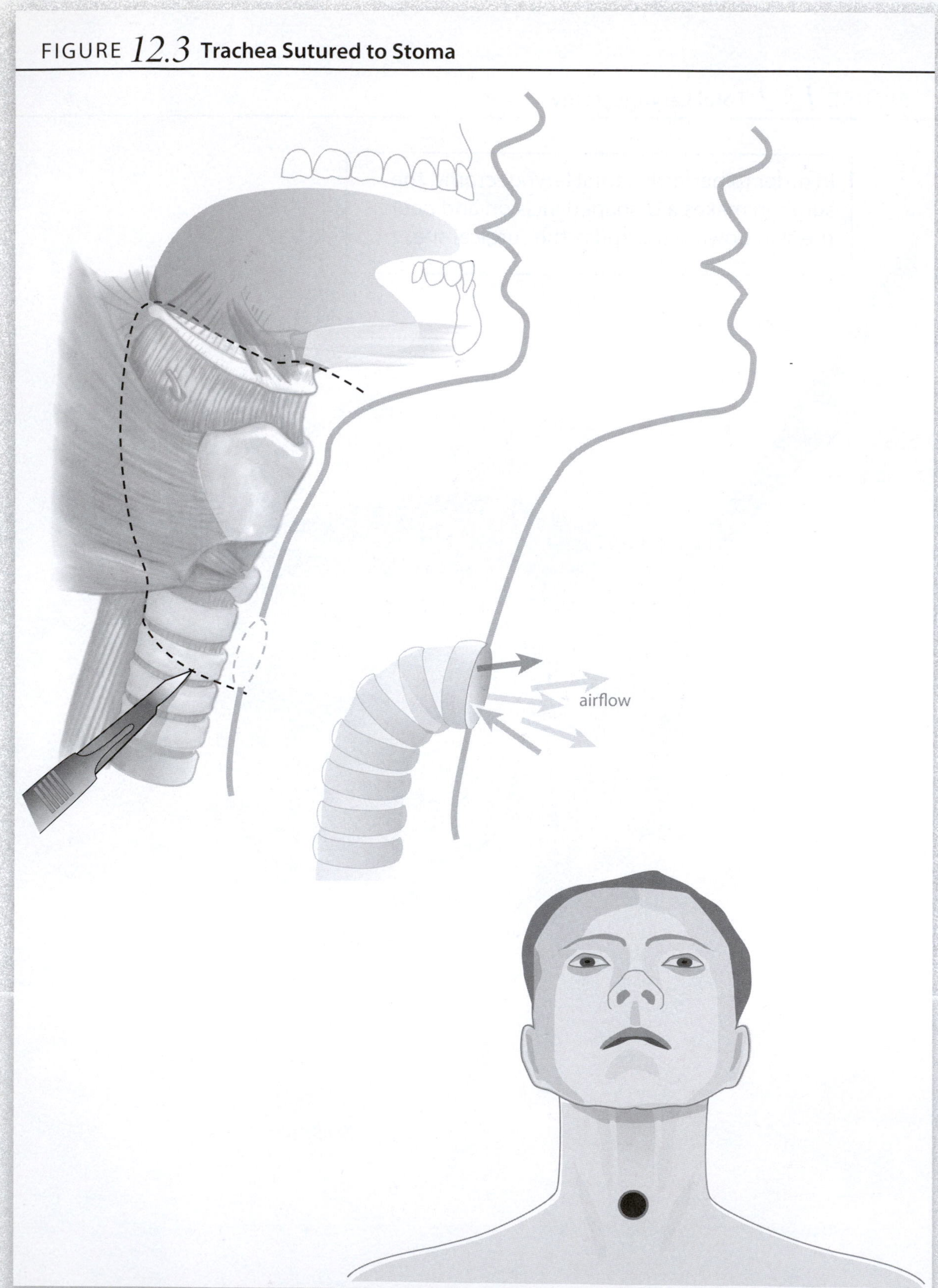

In cases where the cancer has invaded the lymph nodes, a neck dissection is performed to remove the lymph nodes. The basic structure of the respiratory system is changed, and air is transported into and out of the individual's lungs directly from the trachea. In addition, surgical reconstruction of mucosal deficits of the pharynx is sometimes necessary to ensure that the patient is able to swallow safely (Deschler, 2005).

PROBLEMS RELATED TO SURGERY

By its nature, TL has physical, psychosocial, and communicative consequences (Table 12.5). The speech-language pathologist working with a laryngectomized person needs to be aware of these problems and be comfortable in either dealing with them directly or referring the patient to the appropriate professional. A team approach to voice restoration and rehabilitation is crucial to ensure the best possible care for the patient in terms of the entire spectrum of potential difficulties and rehabilitation requirements. Preoperative and postoperative counseling and professional support for the patient and his or her family are integral to the rehabilitative process.

Air Conditioning Functions of the Nasal Passageways. In the normal airway inhaled air is warmed, moistened, and filtered by passage through the nasal cavities (Bien, Okla, van As-Brooks, & Ackerstaff, 2010; Zuur et al., 2009). With the removal of the larynx, the individual breathes solely through the stoma, which adversely affects this air conditioning process. Air inhaled directly into the trachea bypasses the nasal route and is therefore considerably dryer and cooler (Fuller, 2006). Nasal inhalation of air with a temperature of 22 degrees C and

TABLE 12.5 Physical, Psychosocial, and Communication Consequences of Total Laryngectomy

Physical
Stoma irritation
Excess mucus production
Mucous plug
Increased coughing
Stoma care
Stoma size
Reduction in upper body strength
Loss of arm, shoulder, and neck movement
Loss of smell and taste
Dysphagia
Xerostomia
Frequent colds
Chronic pain
Shortness of breath

(continued)

TABLE 12.5 Physical, Psychosocial, and Communication Consequences of Total Laryngectomy (Continued)

Psychosocial
Changed body image
Loss of self-esteem
Changed financial status
Changed family relationships
Fear of cancer return
Depression
Anger
Irritability
Isolation
Communication
Loss of normal voicing
Difficulty acquiring alternative voicing

Sources: Information from Bien et al. (2010); Cady (2002); Depondt & Gehanno (1995); Fuller (2006); Paleri et al. (2006); Pauloski (2008); Risberg-Berlin et al. (2009); Scheenstra et al. (2009); Zuur et al. (2009).

30–40% relative humidity (RH) increases the temperature up to 31–32 degrees C and raises RH up to 95–99% at the level of the pharynx; inhaling air through a tracheostoma increases the temperature only to 27–28 degrees C and 50% RH at the level of the trachea (Bien et al., 2010; Zuur, Muller, de Jongh, van Zandwijk, & Hilgers, 2006). The cool dry air tends to irritate the stoma and trachea, particularly at the beginning stages of recovery. The loss of heat and humidity in the airways results in increased viscosity of mucus within the tracheobronchial tree, thickening and crusting of the mucus, and excess mucus production (Bien et al., 2010; Scheenstra et al., 2009). The result is an increase in the amount, severity and frequency of coughing, increase of forced expectoration of **sputum** (mucus and other matter brought up from the airways), and other pulmonary complaints such as shortness of breath (Bien et al., 2010; Fuller, 2006, Zuur et al., 2009).

There are several ways to deal with this situation. A laryngectomized individual may choose to wear a stoma cover, to prevent debris, dust, and particles from entering the stoma and the trachea. The cover also helps to warm the air within the space between it and the stoma, and it helps absorb mucus. Also available are perforated stoma guards, worn between the stoma and the stoma cover, which prevent the cover from being sucked up against the stoma while the patient is breathing (Deem & Miller, 2000). A "laryngectomy bib" serves a similar function by absorbing mucus and warming inspired air.

Heat and Moisture Exchangers. Commercial heat and moisture exchange (HME) systems are available for filtering and warming the inhaled air. These systems use a piece of foam located in a housing unit, which is kept in place over the stoma by means of adhesive tape. The foam acts as a condensation and absorption surface (Zuur et al., 2006). The patient inhales and exhales through the foam, which pulls air warmed by the body during inhalation and collects moisture from the exhaled air. The subsequent cycle of inhaled air is humidified by the moisture on the tracheal side of the foam (Fuller, 2006). As the patient inhales, the air is filtered and humidified by the natural moisture in the material created by the condensations from the exhalations and warmed by the material. Use of an HME has been reported to increase the temperature of inhaled air to an average of 29–30 degrees C and to add up to 65–70% RH (Acton, 2004; Zuur et al., 2006). An HME system more closely simulates the warming and moistening of air that occurs in normal breathing and reduces the buildup of mucus and the resulting irritation around the stoma and in the trachea. Reportedly, use of an HME reduces water loss from about 500 ml to 250–300 ml per day (Bien et al., 2010). While normal levels of moistening and warming are not reached (Zuur et al., 2009), using an HME has numerous benefits including reduced mucus production, reduction in number of coughs per day, reduced dyspnea, reduction in airway clearing and frequency of expectoration, and decreased incidence of airway infections (Bien et al., 2010; Fuller, 2006; Hilgers & Ackerstaff, 2005; Zuur et al., 2006). Other benefits of using an HME include easier production of alaryngeal voice with less fatigue and improved quality, decreased sleep problems, and decreased levels of anxiety and depression (Fuller, 2006; Hilgers & Ackerstaff, 2005). Breathing through the foam does increase inspiratory and expiratory resistance, but most laryngectomized speakers adapt to the increased resistance within a week.

However, not all laryngectomized individuals are able to tolerate an HME, due to factors such as skin irritation from the cassette, dislodgement of the adhesive that keeps the housing unit in place, increased mucus production, increased coughing, and perceived difficulty of breathing against increased resistance (e.g., Scheenstra et al., 2009).

Stoma Size and Care. The size of the stoma is an important factor. Large stomas can be difficult for the patient to occlude manually for the production of voice, therefore leading to excessive stoma noise and reduced airflow through a speaking valve (Paleri, Wight, Owen, Hurren, & Stafford, 2006). A narrow stoma can be difficult to clean, with the risk of complete airway obstruction (Paleri et al., 2006). A narrow stoma can also create difficulties with the care and replacement of a speech valve and can prevent the individual from using an HME because the device can cause unacceptable airway restriction or swelling of the stoma (Paleri et al., 2006). A stoma that is too narrow may be surgically revised if deemed necessary by the patient and the surgeon.

The cleaning and care of the stoma is a crucial skill that must be learned by the patient and/or by the caregivers in his or her environment. The patient may not be able to clean the stoma if he or she has manual dexterity problems (e.g., arthritis), or lacks the cognitive ability to do so (e.g., dementia). Therefore, people in the individual's environment also need to be familiar with the proper care and maintenance of the stoma. Stoma care is taught either by a nurse and/or a speech-language pathologist while the patient is in the hospital. Part of stoma care is the necessity of avoiding getting water in the stoma. Special stoma covers are available, to prevent water from entering the trachea during showering and bathing.

Feeding and Swallowing Issues. A common difficulty following TL is limited or absent saliva production and xerostomia, particularly if the patient has undergone radiotherapy (Cady, 2002; Depondt & Gehanno, 1995). This may necessitate liquid feeding, which can contribute to loss of appetite and weight loss (Depondt & Gehanno, 1995). Aspiration is not encountered after TL because of the separation between the airway and digestive passageways. However, other problems such as insufficient pressure to move the bolus of food may be present (Pauloski, 2008). Loss of smell and taste that are commonly associated with TL may also contribute to the patient's loss of appetite and feeding difficulties (Cady, 2002; Risberg-Berlin, Ryden, Moller, & Finizia, 2009).

Additional Problems. Loss of smell can create safety problems because the patient may inhale irritating fumes or even toxic gases directly into the lungs without being aware of it (Cady, 2002). Other physical consequences of total laryngectomy are reductions in upper body strength (Fuller, 2006), chronic pain, and possible loss of arm, neck, and shoulder function from neck dissection.

Psychosocial Challenges. Social, emotional, and psychological issues are very likely to arise after total laryngectomy. Voice, self-concept, and personality are closely interwoven, and loss of voice or changed voice can negatively affect the individual's psyche. A difficult adjustment for many patients is the bodily disfigurement that results from the stoma and the neck dissection. These changes can impact the individual's body image, with resulting loss of self-esteem. Additionally, the laryngectomized individual must cope with serious changes that can affect his or her financial status, family relationships, and career. He or she may face concurrent health threats, fear of return or spread of cancer, and a changed role within the family (Graham, 2004). The person may not be able to return to work because of symptoms, fatigue, fear of rejection by colleagues and clients, or because the employer may fire or demote him or her following surgery (Cady, 2002). Patients may experience a variety of negative emotions including depression, anger and irritability, anxiety, loss of self-esteem, suicidal thoughts, feeling useless, shame, fear of recurrence, and a sense of inferiority (Cady, 2002). The person may isolate himself or herself from friends and family (Depondt & Gehanno, 1995). Individuals may feel that they have less control over their lives, and that their vocational or social outlets have become restricted (Salmon, 2005). It is not uncommon for patients to go through a grieving process as they learn to adjust to their changed circumstances. Families of the patient may also experience stress and feel guilt about their perceived role in the illness process (Cady, 2002). An important issue for some laryngectomized individuals is to recognize the influence of alcohol abuse on the patient's coping skills. Many laryngectomized speakers suffer from alcohol abuse, and the stress of diagnosis and treatment or postoperative depression may exacerbate this behavior (Cady, 2002).

Proper counseling and development of a supportive network of family, friends, and other laryngectomized speakers helps the newly laryngectomized individual to cope with these challenges. Patients and families should be supportively counseled preoperatively by the speech-language pathologist as well as by mental health professionals. Strategies should be discussed verbally and written materials provided regarding effective symptom management, symptoms to monitor for and report, safety issues, nutritional and speech therapy support, and support with effective coping strategies (Cady, 2002).

Voice Restoration

Normal voicing is not possible after total laryngectomy, and the aim of treatment is to provide the patient an alternative source of voicing. An important element in the rehabilitation process is pre- and post-surgery counseling by the speech-language pathologist. Before the scheduled surgery, the clinician should meet with the patient and his or her family to discuss the surgical procedure, likely problems postoperatively including communication and swallowing, the rehabilitation process, and different methods of voice restoration. During this visit, the SLP can assess the patient's presurgical communication abilities as a way of preparing for postoperative communication. The clinician should also evaluate the individual's coping skills, level of motivation, interpersonal interactions with family, and other psychosocial factors likely to impact the rehabilitation process. The more prepared the individual, the more likely it is that he or she will respond positively to the surgery and to the voice restoration process. During the preoperative visit, the speech-language pathologist may bring along a laryngectomized speaker, to show the patient that life after the surgery can be productive and fulfilling. Even if not during the preoperative session with the patient, a meeting with a well-adjusted and communicative laryngectomized speaker is crucial during postoperative counseling and rehabilitation. Also during these early sessions, the clinician begins to introduce the various options for communication. The speech-language professional may bring along different types of artificial larynges for the patient to try, if the surgeon finds that there is no medical reason to prevent this. Being able to communicate with an artificial larynx while still in the hospital can be very motivating for the patient. In addition to focusing on communication, the speech language pathologist should provide swallowing exercises for the patient in order to prevent swallowing disorders before they develop (Pauloski, 2008).

There are three main methods of voice restoration: artificial larynx (AL), esophageal speech (ES), and tracheoesophageal speech (TES) (Table 12.6). The patient may use one or a combination of methods, depending on his or her anatomical features, communication needs, motivation, cognitive functioning, hearing status, and individual preference. Research has shown that approximately 44% of individuals who responded to various surveys used AL speech, 22% used ES, and 29% used TES as their primary method of communication (Gelman, 1995; Hillman, Walsh, Wolf, Fisher, & Hong, 1998; Salmon, 2005). Many of the respondents used one primary technique, but they also used other means of voicing as a backup. For example, approximately 40% of TES and ES speakers reported also using AL speech, and around 10% of TE and AL speakers reported using ES.

For each of these voice restoration methods the primary goals are consistent voicing on demand, intelligible speech with good articulatory precision, appropriate intonation with flexible pitch and loudness levels, and minimal visual and/or auditory distractions (Glaze, 2005; Graham, 2006; Salmon, 2005).

TABLE 12.6 **Methods of Voice Restoration: Esophageal Speech (ES), Tracheoesophageal Speech (TE), and Artificial Larynx Speech (AL)**

ES	TE	AL
Air is injected into the esophagus and expelled, causing vibration of the PE segment.	A puncture is created between the trachea and esophagus. A one-way valve allows air from the trachea to pass into the esophagus and be expelled, causing vibration of the PE segment.	Handheld AL is placed against the neck, chin, or cheek. Vibrations from the device pass into the oral cavity and are articulated. Intraoral device has small tube, which is placed in the mouth to conduct vibrations into the oral cavity

ARTIFICIAL LARYNX

The artificial larynx (AL) is probably the quickest and easiest method of voice generation. The AL generates an external sound that can be transferred to the patient's vocal tract and articulated into speech sounds. There are two primary ways of achieving this: pneumatic devices and electronic devices. Pneumatic-type devices are designed to take advantage of the patient's own pulmonary air. The device consists of a tube within which is a reed or membrane that vibrates in response to air passing over it (Slavin, 1997). At one end of the tube is a mouthpiece, and at the other is a stoma cover. The patient inhales through the stoma and covers the stoma during exhalation. Air is thus forced through the tube and into the speaker's oral cavity. The sound that is generated is articulated into speech. The advantage of pneumatic-type devices is that the speech, while low in pitch, is normal in terms of phrasing and does not sound robotic. However, this type of device is inconvenient for everyday functioning since it requires two hands to use: one to cover the stoma, and the other to hold the mouthpiece in place. Pneumatic devices are not currently in frequent use in the United States. They are more commonly used in countries in South and East Asia where intonation and pitch are particularly important linguistic markers in languages such as Mandarin, Cantonese, and Taiwanese (Xu et al., 2009).

Electronic-type devices do not depend on the patient's respiratory system, but generate a tone electronically. Similar to the pneumatic type, the tone is transmitted to the patient's vocal tract either via the neck or the mouth. The mouth (trans-oral) type channels the electronically generated tone into a small plastic tube, which the person holds in the mouth. The generator is contained in a small case, which the patient can clip to an article of clothing or keep in a pocket. The individual uses the on-off switch to coordinate appropriate voicing and articulation. The mouth type is often used immediately after surgery, as it does not interfere with healing of the neck and throat area. This type of device is also useful for patients who are not able to use a neck-type device because of scarred or wasted neck tissue.

The neck-type (trans-cervical) instruments are the most popular (Liu & Ng, 2007). The individual holds the device firmly against his or her neck, and the sound is transmitted through the neck tissues into the vocal tract. Speakers learn to use the on-off switch to coincide with voiced and voiceless sounds. Many different makes are available with different pitch and volume changing capabilities, and different weights, sizes, and shapes. The tone produced does tend to sound mechanical and robotic. However, some devices, particularly more current models, include switches and buttons to regulate pitch and intensity.

Placement of the neck-type artificial larynx is very important. Poor interface between the device and the patient's neck can produce noise, which interferes with intelligibility (Liu & Ng, 2007). The speaker needs to experiment to find the optimal placement for the device so that the electronic buzz is reduced and the sound is perceived as coming from the mouth (Graham, 2006). This is sometimes referred to as the "sweet spot." The speaker should explore which hand to use to hold the AL and which side of the neck provides the best results (Doyle, 2005). Neck devices are suitable for individuals who have neck tissue on at least one side that is healthy, soft, and supple, to facilitate the transmission of the sound (Deem & Miller, 2000; Slavin, 1997).

Some devices can be used either trans-cervically or trans-orally. For example, the SolaTone™ neck-type AL (Griffin Laboratories) can be fitted with an oral adaptor. This is useful, as the patient can utilize the oral adaptor immediately after surgery as his or her neck is healing, and then continue to use the same device trans-cervically when the neck is sufficiently healed.

A prerequisite for successful use of an artificial larynx is that the person must have adequate manual dexterity to be able to use the various switches and to coordinate the sound with the beginning and ending of each utterance. It is more convenient if the individual can learn to use his or her nondominant hand to operate the device, leaving the dominant hand free for normal everyday use.

While the AL is easy to use, intelligibility may be less than optimal due to lack of intonational variability as well as the lack of contrast between voiced and voiceless sounds. Lack of contrast between voiced and voiceless consonants occurs if the device continues to operate during voiceless sounds (Liu & Ng, 2007; Meltzner & Hillman, 2005). Therefore, intelligibility training should focus on helping the speaker to make the adjustments necessary to coordinate the on-off switch on the device with the quick onset and offset of voice needed to distinguish between voiced and voiceless sounds. A slightly slower than normal rate of speech may also help to improve intelligibility. In addition, the patient may benefit from exercises for the lip, tongue, and jaw to improve articulatory strength and precision (Graham, 2006).

Speech breathing patterns also affect intelligibility. AL speakers tend to use atypical speech breathing behaviors including relatively long periods of breath holding interspersed with random inhalations and exhalations, and to speak on inhalation (Bohnenkamp, Stowell, Hesse, & Wright, 2010; Stepp, Heaton, & Hillman, 2008). AL speakers have been reported to demonstrate an elevated resting expiratory level, to use higher values of VC than laryngeal speakers, and to consistently speak into the functional residual capacity (Bohnenkamp et al., 2010). More natural and fluent-sounding speech can be facilitated by modifying the patient's speech breathing patterns. The client is taught to time his or her inhalations with natural linguistic breaks in the utterance and to speak only on exhalations. The person is also encouraged to reduce the forcefulness of exhalation during speech in order to decrease the occurrence of stoma noise (Graham, 2006).

An important component of the rehabilitation process is helping the speaker to eliminate or reduce auditory and visual distractions that can negatively impact the intelligibility and acceptability of his or her speech. A common distractor in AL speech is the delay in the communication interaction if the person has difficulty finding the "sweet spot" on the neck, or has to spend time looking for the device inside a purse or pocket (Salmon, 2005). Another common distractor is the extraneous noise from the device that occurs immediately before or after an utterance, or if the speaker accidentally applies pressure against the activation button (Salmon, 2005).

Advantages and Disadvantages of Artificial Larynges. An important advantage of the AL is that it is easy to use and may be used very soon, or even immediately, after the surgery. Loss of voice is a frightening and disheartening experience, so the sooner the patient is able to communicate the less psychological stress he or she will likely suffer. In addition, the speaker's intelligibility is typically relatively good, even during the beginning of the learning process. Other advantages include the high intensity level that can be very useful in noisy situations and the low maintenance that is required. Some patients use an artificial larynx as their only means of voicing, while others may use one as an adjunct for difficult speaking situations or when they are fatigued.

There are two major disadvantages of this method. The chief one is the inconvenience of having to hold the device, thus leaving only one hand free. The other disadvantage is the unnatural and monotonic sound of the speech (e.g., Meltzner et al., 2005). To combat these problems several commercially available "hands-free" and/or pitch control devices have been developed. For example, the Hands Free™ Electrolarynx Holder (Griffin Laboratories) is designed to hold a TruTone™ or SolaTone™ AL (Griffin). The holder can either be attached to a shirt or hang from the individual's neck on a strap. The top of the holder is positioned against the speaker's neck and is activated when the person moves his or her head down slightly. Tilting the head further up or down also increases or decreases the pitch (www.griffinlab.com/Products/HandsFree-Electrolarynx-Holder.html). Another hands-free device is the JusTalk Digital Audio Larynx (JustMed, Inc.). As described in the product brochure, the individual wears a headset positioned close to or touching the lips (www.axistive.com/justalk-digital-audio-larynx-dal.html). The headset has a small speaker that generates a tone that is directed into the oral cavity. Within the headset there is a small microphone that picks up the speech being produced. The microphone is wired to a signal processing unit and speaker that can be worn around the individual's neck on a lanyard or clipped to a pocket or belt. The device is described as being programmed to recognize voiceless sounds and pauses in speech, which enables it to activate and deactivate itself automatically. This eliminates the need for the speaker to adjust switches during an utterance. Additionally, because the device does not need to press against the individual's neck it can, theoretically, be used immediately after surgery. There are also several pitch selection options.

UltraVoice Ltd. (Newton Square, PA) produces the UltraVoice Plus II, which can be used by hand, but which can also include a hands-free accessory (www.ultravoice.com). The hands-free unit consists of a small loudspeaker, which is embedded in the patient's upper denture or within an orthodontic retainer. The loudspeaker is covered by a flexible membrane to protect it from saliva, food, and liquid. The loudspeaker produces a tone that is directed into the oral cavity. Either a male or female tone can be generated. When the patient is not using the hands-free accessory switch the device is used in the traditional manner in which the individual holds a control unit switch and activates a button to turn the tone on and off. Alternatively, the patient can use a "Hands Free Switch" that is plugged into the control unit, and which can be clipped to a belt. The switch can be positioned on any part of the body that allows the user to press on it. The device has a rechargeable battery that, according to the company, provides for an average day of speaking time.

Other recent developments in hands-free AL speech have focused on detection of pressure levels within the oral cavity. For example, Takahashi, Nakao, Kikuchi, and Kaga (2008) developed and tested an intraoral vibrator with an oral pressure sensor. The device is fixed on the individual's upper jaw similar to a denture. Voiceless consonants are characterized by greater oral pressure than are voiced consonants. The authors used degree of intraoral pressure as a linguistic marker of voicing. They reported that the voicing control achieved by speakers with this device was especially efficient for stop consonants.

Some degree of pitch control is allowed by devices including the TruTone™ (Griffin Laboratories), Servox Intone, and Servox Digital AL. For example, the TruTone has an adjustable baseline pitch and an adjustable frequency range of 300 Hz from baseline (e.g., Watson & Schlauch, 2009). The device is equipped with a single pressure-sensitive button that increases or decreases the F0 within a preset range by responding to changes in the amount of pressure exerted (Liu & Ng, 2007; Searl, 2006). However, synchronizing finger movements for pitch variation with oral articulation is not easy and may result in an excessively slow speaking rate (Liu & Ng, 2007).

In a different approach to hands-free speech, Goldstein, Heaton, Stepp, and Hillman (2007) developed an AL system that utilizes EMG signals from the patient's extrinsic laryngeal muscles to activate the device. Electrical signals from the muscles are detected with a surface electrode. A specified electrical threshold is set to provide on-off control to activate and deactivate the device. In addition to being hands-free, the system allows some degree of pitch control by speaker manipulation of the level of EMG energy above the threshold. The transducer is mounted on a brace that is worn around the base of the neck (under clothing), which holds the transducer head (buzzer) to the neck surface. The advantage of this system is that the user can start and stop the device and vary the F0 solely through muscle contraction. The system is not yet available commercially, but the developers reported that testing to date has shown promising results.

ESOPHAGEAL SPEECH

Esophageal speech (ES) refers to voice that is produced by taking air into the esophagus and then releasing it through the pharynx. As the air is released, it vibrates the ring of muscle that forms a sphincter (upper esophageal sphincter) between the lower portion of the pharynx and upper portion of the esophagus. Muscles that contribute to the sphincter include the cricopharyngeus and inferior pharyngeal constrictors. In the context of voice restoration the sphincter is known as the pharyngoesophageal segment (PE segment), which forms the so-called "neoglottis." When air is taken into the upper esophagus (called **insufflation**) and then released in a controlled manner, the PE segment is vibrated to produce sound (Lombard & Popovich, 2008). However, it is a difficult form of voicing to learn, because the PE segment is ordinarily closed and only opens to allow the passage of food into the esophagus. All methods of ES training focus on teaching the patient to force air into the esophagus through the PE segment.

The PE segment differs from individual to individual in terms of its size, shape, length, mass, and location, so there is wide variability in the resulting voice (Slavin, 1997). Videoradiographic studies of the PE segment and esophagus in ES speakers have demonstrated a widening of the esophagus during voice production, changes in the dimensions of the posterior wall of the pharynx as it closes against the anterior pharyngeal wall, and elevation of the PE segment for voice production (Lundstrom, Hammarberg, Munck-Wikland, & Edsborg, 2008).

The neoglottis differs from the normal vocal folds in important ways. The normal vocal folds are able to vibrate at many different frequencies and amplitudes to regulate pitch and loudness. The neoglottis is a more massive structure with considerably less fine motor control. Thus, the sound that is produced typically has a much lower frequency, ranging from around 69–123 Hz (e.g., Bellandese, 2009; Most, Tobin, & Mimran, 2000; Slavin & Ferrand, 1995; Stajner-Katusic, Horga, Musura, & Globlek, 2006). This corresponds to a drop of a few semitones in pitch for males and around one octave for females. The low pitch is therefore more problematic for females than for males. In addition, amplitude tends to be reduced by an average of 10 dB (Slavin, 1997). It is much harder for the individual to vary the pitch, so often the voice sounds monotonous. Rate of speech is also affected. The normal rate is approximately 150–190 words per minute, while the average rate for esophageal speakers has been found to be around 85–130 words per minute. Several factors account for the slower rate. One is that esophageal speakers need to pause more often to replenish their air supply, because the upper esophagus holds far less air than the lungs. Vital capacity (VC) of the lungs is around 4,000–5,000 ml. The amount of VC used for normal conversational speech is approximately 1,000–2,000 ml, depending on the utterance. The amount of air that the upper esophagus can hold, by comparison, is only around 80 ml. The typical esophageal speaker, therefore, can produce only around 3–5 words per air charge while normal speakers average around 12 words per breath.

Techniques of Air Intake. Techniques of air intake include injection and inhalation. The goal of both methods is to reduce the air pressure within the esophagus relative to that within the vocal tract (Aguiar-Ricz et al., 2007; Lombard & Popovich, 2008). This is necessary so that higher air pressure within the vocal tract overcomes the resistance of the PE segment forcing air into the esophagus. Air pressure within the esophagus is normally lower than that in the vocal tract, and it is often further reduced following a laryngectomy, which can facilitate airflow through the PE segment. The aim of each method is to teach the patient to insufflate and release the air in a controlled manner.

The injection method takes advantage of the fact that oral pressure is normally greater than esophageal pressure. In this method the speaker further increases oral pressure to force air through the PE segment and into the esophagus. The technique is different for high-pressure sounds (obstruents), such as stops, fricatives, and affricates, and resonant sounds (sonorants) that do not require high pressure for their production, such as vowels, diphthongs, glides, liquids, and nasals. Stops, fricatives, and affricates are produced by building up and then releasing oral pressure. The oral pressure achieved during normal production of these sounds may be great enough to overcome the resistance of the PE segment. The patient is taught to time the oral pressure buildup of these consonants with the insufflation that results. Typically, training begins with voiceless consonants, which are easier to produce than voiced sounds. Once the patient has mastered voiceless sounds, they are combined with various vowels. The patient then progresses to increasingly more complex utterances such as words, phrases, sentences, and so on. Voiced stops, fricatives and affricates are learned once the speaker is reliably able to produce the voiceless sounds.

Production of sonorants is achieved by trapping the air within the oral cavity using the lips and/or tongue to form a seal (Graham, 2005). This method is also called the *tongue pump* or *glossopharyngeal press*, because the individual uses his or her tongue to compress and pump the air posteriorly toward the pharynx. As with consonant injection, the higher pressure air is forced through the PE segment. The therapeutic progression for sonorants is similar to that for consonants, with increasingly complex utterances as the speaker gains mastery of the technique. For both obstruents and sonorant sounds it is important for the individual to keep the velopharyngeal passageway closed to prevent air pressure being lost through the nasal cavities.

The inhalation method aims to reduce pressure within the upper esophagus. The individual learns to inhale rapidly and forcefully through the stoma. This increases the volume of the thoracic cavity and substantially decreases the pressure within the esophagus. The air pressure within the vocal tract becomes more positive in relation to esophageal pressure, which has the desired effect of pulling air from the pharynx into the esophagus.

Patients may find one of these techniques easier than the others, but for maximum benefit the individual should attempt to learn both methods and use them as appropriate in connected speech. The injection method for obstruents is only appropriate when the sound occurs in the initial position of words, but the speaker can use either technique for words beginning with sonorant consonants and vowels (Graham, 2005). The patient should be encouraged to avoid swallowing the air. The motoric patterns associated with swallowing are completely different from those associated with fluent esophageal speech (Duguay, 1991). In addition, swallowing air can result in the individual feeling bloated and uncomfortable.

The goal of ES is production of 4–9 syllables per insufflation, with a speaking rate between 85–129 words per minute. Intelligibility should be good, and the individual should be able to speak without auditory and/or visual distractions. He or she must learn to produce voice consistently and on demand, with a quick and efficient air intake and return for speech (Graham, 2006). Good intelligibility requires clear articulatory patterns with recognizable voicing contrasts, natural rate and phrasing, and appropriate use of intonation, stress, and loudness (Graham, 2006). The speaker should also become aware of nonverbal gestures that can facilitate communication, such as appropriate eye contact and facial expressions and effective hand gestures (Graham, 2006).

A large proportion of laryngectomized individuals (around 25–60%) are unable to master ES (Doyle & Eadie, 2005). Difficulties in achieving ES may be due to anatomical changes such as the presence of scar tissue; abnormal muscle contraction patterns of the PE segment; or spasms of the cricopharyngeal and constrictor muscles resulting from an altered neurophysiological response (Doyle & Eadie, 2005). Other physical problems such as paralysis or weakness of the lip and/or tongue muscles, hearing loss, and gastrointestinal problems can also hinder the development of proficient esophageal speech (Duguay, 1991; Slavin, 1997). Psychosocial factors such as the availability of a supportive network of family and friends also factor into the acquisition of ES (Shanks, 1995). The result is considerable individual differences in the ability to acquire esophageal voice.

The most common cause of unsuccessful ES speech is spasms and hypertonicity of the PE segment caused by peripheral nerve changes, fibrosis, recurrent tumors, and surgical healing (Aguiar-Ricz et al., 2007). Individuals may have an esophageal insufflation test to determine whether the PE segment is able to be vibrated by outgoing air. In this procedure a catheter is inserted into the pharynx and upper esophagus. The patient's stoma is occluded with a valve in order to channel the air through the esophagus. Air is then blown into the catheter, and as the air escapes through the PE segment, it is noted whether or not the sphincter goes into spasm or shows any tightening. As the air escapes, the patient is instructed to phonate various sounds, words, and phrases. If the sphincter does tighten or spasm, or if the patient is unable to sustain phonation, he or she may need a myotomy of the pharyngeal constrictor muscles, neurectomy of the pharyngeal plexus, or Botox injection in order to produce voicing more easily. In a myotomy part of the muscle is excised, which disrupts the reflex hypercontraction of the muscle (Doyle & Eadie, 2005). In a neurectomy the nerves that supply the constrictor muscles are sectioned, which disrupts innervation to specific muscles (Doyle & Eadie, 2005). Botox injection into the PE segment has become the most widely used procedure since the mid-1990s. This procedure has been reported to effectively reduce spasms without the disadvantages of surgical intervention such as general anesthesia and risk of complications (Chone 2005, 2008; Krause, Hempel, & Gurkov, 2009; Meleca, 2000; Zormeier et al., 1999).

ES speakers sometimes use facial or bodily gestures to try to facilitate air intake, such as smacking their lips or moving their head and shoulders. These gestures can be distracting, and the speaker must learn to reduce or eliminate them to facilitate effective communication. Individuals also need to avoid "stoma blasts" and "air klunking." Stoma blasts occur when the speaker pushes pulmonary air through the stoma with excess force. He or she must learn to expel the air more slowly to overcome this noisy exhalation, which can interfere with the intelligibility of the speech. Air klunking can occur as the person insufflates the esophagus, and probably results from too much air being used too quickly and with too much effort (Duguay, 1991). Other distractors should also be identified and eliminated, such as double or triple pumping maneuvers to insufflate the esophagus, chin tucking, and facial grimaces (Salmon, 2005).

Many patients learn to produce esophageal voice, but they are unable to develop intelligible, acceptable speech because of difficulty refining aspects of the basic sound such as duration, intensity, pitch, quality, articulation, and prosody (Duguay, 1991). On the other hand, many laryngectomized individuals do learn to manipulate these aspects of speech (e.g., Gandour and Weinberg, 1983; McHenry, Reich, and Minifie, 1982). However, no matter how proficient the ES speaker becomes, his or her voice never sounds normal. Voice quality can be hoarse and harsh with a wet-gurgly sound, volume tends to be reduced, and the pitch is very low, particularly for female speakers (Globlek et al., 2004). Prosody is also affected and ES speakers can benefit from learning to manipulate phrasing rather than pitch to convey prosodic boundaries (Van Rossum, Quene, & Nooteboom, 2008).

TRACHEOESOPHAGEAL SPEECH

Since the 1980s, a form of esophageal voice has become available to many laryngectomized individuals that is considerably easier to produce than regular esophageal speech. Marc Singer, an otolaryngologist, and Eric Blom, a speech-language pathologist, developed a surgical technique to channel air from a laryngectomized patient's lungs directly from the trachea to the esophagus, thus bypassing the need to inject air from the oral cavity into the esophagus. This notion was not new; indeed, many surgeons over many decades had tried unsuccessfully to fashion some kind of shunt from the trachea to the esophagus. The Blom/Singer technique was the first that successfully directed air to the esophagus with minimal complications. The Blom/Singer technique, called *tracheoesophageal puncture (TEP),* involves surgically creating a **fistula** (small hole) in the soft tissue wall that separates the posterior trachea from the anterior esophagus. A cylindrical silicone prosthesis is inserted into this aperture and is fixed securely in place by a flexible retention collar (Sapienza & Ruddy, 2009). At the stomal end, the prosthesis is taped to the skin of the neck to facilitate easy removal and insertion. The prosthesis, called a "duckbill," is a one-way valve that allows air from the trachea to enter the esophagus, but prevents food and liquid from the esophagus from escaping into the trachea. When the patient closes the stoma, either manually with a finger or with a valve that fits into the stoma, exhaled air is directed through the prosthesis into the esophagus. Then, just as with esophageal speech, the air exits via the PE segment, creating vibration and voicing that the individual articulates in the normal way. TEP has become widely accepted as the procedure of choice for voice rehabilitation in many centers around the world (Cantu, Ryan, Tansey, & Johnson, 1998; Pawar, Sayed, Kazi, & Jagade, 2008).

Primary vs. Secondary Puncture. The TE puncture can be performed either at the time of the laryngectomy (primary) or endoscopically at any subsequent time (secondary). Primary puncture is advantageous because it allows for immediate use of TEP speech even when neck dissection and/or radiotherapy are needed (Gultekin, Yelken, Garca, Develioglu, & Kulekci, 2010). Primary TEP often includes a pharyngeal myotomy as part of the procedure, which eliminates potential PE spasms. Primary restoration for appropriate candidates is currently the procedure of choice in many centers both in the United States and other countries (Emerick et al., 2009; Pawar et al., 2008). Primary TEP is contraindicated when the patient has undergone extensive pharyngolaryngeal surgery and separation of the tracheoesophageal tissue; when postoperative radiotherapy may cause difficulties; and if the patient is believed to be inadequately psychologically and/or physically prepared for the procedure (Pawar et al., 2008). In these cases, secondary puncture may be performed. While secondary puncture is usually created under general anesthetic, recently Sidell, Shamouelian, Erman, Gerratt, and Chhetri (2010) reported the successful use of local anesthetic in an office-based setting to create the puncture and insert the voice prosthesis during the same clinical visit.

Primary and secondary procedures have equivalent success rates in terms of voicing production, even subsequent to radiation therapy (e.g., Boscolo-Rizzo et al., 2008; Chone et al., 2005; Emerick et al., 2009). A high degree of satisfaction with both primary and secondary procedures has been reported, with equivalent perceptual and acoustic ratings of voice (Brown, Hilgers, Irish, & Balm, 2003). However, the time to achieve voice is longer for patients undergoing secondary TEP. Emerick et al. (2009) reported that the median time for acquiring fluent speech was 63 days for the patients who received primary TEP, compared to 125 days for those who received secondary TEP.

Prosthesis Insertion. Insertion of the prosthesis is performed when the tissue in the TEP site has healed and is done by an otolaryngologist and/or trained speech-language pathologist. The first step is to measure the length of the puncture tract and to select an appropriately sized prosthesis (Lombard & Popovich, 2008). The puncture is then dilated by inserting catheters of increasing diameter into the site until the puncture is one size larger than the prosthesis (Sapienza & Ruddy, 2009). The prosthesis is inserted and tested for leaks by having the patient drink liquid. Once the device is firmly in place, the patient attempts to phonate by occluding the stoma. Several types of prostheses are available that vary in length, diameter, and airflow resistance (Table 12.7). Factors that determine selection of a prosthesis include degree of

TABLE 12.7 **Tracheoesophageal Puncture Prostheses**

Nonindwelling Duckbill	
Length	6–28 mm
Diameter	16 F, 20 F
Advantages	Good durability
	Can be changed independently
	Inexpensive
Disadvantages	Increased airflow resistance
Nonindwelling Low-Resistance/Pressure Valve	
Length	6–28 mm
Diameter	16 F, 20 F
Advantages	Decreased airflow resistance
	Shorter esophageal extension
	Can be changed independently
Disadvantages	Decreased durability
	Sensitive to esophageal pressure changes
Indwelling Prosthesis	
Length	6–22 mm
Diameter	20 F, 22 F
Advantages	Decreased airflow resistance
	Increased security from dislodgement
	Removable strap
Disadvantages	Clinician dependent
	Potential for gastric distension
	Expensive

Source: Information from Lombard & Popovich (2008).

phonatory effort, ability of the patient and/or caregivers to independently manage the prosthesis, durability of the prosthesis, and cost (Lombard & Popovich, 2008). The speech-language pathologist is responsible for teaching the patient and/or caregivers to insert and remove the device for everyday cleaning.

Indwelling Prosthesis. A low-resistance indwelling prosthesis was developed in 1988, and this type of device is the current method of choice for voice restoration (Makitie et al., 2003). An indwelling prosthesis is a semipermanent device that does not need to be cleaned every day, but can remain in place for a period of several months. The device can be used following either primary or secondary TEP. Thereafter, it is replaced after a period of months by a speech-language pathologist, nurse, or physician in an outpatient setting (Brown et al., 2003). High success rates have been reported with indwelling prostheses (e.g., Brown et al., 2003; Lam et al., 2005; Op de Coul et al., 2000). There are several devices on the market, with the most commonly used being the Provox 1 and Provox 2 (Atos Medical) (e.g., Hilgers et al., 2010; Op de Coul et al., 2000; Tantawy, 2003; Terada et al., 2007). A third generation of the Provox (Provox Vega) is currently undergoing clinical trials (Hilgers et al., 2010). Advantages of an indwelling prosthesis include low airflow resistance, optimum retention in the tracheoesophageal wall, prolonged device lifetime, simple patient maintenance, and comfortable outpatient replacement (Hilgers & Schouwenburg, 1990). An indwelling prosthesis does not preclude postoperative radiotherapy, and the first replacement is usually several months postsurgery, by which time wound healing is complete (Pawar et al., 2008). Replacement of the prosthesis is indicated when fluids begin to leak through or around the valve (Brown et al., 2003). Leakage through the valve usually results from fungal/yeast deposits on the silicone material; leakage outside the device is mostly caused by a prosthesis that is too long (Brown et al., 2003; Searl, 2006). Collagen and autologous fat injection have been reported as successful ways of managing intractable leakage around the TEP site (Luff, Izzat, & Farrington, 1999; Perie, Ming, Dewolf, & St. Guily, 2002; Remacle & Declaye, 1988). Downsizing the prosthesis has also been reported as efficacious (Brown et al., 2003). Other problems that can occur include infections and growth of granulation tissue around the device. However, these are generally easily treated with antibiotics or insertion of a longer device to compensate for the temporary swelling, edema, and granulation formation (Brown et al., 2003). A recent enhancement is the use of yeast-resistant materials for the prosthesis, which has been reported to extend the lifetime of the device by an average of several months (Eerenstein & Schouwenburg, 2003). For example, the Blom-Singer Indwelling Advantage Voice Prosthesis (InHealth Technologies) has a material preservative called silver oxide incorporated into the silicone valve. This has been reported to extend the life of the device for the majority of TE speakers who had experienced early prosthesis failure due to fungal growth on the device (Leder, Acton, Kmiecik, Ganz, & Blom, 2005). The Provox ActiValve (Atos Medical) uses a plastic valve that does not allow yeast to grow into the material itself, although it can grow on the surface and be cleaned off. A reported difficulty with an indwelling prosthesis is that the valve may leak during swallowing because negative pressure generated in the esophagus can suck the valve open as the food passes through the area (Searl, 2006). The ActiValve overcomes this problem as it is fitted with a small magnet that helps to keep it closed.

Speaking Valves. In order to produce voice a speaker may manually occlude the stoma with a finger or thumb to direct air into the esophagus (Figure 12.4). While many individuals choose the manual option, others prefer to use a speaking valve that fits over the stoma. The valve is designed to be sensitive to different degrees of pressure. For normal or heavy breathing it remains open, but it closes when the individual uses the higher pressures

FIGURE 12.4 Voice Prosthesis

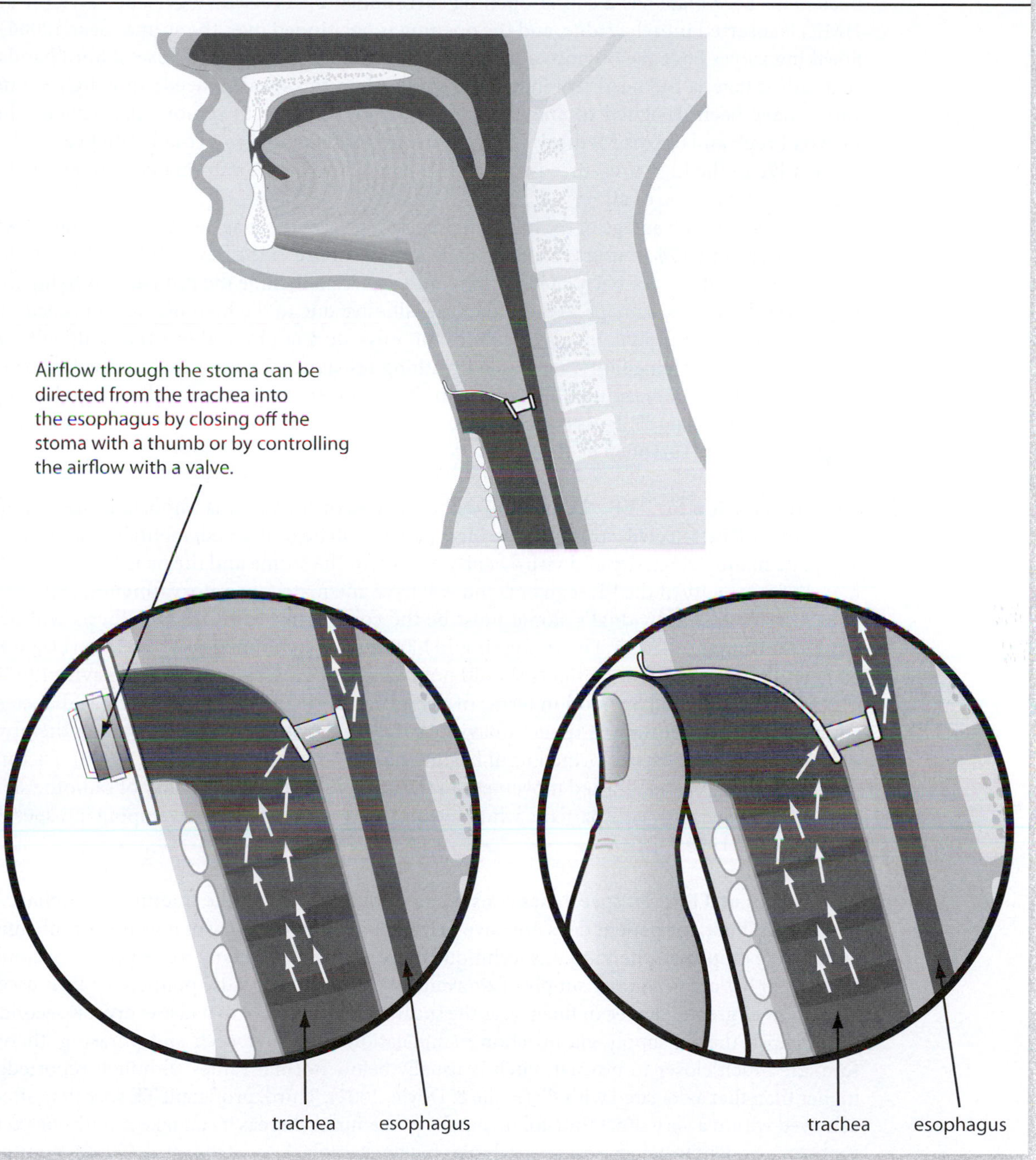

required for speech. Air is thus diverted into the esophagus and released through the PE segment. The valve is usually positioned with a base plate that must be adhered to the neck. This base plate has a center opening surrounded by a raised ridge. The valve (or an HME) is inserted into the ridge, and the opening is positioned over the stoma (Searl, 2006). Speaking valves have the obvious advantage of allowing the speaker full use of both hands. A disadvantage is the need to remove the valve when the speaker needs to cough. Some valves have been designed to allow coughing without having to remove the device. The Provox FreeHands (Atos Medical) incorporates an HME as well as a cough relief valve that is sensitive to the high pressures involved in a cough and opens automatically to allow the high-pressure escape of air.

Despite the advantage of the hands-free speaking valve the long-term success rate is low, with only around 30% of users reporting daily long-term use of the device (Op de Coul et al., 2005). Reasons that have been cited for the limited success include the difficulty of fixing the valve over the stoma, damage to the seal of the adhesive due to the high pressures needed for voicing, inadvertent spontaneous closure of the valve during physical exertion, difficulty in voicing, reduced intelligibility, increased breathing resistance for speaking especially during physical exertion, air escaping from around the housing-skin interface, and difficulty cleaning the valve and housing (Hilgers & Ackerstaff, 2006; Op de Coul et al., 2005; Roxburgh & Perry, 2004; Searl, 2006; Tervonen et al., 2005).

Patient Selection for TEP. To maximize the chances of success it is important that candidates for TEP be selected carefully. The ideal patient will be motivated, mentally stable, have adequate manual dexterity and visual acuity to care for the stoma and the prosthesis, will not have hypertonicity of the PE segment, and will have adequate respiratory function (Elmiyeh et al., 2010). The individual's stoma must be the correct size to fit the prosthesis without compromising the airway. The stoma should have a diameter of no less than 2 cm (Deem & Miller, 2000). In addition, patients should not be alcohol or drug dependent (Slavin, 1997). Physical status should be good in terms of being free of systemic diseases such as diabetes, which impairs the healing of tissues (Slavin, 1997). If the patient has had radiation therapy, the TEP should not be performed until healing has occurred (Elmiyeh et al., 2010). Factors such as reduced vision, limited movement in the arms or hands, and history of radiotherapy have been associated with patients who have not been successful in developing TE speech (Cantu et al., 1998).

Advantages of TEP. TE speech has considerable advantages over the traditional esophageal techniques. First, the patient does not have to learn a difficult new way of injecting or inhaling air into the esophagus, making this technique more accessible to many more people. Second, the patient has a much larger supply of air available for speech, because pulmonary air is used. This allows a greater degree of fluency, as the speaker does not have to pause every few seconds to replenish the air supply via injection or inhalation. Rate of speech and phrasing, therefore, are much closer to normal. Pitch is usually below normal values, although reportedly higher than that associated with ES (Eadie & Doyle, 2002). Third, proficient TE speech is often achieved within a very short time following the procedure, whereas it can take months or even years for a patient to achieve esophageal speech. For example, Lundstrom et al. (2008) reported that the TE speakers in their study were able to speak fluently 2–7 weeks after laryngectomy, compared to proficient ES speakers whose rehabilitation lasted around 3 months before they could use shorter phrases.

Problems with TEP. While the advantages of TE speech are evident, there are some difficulties that may be encountered by speakers. Some of these are related to the individual's specific anatomical and physical features; others are related to the prosthesis or to the speaking valve. Speaker-related problems include narrowing or closure of the tracheoesophageal puncture; hypertonicity or spasm of the PE segment; problems with stoma occlusion or scarring or radiation fibrosis; and growth of granulation tissue around the tracheoesophageal puncture from an improperly fitted prosthesis (Klaben, 2006). Problems related to the prosthesis include the valve getting stuck in a closed position; encrusted material within the prosthesis that prevents airflow through to open the valve; incorrect length of the prosthesis that may press on the posterior wall of the esophagus and prevent airflow to vibrate the PE segment; and leakage around or through the prosthesis while drinking (Elmiyeh et al., 2010; Kazi et al., 2005; Klaben, 2006).

Hypertonicity or spasms of the PE segment may hinder the acquisition of fluent TE speech in patients who undergo TEP as a secondary procedure (Chone et al., 2008). This is not usually a problem in primary TEP because myotomy of the middle and inferior constrictor muscles is one of the surgical steps in the procedure (Chone et al., 2005). PE segment spasms result in difficulties with the onset of TEP speech, phonatory breaks during speech, strangled sounding voice, and/or inability to produce any phonation (Meleca et al., 2000).The most widely used procedure currently for reducing or eliminating the spasms is Botox injection, which has been reported to be very successful in facilitating relaxation of the muscles and improved volitional control of the PE segment (e.g., Chone et al., 2005; Chone et al., 2008; Elmiyeh et al., 2010; Krause et al., 2009; Lewin, Bishop-Leone, Forman, & Diaz, 2001; Meleca et al., 2000; Tantawy, 2003; Zormeier et al., 1999).

Intelligibility and Quality of TE Speech. Intelligibility of TE speech is usually relatively high, although less so than normal laryngeal speech (Searl, 2007). Intelligibility values for TE speakers range from around 50–90% (e.g., Bohnenkamp et al., 2010). Much of the decrease in intelligibility has been shown to result from voicing errors, primarily the replacement of voiceless sounds by voiced sounds (e.g., Evitts, Portugal, Van Dine, & Holler, 2009; Jongmans, Hilgers, Pols, & Van As-Brooks, 2006; Searl, Carpenter, & Banta, 2001). The voicing confusion has been attributed to the characteristics of the PE segment, which does not have sufficiently fine motor control to initiate and cease vibration in coordination with the articulatory gesture for a voiceless sound (Jongmans et al., 2010; Lundstrom & Hammarberg, 2004; Searl & Carpenter, 2002; Searl & Ousley, 2004). When judging intelligibility, listeners have been reported to make most errors in perceiving voiceless phonemes as voiced and fewer related to place and manner of articulation (Searl et al., 2001). The speaker's intelligibility tends to decrease further when speaking in noisy environments (McColl, 2006).

Acoustically, most studies have found that F0 in both males and females is substantially lower than in normal laryngeal speech (e.g., Bellandese, Lerman, & Gilbert, 2001; Eadie, Doyle, Hansen, & Beaudin, 2008; Kazi et al., 2006). This is to be expected, given that the relatively massive neoglottis forms the vibratory source of sound. However, some researchers have reported that F0 for male TE speakers is essentially comparable to that of male laryngeal speakers, around 98–104 Hz (e.g., Kazi et al., 2009; Van As-Brooks, Koopmans-van Beinum, Pols, & Hilgers, 2006). Similar to esophageal speech, F0 for female TE speakers is around an octave lower than for normal female speakers, around 115–120 Hz (e.g., Bellandese et al., 2001; Kazi et al., 2006, 2009; Van As-Brooks et al., 2006). However, average F0 in female TE speakers is higher than that of male TE speakers, suggesting that the PE segment in females may be smaller and thinner than in males (Kazi et al., 2008). There is also a large amount of variability in TE speakers' F0 values, resulting from anatomical and physiological differences in the PE segment (Van As-Brooks et al., 2006). Kazi et al. (2009) reported that patients who underwent reconstruction of the pharynx demonstrated a significantly lower F0 than those who did not. Other acoustic aspects that have been studied include intensity, jitter, shimmer, and harmonics-to-noise/signal-to-noise ratio (e.g., Bellandese et al., 2001; Kazi et al., 2009; McColl, 2006). Not unexpectedly, acoustic analysis confirms the less stable, less periodic, and less intense voice resulting from vibration of the neoglottis. These characteristics tend to become worse when the speaker is in a noisy environment (McColl, 2006). Rate of speech is also somewhat slower in TE speakers, probably because TE speech requires greater airflow rates so speakers need to pause more often to replenish the air supply (e.g., Kazi et al., 2009; McColl, 2006).

Perceptually, TE speech has been evaluated in terms of dimensions such as intelligibility, acceptability naturalness, pleasantness, and overall voice quality. Acceptability is defined in terms of pitch, rate of speech, understandability, and voice quality; naturalness is determined on the basis of rate, rhythm, intonation, and stress (e.g., Eadie et al., 2008). These factors are likely related to the listener's perception of the overall voice and communication abilities of the speaker in comparison to normal laryngeal speech. TE speech is judged perceptually as being deviant from normal speech in terms of voice quality, pitch, and tempo (Van As, Koopmans-van Beinum, & Hilgers, 2003). Vibration of the PE segment is often inconsistent and chaotic, giving rise to the typical rough voice quality (Lundstrom & Hammarberg, 2004). Studies that have attempted to correlate acoustic variables and acceptability ratings have demonstrated that better ratings are associated with greater intensity, higher F0, faster rate, and improved fluency (Eadie et al., 2008).

GENERAL CONSIDERATIONS FOR VOICE RESTORATION

In general, although all three forms of alaryngeal speech tend to be viewed by listeners as abnormal, any of these methods can be effective in facilitating functional communication for laryngectomized individuals. The more the alaryngeal speech resembles normal laryngeal speech, both acoustically and/or perceptually, the more the speech is perceived as acceptable, natural, and proficient (Evitts, Gabel, & Searl, 2007). Which one (or combination) the speaker chooses depends on his or her physical characteristics, communication needs, mental and emotional status, and sociocultural background. Clinicians should be aware of the advantages and disadvantages of each type of voice restoration method and be open to helping the patient acquire the best voice possible using any or a combination of techniques. See Table 12.8 for reported difficulties related to each method of voice restoration. It should be noted that 5–15% of laryngectomized individuals are not able to acquire any method of voicing (Singer, Merbach, Dictz, & Scwarz, 2007).

Individual vs. Group Treatment. The laryngectomized speaker can benefit from both individual therapy sessions to learn and maximize performance of the new voicing method, as well as from group therapy sessions, which provide the opportunity to practice newly learned techniques in a safe and protected environment. Individual treatment is important because it focuses on specific aspects of performance, provides the opportunity to

TABLE 12.8 **Reported Difficulties with Artificial Larynx Speech (AL), Esophageal Speech (ES), and Tracheoesophageal Speech (TES)**

AL	ES	TES
Difficulty being heard in a noisy environment	Difficulty being heard in a noisy environment	Stoma secretions
Battery problems	Difficulty speaking after eating	Speaking valve needs to be manually adjusted for loud speech or coughing
Speech unclear to strangers	Difficulty enunciating words	Leakage around prosthesis
Need one hand to speak	Tightness/stiffness in neck after a lot of talking	
Device is heavy		
Cannot speak quickly		
Cannot sing		
Difficulty finding sweet spot		

Source: Information from Carr, Schmidbauer, Majaess, & Smith (2000).

obtain the maximum number of responses, and allows the clinician and client to try different activities and change them as necessary (Graham, 2006). Group treatment is helpful in transferring the skills learned in individual therapy sessions to communication situations with many different individuals (Graham, 2006). Other benefits of group therapy include opportunities for constructive clinician, peer, and client self-evaluation; social and emotional support; and the chance for individuals to observe other group members at various stages of rehabilitation and who are using a variety of different voicing methods (Graham, 2004, 2006). In addition, family members and friends are often able to participate and observe the learning process, ask questions, contribute to the discussions, and become effective partners in the transition of the newly learned communication skills to the home environment (Graham, 2004).

Quality of Life. The experience of cancer, the surgery, and numerous postsurgery issues can have a profound effect on the patient's quality of life (QOL) after total laryngectomy. Cancer survivors often experience multiple physical, psychological, and social problems concurrently (Sayed et al., 2009) (Table 12.9).

Specific aspects that contribute to QOL following total laryngectomy include physical factors related to the surgery including the extent of the neck dissection, side effects of radiation and chemotherapy, loss of arm and shoulder function, chronic pain, dysphagia, xerostomia, and loss of smell and taste (Eadie et al., 2006; Graham, 2004; Terrell, Fisher, & Wolf, 1998). In terms of psychological factors, depression is common as is a loss of self-esteem, feelings of inferiority, fear of rejection, vulnerability, sadness, fear, and social isolation (Penner, 2009; Sharma, Nagarkar, Jindal, Kaur, & Gupta, 2008; Terrell et al., 1998).

TABLE 12.9 Physical, Psychological, and Environmental Factors That Influence Quality of Life Following Total Laryngectomy

Physical
Extent of neck dissection
Side effects of radiation and/or chemotherapy
Loss of arm and shoulder function
Presence and degree of chronic pain
Presence and degree of dysphagia
Xerostomia
Loss of smell and taste
Loss of sexual function
Psychological
Depression
Loss of self-esteem
Feelings of inferiority
Fear of rejection
Sense of vulnerability
Sadness
Environmental
Social isolation
Level of support
Socioeconomic status
Educational level
Communicative abilities
Gender
Community attitudes toward illness and disability
Financial considerations

Sources: Information from Bellandese (2009); Eadie & Doyle (2005); Eadie et al. (2006); Farrand & Duncan (2007); Graham (2004); Llewellyn et al. (2005); Penner (2009); Sharma et al. (2008); Terrell et al. (1998).

The level of support available to the individuals from family members, friends, medical personnel, and other laryngectomized speakers contributes to the patient's quality of life (Farrand & Duncan, 2007). Active involvement in support groups can be an effective means of obtaining information, as well as social and emotional support that can facilitate good coping and adjustment skills (Eadie & Doyle, 2005). Socioeconomic status (SES) and educational level have also been found to influence QOL. Eadie and Doyle (2005) suggested that education and SES may affect an individual's knowledge of the health care system, access to services, and level of involvement in treatment decisions and care. In addition, they proposed that patients who are better educated may ask more questions and be more compliant with the recommendations of health care providers. QOL for laryngectomized speakers may also be related to gender. Female alaryngeal speakers report higher levels of distress regarding their voice, typically because the pitch is so low (e.g., Bellandese, 2009). Other factors influencing QOL include the person's interpersonal relationships, financial considerations, sexual function, depression, communication abilities, and their community's attitudes toward illness and disability (e.g., Eadie & Doyle, 2005; Eadie, Myers, Beaudin, & Doyle, 2006; Graham, 2004; Llewellyn, McGurk, & Weinman, 2005; Terrell et al., 1998).

The ability to communicate is obviously extremely important to a patient's quality of life and can have a substantial impact on the individual's vocational/professional and social life (Graham, 2004).

However, while communication is clearly an integral factor in quality of life, speech-language pathologists may sometimes overestimate the importance of communication compared to patients' own perceptions. Farrand and Duncan (2007) surveyed laryngectomized speakers and reported that communication was ranked as only the third most important factor affecting their QOL. The respondents identified physical consequences and interference with social activities resulting from treatment as more important than the quality of their communicative skills. Kazi et al. (2007) reported that two-thirds of the participants in their survey noted moderate to severe levels of voice handicap on the VHI and V-RQOL. Despite this, the majority of respondents reported a range of QOL from fair to excellent.

The individual's cultural attitudes and beliefs can also affect QOL and must be taken into account by all professionals working with a laryngectomized speaker. Mitchell (2002) pointed out that while the medical community in the United States is increasingly emphasizing full truthful disclosure of cancer diagnoses, other cultures consider complete and accurate disclosure of cancer undesirable (e.g., European, Japanese, Native American, and various ethnic American groups including Korean, Chinese, Mexican, Hispanic, African, and European American). All members of the team should be aware of how the patient would like to be informed of a diagnosis, and how involved he or she would like family members to be (Mitchell, 2002). The way that the diagnosis is worded is another factor, as the term *cancer* can have extremely negative social connotations. Mitchell (2002) noted that phrases such as "malignant tumor" or "growth" are more readily accepted by the patient and his or her family. Even in mainstream United States, there is often a stigma attached to the diagnosis of cancer, and Eadie et al. (2006) noted that the diagnosis of cancer and how it is treated may pose clear social barriers.

Because of all the physical, emotional, and psychological issues surrounding the experience of cancer, the surgery, and postsurgical issues, psychological counseling both before and after surgery is crucial for laryngectomized individuals (Penner, 2009; Sharma et al., 2008).

Support Groups. Many laryngectomized speakers opt to join local, regional, national, and international support groups such the International Association of Laryngectomees, Web Whispers, Lost Chord clubs, and New Voice clubs. These groups are an invaluable resource for laryngectomized persons, providing educational and emotional support from people in a similar situation. Many clubs, such as the Florida Laryngectomy Association, have members who are trained in pre- and postoperative counseling, with different members illustrating different voicing options. The groups provide the opportunity to socialize with other laryngectomized individuals, family, and friends, and to make new friends in a supportive and caring atmosphere.

chapter SUMMARY

WORLDWIDE, APPROXIMATELY 182,000 new cases of laryngeal cancer are diagnosed annually, of which around 22,000 are women. The number of new cases of cancer of the larynx in the United States in 2009 was 12,290. Of those, 9,920 were male and 2,370 were female. The survival rate for laryngeal cancer depends on the site of the tumor (glottic, subglottic, or supraglottic) and how early the disease is detected and treated. In the very early stages the prognosis for glottic cancer is very good, with survival rates of 90%. Glottic cancers are often detected at an early stage because hoarseness is an early symptom that acts as a warning signal. The location and extent of disease is staged in the TNM classification developed by the American Joint Cancer Committee. The main risk factors for developing laryngeal cancer are tobacco and alcohol consumption.

Symptoms of laryngeal cancer vary depending on the location and stage of the disease. Glottic tumors result in hoarseness, breathiness, reduced loudness, increased vocal effort, and/or pain on phonation. Supraglottic tumors tend to produce dysphagia, otalgia, globus sensation, and swelling of the neck. Tumors in the subglottal area may result in pain and airway obstruction. Other symptoms can include persistent throat-clearing and coughing, persistent sore throat, halitosis, and unexplained weight loss.

Cancer is diagnosed using a number of techniques including a physical examination by the physician to check for abnormal lumps and/or swelling of the lymph nodes in the neck, laryngeal endoscopy, CT scans and MRI, x-rays, modified barium swallow, and PET scans. There are two primary modes of treatment for laryngeal cancer: radiation and/or chemotherapy, either alone or in combination, and surgery. Surgical techniques include various methods of tumor removal and resection of the whole or portions of the laryngeal structure, as well as neck dissection where indicated. Surgeries include laser resection, vertical partial laryngectomy, supraglottic laryngectomy, supracricoid laryngectomy, near total laryngectomy, and total laryngectomy. Choice of treatment is determined based on stage of cancer, potential side effects, probable functional outcomes in terms of voice and swallowing, patient needs and expectations, and quality of life considerations.

Total laryngectomy is associated with many physical, psychosocial, and communicative consequences. Normal voicing is not possible after total laryngectomy, and the aim of treatment is to provide the patient an alternative source of voicing. There are three main methods of voice restoration: artificial larynx, esophageal speech, and tracheoesophageal speech. Each of these has advantages and disadvantages. The patient may use one or a combination of methods, depending on his or her anatomical features, communication needs, motivation, cognitive functioning, hearing status, and individual preference. Although all three forms of alaryngeal speech tend to be viewed by listeners as abnormal, any of these methods can be effective in facilitating functional communication for laryngectomized individuals. Many laryngectomized speakers opt to join local, regional, national, and international support groups such the International Association of Laryngectomees, Web Whispers, Lost Chord clubs, and New Voice clubs.

review QUESTIONS

1. Explain why the prognosis for laryngeal cancer is good at early stages of the disease.
2. Describe the TMN staging system for laryngeal cancer. Why is it important to differentiate between glottal, supraglottal, and subglottal sites?
3. Describe advantages and disadvantages of radiation therapy in terms of vocal production.
4. Compare and contrast partial laryngectomy procedures in terms of their effects on voice.
5. Describe the main functions and advantages, and disadvantages of a heat and moisture exchange system.
6. Identify the main difficulties with artificial larynges, and describe how these are addressed by current devices.
7. Discuss similarities and differences between esophageal and tracheoesophageal speech. What are the benefits and drawbacks associated with each?
8. Comment on the fact that there is often a disconnect between speech-language pathologists' and laryngectomized patients' perception of the importance of communication in quality of life.

PREPARING FOR THE PRAXIS

CASE STUDY 12.1: Laryngeal Cancer

Directions: Please read the case study and answer the five questions that follow. The answers can be found at the bottom of the page.

Don Jeffrey is a 54-year-old police officer. He has been a heavy smoker for 36 years. He recently went to his doctor complaining that he had lost his appetite and was losing weight. The doctor noticed that his voice was noticeably hoarse, and recommended that Don consult an otolaryngologist. The otolaryngologist diagnosed T4 tumors on both vocal folds.

1. Based on the description of the cancer, the least invasive treatment approach that could control the disease is
   a. radiation and chemotherapy followed by resection
   b. vertical partial laryngectomy
   c. supraglottic laryngectomy
   d. supracricoid laryngectomy
   e. near total laryngectomy

2. If the approach selected in question 1 is not successful, Don may need to undergo a total laryngectomy. Following the procedure, he may experience an increase in the amount, severity, and frequency of coughing and increased mucus production. These problems arise due to
   a. disruption in sleeping habits
   b. disruption in dietary intake
   c. lack of warming and moistening of inhaled air
   d. emotional distress
   e. all of the above

3. Which of the following types of swallowing difficulties (if any) does NOT occur following total laryngectomy?
   a. aspiration
   b. decrease in saliva production and xerostomia
   c. insufficient pressure to move the bolus of food
   d. loss of smell and taste
   e. all of these problems can occur

4. The most important factors in choice of voice restoration method are Don's
   a. anatomical features following surgery
   b. cognitive status
   c. hearing status
   d. communication needs
   e. all of the above

5. An indwelling prosthesis used for tracheoesophageal speech
   a. is a permanent device that never needs to be removed
   b. cannot be used if the patient needs postoperative radiation therapy
   c. can only be used in primary tracheoesophageal puncture
   d. must be replaced after a period of months by a speech-language pathologist, nurse, or physician in an outpatient setting
   e. none of the above

Answers for Case Study 12.1: 1. (d); 2. (c); 3. (a); 4. (e); 5. (d)

Glossary

Abdominal trussing process of fixing the abdomen inward relative to its rest position using abdominal binders or corsets, abdominal wraps, and pneumobelts

Abduction posterior cricoarytenoid muscle contraction that opens the glottis

Abductor spasmodic dysphonia laryngeal disorder characterized by involuntary spasms of the abductor muscles during phonation

Acetylcholine excitatory neurotransmitter involved in facilitation of nerve impulses across the synaptic gap

Acquired subglottic stenosis narrowing of the cricoid region resulting from infection, trauma, or other causes

Acute supraglottitis (epiglottitis) viral infection associated with severe throat pain, difficulty swallowing, drooling, high fever; epiglottis and aryepiglottic folds are swollen and red

Adaptation period period during which child's efficiency in breathing for speech continues to become increasingly adultlike as he or she continues to grow physically and becomes more linguistically adept

Adduction lateral cricoarytenoid and interarytenoid muscle contraction that closes the glottis

Adductor paralysis paralysis of the vocal folds in an abducted position; can be unilateral or bilateral

Adductor spasmodic dysphonia laryngeal disorder characterized by laryngospasms of the adductor muscles during phonation

Air hunger sensation of an inability to obtain adequate air on inhalation, with the resulting strong urge to breathe more deeply; also known as uncomfortable urge to breathe, breathlessness, shortness of breath

Amplitude measured in dB SLP (sound pressure level); corresponds perceptually to loudness

Amyotrophic lateral sclerosis progressive neurological disease that strikes the lower and upper motor neurons; also known as Lou Gehrig's disease

Anastomosis connection between two structures

Androgens male sex hormones

Ankylosis stiffening or fixation of a joint

Ansa cervicalis loop of nerves in the neck attached to the hypoglossal nerve and to the first two to three cervical spinal nerves; branches of the ansa cervicalis innervate the infrahyoid muscles

Anterior corticospinal tract 20% of fibers in the corticospinal tract that continue ipsilaterally to the spinal cord

Anterior cricoid split surgical procedure to widen the cricoid cartilage by making an incision through the first two tracheal rings, cricoid cartilage, and the bottom one-third of the thyroid cartilage

Anterior macula flava extension of the intermediate layer of the lamina propria; inserts into Broyle's ligament at the anterior commissure

Anticholinesterase agent that prevents the breakdown of acetylcholine

Antispasmodic drugs agents used to alleviate muscle spasms

Aphonia complete lack of voicing

Apnea of infancy unexplained cessation of breathing for 20 seconds or longer or a shorter respiratory pause in breathing; accompanied by slowness of the heartbeat, purplish coloration of the skin and mucous membrane, pallor, and/or marked hypotonia

Apoptosis programmed cell death

Aryepiglottic folds bundles of connective tissue and muscle; extend from the superior and lateral margins of the epiglottis to the apex of each arytenoid cartilage

Aryepiglottic muscle extension of oblique interarytenoid muscle; contraction causes epiglottis to be pulled downward and backward to cover the entrance to the larynx

Arytenoid adduction surgical procedure in which the muscular process of the arytenoid of the affected fold is sutured to another point in the larynx

Arytenoid cartilage paired cartilages of the larynx located on the superior aspect of the quadrate lamina

Arytenoidectomy surgical procedure in which the whole or a portion of the arytenoid cartilage is removed in order to widen the airway

Ataxic dysarthria lack of coordination of structures involved in speech production; results from damage to the cerebellum and/or its sensory and motor nerve pathways

Auditory-perceptual evaluation subjective judgment of voice on the part of a speaker or listener; influenced by an individual's experience, expectations of what a normal voice should sound like, cultural factors, geographic location, and age and gender of the listener and of the speaker

Augmentation procedures surgical procedures that involve splitting the laryngotracheal framework and expanding the narrowed segment using various combinations of grafts and stents

Autoimmune diseases result from aberrant response of the immune system to healthy cells in the body

Autologous cellular therapy surgical procedure to repair vocal fold defects in which cells are taken from an individual, expanded in the laboratory, and then injected back into the individual

Average intensity vocal intensity measured over an utterance

Balloon dilation technique used to enlarge/dilate/stretch a narrow opening or passage using a soft hollow tube with an inflatable balloon at its tip

Basal ganglia also called basal nuclei; collection of subcortical nerve cells involved in the regulation of voluntary movement

Basement membrane zone attachment between the epithelium and superficial lamina propria; composed of two types of collagen

Bernoulli's principle states that as a fluid flows through a narrow channel the speed of flow increases, resulting in decrease of pressure

Biofeedback provision of information to an individual regarding some aspect of his or her physiological behavior

Biphasic stridor occurs during both phases of respiration; associated with glottic or subglottic anomalies

Blepharospasm involuntary contractions of the eye muscles resulting in uncontrolled squinting and/or eye closing

Botox medical form of botulinum toxin; neurotoxin that prevents the transmission of nerve impulses

Bradycardia slowness of the heartbeat

Bradykinesia slowness in initiating and executing movement

Breathy whispery voice quality due to excess air escaping during vocal fold vibration

Calcium hydroxylapatite compound of phosphate and calcium used for vocal fold injection

Cartilaginous glottis posterior two-fifths of the glottis bounded by the vocal processes

Cartilaginous stenosis thickening or deformation of the cricoid cartilage creating a shelf-like plate of cartilage that leaves only a small opening at the posterior margin

Caseness term used to refer to the presence of clinically significant psychological distress that is indicative of an active psychiatric disorder

Central fatigue reduction of neural stimulation to muscles by the central nervous system as a protective strategy to avoid muscle damage

Cerebellum part of the brain that regulates the force, speed, range, timing, direction, and amount of displacement of movements so that smooth synergistic muscle patterns are maintained

Cholinesterase inhibitor agent that prevents acetylcholine from being reabsorbed by the presynaptic neuron too soon

Chorea quick and jerky involuntary movements; occur in the limbs and/or the muscles of the face, jaw, tongue, and larynx

Cidofovir antiviral agent used in the treatment of recurrent respiratory papillomatosis

CO_2 laser supraglottoplasty procedure in which the aryepiglottic folds are divided and the excess arytenoid tissue is vaporized

Collagen fibrous protein forming the main component of connective tissue

Combination laryngocele most common type of laryngocele; has features of both internal and external types

COMT (catechol-O-methyltransferase) inhibitor agent that prolongs the availability of levadopa

Congenital subglottic stenosis narrowing of the cricoid cartilage due to a problem in embryological development

Conus elasticus inferior portion of the elastic membrane lining the interior of the larynx; composed of the paired triangular membranes

Conversion disorder see somatoform disorder

Corniculate cartilages paired cartilages located on the apex of each arytenoid cartilage

Corticobulbar pathway also called corticonuclear pathway; nerve pathway originating in the motor cortex and synapsing directly with motor nuclei of cranial nerves V, VII, X, and XII in the medulla

Corticospinal pathway nerve pathway originating in the motor and parietal cortex and synapsing directly with motor nerve cells in the spinal cord; 80% of fibers decussate at the medulla

Cover-body model explains the biomechanical properties of the vocal folds in terms of stiffness characteristics of the cover, transition, and body

Cricoarytenoid joint laryngeal joint permitting rocking and gliding motion of the arytenoid cartilages; regulates vocal fold adduction and abduction

Cricoid cartilage unpaired cartilage of the larynx; located immediately superior to the first tracheal ring

Cricothyroid approximation surgical procedure in which the cricoid and thyroid cartilages are brought closer together; elongates and stretches the vocal folds to create a higher pitch

Cricothyroid joint laryngeal joint permitting movement of the cricoid and thyroid cartilages; regulates pitch change

Cricothyroid membrane connects the external, anterior surfaces of the thyroid and cricoid cartilages

Cricothyroid muscle intrinsic laryngeal muscle; regulates longitudinal tension of the vocal folds

Cricotracheal membrane connects the cricoid cartilage to the first tracheal ring

Cricotracheal resection surgical procedure in which the anterior cricoid arch and the narrowed portion of the subglottic/tracheal region are sectioned; remaining healthy trachea is connected to the thyroid lamina

Croup viral infection affecting very young children; also known as acute laryngotracheitis

Cul de sac resonance voice quality that sounds muffled and low in volume

Cuneiform cartilage paired elastic cartilages embedded in the aryepiglottic folds

Cyanosis a condition in which the skin turns blue or purplish due to lack of oxygen

Cyst sac filled with fluid or a semisolid substance

Cytokines small protein molecules that regulate the inflammatory process by facilitating communication between different types of cells and by influencing cell behavior and interactions

Decibels (dB) measure of loudness or intensity of a sound

Decorin interstitial protein that regulates the thickness of collagen fibers

Deep layer of the lamina propria innermost layer of the lamina propria; mostly made up of collagen

Dilation process of enlarging an opening or the lumen of a hollow structure

Diplophonia perception of two different pitches being produced simultaneously

Diplopia double vision

Dopamine inhibitory neurotransmitter manufactured in the substantia nigra; inhibits nerve impulses from crossing the synaptic gap

Duty cycle phases of opening and closing in one cycle of vocal fold vibration

Dynamic range complete range of intensities a person is capable of generating, from the softest phonation produced without whispering to the loudest

Dysarthria umbrella term referring to neurological disorders affecting muscles of respiration, phonation, articulation, and resonance

Dysphonia impairment of speaking or singing voice in terms of pitch, loudness, and/or quality; generic term for any disruption of vocal quality; sometimes used interchangeably with the term hoarseness

Dysplasia abnormal tissue development

Dyspnea subjectively perceived discomfort in breathing; shortness of breath

Dystonia neurological disorder characterized by involuntary and uncontrollable movements

Ecchymosis purplish patch caused by leaking out of blood into the skin

Ectasia dilation or expansion of blood vessels

Elastic membrane extensive intrinsic laryngeal membrane; connects the entire inner framework of the larynx

Elastin type of highly flexible fibrous protein

Electromyography process in which electrical activity is recorded from individual or aggregated muscle fibers

End-expiratory level endpoint of a tidal exhalation

Eosinophils type of white blood cells that are components of the immune system

Epiglottis unpaired elastic cartilage of the larynx

Epiglottopexy surgical fixation of the epiglottis to prevent it from being pulled inward

Epithelium tissue that covers all free surfaces and lines the cavities within the body, including the oral and nasal cavities, pharynx, and respiratory passages

Erythema redness of tissue resulting from inflammation

Esophagitis inflammation of the esophagus

Essential tremor neurological disorder characterized by tremor

Estrogens female sex hormones

Evidence-based practice (EBP) three-pronged approach to clinical management that involves providing patients with the best possible services based on combining evidence from the research literature with clinical expertise and the individual's specific needs, wishes, and values

Expiratory stridor stridor occurring on exhalation associated with obstruction of the lower airways

External intercostal muscles muscles of the ribcage; contract to pull the ribcage in an upward and outward direction resulting in the expansion of the thoracic cavity

External laryngocele laryngocele that protrudes through the thyrohyoid membrane; forms a bulge or swelling on the side of the neck

Extracellular matrix part of connective tissue in which fibroblasts are embedded; composed of fibrous and interstitial proteins

Extrinsic laryngeal muscles have one attachment to the larynx or hyoid bone and another attachment to a structure external to the larynx

False vocal folds see ventricular vocal folds

Fetal cell transplantation surgical procedure to increase the production of dopamine by implanting fetal cells directly into the basal ganglia

Fibroblast connective tissue cell that produces fibrous and interstitial proteins such as collagen, hyaluronic acid (HA), fibronectin (FN), and decorin

Fibronectin interstitial protein located in extracellular matrix; promotes migration of fibroblasts into a wound

Fibrotic/hyaline polyp polyp filled with thick fluid and connective tissue stroma

Fibrous proteins located in extracellular matrix; include collagen and elastin

Fistula small tear or hole in a tissue

Focal dystonia task-specific dystonia limited to one structure

Frequency variability changes in fundamental frequency either in connected speech or in an isolated vowel; measured by the standard deviation of F0 (F0SD) or pitch sigma

Functional dysphonia voice disorder existing in the absence of any organic or neurogenic cause

Fundamental frequency (F0) rate at which the vocal folds vibrate; measured in Hertz (Hz); acoustic correlate of vocal pitch

Gastroesophageal reflux disease (GERD) chronic symptoms or mucosal damage resulting from abnormal reflux of stomach fluids into the esophagus

Glottis space between the true vocal folds

Glottoplasty surgical procedure in which the deepithelialized anterior portion of the vocal folds is sutured at the anterior commissure

Glycoproteins molecules that have short chains of carbohydrates attached to them

Graft surgical procedure in which cartilage is taken from elsewhere in the patient's body to fill in a defect

Granulation tissue specialized tissue formed during the wound healing process; contains myofibroblasts

Granuloma mass of tissue consisting of inflammation, a large amount of blood cells and connective tissue; covered by squamous epithelium

H_2 blockers histamine receptor antagonists that block histamine receptors on the acid-producing cells in the stomach

Harmonics-to-noise ratio (HNR) measure of spectral noise that quantifies the ratio between the harmonic (periodic) and inharmonic (aperiodic) components of the voice; measured in dB

Harshness low-pitched and rough voice quality resulting from hyperadducted vocal folds

Heat shock protein molecules that rigger an immune response in the body

Hemorrhagic polyps polyps characterized by vascular changes

Hemosiderin yellow or brown protein

Hemosiderosis accumulation of hemosiderin

Hernia protrusion of a part or structure through the tissue that normally contains it

Hertz measure of frequency in cycles per second

Hoarseness breathy and harsh voice quality

Hoehn and Yahr Staging of Parkinson's disease commonly used five-level staging system for Parkinson's disease

Human papillomavirus DNA virus; can induce uncontrolled cellular proliferation resulting in a broad range of diseases characterized by epithelial cell proliferation

Huntington's disease progressive genetic neurological disease cause by a problem with a specific gene protein called huntingtin on chromosome 4

Hyaluronic acid interstitial protein that attracts water and creates a gel-like substance; found in connective tissue

Hyoid bone forms location of suspension of the larynx; attachment for the root of the tongue

Hyperalgesia increased sensitivity to pain

Hypercapnia abnormally high carbon dioxide levels in the blood

Hyperkeratosis thickening of a mucous membrane

Hyperkinetic dysarthria dysarthria resulting from damage to the basal ganglia and/or its connections to other brain regions

Hypernasality voice sounds overly nasalized, usually due to problems with velopharyngeal function

Hyperplasic excessive tissue growth

Hypokinesia movements that are abnormally reduced in amplitude

Hypoxia abnormally low oxygen levels in the blood

Immunoglobulin antibodies produced by the immune system

Indole-3-carbinol nutritional supplement found in vegetables such as cabbage, broccoli, and cauliflower; used as an adjuvant therapy for recurrent respiratory papillomatosis

Inflammation regulatory process in which cellular and chemical reactions occur in blood vessels and connective tissues in response to injury and defense against harmful stimuli

Infrahyoid muscles extrinsic laryngeal muscles attaching from the hyoid bone to structures below the hyoid

Injection augmentation surgical procedure used to enlarge a vocal fold and maximize glottal closure

Insufflation taking air into the esophagus for voice production

Intensity variability changes in intensity occurring within an utterance; measured in dB as the standard deviation of average intensity

Interarytenoid muscle unpaired intrinsic laryngeal muscle; adduction closes the posterior glottis

Interferon naturally produced protein with antiviral and antiproliferative actions

Intermediate layer of the lamina propria deeper than the superficial layer; composed of densely organized elastin

Internal laryngocele laryngocele in which the inflated tissue does not penetrate the thyrohyoid membrane, but pushes against the false vocal folds and/or aryepiglottic folds

International Classification of Functioning, Disability, and Health (ICF) model developed by the World Health Organization that takes into account the individual's physical (or mental) impairment, the limitation of activities resulting from the impairment, and the restrictions in participation effected by the disability; the model also takes into account the individual's environment, cultural values and beliefs, goals, expectations, standards, and concerns

Interstitial proteins include hyaluronic acid, decorin, fibronectin, and others; influence tissue viscosity, fluid content thickness, and amount of collagen

Intrinsic laryngeal muscles have both of their attachments to or within the larynx

Jitter Cycle-to-cycle frequency variations in vocal fold vibration; measured as a percentage or in milliseconds

Keratin a type of strengthening and waterproofing protein

La belle indifference surprising indifference to symptoms demonstrated by some patients with conversion disorders

Lamina densa layer of the basement membrane zone composed of collagen fibers

Lamina lucida layer of the basement membrane zone composed of collagen fibers

Lamina propria three-part layer of mucous membrane deep to the vocal fold epithelium

Laryngeal atresia complete fusion of the vocal folds

Laryngeal cyst closed sac filled with fluid or semi-solid substance

Laryngeal saccule part of the laryngeal ventricle containing glands that secrete fluids to keep vocal folds moist and lubricated

Laryngeal ventricle separates false and true vocal folds

Laryngeal web also called glottic stenosis; condition that occurs when abnormal tissue forms between the vocal folds; can be congenital or acquired

Laryngectomy partial or total removal of the larynx

Laryngitis umbrella term for inflammation of the larynx

Laryngocele dilation or herniation of the saccule extending upward within the false vocal fold

Laryngofissure surgical split that separates the vocal folds at the anterior commissure

Laryngomalacia a congenital laryngeal disorder characterized by pathologically soft and flexible supraglottic cartilages

Laryngopharyngeal reflux laryngeal inflammation resulting from the backflow of stomach acid and pepsin into the laryngopharyngeal area

Laryngotracheal reconstruction group of surgical procedures that include a variety of techniques such as resection (cutting or excising) of various portions of cartilage, with or without the incorporation of grafts and stents

Larynx complex structure formed by interlinked cartilages, membranes, ligaments, and muscles

Lateral corticospinal tract composed of 80% of fibers of the corticospinal tract that decussate at the level of the medulla and continue contralaterally to the spinal cord

Lateral cricoarytenoid muscle paired intrinsic laryngeal muscle; vocal fold adductor

Lateral thyrohyoid ligaments thickened lateral margins of the thyrohyoid membrane

Lateral thyrotomy surgical procedure in which the thyroid cartilage is divided vertically

Lee Silverman Voice Treatment systematic program of behavioral voice therapy designed to help patients recalibrate a higher level of vocal effort

Leukoplakia a clinical descriptor indicating the presence of keratin on an epithelial surface

Levodopa (L-dopa) drug used to treat motor symptoms in Parkinson's disease

Loft register highest range of fundamental frequencies; also called falsetto

Longitudinal phase difference slight time lag between opening and closing of the anterior and posterior margins of the vocal folds during vibration

Loudness perceptual counterpart to vocal intensity

Lower motor neuron includes the spinal and cranial nerves as well the myoneural junction between the nerve ending and the muscle fibers that it innervates

Lumen inside of a tube

Lysis surgical division of adhesions

Macrophage type of white blood cell that ingests foreign material

Marsupialization procedure in which a surgical incision is made in a cyst with a few stitches on either side creating a permanent opening through which the cyst can drain

Masked facies inability to move the facial muscles

Maximum phonational frequency range complete range of F0s a person is able to generate from the lowest to highest including falsetto; measured in Hz or in octaves

Medial arytenoidectomy surgical procedure to widen the airway; creates a concavity along the glottic edge of the body of the arytenoid cartilage

Medial compression force exerted by the lateral cricoarytenoid and interarytenoid muscles that adducts the vocal folds to initiate the vibratory cycle

Medial thyrohyoid ligament thickened central portion of the thyrohyoid membrane

Medulla part of the brainstem

Meige's syndrome combination of blepharospasm and oromandibular dystonia

Membranous glottis anterior three-fifths of the glottis bounded by the membranous vocal folds

Membranous stenosis caused when the soft mucosal tissue that lines the inside of the cartilage thickens due to an increase in fibrous connective tissue, hyperplasia of the mucous glands, or presence of granulation tissue

Metastasis spread of a disease from one part of the body to another

Modal register middle range of frequencies most often used in conversational speech

Monoamine oxidase inhibitors used for symptom relief in Parkinson's disease by prolonging the effects of dopamine in the brain

Motivational interviewing systematic approach to increasing patient motivation and compliance by increasing motivation to engage in change

Mucosal wave wavelike fashion in which the vocal folds approximate and separate from each other during a cycle of vibration

Multiple sclerosis autoimmune disorder in which antibodies attack the myelin coating surrounding nerve axons, resulting in inflammation and scarring

Muscle tension dysphonia dysphonia that results from hypercontraction of the intrinsic and extrinsic laryngeal muscles as well as muscles in the face, jaw, tongue, neck, and shoulders

Mutational falsetto also called puberphonia or mutational dysphonia; characterized by an inappropriately high pitch in postadolescent males

Myasthenia gravis nervous system disorder that results in flaccid dysarthria; characterized by an individual's movements in the affected structures becoming progressively weaker with repetition in an extremely short period of time

Myer-Cotton system staging system used to categorize degree of subglottic stenosis

Myoelastic-aerodynamic theory describes one cycle of vocal fold vibration as an interaction of muscle forces, elastic recoil forces, and aerodynamic forces

Myofibroblasts cells that have characteristics of both fibroblasts and smooth muscle cells

Myofilaments muscle fibers that contract and allow the muscle to contract and shorten

Myxomatous material benign neoplasm derived from connective tissue

Nasal emission audible release of air through the nose occurring on stops and fricatives

Nasoendoscopy endoscopic procedure done with a flexible fiberscope passed through the nose and pharynx; allows visualization of vocal fold structure and function

Neuroleptics drugs used to treat certain psychiatric illnesses

Nissen fundoplication surgical procedure to eliminate gastric reflux; the gastric fundus is wrapped around the lower portion of the esophagus and sutured in place

Nodule benign growth that develops on the epithelium of the vocal folds as a consequence of vocal hyperfunction and resulting inflammation

Nucleus ambiguus collection of nerve cells in the medulla that house the motor neurons of the vagus nerve

Nucleus retroambiguus collection of nerve cells in the medulla that house the motor neurons that innervate the muscles of the tongue, pharynx, soft palate, muscles of exhalation, and larynx

Odynophagia painful swallowing

Odynophonia pain upon phonation

Oromandibular dystonia focal dystonia resulting in spasms of the tongue, mouth, and pharyngeal muscles

Otolaryngologist physician who specializes in diseases of the ear, nose, larynx, and pharynx

Papilloma benign wartlike growth of the epithelium

Papillomatosis development of numerous papillomas

Paradoxical vocal fold motion respiratory/laryngeal disorder characterized primarily by inappropriate vocal fold adduction during the inhalation phase of breathing

Paresis slight or partial paralysis resulting in partial loss of muscle strength and movement

Parietal pleura membrane that lines the inside surface of the thoracic cavity

Parkinson's disease central nervous system disease in which dopamine is reduced

Periaqueductal grey a diffuse area of gray matter surrounding the cerebral aqueduct

Peripheral fatigue muscular fatigue resulting from chemical changes in muscles and tissues

Petiole narrowest part of the epiglottis

Pexy surgical fixation of structures

Phonation process whereby exhaled air is converted to voiced sound by vocal fold vibration

Phonation threshold pressure minimum amount of subglottal pressure necessary to set the vocal folds into vibration

Phonation time quantification of voice use measured in terms of phonation per hour

Phonosurgery name for a group of different types of surgical procedures that have as their aim the preservation or restoration of the patient's best possible voice

Phonotrauma inflammatory response of the vocal fold mucosa to the biomechanical stresses that the vocal folds undergo during hyperfunctional phonation

Physiological sulcus groove on the epithelial surface of the vocal fold; normal lamina propria

Pitch perceptual correlate of fundamental frequency

Plasmaphoresis plasma exchange; used for severe cases of myasthenia gravis

Pleural fluid fluid within the pleural space; has consistent negative pressure that keeps the lungs and thorax closely approximated

Pleural linkage mechanism by which the lungs and thorax act as an integrated unit

Pleural space potential space between the visceral pleura and parietal pleura

Polyps benign growths on the vocal fold mucosa that may result from laryngeal hyperfunction, smoking, and/or allergies; may be sessile, pedunculated, or polypoid degeneration

Posterior cricoarytenoid muscle paired intrinsic laryngeal muscle; vocal fold abductor

Potential energy stored energy that could be released in the form of kinetic energy

Presbyphonia term used to characterize the aging of the laryngeal mechanism

Primary prevention aims to entirely eliminate or prevent the onset of a disorder by reducing a person's susceptibility to the disorder, or by reducing exposure of a susceptible individual to that disorder

Primary progressive multiple sclerosis form of multiple sclerosis characterized by the gradual but steady loss of function over a period of years, with no remissions in between

Progressive-relapsing multiple sclerosis form of multiple sclerosis characterized by steady worsening from the onset, in conjunction with acute relapses

Prokinetics agents that enhance esophageal motility; increase the movement of food and liquid through the gastrointestinal tract

Prolonged intubation endotracheal intubation for a period of greater than 14 days

Proteoglycans molecules containing more carbohydrate than protein

Proton pump inhibitors agents that prevent acid-producing cells in the stomach from discharging the acid

Ptosis drooping of the eyelid

Pulmonary stretch receptors sense the airway smooth muscle tone and project to the medullary respiratory neural network through the vagus

Pulsed dye laser angiolytic laser that obliterates blood vessels

Pulse register lowest range of fundamental frequencies; also called glottal fry, vocal fry, or creak

Pyramidal tract made up of the corticospinal and corticobulbar pathways

Quadrangular membrane superior portion of the elastic membrane

Quadrate lamina posterior portion of the cricoid cartilage

Radiofrequency ablation technique used for tumor removal

Rapidly adapting receptors sensory nerve receptors located in the smooth muscles of the tracheobronchial tree; sensitive to both mechanical and chemical changes in the muscles

Recurrent respiratory papillomatosis disease characterized by proliferation of papilloma within and/or outside aerodigestive tract

Reflux finding score evaluation tool that uses laryngoscopy to rate the most prevalent signs of LPR including subglottic edema, ventricular obliteration, erythema/hyperemia, vocal fold edema, diffuse laryngeal edema, posterior laryngeal hypertrophy, granulomas/granulation tissue, and thick endolaryngeal mucus

Reflux Symptom Index questionnaire probing the types and degree of severity of patient-perceived symptoms of reflux

Reinke's edema a condition of polypoid degeneration of the vocal fold characterized as a chronic inflammatory disease in which the entire membranous portion of the vocal folds becomes infiltrated with thick, gelatinous fluid

Relapsing polychondritis disorder characterized by recurring episodes of inflammation of connective tissues; particularly affects the cartilages of the ears, nose, larynx, trachea, eyes, heart valves, kidneys, and blood vessels

Relapsing-remitting multiple sclerosis nervous system disease characterized by periods of remission interspersed with relapses of symptoms

Repetitive stimulation test diagnostic procedure in which a motor nerve is repeatedly stimulated at a rate of 2–3 times per second

Resonant voice term used to describe a voice produced with the least possible muscular effort and lowest possible collision forces between the vocal folds

Resting expiratory level state of equilibrium in the respiratory system in which alveolar pressure and atmospheric pressure are equalized

Retention cysts result from an obstruction to the excretory duct of a gland; contain mucus

Rheumatoid arthritis chronic inflammatory autoimmune disease affecting joints

Scanning speech abnormally slow speech in which all syllables are stressed equally

Scar end result of wound healing process characterized by increased collagen, decreased and fragmented elastin fibers, and changes in the proportion of other interstitial proteins

Scar remodeling wound healing process whereby extracellular matrix components continue to be deposited and reorganized

Sebum oily substance secreted by sebaceous glands

Secondary prevention early detection and treatment of disorders

Secondary progressive multiple sclerosis nervous system disease characterized by relapses and remissions, but the relapses start to predominate, and the remissions become less frequent

Shimmer cycle-to-cycle variation in vocal fold amplitude measured in dB or as a percentage

Signal-to-noise ratio (SNR) measure of spectral noise; quantifies the ratio between the harmonic (periodic) and inharmonic (aperiodic) components of the voice; measured in dB

Somatic compliance cooccurrence of a neurological and psychological disorder

Somatoform disorder disorder in which symptoms suggest a physical etiology such as a medical condition, disease, or injury; no evident physical cause is found, and the condition is thought to be an expression of psychological conflict

Spasmodic dysphonia focal dystonia resulting in a voice disorder characterized by spasms of either the adductor and/or abductor intrinsic laryngeal muscles

Spasmodic torticollis focal dystonia involving involuntary spasms of the cervical neck muscles

Spastic dysarthria neurological disorder resulting from damage to the corticobulbar tracts of the upper motor neuron; characterized by weakness and spasticity of affected muscles

Speaking fundamental frequency average fundamental frequency measured in a segment of connected speech

Sputum mucus and other matter brought up from the airways

Stenosis narrowing or constriction of an orifice

Stress set of emotional, cognitive, and physiological reactions to psychological demands and challenges; influenced by an individual's coping ability

Stridor noisy inhalation and/or exhalation; audible sound generated during respiration indicating airway obstruction

Stroma connective tissue framework of an organ

Subglottal pressure air pressure underneath the vocal folds

Subglottic stenosis narrowing of the airway between the glottis and the first tracheal ring; can be congenital or acquired

Substantia nigra subcortical structure that produces dopamine

Sulcus vergeture loss of the superficial layer of the lamina propria with a linear depression or vergeture along the free edge of the fold resulting in an abnormally thin layer of tissue between the epithelium and the vocal ligament

Sulcus vocalis pit in the vocal fold epithelium, with severe loss of lamina propria tissue that extends into the vocal ligament or thyroarytenoid muscle

Superficial layer of the lamina propria outermost layer of the lamina propria; composed mostly of loosely organized elastin fibers

Supraglottis portion of the larynx superior to the true vocal folds

Supraglottoplasty endoscopic techniques that fixate the epiglottis to prevent the aryepiglottic folds from being pulled inward and/or remove excess tissue to enlarge the airway

Suprahyoid muscles extrinsic laryngeal muscles attaching from the hyoid bone to superior structures

Synechia adhesion between the margins of the vocal folds; occurs when the anterior commissure is irritated and heals with excess tissue

Synkinesis involuntary movement that occurs in conjunction with a voluntary movement; results when a damaged nerve regenerates and reinnervates an incorrect muscle

Systemic lupus erythematosus progressive disorder of connective tissues, blood vessels, and mucous membranes

Tachypnea rapid breathing

Tardive dyskinesia abnormal movements resulting as a side effect of some medications

Tensile strength force required to pull on a structure to its breaking point

Tertiary prevention clinical management techniques aimed at restoring normal functioning to the extent possible

Thalamus subcortical structure responsible for level of arousal and alertness; involved in integrating emotional expression into motor activity

Thoracic cavity area bounded by the sternum, ribs, and vertebrae

Thymectomy surgical removal of the thymus gland

Thymoma tumor on the thyroid gland

Thyroarytenoid muscle intrinsic laryngeal muscle made up of the medial thyrovocalis fibers and the lateral thyromuscularis fibers; forms the body of the vocal folds

Thyroarytenoid myectomy/myotomy surgical procedure that involves resecting the thyroarytenoid muscle; creates permanent muscular weakness that prevents the vocal folds from hyperadducting during laryngospasms

Thyrohyoid membrane sheet of membrane connecting the hyoid bone and larynx

Thyroid cartilage largest unpaired cartilage in the larynx

Thyroplasty group of surgical procedures designed to modify the position and tension of the vocal folds by altering the relationships between the thyroid and other laryngeal cartilages

Trachea hollow air-conducting tube situated beneath the larynx

Tracheobronchial tree air-conducting system formed by the trachea, bronchi, bronchioles, and alveolar sacs

Tracheomalacia disorder characterized by the collapse of the tracheal walls

Transgender term describing all persons whose identities, behavior, or dress vary from traditional gender norms, including transsexuals, transgenderists, cross dressers, and drag queens

Translucent polyp polyp filled with edematous-appearing fluid

Transsexual condition in which an individual wishes to manifest the primary and secondary sex characteristics of the non-natal sex and live as a member of that sex, and who modifies his or her body with hormones and surgery to achieve that end

Transverse cordotomy surgical procedure to enlarge the posterior part of the glottis

Triangular membranes intrinsic laryngeal membranes; attach anteriorly to the thyroid and cricoid cartilages, inferiorly to the cricoid cartilage, and posteriorly to the vocal processes of the arytenoids

Triticeal cartilages small cartilages within the lateral thyrohyoid ligaments

True vocal folds complex five-layered musculomembranous structure; forms inferior valve of the larynx

Ulcer lesion on a mucous surface caused by superficial loss of tissue; usually occurs in conjunction with inflammation

Unified Parkinson Disease Rating Scale comprehensive classification system that categorizes the assortment of problems associated with Parkinson's disease in terms of cognition, personality, everyday living ability, and movement

Vallecula space between the epiglottis and the tongue

Varix prominent dilated vein on the surface of the vocal fold

Ventilation process of moving air into and out of the airways and lungs in order to exchange oxygen entering the lungs and carbon dioxide leaving the lungs

Ventricular vocal folds also called false vocal folds; located superior to the true vocal folds and separated from them by the laryngeal ventricle

Vertical phase difference slight time lag between the opening and closing of the inferior and superior margins of the vocal folds during vibration

Videostroboscopy method of visualization based on the synchronization of a light source with fundamental frequency; allows observation of vibratory function including mucosal wave, vibratory amplitude, periodicity, and symmetry of vibration

Visceral pleura airtight membrane that encases each lung

Viscosity describes a fluid's resistance to flow

Vital capacity maximum amount of air that one is able to voluntarily breathe in and out

Vocal fatigue physiological decline in the force of muscle contraction via central and peripheral factors; results in the subjective perception of increased effort to produce voice

Vocal fold hemorrhage diffuse subepithelial bleeding

Vocal fold paralysis neurological disorder; may be unilateral or bilateral, abductor or adductor

Vocal hyperfunction hypertonic state of both intrinsic and extrinsic laryngeal musculature

Vocal intensity the strength of a sound wave measured in decibels

Vocal register particular range of vocal fundamental frequencies that have a specific quality associated with that register

Vocal tremor rhythmic fluctuations in voice frequency or intensity

Voice arrest complete cessation of voicing for a brief period of time

Voice quality the tone of the voice in terms of clarity, acceptability, and pleasantness

Wound healing complex physiological mechanism encompassing stages of inflammation, extracellular matrix cell proliferation, and scar remodeling

Xerostomia condition in which mucous membranes dry out; also called dry mouth

References

Abaza, M. M., Levy, S., Hawkshaw, M. J., & Sataloff, R. T. (2007). Effects of medications on the voice. *Otolaryngologic Clinics of North America, 40,* 1081–1090.

Abitbol, J., Abitbol, P., & Abitbol, B. (1999). Sex hormones and the female voice. *Journal of Voice, 13,* 424–446.

Abrahams, J. J., & Caceres, C. (1998). Mandibular erosion from Silastic implants: Evaluation with a dental CT software program. *American Journal of Neuroradiology, 19,* 519–522.

Ackermann, H., & Hertrich, I. (2000). The contribution of the cerebellum to speech processing. *Journal of Neurolinguistics, 13,* 95–116.

Acton, L. (2004). Heat and moisture exchange: Laryngectomy, issues and answers. Available from SpeechPathology.com, www.speechpathology.com/articles/article_detail.asp?article_id=224

Adler, R. K. (2006). Vocal misuse and vocal hygiene. In R. K. Adler, S. Hirsch, & M. Mordaunt (Eds.), *Voice and communication therapy for the transgender/transsexual client: A comprehensive clinical guide* (pp. 127–138). San Diego, CA: Plural Publishing.

Adler, R. K., & Van Borsel, J. (2006). Female-to-male considerations. In R. K. Adler, S. Hirsch, & M. Mordaunt (Eds.), *Voice and communication therapy for the transgender/transsexual client: A comprehensive clinical guide* (pp. 139–167). San Diego, CA: Plural Publishing.

Agada, F. O., Bell, J., & Knight, L. (2006). Subglottic cysts in children: A 10-year review. *International Journal of Pediatric Otorhinolaryngology, 70,* 1485–1488.

Agarwal, J. P., Baccher, G. K., Waghmare, C. M., Mallick, I., Ghosh-Laskar, S., Budrukkar, A., Pai, P., Chaturvedi, P., . . . Dinshaw, K. A. (2009). Factors affecting the quality of voice in the early glottic cancer treated with radiotherapy. *Radiotherapy and Oncology, 90,* 177–182.

Agarwal, M., Scherer, R. C., & Hollien, H. (2003). The false vocal folds: Shape and size in frontal view during phonation based on laminagraphic tracings. *Journal of Voice, 17,* 97–113.

Agrawal, N., Black, M., & Morrison, G. (2007). Ten-year review of laryngotracheal reconstruction for paediatric airway stenosis. *International Journal of Pediatric Otorhinolaryngology, 71,* 699–703.

Aguiar-Ricz, L., Dantas, R. O., Ricz, H., Gielow, I., Mamede, R. C. M., & Perdona, G. C. (2007). Behavior of the cricopharyngeal segment during esophageal phonation in laryngectomized patients. *Journal of Voice, 21,* 248–256.

Ahmad, S. M., & Soliman, A. M. S. (2008). Airway obstruction: A rare complication of benign vocal fold polyps. *Annals of Otology, Rhinology, & Laryngology, 117,* 106–109.

Ahn, S.-H., Sung, M.-W., & Kim, K. H. (2004). Factors associated with staged reconstruction and successful stoma closure in tracheal resection and end-to-end anastomosis. *Archives of Otolaryngology—Head and Neck Surgery, 130,* 57–62.

Alexander, R. A., & Fried, M. P. (2007). Surgical therapy for recurrent respiratory papillomatosis. *Ear, Nose and Throat Journal, 86,* 68–71.

Ali, S. O., Thomassen, M., Schulz, G. M., Hosey, L. A., Varga, M., Ludlow, C. L., & Braun, A. R. (2006). Alterations in CNS activity induced by botulinum toxin treatment in spasmodic dysphonia: An $H_2{}^{15}O$ PET study. *Journal of Speech, Language and Hearing Research, 49,* 1127–1146.

Allan, P. F., Abouchahine, S., Harvis, L., & Morris, M. J. (2006). Progressive vocal cord dysfunction subsequent to a chlorine gas exposure. *Journal of Voice, 20,* 291–296.

Allen, K. D. (2007, June 22). EMG biofeedback treatment of dysphonias and related voice disorders. The Free Library. (2007). Retrieved April 4, 2010 from www.thefreelibrary.com/EMG biofeedback treatment of dysphonias and related voice disorders. -a0170157272

Allison, R. (2010). Aligning bodies with minds: The case for medical and surgical treatment of gender dysphoria. *Journal of Gay and Lesbian Mental Health, 14,* 139–144.

Alpert, M., Pouget, E. R., & Silva, R. R. (2001). Reflections of depression in acoustic measures of the patient's speech. *Journal of Affective Disorders, 66,* 59–69.

Altenberg, E. P., & Ferrand, C. T. (2006). Fundamental frequency in monolingual English, bilingual English/Russian, and bilingual English/Cantonese young adult women. *Journal of Voice, 20,* 89–96.

Altenberg, E. P., & Ferrand, C. T. (2006). Perception of individuals with voice disorders by monolingual English, bilingual Cantonese-English, and bilingual Russian-English women. *Journal of Speech, Language, and Hearing Research, 49,* 879–887.

Altieri, A., Garavello, W., Bosetti, C., Gallus, S., & La Vecchia, C. (2005). Alcohol consumption and risk of laryngeal cancer. *Oral Oncology, 41,* 956–965.

Altman, K. W., Atkinson, C., & Lazarus, C. (2005). Current and emerging concepts in muscle tension dysphonia: A 30-month review. *Journal of Voice, 19,* 261–267.

Altman, K. W., Simpson, C. B., Amin, M. R., Abaza, M., Balkissoon, R., & Casiano, R. R. (2002). Cough and paradoxical vocal fold motion. *Otolaryngology—Head and Neck Surgery, 127,* 501–511.

Alvarez-Neri, H., Penchyna-Grub, J., Porras-Hernandez, J. D., Blanco-Rodriguez, G., Gonzalez, R., & Rutter, M. J. (2005). Primary cricotracheal resection with thyrotracheal anastomosis for the treatment of severe subglottic stenosis in children and adolescents. *Annals of Otology, Rhinology, & Laryngology, 114,* 2–6.

American Cancer Society. (2009). *Cancer facts and figures—2009.* Atlanta, GA: Author.

American Joint Committee on Cancer. (2002). *AJCC cancer staging handbook* (6th ed.). New York: Springer.

American Psychiatric Association (1994). *Diagnostic and statistical manual of mental disorders* (4th ed.). American Psychiatric Association, Washington DC.

American Speech-Language-Hearing Association. (1988). *Prevention of communication disorders* [Position Statement]. Available from www.asha.org/policy

American Speech-Language-Hearing Association. (1991). *Prevention of communication disorders tutorial* [Relevant Paper]. Available from www.asha.org/policy

American Speech-Language-Hearing Association. (2004). *Knowledge and skills needed by speech-language pathologists and audiologists to provide culturally and linguistically appropriate services* [Knowledge and Skills]. Available from www.asha.org/policy

American Speech-Language-Hearing Association. (2004). *Knowledge and skills for speech-language pathologists with respect to vocal tract visualization and imaging* [Knowledge and Skills]. Available from www.asha.org/policy

American Speech-Language-Hearing Association. (2004). *Preferred practice patterns for the profession of speech-language pathology* [Preferred Practice Patterns]. Available from www.asha.org/policy

American Speech-Language-Hearing Association. (2004). *Roles and responsibilities of speech-language pathologists with respect to evaluation and treatment for tracheoesophageal puncture and prosthesis* [Position Statement]. Available from www.asha.org/policy

American Speech-Language-Hearing Association. (2004). *Vocal tract visualization and imaging: Position statement* [Position Statement]. Available from www.asha.org/policy

American Speech-Language-Hearing Association. (2005). *Evidence-based practice in communication disorders* [Position Statement]. Available from www.asha.org/policy

American Speech-Language-Hearing Association. (2005a). *The role of the speech-language pathologist, the teacher of singing, and the speaking voice trainer in voice habilitation* [Technical Report]. Available from www.asha.org/policy

American Speech-Language-Hearing Association. (2005b). *The use of voice therapy in the treatment of dysphonia* [Technical Report]. Available from www.asha.org/policy

American Thoracic Society. (1999). Dyspnea. Mechanisms, assessment, and management: a consensus statement. *American Journal of Respiratory Critical Care Medicine, 159,* 321–340.

Amir, O., Ashkenazi, O., Leibovitzh, T., Michael, O., Tavor, Y., & Wolf, M. (2006). Applying the Voice Handicap Index (VHI) to dysphonic and nondysphonic Hebrew speakers. *Journal of Voice, 20,* 318–324.

Amir, O., Biron-Shental, T., Tzenker, O., & Barer, T. (2005). Different oral contraceptives and voice quality—an observational study. *Contraception, 71,* 348–352.

Amir, O., Dukas, M., & Shnaps-Baum, R. (2005). The effect of a 'voice course' on the voices of people with and without pathologies: Preliminary observations. *Logopedics, Phoniatrics, Vocology, 30,* 63–71.

Anderson, T. D., & Sataloff, R. T. (2004). Complications of collagen injection of the vocal fold: Report of several unusual cases and review of the literature. *Journal of Voice, 18,* 392–397.

Andersson, K., & Schalen, L. (1998). Etiology and treatment of psychogenic voice disorder: Results of a follow-up study of thirty patients. *Journal of Voice, 12,* 96–106.

Andrade, D. F., Heuer, R., Hockstein, N. E., Castro, E., Spiegel, J. R., & Sataloff, R. T (1999). The frequency of hard glottal attacks in patients with muscle tension dysphonia, unilateral benign masses and bilateral benign masses. *Journal of Voice, 14,* 240–246.

Andrews, B. T., Van Daele, D. J., Karnell, M. P., McCulloch, T. M., Graham, S. M., & Hoffman, H. T. (2008). Evaluation of open approach and injection laryngoplasty in revision thyroplasty procedures. *Otolaryngology—Head and Neck Surgery, 138,* 226–232.

Andrews, M. L. (1995). Manual of voice treatment: Pediatrics through geriatrics. San Diego, CA: Singular Publishing Group.

Andrews, M. L., & Schmidt, C. P. (1995). Congruence in personality between clinician and client: Relationship to ratings of voice treatment. *Journal of Voice, 9,* 261–269.

Andrews, S., Warner, J., & Stewart, R. (1986). EMG biofeedback and relaxation in the treatment of hyperfunctional dysphonia. *International Journal of Language & Communication Disorders, 21,* 353–369.

Andrianopoulos, M. V., Darrow, K. N., & Chen, J. (2001a). Multimodal standardization of voice among four multicultural populations: Fundamental frequency and spectral characteristics. *Journal of Voice, 15,* 194–219.

Andrianopoulos, M. V., Darrow, K. N., & Chen, J. (2001b). Multimodal standardization of voice among four multicultural populations: Formant structures. *Journal of Voice, 15,* 61–77.

Andrianopoulos, M. V., Gallivan, G. J., & Gallivan, K. H. (2000). PVCM, PVCD, EPL, and irritable larynx syndrome: What are we talking about and how do we treat it? *Journal of Voice, 14,* 607–618.

Angsuwarangsee, T., & Morrison, M. (2002). Extrinsic laryngeal muscular tension in patients with voice disorders. *Journal of Voice, 16,* 333–343.

Argiris, A., Karamouzis, M., Raben, D., & Ferris, R. (2009). Head and neck cancer. *The Lancet, 371,* 1695–1709.

Arsura, E. L., Brunner, N. G., & Grob, D. (1988). Effects of repeated doses of intravenous immunoglobulin in myasthenia gravis. *The American Journal of Medical Sciences, 295.*

Ashraf, V. V., Taly, A. B., Veerendrakumar, M., & Rao, S. (2006). Myasthenia gravis in children: A longitudinal study. *Acta Neurologica Scandinavia, 114,* 119–123.

Aubry, K., Leboulanger, N., Harris, R., Gentry, E., Denoyelle, F., & Garabedian, E-N. (2010). Laser arytenoidectomy in the management of bilateral vocal cord paralysis in children. *International Journal of Pediatric Otorhinolaryngology, 74,* 451–455.

Aviv, J. E., Martin, J. H., Kim, T., Sacco, R. L., Thomson, J. E., Diamond, B., & Close, L. G. (1999). Laryngopharyngeal sensory discrimination testing and the laryngeal adductor reflex. *Annals of Otology, Rhinology, & Laryngology, 108,* 725–730.

Awan, S. N. (2001). *The voice diagnostic protocol: A practical guide to the diagnosis of voice disorders.* Gaithersburg, MD: Aspen.

Awan, S. N., & Mueller, P. B. (1996). Speaking fundamental frequency characteristics of White, African-American, and Hispanic kindergartners. *Journal of Speech and Hearing Research, 39,* 573–577.

Awan, S. N., & Roy, N. (2005). Acoustic prediction of voice type in women with functional dysphonia. *Journal of Voice, 19,* 268–282.

Axon, P. R., Hartley, C., & Rothera, M. P. (1995). Endoscopic balloon dilatation of subglottic stenosis. *The Journal of Laryngology & Otology, 109,* 876–879.

Azadarmaki, R., Mirza, N., & Soliman, A. M. S. (2010). Unilateral true vocal fold synkinesis presenting with airway obstruction. *Annals of Otology, Rhinology, & Laryngology, 118,* 587–591.

Aziz, L., & Ejnell, H. (2003). Obstructive sleep apnea caused by bilateral vocal fold paralysis. *Ear, Nose, & Throat Journal, 82,* 326–327.

Bach, K. K., Belafsky, P. C., Wasylik, K., Postma, G. N., & Koufman, J. A. (2005). Validity and reliability of the Glottal Function Index. *Archives of Otolaryngology—Head and Neck Surgery, 131,* 961–964.

Baeck, H. E., & de Souza, M. N. (2007). Longitudinal study of the fundamental frequency of hunger cries along the first 6 months of healthy babies. *Journal of Voice, 21,* 551–559.

Bailey, C. M., Clary, R. A., Pengilly, A., & Albert, D. M. (1995). Voice quality following laryngotracheal reconstruction. *International Journal of Pediatric Otorhinolaryngology, 32* (Suppl.), 593–595.

Bailey, E. F., & Hoit, J. D. (2002). Speaking and breathing in high respiratory drive. *Journal of Speech, Language, and Hearing Research, 45,* 89–99.

Bajaj, Y., Sethi, N., Shayah, A., Harris, A.T., Henshaw, P., Coatesworth, A. P., & Nicolaides, A. R. (2009). Vocal fold paralysis: Role of bilateral transverse cordotomy. *The Journal of Laryngology & Otology, 122,* 1348–1351.

Baken, R. J. (1992). Electroglottography. *Journal of Voice, 6,* 98–110.

Baken, R. J. (2005). The aged voice: A new hypothesis. *Journal of Voice, 19,* 317–325.

Baken, R. J. (2005). An overview of laryngeal function for voice production. In R. T. Sataloff (Ed.), *Voice science* (pp. 147–165). San Diego, CA: Plural Publishing.

Baker, J. (1998). Psychogenic dysphonia: Peeling back the layers. *Journal of Voice, 12,* 527–535.

Baker, J. (2003). Psychogenic voice disorders and traumatic stress experience: A discussion paper with two case reports. *Journal of Voice, 17,* 308–318.

Baker, K., Ramig, L., Luschei, E., & Smith, M. (1998). Thyroarytenoid muscle activity associated with hypophonia in Parkinson disease and aging. *Neurology, 51,* 1592–1598.

Baker, K. K., Ramig, L. O., Sapir, S., Luschei, E. S., & Smith, M. E. (2001). Control of vocal loudness in young and old adults. *Journal of Speech, Language, Hearing Research, 44,* 297–305.

Baker, S., Kelchner, L., Weinrich, B., Lee, L., Willging, P., Cotton, R., & Zur, K. (2006). Pediatric laryngotracheal stenosis and airway reconstruction: A review of voice outcomes, assessment, and treatment issues. *Journal of Voice, 20,* 631–641.

Bakthavachalam, S., & McClay, J. E. (2008). Endoscopic management of subglottic stenosis. *Otolaryngology—Head and Neck Surgery, 139,* 551–559.

Balter, M. S., Adams, S. C., & Chapman, K. R. (2001). Inhaled Beclomethasone Dipropionate improves acoustic measures of voice in patients with asthma. *Chest, 120,* 1829–1834.

Bandi, V., Munnur, U., & Braman, S. S. (2002). Airway problems in patients with rheumatologic disorders. *Critical Care Clinics, 18,* 749–765.

Barkmeier, J. M., Case, J. L., & Ludlow, C. L. (2001). Identification of symptoms for spasmodic dysphonia and vocal tremor: A comparison of expert and nonexpert judges. *Journal of Communication Disorders, 34,* 21–37.

Barrichelo-Lindstrom, V., & Behlau, M. (2009). Resonant voice in acting students: Perceptual and acoustic correlates of the trained Y-Buzz by Lessac. *Journal of Voice, 23,* 603–609.

Bass, H. (1973). The flow volume loop: Normal standards and abnormalities in chronic obstructive pulmonary disease. *Chest, 63,* 171–176.

Bassiouny, S. (1998). Efficacy of the accent method of voice therapy. *Folia Phoniatrica et Logopedica, 50,* 146–164.

Baylor, C. R., Yorkston, K. M., Eadie, T. L., & Maronian, N. C. (2007). The psychosocial consequences of Botox injections for spasmodic dysphonia: A qualitative study of patients' experiences. *Journal of Voice, 21,* 231–247.

Baylor, C. R., Yorkston, K. M., Eadie, T. L., Strand, E. A., & Duffy, J. (2006). A systematic review of outcome measurement in unilateral vocal fold paralysis. *Journal of Medical Speech-Language Pathology, 14,* xxvii–lvii.

Behrman, A. (2005). Common practices of voice therapists in the evaluation of patients. *Journal of Voice, 19,* 454–469.

Behrman, A. (2006). Facilitating behavioral change in voice therapy: The relevance of motivational interviewing. *American Journal of Speech-Language Pathology, 15,* 215–225.

Behrman, A., Dahl, L. D., Abramson, A. L., & Schutte, H. K. (2003). Anterior-posterior and medial compression of the supraglottic: Signs of nonorganic dysphonia or normal postures? *Journal of Voice, 17,* 403–410.

Behrman, A., Rutledge, J., Hembree, A., & Sheridon, S. (2008). Vocal hygiene education, voice production therapy, and the role of patient adherence: A treatment effectiveness study in women with phonotrauma. *Journal of Speech, Language, and Hearing Research, 51,* 350–366.

Behrman, A., & Sulica, L. (2003). Voice rest after microlaryngoscopy: Current opinion and practice. *The Laryngoscope, 113,* 2182–2186.

Belafsky, P. C., Postma, G. M., Amin, M. R., & Koufman, J. A. (2002). Symptoms and findings of laryngopharyngeal reflux. *Ear Nose Throat Journal, 81* (Suppl. 2), 10–13.

Belafsky, P. C., Postma, G. N., Reulbach, T. R., & Holland, B. W. (2002). Muscle tension dysphonia as a sign of underlying glottal insufficiency. *Otolaryngology—Head and Neck Surgery, 127,* 448–451.

Belafsky, P. C., Postma, G. N., & Koufman, J. A. (2001). The validity and reliability of the Reflux Finding Score (RFS). *The Laryngoscope, 111,* 1313–1317.

Belafsky, P. C., Postma, G. N., Reulbach, T. R., & Holland, B. W. (2002). Muscle tension dysphonia as a sign of underlying glottal insufficiency. *Otolaryngology—Head and Neck Surgery, 127,* 448–451.

Bellandese, M. H. (2009). Fundamental frequency and gender identification in standard esophageal and tracheoesophageal speakers. *Journal of Communication Disorders, 42,* 89–99.

Bellandese, M. H., Lerman, J. W., & Gilbert, H. R. (2001). An acoustic analysis of excellent female esophageal, tracheoesophageal, and laryngeal speakers. *Journal of Speech, Language, and Hearing Research, 44,* 1315–1320.

Bennett, S. (1983). A 3-year longitudinal study of school-aged children's F0s. *Journal of Speech and Hearing Research, 26,* 137–142.

Benninger, M. S. (2000). Microdissection or microspot CO_2 laser for limited vocal fold benign lesions: A prospective randomized trail. *Laryngoscope, 110,* 1. doi:10.1097/00005537-200002009-00001

Benninger, M. S., Alessi, D., Archer, S., Bastian, R., Ford, C., Koufman, J., . . . Spiegel, J. R. (1996). Vocal fold scarring: Current concepts and management. *Otolaryngology—Head and Neck Surgery, 115,* 474–482.

Benson, B. E., Baredes, S., Schwartz, R. A., & Kumar, M. (2006). Stridor. http://emedicine.medscape.com/article/995267-diagnosis

Berardelli, A., Rothwell, J. C., Hallett, M., Thompson, P. D., Manfredi, M., & Marsden, C. D. (1998). The pathophysiology of primary dystonia. *Brain, 121,* 1195–1212.

Bergamini, G., Alicandri-Ciufelli, M., Molteni, G., Villari, D., Luppi, M. P., Genovese, E., & Presutti, L. (2010). Therapy of unilateral vocal fold paralysis with polydimethylsiloxane injection laryngoplasty: Our experience. *Journal of Voice, 24,* 119–125.

Berjawi, G., Uthman, I., Mahfoud, L., Husseini, S. Y., Nassar, J., Kotobi, A., & Hamdan, A.-L. H. (2009). Cricoarytenoid joint abnormalities in patients with rheumatoid arthritis. *Journal of Voice.*

Berliti, S., Omidi, M., & Wenig, B. (2005). Chronic laryngitis, infectious or allergic. www.emedicine.com/ent/topic354.htm

Bernaldez, R., Garcia-Pallares, M., Morera, E., Lassaletta, L., Del Palacio, A., & Gavilan, J. (2003). Oncologic and functional results of near-total laryngectomy. *Otolaryngology—Head and Neck Surgery, 128,* 700–705.

Bernstein Ratner, N. (2006). Evidence-based practice: An examination of its ramifications for the practice of speech-language pathology. *Language, Speech, and Hearing Services in Schools, 37,* 257–267.

Berry, D. A., Montequin, D. W., Chan, R. W., Titze, I. R., & Hoffman, H. T. (2003). An investigation of cricoarytenoid joint mechanics using simulated muscle forces. *Journal of Voice, 17,* 47–62.

Bertino, G., Bellomo, A., Ferrero, F. E., & Ferlito, A. (2001). Acoustic analysis of voice quality with or without false vocal fold displacement after cordectomy. *Journal of Voice, 15,* 131–140.

Bestall, J. C., Paul, E. A., Garrod, R., Garnham, R., Jones, P. W., & Wedzicha, J. A. (1999). Usefulness of the Medical Research Council (MRC) dyspnoea scale as a measure of disability in patients with chronic obstructive pulmonary disease. *Thorax, 54,* 581–586.

Bhalla, R. K., Watson, G., Taylor, W., Jones, A. S., & Roland, N. J. (2008). Acoustic analysis in asthmatics and the influence of inhaled corticosteroid therapy. doi:10.1016/j.jvoice.11.001

Bhuta, T., Patrick, L., & Garnett, J. D. (2004). Perceptual evaluation of voice quality and its correlation with acoustic measurements. *Journal of Voice, 18,* 299–304.

Biary, N., Pimental, P. A., & Langenberg, P. W. (1988). A double-blind trial of clonazepam in the treatment of parkinsonian dysarthria. *Neurology, 38,* 255–258.

Bielamowicz, S., Stager, S. V., Badillo, A., & Godlewski, A. (2002). Unilateral versus bilateral injections of botulinim toxin in patients with adductor spasmodic dysphonia. *Journal of Voice, 16,* 117–123.

Bielecki, I., Mniszek, J., & Cofala, M. (2009). Intralesional injection of cidofovir for recurrent respiratory papillomatosis in children. *International Journal of Pediatric Otorhinolaryngology, 73,* 681–684.

Bien, S., Okla, S., van As-Brooks, C. J., & Ackerstaff, A. H. (2010). The effect of a heat and moisture exchanger (Provox HME) on pulmonary protection after total laryngectomy: A randomized controlled study. *European Archives of Otorhinolaryngology, 267,* 429–435.

Biever, D. M., & Bless, D. M. (1989). Vibratory characteristics of the vocal folds in young adult and geriatric women. *Journal of Voice, 3,* 120–131.

Billante, C. R., Clary, J., Sullivan, C., & Netterville, J. L. (2002). Voice outcome following thyroplasty in patients with longstanding vocal fold immobility. *Auris Nasus Larynx, 29,* 341–345.

Birkent, H., Maronian, N., Waugh, P., Merati, A. L., Perkel, D., & Hillel, A. D. (2009). Dosage changes in patients with long-term botulinum toxin use for laryngeal dystonia. *Otolaryngology—Head and Neck Surgery, 140,* 43–47.

Bisetti, M. S., Segala, F., Zappia, F., Albera, R., Ottaviani, F., & Schindler, A. (2009). Non-invasive assessment of benign vocal folds lesions in children by means of ultrasonography. *International Journal of Pediatric Otorhinolaryngology, 73,* 1160–1162.

Bitar, M., Baz, R., Fuleihan, N., & Muallem, M. (2007). Can zinc be an adjuvant therapy for juvenile onset recurrent respiratory papillomatosis? *International Journal of Pediatric Otorhinolaryngology, 71,* 1163–1173.

Blager, F. B. (2006). Vocal cord dysfunction. *Perspectives on Voice and Voice Disorders, 16,* 7–10.

Blalock, P. D. (1992). Breath support. *The Visible Voice, 1,* 6–7.

Blaugrund, S. M., Isshiki, N., & Taira, T. (1992). Phonosurgery. In A. Blitzer, M. E. Brin, C. T. Sasaki, S. Fahn, & K. S. Harris (Eds.), *Neurologic disorders of the larynx.* New York: Thieme Medical.

Bliss-Moreau, E., Owren, M. J., & Barrett, L. F. (2010). I like the sound of your voice: Affective learning about vocal signals. *Journal of Experimental Social Psychology, 46,* 557–563.

Blitzer, A. (2010). Spasmodic dysphonia and botulinum toxin: Experience from the largest treatment series. *European Journal of Neurology, 17* (Suppl. 1), 28–30.

Blitzer, A., Brin, M. F., & Stewart, C. F. (1998). Botulinum toxin management of spasmodic dysphonia: A 12-year experience in more than 900 patients. *Laryngoscope, 108,* 1435–1441.

Block, B. B., & Brodsky, L. (2007). Hoarseness in children: The role of laryngopharyngeal reflux. *International Journal of Pediatric Otorhinolaryngology, 71,* 1361–1369.

Blomgren, M., Chen, Y., Ng, M. L., & Gilbert, H. R. (1998). Acoustic, aerodynamic, physiologic, and perceptual properties of modal and vocal fry registers. *Journal of the Acoustical Society of America, 103,* 2649–2658.

Blood, G. W. (1993). Development and assessment of a scale addressing communication needs of patients with laryngectomees. *American Journal of Speech-Language Pathology, 2,* 82–90.

Bluestone, C. D. (2005). Humans are born too soon: Impact on pediatric otolaryngology. *International Journal of Pediatric Otorhinolaryngology, 69,* 1–8.

Blumin, J. H., & Berke, G. S. (2002). Bilateral vocal fold paresis and multiple system atrophy. *Archives of Otolaryngology—Head and Neck Surgery, 128,* 1404–1407.

Blumin, J. H., Keppel, K. L., Braun, N. M., Kerschner, J. E., & Merati, A. L. (2008). The impact of gender and age on voice related quality of life in children: Normative data. *International Journal of Pediatric Otorhinolaryngology, 72,* 229–234.

Blumin, J. H., & Merati, A. L. (2008). Laryngeal reinnervation with nerve-nerve anastomosis versus laryngeal framework surgery alone: A comparison of safety. *Otolaryngology—Head and Neck Surgery, 138,* 217–220.

Blumin, J. H., Poolinsky, D. E., & Atkins, J. P. (2004). Laryngeal findings in advanced Parkinson's disease. *Annals of Otology, Rhinology, & Laryngology, 113,* 253–258.

Boers, J., Klop, E. M., Hulshoff, A. C., de Weerd, H., & Holstege, G. (2007). Direct projections from the nucleus retroambiguus to cricothyroid motoneurons in the cat. *Neuroscience Letters, 319,* 5–8. Retrieved from http://keur.eldoc.ub.rug.nl/wetenschappers/1/17537/

Bohnenkamp, T. A., Stowell, T., Hesse, J., & Wright, S. (2010). Speech breathing in speakers who use an electrolarynx. *Journal of Communication Disorders, 43,* 199–211.

Boliek, C. A., Hixon, T. J., Watson, P. J., & Jones, P. B. (2009). Refinement of speech breathing in healthy 4- to 6-year-old children. *Journal of Speech, Language, and Hearing Research, 52,* 990–1007.

Boliek, C., Hixon, T., Watson, P., & Morgan, W. (1996). Vocalization and breathing during the first years of life. *Journal of Voice, 10,* 1–22.

Boliek, C., Hixon, T., Watson, P., & Morgan, W. (1997). Vocalization and breathing during the second and third years of life. *Journal of Voice, 11,* 373–390.

Bonelli, R. M., Wenning, G. K., & Kapfhammer, H. P. (2004). Huntington's disease: Present treatments and future therapeutic modalities. *International Clinical Psychopharmacology, 19,* 51–62.

Bonner, J. A., Harari, P. M., Giralt, J., Azarnia, N., Shin, D. M., Cohen, R. B., . . . Ang, K. K. (2006). Radiotherapy plus cetuximab for squamous-cell carcinoma of the head and neck. *The New England Journal of Medicine, 354,* 567–578.

Boone, D. R. (1974). Dismissal criteria in voice therapy. *Journal of Speech and Hearing Disorders, 39,* 133–139.

Boone, D. R., & McFarlane, S. C. (1993). A critical view of the yawn-sigh as a voice therapy technique. *Journal of Voice, 7,* 75–80.

Borg, G. A. (1982). Psychophysical bases of perceived exertion. *Medicine and Science in Sports and Exercise, 14,* 377–381.

Boscolo-Rizzo, P., Zanetti, F., Carpene, S., & Da Mosto, M. C. (2008). Long-term results with tracheoesophageal voice prosthesis: Primary versus secondary TEP. *European Archives of Otorhinolaryngology, 265,* 73–77.

Bosely, M. E., Cunningham, M. J., Volk, M. S., & Hartnick, C. J. (2006). Validation of the Pediatric Voice-Related Quality of Life Survey. *Archives of Otolaryngology—Head and Neck Surgery, 132,* 717–720.

Boshoff, P. (1945). The anatomy of the South African Negro larynges. *South African Journal of Medical Sciences, 10,* 35–50.

Bosley, B., Rosen, C. A., Simpson, C. B., McMullin, B.T., Gartner-Schmidt, J. L. (2005). Medial arytenoidectomy versus transverse cordotomy as a treatment for bilateral vocal fold paralysis. *Annals of Otology, Rhinology, & Laryngology, 114,* 922–926.

Boucher, V. J. (2008). Acoustic correlates of fatigue in laryngeal muscles: Findings for a criterion-based prevention of acquired voice pathologies. *Journal of Speech, Language, and Hearing Research, 51,* 1161–1170.

Boucher, V. J., & Ayad, T. (2010). Physiological attributes of vocal fatigue and their acoustic effects: A synthesis of findings for a criterion-based prevention of acquired voice disorders. *Journal of Voice, 24,* 324–336.

Boutsen, F., Cannito, M. P., Taylor, M., & Bender, B. (2002). Botox treatment in adductor spasmodic dysphonia: A meta-analysis. *Journal of Speech, Language, and Hearing Research, 45,* 469–481.

Bovo, R., Galceran, M., Petrucelli, J., & Hatzopoulos, S. (2007). Vocal problems among teachers: Evaluation of a preventive voice program. *Journal of Voice, 21,* 705–722.

Braden, M. N., Johns III, M. M., Klein, A. M., Delgaudio, J. M., Gilman, M., & Hapner, E. R. (2010). Assessing the effectiveness of botulinum toxin injections for adductor spasmodic dysphonia: Clinician and patient perception. *Journal of Voice, 24,* 242–249.

Branco, A., Behlau, M., & Rehder, M. I. (2005). The neonate cry after cesarean section and vaginal delivery during the first minutes of life. *International Journal of Pediatric Otorhinolaryngology, 69,* 681–689.

Branco, A., Fekete, S. M. W., Rugolo, L. M. S. S., & Rehder, M. I. (2007). The newborn pain cry: Descriptive acoustic spectrographic analysis. *International Journal of Pediatric Otorhinolaryngology, 71,* 539–546.

Brandon, C. A., Rosen, C., Georgelis, G., Horton, M. J., Mooney, M. P., & Sciote, J. J. (2003). Staining of human thyroarytenoid muscle with myosin antibodies reveals some unique extrafusal fibers, but no muscle spindles. *Journal of Voice, 17,* 245–254.

Branski, R. C., Cukier-Blaj, S., Pusic, A., Cano, S. J., Klassen, A., Mener, D., . . . Kraus, D. H. (2009). Measuring quality of life in dysphonic patients: A systematic review of content development in patient-reported outcome measures. *Journal of Voice,* doi:10.1016/j.jvoice.2008.05.006

Branski, R. C., Murry, T., & Rosen, C. A. (2005). Voice therapy. Available from www.emedicine.com/ent/topic683.htm

Branski, R., & Sivasankar, M. (2006). An update on voice research in the United States. *The ASHA Leader, 11,* 10–11.

Branski, R. C., Verdolini, K., Sandulache, V., Rosen, C. A., & Hebda, P. A. (2006). Vocal fold wound healing: A review for clinicians. *Journal of Voice, 20,* 432–442.

Breatnach, E., Abbott, G. C., & Fraser, R. G. (1984). Dimensions of the normal human trachea. *American Journal of Roentgenology, 142,* 903–906.

Breiss, B. (1957). Voice therapy. Part I. Identification of specific laryngeal muscle dysfunction by voice testing. *Archives of Otolaryngology, 66,* 375–382.

Breiss, B. (1959). Voice therapy. Part II. Essential treatment phases of specific laryngeal muscle dysfunction. *Archives of Otolaryngology, 69,* 61–69.

Brigger, M. T., & Hartnick, C. J. (2009). Laryngotracheal reconstruction. *Operative Techniques in Otolaryngology, 20,* 229–235.

Bristol, L. A., & Rothstein, J. D. (1996). Glutamate transporter gene expression in amyotrophic lateral sclerosis motor cortex. *Annals of Neurology, 39,* 676–679.

Brondbo, K., & Benninger, M. S. (2004). Laser resection of T1a glottic carcinomas: Results and postoperative voice quality. *Acta Otolaryngologica, 124,* 976–979.

Brooks, B. R., Miller, E. G., & Swash, M. (2000). El Escorial revisited: Revised criteria for the diagnosis and amyotrophic lateral sclerosis. *Amyotrophic Lateral Sclerosis and Other Motor Neuron Disorders, 5,* 293–299.

Brown, D. H., Hilgers, F. J. M., Irish, J. C., & Balm, A. J. M. (2003). Postlaryngectomy voice rehabilitation: State of the art at the millennium. *World Journal of Surgery, 27,* 824–831.

Brown, M., Perry, A., Cheesman, A. D., & Pring, T. (2000). Pitch change in male-to-female transsexuals: Has phonosurgery a role to play? *International Journal of Language and Communication Disorders, 35,* 129–136.

Brown, W. S. Jr., Morris, R. J., & Michel, J. F. (1989). Vocal jitter in young adult and aged female voices. *Journal of Voice, 3,* 113–119.

Brown, W. S. Jr., Morris, R. J., & Murry, T. (1996). Comfortable effort level revisited. *Journal of Voice, 10,* 299–305.

Brown, M. L., & Rounsley, C. A. (1996). *True selves: Understanding transsexualism.* San Francisco: Jossey Bass Publishers.

Brown, S., Ngan, E., & Liotti, M. (2007). A larynx area in the human motor cortex. *Cerebral Cortex,* doi:10.1093/cercor/bhm131 Downloaded from http://cercor.oxfordjournals.org on May 8, 2010.

Buckmire, R. A. (2006). Arytenoid fixation. www.emedicine.com/ent/topic609.htm

Buckmire, R. A., Bryson, P. C., & Patel, M. R. (2010). Type I Gore-Tex laryngoplasty for glottic incompetence in mobile vocal folds. *Journal of Voice,* doi:10.1016/j.jvoice.2009.12.003

Buddiga, P. (2010). Vocal cord dysfunction: Differential diagnosis and workup. Available from http://emedicine.medscape.com/article/137782-diagnosis

Burns, J. A., Har-El, G., Shapshay, S., Maune, S., & Zeitels, S. M. (2009). Endoscopic laser resection of laryngeal cancer: Is it oncologically safe? Position Statement from the American Broncho-Esophagological Association. *Annals of Otology, Rhinology, & Laryngology, 118,* 399–404.

Cady, J. (2002). Laryngectomy: Beyond loss of voice—Caring for the patient as a whole. *Clinical Journal of Oncology Nursing, 6,* 1–5.

Camphina-Bacote, J. (1993). Cultural competence in psychiatric-mental health nursing: A conceptual model. In J. Campinha-Bacote (Ed.), *Readings in transcultural health care* (4th ed., pp. 147–165). Wyoming, OH: Transcultural C.A.R.E. Associates.

Cannito, M. P., & Woodson, G. E. (2000). The spasmodic dysphonias. In R. D. Kent & M. J. Ball (Eds.), *Voice quality measurement.* San Diego, CA: Singular Publishing Group.

Cantu, E., Ryan, W. J., Tansey, S., & Johnson, C. S., Jr. (1998). Tracheoesophageal speech: Predictors of success and social validity ratings. *American Journal of Otolaryngology, 19,* 12–17.

Caputo-Rosen, D., & Sataloff, R. T. (1998). Psychological aspects of voice disorders. In R. T. Sataloff (Ed.), *Vocal Health and Pedagogy* (pp. 243–255). San Diego, CA: Singular Publishing Group, Inc.

Carding, P., Carison, E., Epstein, R., Mathieson, L., & Shewell, C. (2000). Formal perceptual evaluation of voice quality in the United Kingdom. *Logopedics Phoniatrics Vocology, 25,* 133–138.

Carding, P. N., Horsley, I. A., & Docherty, G. J. (1998). The effectiveness of voice therapy for patients with non-organic dysphonia. *Clinical Otolaryngology, 23,* 310–318.

Carew, L., Dacakis, G., & Oates, J. (2007). The effectiveness of oral resonance therapy on the perception of femininity of voice in male-to-female transsexuals. *Journal of Voice, 21,* 591–603.

Carleton, R. N., Peluso, D. L., Collimore, K. C., & Asmundson, G. J. G. (2011). Social anxiety and posttraumatic stress symptoms: The impact of distressing social events. *Journal of Anxiety Disorders, 25,* 49–57.

Carney, I. K., Gibson, P. G., Murree-Allen, K., Saltos, N., Olson, L. G., & Hensley, M. J. (1997). A systematic evaluation of mechanisms in chronic cough. *American Journal of Respiratory Critical Care Medicine, 156,* 211–216.

Carr, M. M., Schmidbauer, J. A., Majaess, L., & Smith, R. L. (2000). Communication after laryngectomy: An assessment of quality of life. *Otolaryngolog—Head and Neck Surgery, 122,* 39–43.

Carrau, R. L., Khidr, A., Crawley, J. A., Hillson, E. M., Davis, J. K., & Pashos, C. L. (2004). The impact of laryngopharyngeal reflux on patient-reported quality of life. *The Laryngoscope, 114,* 670–674.

Carrau, R. L., Khidr, A., Gold, K. F., Crawley, J. A., Hillson, E. M., Koufman, J. A., & Pashos, C. L. (2005). Validation of a Quality-of-Life instrument for laryngopharyngeal reflux. *Archives of Otolaryngology—Head and Neck Surgery, 131,* 315–320.

Carroll, T. L., & Rosen, C. A. (2010). Trial vocal fold injection. *Journal of Voice,* 24, 494–498.

Case, J. L. (2002). *Clinical management of voice disorders* (4th ed.). Austin, TX: Pro-Ed.

Casiano, R. R., Ruiz, P. J., & Goldstein, W. (2010). Histopathologic changes in the aging human cricoarytenoid joint. *Laryngoscope, 104,* 533–538.

Casper, M. A., Raphael, L. J., Harris, K. S., & Geibel, J. M. (2007). Speech prosody in cerebellar ataxia. *International Journal of Language and Communication Disorders, 42,* 407–426.

Catten, M., Gray, S. D., Hammond, T. H., Zhou, R., & Hammond, E. (1998). Analysis of cellular location and concentration in vocal fold lamina propria. *Otolaryngology—Head and Neck Surgery, 118,* 663–667.

Chang, A., & Karnell, M. P. (2004). Perceived phonatory effort and phonation threshold pressure across a prolonged voice loading task: A study of vocal fatigue. *Journal of Voice, 18,* 454–466.

Chang, C.-H., Lee, K.-W., & Kuo, W.-R. (2004). Dysphonia as the initial symptom of myasthenia gravis. *Journal of Otolaryngology, 33,* 57–59.

Chang, C. Y., Chabot, P., & Walz, C. M. (2009). A survey of current practices of physicians who treat adductor spasmodic dysphonia in the U.S. *ENT: Ear, Nose & Throat Journal, 88,* E. 18.

Chang, Y., Brewer, N. T., Rinas, A. C., Schmitt, K., & Smith, J. S. (2009). Evaluating the impact of human papillomavirus vaccines. *Vaccine, 27,* 4355–4362.

Chatham, M., Bleecker, E. R., Norman, P., Smith, P. L., & Mason, P. (1982). A screening test for airways reactivity: An abbreviated methacholine inhalation challenge. *Chest, 82,* 15–18.

Chawla, S., & Carney, A. S. (2009). Organ preservation surgery for laryngeal cancer. *Head and Neck Oncology,* doi:10.1186/1758-3284-1-12

Cheang, H. S., & Pell, M. D. (2007). An acoustic investigation of Parkinsonian speech in linguistic and emotional contexts. *Journal of Neurolinguistics, 20,* 221–241.

Chen, A., & Garrett, C. G. (2005). Otolaryngologic presentations of amyotrophic lateral sclerosis. *Otolaryngology—Head and Neck Surgery, 132,* 500–504.

Chen, J.-J. (2007). Laryngeal lesions in patients with chronic cough and normal chest radiographs and auscultation. *Tzu Chi Medical Journal, 19,* 145–151.

Chen, S. H., Chiang, S.-C., Chung, Y.-M., Hsiao, L.-C., & Hsiao, T.-Y. (2010). Risk factors and effects of voice problems for teachers. *Journal of Voice, 24,* 183–192.

Chen, S. H., Hsiao, T.-Y., Hsiao, L.-C., Chung, Y.-M., & Chiang, S.-C. (2007). Outcome of resonant voice therapy for female teachers with voice disorders: Perceptual, physiological, acoustic, aerodynamic, and functional measurements. *Journal of Voice, 21,* 415–425.

Chen, Y., Kimelman, M. D. Z., & Micco, K. (2009). Investigation of habitual pitch during free play activities for preschool-aged children. *International Journal of Pediatric Otorhinolaryngology, 73,* 73–80.

Cheng, A. T. L., & Beckenham, E. J. (2009). Congenital anterior glottic webs with subglottic stenosis: Surgery using perichondrial keels. *International Journal of Pediatric Otorhinolaryngology, 73,* 945–949.

Chernobelsky, S. (2002). The use of electroglottography in the treatment of deaf adolescents with puberphonia. *Logopedics, Phoniatrics, Vocology, 27,* 63–65.

Cheung, Y. L., Molassiotas, A., & Chang, A. M. (2003). The effect of progressive muscle relaxation training on anxiety and quality of life after stoma surgery in colorectal cancer patients. *Psycho-Oncology, 12,* 254–266.

Chhetri, D. K., Head, C., Revazova, E., Hart, S., Bhuta, S., & Berke, G. S. (2004). Lamina propria replacement therapy with cultured autologous fibroblasts for vocal fold scars. *Otolaryngology—Head and Neck Surgery, 131,* 864–870.

Chhetri, D. K., Merati, A. L., Blumin, J. H., Sulica, L., Damrose, E. J., & Tsai, V. W. (2008). Reliability of the perceptual evaluation of adductor spasmodic dysphonia. *Annals of Otology, Rhinology, & Laryngology, 117,* 159–165.

Chiang, W. C., Goh, A., Tang, J. P. L., & Chay, O. M. (2008). Paradoxical vocal cord dysfunction: When a wheeze is not asthma. *Singapore Medical Journal, 49,* e110–e112.

Chitose, S., Umeno, H., & Nakashima, T. (2009). Endoscopic surgical treatment of posterior glottic stenosis. *Journal of Laryngology and Otology, 31* (Suppl.), 68–71.

Chone, C. T., Gripp, F. M., Spina, A. L., & Crespo, A. N. (2005). Primary versus secondary tracheoesophageal puncture for speech rehabilitation in total laryngectomy: Long-term results with indwelling voice prosthesis. *Otolaryngology—Head and Neck Surgery, 133,* 89–93.

Chone, C. T., Seixas, V. O., Paes, L. A., Gripp, F. M., Teixeira, C., Andreollo, N. A., . . . Crespo, A. N. (2008). Use of computerized manometry for the detection of pharyngoesophageal spasm in tracheoesophageal speech. *Otolaryngology—Head and Neck Surgery, 139,* 449–452.

Christopher, K. L., & Morris, M. J. (2010). Vocal cord dysfunction, paradoxic vocal fold motion, or laryngomalacia? Our understanding requires an interdisciplinary approach. *Otolaryngology Clinics of North America, 43,* 43–66.

Chun, J. Y., Kim, Y. H., Choi, E. C., Byeon, H. K., Jung, J., & Kim, S.-H. (2010). The oncologic safety and functional preservation of supraglottic partial laryngectomy. *American Journal of Otolaryngology, 31,* 246–251.

Chung, B. J., Akst, L. M., & Koltai, P. J. (2006). 3.5 year follow-up of intralesional cydofovir protocol for pediatric recurrent respiratory papillomatosis. *International Journal of Pediatric Otorhinolaryngology, 70,* 1911–1917.

Chung, J. H., Tae, K., Lee, Y. S., Jeong, J., Cho, S. H., Kim, K. R., . . . Han, D. S. (2009). The significance of laryngopharyngeal reflux in benign vocal mucosal lesions. *Otolaryngology—Head and Neck Surgery, 141,* 369–373.

Chung, K. F. (2006). Measurement of cough. *Respiratory Physiology and Neurobiology, 152,* 329–339.

Chung, K. F., & Pavord, I. D. (2008). Prevalence, pathogenesis, and causes of chronic cough. *Lancet, 371,* 1364–1374.

Clary, R. A., Pengilly, A., Bailey, M., Jones, N., Albert, D., Comins, J., et al. (1996). Analysis of voice outcomes in pediatric patients following surgical procedures for laryngotracheal stenosis. *Archives of Otolaryngology—Head and Neck Surgery, 122,* 1189–1194.

Cohen, S. M., & Garrett, C. G. (2007). Utility of voice therapy in the management of vocal fold polyps and cysts. *Otolaryngology—Head and Neck Surgery, 136,* 742–746.

Cohen, S. M., Garrett, C. G., Dupont, W. D., Ossoff, R. H., & Courey, M. S. (2006). Voice-related quality of life in T1 glottic cancer: Irradiation versus endoscopic excision. *Annals of Otology, Rhinology, & Laryngology, 115,* 581–586.

Cohen, S. M., Garrett, C. G., Netterville, J. L., & Courey, M. S. (2006). Laryngoscopy in bilateral vocal fold immobility: Can you make a diagnosis? *Annals of Otology, Rhinology, & Laryngology, 115,* 439–443.

Cohen-Kettenis, P. T., & Pfafflin, F. (2010). The DSM diagnostic criteria for gender identity disorders in adolescents and adults. *Archives of Sexual Behavior, 39,* 499–513.

Cohn, J. R., Sataloff, R. T., & Branton, C. (2001). Response of asthma-related voice dysfunction to allergen immunotherapy: A case report of confirmation by methacholine challenge. *Journal of Voice, 15,* 558–560.

Colton, R. H., Casper, J. K., & Leonard, R. (2006). *Understanding voice problems: A physiological perspective for diagnosis and treatment* (3rd ed.). Philadelphia, PA: Lippincott Williams & Wilkins.

Comar, M., Fabris, A., Vatta, S., Pelos, G., Zocconi, E., & Campello, C. (2006). HPV genotyping and HLA II analysis in a pedigree study of pediatric RRP: Preliminary results. *International Journal of Pediatric Otorhinolaryngology, 70,* 1935–1939.

Comins, R. (1992). Voice forum: Voice in the curriculum. *Voice, 1,* 67–73.

Connaghan, K. P., Moore, C. A., & Higashakawa, M. (2004). Respiratory kinematics during vocalization and nonspeech respiration in children from 9 to 48 months. *Journal of Speech, Language, and Hearing Research, 47,* 70–84.

Connelly, A., Clement, W. A., & Kubba, H. (2009). Management of dysphonia in children. *Journal of Laryngology and Otology, 123,* 642–647.

Connor, N. P., Cohen, S. B., Theis, S. M., Thibeault, S. L., Heatley, D., & Bless, D. M. (2008). Attitudes of children with dysphonia. *Journal of Voice, 22,* 197–209.

Connor, N. P., Palazzi-Churas, K. L. P., Cohen, S. B., Leverson, G. E., & Bless, D. M. (2007). Symptoms of extraesophageal reflux in a community-dwelling sample. *Journal of Voice, 21,* 189–202.

Constantinescu, G. A., Theodoros, D. G., Russell, T. G., Ward, E. C., Wilson, S. J., & Wootton, R. (2010). Home-based speech treatment for Parkinson's disease delivered remotely: A case report. *Journal of Telemedicine and Telecare, 16,* 100–104.

Cooksey, J. M. (2000). Voice transformation in male adolescents. In L. Thurman & G. Welch (Eds.), *Body mind and voice—Foundations of voice education* (pp. 718–738). Iowa City, IA: The Voice Care Network.

Coppens, P. (2007). Speech therapy for patients with myasthenia gravis. Available from www.speechpathology.com/askexpert/display_question.asp?question_id=251

Cornwell, P. L., Murdoch, B. E., Ward, E. C., & Kellie, S. (2003). Perceptual evaluation of motor speech following treatment for childhood cerebellar tumour. *Clinical Linguistics and Phonetics, 17,* 597–615.

Corrao, W. M., Braman, S. S., & Irwin, R. S. (1979). Chronic cough as the sole presenting manifestation of bronchial asthma. *New England Journal of Medicine, 300,* 633–637.

Costa, D. J., & Stith, J. A. (2009). Posterior glottic web in a 6-year-old boy. *Ear, Nose, & Throat Journal, 88,* 1154–1156.

Craig, S., & Derkay, C. S. (2001). Recurrent respiratory papillomatosis. *The Laryngoscope, 111,* 57–69.

Dacakis, G. (2000). Long-term maintenance of fundamental frequency increases in male-to-female transsexuals. *Journal of Voice, 14,* 549–556.

Dacakis, G. (2006). Assessment and goals. In R. K. Adler, S. Hirsch, & M. Mordaunt (Eds.), *Voice and communication therapy for the transgender/transsexual client* (pp. 101–126). San Diego, CA: Plural Publishing.

Dagli, M., Acar, A., Stone, R. E. Jr., Dursun, G., & Eryilmaz, A. (2008). Mutational falsetto: Intervention outcomes in 45 patients. *Journal of Laryngology and Otology, 122,* 277–281.

Dailey, S. H., & Ford, C. N. (2006). Surgical management of sulcus vocalis and vocal fold scarring. *Otolaryngologic Clinics of North America, 39,* 23–42.

D'Alatri, L., Paludetti, G., Contarino, M. F., Galla, S., Marchese, M. R., & Bentivoglio, A. R. (2008). Effects of bilateral subthalamic nucleus stimulation and medication on Parkinsonian speech impairment. *Journal of Voice, 22,* 365–372.

Damrose, E. J. (2008). On the development of idiopathic subglottic stenosis. *Medical Hypotheses, 71,* 122–135.

Damrose, E. J. (2008). Quantifying the impact of androgen therapy on the female larynx. *Auris Nasus Larynx,* doi:10.1016/j.anl.2008.03.002

Damrose, J. F., Goldman, S. N., Groessl, E. J., & Orloff, L. A. (2004). The impact of long-term botulinum toxin injections on symptom severity in patients with spasmodic dysphonia. *Journal of Voice, 18,* 415–422.

Damste, H., Hollien, H., Moore, G. P., & Murry, T. (1968). An X-ray study of vocal fold length. *Folia Phoniatrica, 20,* 349–359.

Daneshi, A., Mohammadi, S., & Hassannia, F. (2009). Delayed laryngotracheal reconstruction with titanium plate: Report of 10 cases. *Journal of Voice.* doi:10.1016/j.voice.2009.06.002

Daniilidou, P., Carding, P., Wilson, J., Drinnan, M., & Deary, V. (2007). Cognitive behavioral therapy for functional dysphonia: A pilot study. *Annals of Otology, Rhinology, & Laryngology, 116,* 717–722.

Darley, F. L., Aronson, A. E., & Brown, J. R. (1969). Clusters of deviant speech dimensions in the dysarthrias. *Journal of Speech and Hearing Research, 12,* 462–496.

Davenport, P. W. (2008). Urge-to-cough: What can it teach us about cough? *Lung, 186* (Suppl. 1), S107–111.

Davis, R. K., Hadley, K., & Smith, M. E. (2004). Endoscopic vertical partial laryngectomy. *Laryngoscope, 114,* 236–240.

Davis, P. J., Zhang, S. P., & Bandler, R. (1996). Midbrain and medullary regulation of respiration and vocalization. *Progress in Brain Research, 107,* 315–325.

Deal, L. V., & Oyer, H. J. (1991). Ratings of vocal pleasantness and the aging process. *Folia Phoniatrica (Basel), 43,* 44–48.

De Alarcon, A., Brehm, S. B., Kelchner, L. K., Meinzen-Derr, J., Middendorf, J., & Weinrich, B. (2009). Comparison of Pediatric Voice Handicap Index scores with perceptual voice analysis in patients following airway reconstruction. *Annals of Otology, Rhinology, & Laryngology, 118,* 581–586.

Deary, I. J., Wilson, J. A., Carding, P. N., & Mackenzie, K. (2003). The dysphonic voice heard by me, you and it: Differential associations with personality and psychological distress. *Clinical Otolaryngology, 28,* 374–378.

Debnath, I., Rich, J. T., & Paniello, R. C. (2008). Intrinsic laryngeal muscle reinnervation using the muscle-nerve-muscle technique. *Annals of Otology, Rhinology, & Laryngology, 117,* 382–388.

De Bodt, M. S., Ketelslagers, K., Peeters, T., Wuyts, F. L., Mertens, F., Pattyn, J., . . . Van de Heyning, P. (2007). Evolution of vocal fold nodules from childhood to adolescence. *Journal of Voice, 21,* 151–156.

Debruyne, F., & Decoster, W. (1999). Acoustic differences between sustained vowels perceived as young or old. *Logopedics, Phoniatrics, Vocology, 24,* 1–5.

Debruyne, F., De Jong, F., & Oosterlinck, K. (1995). Changes in fundamental frequency and spectrum of the voice after cricothyroid approximation. *Scandinavian Journal of Logopedics and Phoniatrics, 20,* 103–106.

Dedivitis, R. A., Queija, D. S., Barros, A. P. B., Pfuetzenreiter, E. G., Felippu, A., Salvia, V. F., . . . Nishimoto, S. N. (2008). The impact of the glottic configuration after frontolateral laryngectomy on the perceptual voice analysis: A preliminary study. *Journal of Voice, 22,* 760–764.

Dedivitis, R. A., Pfuetzenreiter, E. G., Castro, M. A. F., & Curioni, O. A. (2011). Structures constituting the sound course after the treatment of early glottic cancer. *Journal of Voice, 25,* 47–51.

Deem, J. F., & Miller, L. (2000). *Manual of voice therapy* (2nd ed.). Austin, TX: Pro-Ed.

De Jong, F. I. C. R. S., & Norbart, T. C. J. (1996). Cricothyroid approximation for the raise of vocal pitch in androphonia. In O. Kleinsasser, H. Glanz, J. Oloffsson (Eds.). *Advances in laryngology in Europe.* Proceedings of the 1st Scientific Conference of the European Laryngological Society, Marburg, Germany.

DeLeo LeBorgne, W. (2007). Clinical applications and use of the voice range profile. *Perspectives on Voice and Voice Disorders, 17,* 18–24.

DeLeo LeBorgne, W., & Weinrich, B. D. (2002). Phonetogram changes for trained singers over a nine-month period of vocal training. *Journal of Voice, 16,* 37–43.

De Letter, M., Santens, P., Estercam, I., Van Maele, G., De Bodt, M., Boon, P., & Van Borsel, J. (2007). Levadopa-induced modifications of prosody and comprehensibility in advanced Parkinson's disease as perceived by professional listeners. *Clinical Linguistics and Phonetics, 21,* 783–791.

De Letter, M., Santens, P., & van Borsel, J. (2005). The effects of levadopa on word intelligibility in Parkinson's disease. *Journal of Communication Disorders, 38,* 187–196.

DelGaudio, J. M. (2002). Steroid inhaler laryngitis: Dysphonia caused by inhaled fluticasone therapy. *Archives of Otolaryngology—Head and Neck Surgery, 128,* 677–681.

Deliyski, D. D. (2007). Clinical feasibility of high-speed videoendoscopy. *Perspectives on Voice and Voice Disorders, 17*(1), 12–16.

Deliyski, D. D., Evans, M. K., & Shaw, H. S. (2005). Influence of data acquisition environment on accuracy of acoustic voice quality measurements. *Journal of Voice, 19,* 176–186.

De Medeiros, A. M., Barreto, S. M., & Assuncao, A. A. (2007). Voice disorders (dysphonia) in public school female teachers working in Belo Horizonte: Prevalence and associated factors. *Journal of Voice 22*(6), 676–687.

De Menezes, L. N., & Vicente, L. C. C. (2007). Vocal aging of institutionalized elderly people. *Revista CEFAC, 9,* 90–98.

Demmink-Geertman, L., & Dejonckere, P. H. (2002). Nonorganic habitual dysphonia and autonomic dysfunction. *Journal of Voice, 16,* 549–559.

Denny, D. (2004). Changing models of transsexualism. In U. Leli & J. Drescher (Eds.), *Transgender subjectives: A clinician's guide* (pp. 25–40). Binghamton, NY: Haworth.

de Paula, A. A. D., de Carvalho, E. C., & dos Santos, C. B. (2002). The use of the "Progressive Muscle Relaxation" technique for pain relief in gynecology and obstetrics. *Revista Latino-Americana de Enfermagem, 10,* doi:10.1590/S0104-11692002000500005

De Peuter, S., Van Diest, I., Lemaigre, V., Verleden, G., Demedts, M., & Van den Bergh, O. (2004). Dyspnea: The role of psychological processes. *Clinical Psychology Review, 24,* 557–581.

De Pinto, O., & Hollien, H. (1982). Speaking fundamental frequency characteristics of Australian women: Then and now. *Journal of Phonetics, 10,* 367–375.

Depondt, J., & Gehanno, P. (1995). Laryngectomized patients' education and follow-up. *Patient Education and Counseling, 26,* 33–36.

Derkay, C. S. (1995). Task force on recurrent respiratory papillomatosis. *Archives of Otolaryngology Head and Neck Surgery, 121,* 1386–1391.

Derkay, C. S. (2005). Cydofovir for recurrent respiratory papillomatosis (RRP): A re-assessment of risks. Editorial, *International Journal of Pediatric Otorhinolaryngology, 69,* 1465–1467.

Derkay, C. S., & Darrow, D. H. (2006). Recurrent respiratory papillomatosis. *Annals of Otology, Rhinology & Laryngology, 115,* 1–11.

Derkay, C. S., Hester, R. P., Burke, B., Carron, J., & Lawson, L. (2004). Analysis of a staging assessment system for prediction of surgical interval in recurrent respiratory papillomatosis. *International Journal of Pediatric Otorhinolaryngology, 68,* 1493–1498.

Derkay, C. S., Smith, R. J. H., McClay, J., van Burik, J.-A. H., Wiatrak, B. J., Arnold, J., . . . Neefe, J. R. (2005). HspE7 treatment of pediatric recurrent respiratory papillomatosis: Final results of an open-label trial. *Annals of Otology, Rhinology & Laryngology, 114,* 730–737.

Deschler, D. G. (2005). Surgical reconstruction following total laryngectomy with extended or total pharyngectomy. In P. C. Doyle & R. L. Keith (Eds.), *Contemporary considerations in the treatment and rehabilitation of head and neck cancer: Voice, speech, and swallowing* (pp. 237–260). Austin, TX: Pro-Ed.

De Stefani, E., Correa, P., Oreggia, F., Leiva, J., Rivero, S., Fernandez, G., . . . Fontham, E. (1987). Risk factors for laryngeal cancer. *Cancer, 60,* 3087–3091.

Dettmar, P. W., Strugala, V., Fathi, H., Dettmar, H. J., Wright, C., & Morice, A. H. (2009). The online cough clinic—Developing guideline-based diagnosis and advice. *European Respiratory Journal, 34,* 819–824.

Devaney, K. O., Rinaldo, A., & Ferlito, A. (2005). Vocal process granuloma of the larynx—recognition, differential diagnosis and treatment. *Oral Oncology, 41,* 666–669.

Devesa, P. M., Ghufoor, K., & Lloyd, S. (2002). Endoscopic CO_2 laser management of laryngocele. *Laryngoscope, 112,* 1426–1430.

D'haeseleer, E., Depypere, H., Claeys, S., Van Borsel, J., & Van Lierde, K. (2009). The menopause and the female larynx, clinical aspects and therapeutic options: A literature review. *Maturitas, 64,* 27–32.

D'haeseleer, E., Depypere, H., Claeys, S., Wuyts, F. L., Baudonck, N., & Van Lierde, K. M. (2011). Vocal characteristics of middle-aged premenopausal women. *Journal of Voice, 25,* 360–366.

Dietrich, M., Verdolini Abbott, K., Gartner-Schmidt, J., & Rosen, C. A. (2008). The frequency of perceived stress, anxiety, and depression in patients with common pathologies affecting voice. *Journal of Voice, 22,* 472–488.

Dikkers, F. G., Hulstaert, C. E., Oosterbaan, J. A., & Cervera-Paz, F. J. (1993). Ultrastructural changes of the basement membrane zone in benign lesions of the vocal folds. *Acta Otolaryngologica, 113,* 98–101.

Di Nicola, V., Fiorella, M. L., Spinelli, D. A., & Fiorella, R. (2006). Acoustic analysis of voice in patients treated by reconstructive subtotal laryngectomy: Evaluation and critical review. *Acta Otorhinolaryngologica Ital, 26,* 59–68.

Dogan, M., Eryuksel, E., Kocak, I., Celikel, T., & Sehitoglu, M. A. (2007). Subjective and objective evaluation of voice quality in patients with asthma. *Journal of Voice, 21,* 224–230.

Dogan, M., Midi, I., Yazici, M. A., Kocak, I., Gunal, D., & Sehitoglu, M. A. (2007). Objective and subjective evaluation of voice quality in multiple sclerosis. *Journal of Voice, 21,* 735–740.

Donne, A. J., Hampson, L., Homer, J. J., & Hampson, L. N. (2010). The role of HPV type in recurrent respiratory papillomatosis. *International Journal of Pediatric Otorhinolaryngology, 74,* 7–14.

Donne, A. J., Rothera, M. P., & Homer, J. J. (2008). Scientific and clinical aspects of the use of cidofovir in recurrent respiratory papillomatosis. *International Journal of Pediatric Otorhinolaryngology, 72,* 939–944.

Donzelli, G., Rapisardi, G., Moroni, M., Zani, S., Tomasini, B., Ismaelli, A., & Bruscaglioni, P. (1994). Computerized cry analysis in infants affected by severe protein energy malnutrition. *Acta Pediatrica, 83,* 204–211.

Doshi, D. R., & Weinberger, M. M. (2006). Long-term outcome of vocal cord dysfunction. *Annals of Allergy, Asthma, & Immunology, 96,* 794–799.

Doyle, P. C. (2005). Clinical procedures for training use of the electronic artificial larynx. In P. C. Doyle & R. L. Keith (Eds.), *Contemporary considerations in the treatment and rehabilitation of head and neck cancer: Voice, speech, and swallowing* (pp. 545–570). Austin, TX: Pro-Ed.

Doyle, P. C., & Eadie, T. L. (2005). Pharyngoesophageal segment function. In P. C. Doyle & R. L. Keith (Eds.), *Contemporary considerations in the treatment and rehabilitation of head and neck cancer: Voice, speech, and swallowing* (pp. 521–543). Austin, TX: Pro-Ed.

Draganov, P., Todorov, S., Todorov, I., Karchev, T., & Kalvatchev, Z. (2006). Identification of HPV DNA in patients with juvenile-onset recurrent respiratory papillomatosis using SYBR Green real-time PCR. *International Journal of Pediatric Otorhinolaryngology, 70,* 469–473.

Dreary, I. J., Wilson, J. A., Carding, P. N., & MacKenzie, K. (2003). VoiSS: A patient-derived voice symptom scale. *Journal of Psychosomatic Research, 54,* 483–489.

Dromey, C., Nissen, S. L., Roy, N., & Merrill, R. M. (2008). Articulatory changes following treatment of muscle tension dysphonia: Preliminary acoustic evidence. *Journal of Speech, Language, and Hearing Research, 51,* 196–208.

Dromey, C., Ramig, L. O., & Johnson, A. B. (1995). Phonatory and articulatory changes associated with increased vocal intensity in Parkinson disease: A case study. *Journal of Speech & Hearing Research, 38,* 751–764.

Dromey, C., Stathopoulos, E. T., & Sapienza, C. M. (1992). Glottal airflow and electroglottographic measures of vocal function at multiple intensities. *Journal of Voice, 6,* 44–54.

Dromey, C., Warrick, P., & Irish, J. (2002). The influence of pitch and loudness changes on the acoustics of vocal tremor. *Journal of Speech, Language, and Hearing Research, 45,* 879–890.

Duff, M. C., Proctor, A., & Yairi, E. (2004). Prevalence of voice disorders in African American and European American preschoolers. *Journal of Voice, 18,* 348–353.

Duffy, J. (2005). *Motor speech disorders: Substrates, differential diagnosis, and management* (2nd ed.). St. Louis, MO: Elsevier Mosby.

Duffy, J. (2008). Psychogenic speech disorders in people with suspected neurologic disease: Diagnosis and management. Paper presented at the American Speech-Language-Hearing Association Annual Convention, Chicago.

Duguay, M. J. (1991). Esophageal speech training: The initial phase. In S. J. Salmon & K. H. Mount (Eds.), *Alaryngeal speech rehabilitation* (pp. 47–78). Austin, TX: Pro-Ed.

Dursun, G., Boynukalin, S., Ozgursoy, O. B., & Coruh, I. (2008). Long-term results of different treatment modalities for glottic insufficiency. *American Journal of Otolaryngology—Head and Neck Medicine and Surgery, 29,* 7–12.

Duynstee, M. L. G., De Krijger, R. R., Monnier, P., Verwoerd, C. D. A., & Verwoerd-Verhof, H. L. (2002). Subglottic stenosis after endolaryngeal intubation in infants and children: Result of wound healing processes. *International Journal of Pediatric Otorhinolaryngology, 62,* 1–9.

Dworkin, J. P. (1991). *Motor speech disorders—A treatment guide.* St. Louis, MO: Mosby Year Book.

Dworkin, J. P. (2008). Laryngitis: Types, causes, and treatments. *Otolaryngologic Clinics of North America, 41,* 419–436.

Dworkin, J. P., Meleca, R. J., Simpson, M. L., & Garfield, I. (2000). Use of topical lidocaine in the treatment of muscle tension dysphonia. *Journal of Voice, 14,* 567–574.

Dworkin, J. P., Meleca, R. J., Zacharek, M. A., Stachler, R. J., Pasha, R., Abkarian, G. G., . . . Jacobs, J. R. (2003). Voice and deglutition functions after the supracricoid and total laryngectomy procedures for advanced state laryngeal carcinoma. *Otolaryngology-Head and Neck Surgery, 129,* 311–320.

Dworkin, J. P., Shah, A. G., Stachler, R. J., & Meleca, R. J. (2006). Medialization thyroplasty versus injection laryngoplasty for unilateral vocal fold paralysis: A comparative analysis of functional outcomes. *Journal of Medical Speech-Language Pathology, 14,* 1–11.

Dworkin, J. P., & Treadway, C. (2009). Idiopathic vocal fold paralysis: Clinical course and outcomes. *Journal of the Neurological Sciences 284*(1), 56–62.

Eadie, T. L. (2003). The ICF: A proposed framework for comprehensive rehabilitation of individuals who use alaryngeal speech. *American Journal of Speech Language Pathology, 12,* 189–197.

Eadie, T. L., & Doyle, P. C. (2002). Direct magnitude estimation and interval scaling of naturalness and severity in tracheoesophageal (TE) speakers. *Journal of Speech, Language, and Hearing Research, 45,* 1088–1096.

Eadie, T. L., & Doyle, P. C. (2005). Classification of dysphonic voice: Acoustic and auditory-perceptual measures. *Journal of Voice, 19,* 1–14.

Eadie, T. L., & Doyle, P. C. (2005). Quality of life in male tracheoesophageal (TE) speakers. *Journal of Rehabilitation Research and Development, 42,* 115–124.

Eadie, T. L., & Doyle, P. C. (2005). Scaling of voice pleasantness and acceptability in tracheoesophageal speakers. *Journal of Voice, 19,* 373–383.

Eadie, T. L., Doyle, P. C., Hansen, K., & Beaudin, P. G. (2008). Influence of speaker gender on listener judgments of tracheoesophageal speech. *Journal of Voice, 22,* 43–57.

Eadie, T. L., Kapsner, M., Rosenzweig, J., Waugh, P., Hillel, A., & Merati, A. (2010). The role of experience on judgments of dysphonia. *Journal of Voice, 24,* 564–573.

Eadie, T. L., Myers, C., Beaudin, P. F., & Doyle, P. C. (2006). Factors influencing quality of life in individuals with head and neck cancer. *Perspectives on Voice and Voice Disorders, 16,* 19–24.

Eadie, T. L., Nicolici, C., Baylor, C., Almand, K., Waugh, P., & Maronian N. (2007). Effect of experience on judgments of adductor spasmodic dysphonia. *Annals of Otology, Rhinology & Laryngology, 116,* 695–701.

Eaton, D. A., & Murray, A. D. (2006). Laryngeal stenosis. Available from www.emedicine.com/ent/topic747.htm

Echternach, M., Sundberg, J., Arndt, S., Markl, M., Schumacher, M., & Richter, B. (2010). Vocal tract in female registers—A dynamic real-time MRI study. *Journal of Voice, 24,* 133–139.

Eckley, C. A., Corvo, M. A., Yoshimi, R., Swensson, J., & Duprat, A. D. C. (2009). Unsuspected intraoperative finding of structural abnormalities associated with vocal fold polyps. *Journal of Voice.*

Edgar, J. D., Sapienza, C. M., Bidus, K., & Ludlow, C. L. (2001). Acoustic measures of symptoms in abductor spasmodic dysphonia. *Journal of Voice, 15,* 362–372.

Edmondson, N. E., & Bent III, J. (2010). Serial intralesional steroid injection combined with balloon dilation as an alternative to open repair of subglottic stenosis. *International Journal of Pediatric Otorhinolaryngology.* doi:10.1016/ijport.2010.05.027

Edmunds, A. L., Mudd, P. A., Jailwala, J., Shaker, R., & Amirlak, B. (2007). Reflux laryngitis. Available from www.emedicine.com/ent/topic355.htm

Eerenstein, S. E. J., & Schouwenburg, P. F. (2003). Long-term results of VoiceMaster voice prosthesis use in laryngectomized patients. *Acta Otolaryngologica, 123,* 655–660.

Eguchi, S., & Hirsh, L. J. (1969). Development of speech sounds in children. *Acta Otolaryngologica Supplement, 257,* 1–51.

Eksteen, E. C., Rieger, J., Nesbitt, M., & Seikaly, H. (2003). Comparison of voice characteristics following three different methods of treatment for laryngeal cancer. *The Journal of Otolaryngology, 32,* 250–253.

El-Hakim, H. (2008). Injection of botulinim toxin into external laryngeal muscles in pediatric laryngeal paralysis. *Annals of Otology, Rhinology, & Laryngology, 117,* 614–620.

Eller, R., Hawkshaw, M., & Sataloff, R. T. (2006, October). Bilateral sulcus vocalis. *ENT—Ear, Nose and Throat Journal.*

Elmiyeh, B., Dwivedi, R. C., Jallali, N., Chisholm, E. J., Kazi, R., Clarke, P. M., & Rhys-Evans, P. H. (2010). Surgical voice restoration after total laryngectomy: An overview. *Indian Journal of Cancer, 47,* 239–247.

Elmiyeh, B., Prasad, V. M. N., Upile, T., Saunders, N., Youl, B. D., Epstein, R., & Rubin, J. S. (2010). A single-centre retrospective review of unilateral and bilateral Dysport injections in adductor spasmodic dysphonia. *Logopedics Phoniatrics Vocology, 35,* 39–44.

El-Serag, H. B., Hepworth, E. J., Lee, P., & Sonnenberg, A. (2001). Gastroesophageal reflux disease is a risk factor for laryngeal and pharyngeal cancer. *The American Journal of Gastroenterology, 97,* 2013–2018.

El Sharkawi, A., Ramig, L. O., Logemann, J. A., Pauloski, B. R., Rademaker, A. W., Smith, C. H., Paulas, A., Baum, S., & Werner, C. (2002). Swallowing and voice effects of Lee Silverman Voice Treatment (LSVT®): A pilot study. *Journal of Neurology, Neurosurgery, and Psychiatry, 71,* 31–36.

Emami, A. J., Morrison, M., Rammage, L., & Bosch, D. (1999). Treatment of laryngeal contact ulcers and granulomas: A 12-year retrospective analysis. *Journal of Voice, 4,* 612–617.

Emerick, K. S., Tomycz, L., Bradford, C. R., Lyden, T. H., Chepeha, D. B., Wolf, G. T., & Teknos, T. N. (2009). Primary versus secondary tracheoesophageal puncture in salvage total laryngectomy following chemoradiation. *Otolaryngology—Head and Neck Surgery, 140,* 386–390.

Enright, P. L., Lebowitz, M. D., & Cockroft, D. W. (1994). Physiologic measures: Pulmonary function tests. Asthma outcome. *American Journal of Respiratory and Critical Care Medicine. 149,* S9–18.

Epstein, R., Hirani, S. P., Stygall, J., & Newman, S. P. (2009). How do individuals cope with voice disorders? Introducing the Voice Disability Coping Questionnaire. *Journal of Voice, 23,* 209–217.

Erickson, E., & Sivasankar, M. (2010). Evidence for adverse phonatory change following an inhaled combination treatment. *Journal of Speech, Language, and Hearing Research, 53,* 75–83.

Erickson, J. G., Devlieger, P. J., & Moon Sung, J. (1999). Korean-American female perspectives on disability. *American Journal of Speech-Language Pathology, 8,* 99–108.

Ettema, S. L., Tolejano, C. J., Thielke, R. J., Toohill, R. J., & Merati, A. L. (2006). Perceptual voice analysis of patients with subglottic stenosis. *Otolaryngology—Head and Neck Surgery, 135,* 730–735.

Eustace, C. S., Stemple, J. C., & Lee, L. (1996). Objective measures of voice production in patients complaining of laryngeal fatigue. *Journal of Voice, 10,* 146–154.

Evans, M. K., & Deliyski, D. D. (2007). Acoustic voice analysis of prelingually deaf adults before and after cochlear implantation. *Journal of Voice, 21,* 669–682.

Evans, S., Neave, N., Wakelin, D., & Hamilton, C. (2008). The relationship between testosterone and vocal frequencies in human males. *Physiology and Behavior, 93,* 783–788.

Everett, C. F., Kastelik, J. A., Thompson, R. H., & Morice, A. H. (2007). Chronic persistent cough in the community: A questionnaire survey. *Cough, 3,* 5; doi:10.1186/1745-9974-3-5

Everett, C. F., & Morice, A. H. (2007). Clinical history in gastroesophageal cough. *Respiratory Medicine, 101,* 345–348.

Evitts, P. M., Gabel, R., & Searl, J. (2007). Listeners' perceptions of the personality of male alaryngeal speakers. *Logopedics, Phoniatrics, Vocology, 32,* 53–59.

Evitts, P. M., Portugal, L., Van Dine, A., Holler, A. (2009). Effects of audio-visual information on the intelligibility of alaryngeal speech. *Journal of Communication Disorders,* doi:10.1016/j.jcomdis.2009.10.002

Fajdiga, I., Beden, A. B., Krivec, U., & Iglic, C. (2008). Epiglottic suture for treatment of laryngomalacia. *International Journal of Pediatric Otorhinolaryngology, 72,* 1345–1351.

Fanta, C. H. (2009). Asthma. *New England Journal of Medicine, 360,* 1002–1014.

Farrand, P., & Duncan, F. (2007). Generic health-related quality of life amongst patients employing different voice restoration methods following total laryngectomy. *Psychology, Health & Medicine, 12,* 255–265.

Farrell, A., Theodoros, D., Ward, E., Hall, B., & Silburn, P. (2005). Effects of neurosurgical management of Parkinson's disease on speech characteristics and oromotor function. *Journal of Speech, Language, and Hearing Research, 48,* 5–20.

Fatterpekar, G. M., Mukherji, S. K., Rajgopalan, P., Lin, Y., & Castillo, M. (2004). Normal age-related signal change in the laryngeal cartilages. *Neuroradiology, 46,* 678–681.

Fayoux, P., Vachin, F., Merrot, O., & Bernheim, N. (2006). Thyroid alar cartilage graft in paediatric laryngotracheal reconstruction. *International Journal of Pediatric Otorhinolaryngology, 70,* 717–724.

Feijo, A. V., Parente, M. A., Behlau, M., Haussen, S., De Veccino, M. C., & Martignago, B. C. dF. (2004). Acoustic analysis of voice in multiple sclerosis patients. *Journal of Voice, 18,* 341–347.

Feehery, J. M., Pribitkin, E. A., Heffelfinger, R. N., Lacombe, V. G., Lee, D. , Lowry, L. D., . . . Sataloff, R. T. (2003). The evolving etiology of bilateral vocal fold immobility. *Journal of Voice, 17,* 76–81.

Ferlito, A., Shaha, A. R., Lefebvre, J.-L., Silver, C. E., & Rinaldo, A. (2002). Organ and voice preservation in advanced laryngeal cancer. *Acta Otolaryngologica, 122,* 438–442.

Ferrand, C. T. (2000). Harmonics-to-noise ratios in normally speaking prepubescent girls and boys. *Journal of Voice, 14,* 17–21.

Ferrand, C. T. (2002). Harmonics-to-noise ratio: An index of vocal aging. *Journal of Voice, 16,* 480–487.

Ferrand, C. T. (2007). *Speech science: An integrated approach to theory and clinical practice* (2nd ed.). Boston, MA: Pearson Education.

Ferrand, C. T., & Bloom, R. L. (1996). Gender differences in children's intonational patterns. *Journal of Voice, 10,* 284–291.

Fex, B., Fex, S., Shiromoto, O., & Hirano, M. (1994). Acoustic analysis of functional dysphonia before and after voice therapy (Accent Method). *Journal of Voice, 8,* 163–167.

Filho, P. A. A., & Rosen, C. A. (2004). Bilateral vocal fold paralysis: An unusual treatment with botulinim toxin. *Journal of Voice, 18,* 254–255.

Finck, C. L., Harmegnies, B., Remacle, A., & Lefebvre, P. (2010). Implantation of esterified hyaluronic acid in the microdissected Reinke's space after vocal fold microsurgery: Short- and long-term results. *Journal of Voice, 24,* 626–635.

Finizia, C., Palme, C., & Bergman, B. (2002). A longitudinal study of the Swedish Self-Evaluation of Communication Experiences after Laryngeal Cancer questionnaire in patients treated for laryngeal cancer. *Acta Oncologica, 41,* 262–268.

Finnegan, E. M., Luschei, E. S., & Hoffman, H. T. (2000). Modulations in respiratory and laryngeal activity associated with changes in vocal intensity during speech. *Journal of Speech, Language, and Hearing Research, 43,* 934–950.

Fitch, J. L. (1990). Consistency of fundamental frequency and perturbation in repeated phonations of sustained vowels, reading, and connected speech. *Journal of Speech and Hearing Disorders, 55,* 360–363.

Flynn, P. T. (1983). Speech-language pathologists and primary prevention: From ideas to action. *Language, Speech, and Hearing Services in Schools, 14,* 99–104.

Ford, C. N. (2005). Evaluation and management of laryngopharyngeal reflux. *Journal of the American Medical Association, 294,* 1534–1540.

Ford, C. N., & Bless, D. M. (1996). Muscle tension dysphonia and spasmodic dysphonia: The role of manual laryngeal tension reduction in diagnosis and management. Paper presented at the American Laryngological Association, Orlando, Florida.

Forte, V., Fuocco, G., & James, A. (2004). A new classification system for congenital laryngeal cysts. *Laryngoscope, 114,* 1123–1127.

Fox, C. M., Morrison, C. E., Ramig, L. O., & Sapir, S. (2002). Current perspectives on the Lee Silverman Voice Treatment (LSVT) for individuals with idiopathic Parkinson disease. *American Journal of Speech-Language Pathology, 11,* 111–123.

Franco, R. A. (2007). Aminolevulinic acid 585 nm pulsed dye laser photodynamic treatment of laryngeal keratosis with atypia. *Otolaryngology—Head and Neck Surgery, 136,* 882–887.

Franco, R. A., & Andrus, J. G. (2009). Aerodynamic and acoustic characteristics of voice before and after adduction arytenopexy and medialization laryngoplasty with Gore-Tex in patients with unilateral vocal fold immobility. *Journal of Voice, 23,* 261–267.

Francois, M., Dumont, A., & Narcy, P. (1997). Longitudinal survey of voice quality after pediatric laryngotracheoplasty. *International Journal of Pediatric Otorhinolaryngology, 40,* 163–172.

Franic, D., Bramlett, R. E., & Bothe, A. C. (2005). Psychometric evaluation of disease specific quality of life instruments in voice disorders. *Journal of Voice, 19,* 300–315.

Freed, G. L., & Derkay, C. S. (2006). Prevention of recurrent respiratory papillomatosis: Role of HPV vaccination. *International Journal of Pediatric Otorhinolaryngology, 70,* 1799–1803.

French, C. T., Irwin, R. S., Fletcher, K. E., & Adams, T. M. (2002). Evaluation of a Cough-Specific Quality-of-Life questionnaire. *Chest, 121,* 1123–1131.

Friedrich, G. (1999). Titanium vocal fold medializing implant: Introducing a novel implant system for external vocal fold medialization. *Annals of Otology, Rhinology, & Laryngology, 108,* 79–86.

Fritzell, B. (1996). Voice disorders and occupations. *Logopedics Phoniatrics Vocology, 21,* 7–11.

Froeschels, E. (1952). Chewing method as therapy. *Archives of Otolaryngology, 56,* 427–434.

Froeschels, E., Kastein, S., & Weiss, D. A. (1955). A method of therapy for paralytic conditions of the mechanisms of phonation, respiration, and glutination. *Journal of Speech and Hearing Disorders, 20,* 365–370.

Fuchs, M., Froehlich, M., Hentschel, B., Stuermer, I. W., Kruse, E., & Knauft, D. (2007). Predicting mutational change in the speaking voice of boys. *Journal of Voice, 21,* 169–178.

Fujimura, M., Ogawa, H., Nishizawa, Y., & Nishi, K. (2003). Comparison of atopic cough with cough variant asthma: Is atopic cough a precursor of asthma? *Thorax, 58,* 14–18.

Fulcher, R., Cellucci, T. (1997). Case formulation and behavioral treatment of chronic cough. *Journal of Behavioral Therapy & Experimental Psychiatry, 28,* 291–296.

Fuller, D. (2006). Pulmonary functioning following total laryngectomy. *Perspectives on Voice and Voice Disorders, 16,* 9–12.

Fung, F., & Roseberry-McKibbin, C. (1999). Service delivery considerations in working with clients from Cantonese-speaking backgrounds. *American Journal of Speech-Language Pathology, 8,* 309–318.

Fung, K., Lyden, T. H., Lee, J., Urba, S. G., Worden, F., Eisbruch, A., . . . Wolf, G. T. (2005). Voice and swallowing outcomes of an organ-preservation trial for advanced laryngeal cancer. *International Journal of Radiation Oncology, Biology, Physics, 63,* 1395–1399.

Gaafar, A. H., & Fasyh, N. A. (2011). Vocal cord dysfunction: A rare cause of stridor in children. *International Journal of Pediatric Otorhinolaryngology Extra, 6,* 13–16.

Gajdos, P., Chevret, S., Clair, B., Tranchant, C., & Chastang, C. (1997). Clinical trial of plasma exchange and high-dose intravenous immunoglobulin in myasthenia gravis. *Annals of Neurology, 41,* 789–796.

Galgano, J., & Froud, K. (2008). Evidence of the voice-related cortical potential: An electroencephalographic study. *NeuroImage, 41,* 1313–1323.

Galgano, J. F., Peck, K. K., Branski, R. C., Bogomolny, D., Mener, D., Ho, M., . . . Kraus, D. H. (2009). Correlation between functional MRI and voice improvement following Type I thyroplasty in unilateral vocal fold paralysis—A case study. *Journal of Voice, 23,* 639–645.

Gallena S. K. (2007). *Voice and laryngeal disorders: A problem-based clinical guide with voice samples.* St. Louis, MO: Mosby Elsevier.

Gallivan, G. J., Gallivan, H. K., & Eitnier, C. M. (2008). Dual intracordal vocal fold cysts: A perplexing diagnostic and therapeutic challenge. *Journal of Voice, 22,* 119–124.

Gallivan, G. J., Gallivan, K. H., & Gallivan, H. K. (2007). Inhaled corticosteroids: Hazardous effects on voice—an update. *Journal of Voice, 21,* 101–111.

Gamboa, J., Jimenez-Jimenez, F. J., Nieto, A., Montojo, J., Orti-Pareja, M., Molina, J. A., Garcia-Albia, E., &

Cobeta, I. (1997). Acoustic voice analysis in patients with Parkinson's disease treated with dopaminergic drugs. *Journal of Voice, 11,* 314–320.

Gandour, J., & Weinberg, B. (1983). Perception of intonational contrasts in alaryngeal speech. *Journal of Speech and Hearing Research, 26,* 142–148.

Garabedian, E.-N., Nicollas, R., Roger, G., Delattre, J., Froelich, P., & Triglia, J.-M. (2005). Cricotracheal resection in children weighing less than 10 kg. *Archives of Otolaryngology—Head and Neck Surgery, 131,* 505–508.

Garavello, W., Lucenteforte, E., Bosetti, C., Talamini, R., Levi, F., Tavani, A., . . . La Vecchia, C. (2009). Diet diversity and the risk of laryngeal cancer: A case-control study from Italy and Switzerland. *Oral Oncology, 45,* 85–89.

Garcia, M. J. V., Cobeta, I., Martin, G., Alonso-Navarro, H., & Jimenez-Jimenez, F. J. (2011). Acoustic analysis of voice in Huntington's disease patients. *Journal of Voice, 25,* 208–217.

Garnett, J. D. (2001). Contact granulomas. Available from www.emedicine.com/ent/topic603.htm

Garnett, J. D. (2005). Subglottic stenosis in adults. Available from www.emedicine.com/ent/topic499.htm

Gartner-Schmidt, J. L., & Rosen, C. A. (2009). The evolution of diagnosing benign vocal fold lesions: From vague to specific. *Perspectives on Voice and Voice Disorders, 19*(1), 8–14.

Gasparini, G., & Behlau, M. (2007). Quality of life: Validation of the Brazilian version of the Voice-Related Quality of Life (V-RQOL) measure. *Journal of Voice;* doi:10.1016/j.jvoice.2007.04.005

Gavin, L. A., Wamboldt, M., Brugman, S., Roesler, T. A., & Wamboldt, F. (1998). Psychological and family characteristics of adolescents with vocal cord dysfunction. *Journal of Asthma, 35,* 409–417.

Gay, M., Blager, F., Bartsch, K., Emery, C. F., Rosenstiel-Gross, A. K., & Spears, J. (1987). Psychogenic habit cough: Review and case reports. *Journal of Clinical Psychiatry, 48,* 483–486.

Gay, T., Hirose, H., Strome, M., & Sawashima, M. S. (1972). Electromyography of the intrinsic laryngeal muscles during phonation. Reprinted from the *Annals of Otology, Rhinology, and Laryngology, 81,* 401. Retrieved 5/1/2010 from http://web.haskins.yale.edu/Reprints/HLO118.pdf

Gelfer, M. P. (1999). Voice treatment for the male-to-female transgendered client. *American Journal of Speech-Language Pathology, 8,* 201–208.

Gelfer, M. P., & Mikos, V. A. (2005). The relative contributions of speaking fundamental frequency and formant frequencies to gender identification based on isolated vowels. *Journal of Voice, 19,* 544–554.

Gelfer, M. P., & Pazera, J. F. (2006). Maximum duration of sustained /s/ and /z/ and the s/z ratio with controlled intensity. *Journal of Voice, 20,* 369–379.

Gelfer, M. P., & Schofield, K. J. (2000). Comparison of acoustic and perceptual measures of voice in male-to-female transsexuals perceived as female versus those perceived as male. *Journal of Voice, 14,* 22–33.

Gelman, J. (1995, November 20). Trends in alaryngeal speech: Use of artificial larynx, prosthetic-assisted speech on the rise. *Advance for Speech-Language Pathologists and Audiologists,* 5–15.

George, M., Ikonomidis, C., Jaquet, Y., & Monnier, P. (2009). Partial cricotracheal resection for congenital subglottic stenosis in children: The effect of concomitant anomalies. *International Journal of Pediatric Otorhinolaryngology, 73,* 981–985.

George, M., & Monnier, P. (2010). Long-term voice outcome following partial cricotracheal resection in children for severe subglottic stenosis. *International Journal of Pediatric Otorhinolaryngology, 74,* 154–160.

Gerber, M. E., & Chen, J. L. (2009). Laryngeal stenosis. Available from http://emedicine.medscape.com/article/867177-overview

Gerein, V., Rastorguev, E., Gerein, J., Jecker, P., & Pfister, H. (2005). Use of interferon-alpha in recurrent respiratory papillomatosis: 20-year follow-up. *Annals of Otology, Rhinology & Laryngology, 114,* 463–471.

Gerein, V., Schmandt, S., Babkina, N., Barysik, N., Coerdt, W., & Pfister, H. (2007). Human papilloma virus (HPV)-associated gynecological alteration in mothers of children with recurrent respiratory papillomatosis during long-term observation. *Cancer Detection and Prevention, 31,* 276–281.

Gerein, V., Soldatski, I. L., Babkina, N., Onufrieva, E. K., Barysik, N., & Pfister, H. (2006). Children and partners of patients with recurrent respiratory papillomatosis have no evidence of the disease during long-term observation. *International Journal of Pediatric Otorhinolaryngology, 70,* 2061–2066.

Ghafari, S., Ahmadi, F., Nabavi, M. D., Anoshirvan, K., Memarian, R., & Rafatbakhsh, M. (2009). Effectiveness of applying progressive muscle relaxation technique on quality of life of patients with multiple sclerosis. *Journal of Clinical Nursing, 18,* 2171–2179.

Giannoni, C., Sulck, M., Friedman, E. M., & Duncan, N. O. (1998). Gastroesophageal reflux association with laryngomalacia: A prospective study. *International Journal of Pediatric Otorhinolaryngology, 43,* 11–20.

Gibson, P. G., & Vertigan, A. E. (2009). Speech pathology for chronic cough: A new approach. *Pulmonary Pharmacology & Therapeutics, 22,* 159–162.

Gilbert, H. R., & Robb, M. P. (1996). Vocal fundamental frequency characteristics of infant hunger cries: Birth to 12 months. *International Journal of Pediatric Otorhinolaryngology, 34,* 237–243.

Gildea, T. R., & McCarthy, K. (2003). Pulmonary function testing. Retrieved from www.clevelandclinicmeded.com/medicalpubs/diseasemanagement/pulmonary/pulmoary-function-test

Gillivan-Murphy, P., Drinnan, M. J., O'Dwyer, T. P., Ridha, H., & Carding, P. (2006). The effectiveness of a voice treatment approach for teachers with self-reported voice problems. *Journal of Voice, 20,* 423–431.

Gilman, F., & Hapner, M. (2006). The listening and looking worksheet for evaluating the voice. Presented at the Annual Convention of the American Speech-Language-Hearing Association.

Gilman, M. (2010). Learning to see: The role of posture in vocal rehabilitation. Presented at the Annual Convention of the American Speech-Language-Hearing Association, Philadelphia, PA, November.

Glaze, L. E. (2005). Peer group support in laryngectomy rehabilitation. In P. C. Doyle & R. L. Keith (Eds.), *Contemporary considerations in the treatment and rehabilitation of head and neck cancer: Voice, speech, and swallowing* (pp. 625–638). Austin, TX: Pro-Ed.

Glaze, L. E., Bless, D. M., Milenkovic, P., & Susser, R. D. (1988). Acoustic characteristics of children's voice. *Journal of Voice, 2,* 312–319.

Gliklich, R. E., Glovsky, R. M., Montgomery, W. W. (1999). Validation of a voice outcome survey for unilateral vocal cord paralysis. *Otolaryngology—Head and Neck Surgery, 120,* 153–158.

Globlek, D., Simunjak, B., Ivkic, M., & Hedjever, M. (2004). Speech and voice analysis after near-total laryngectomy and tracheoesophageal puncture with implantation of Provox 2 prosthesis. *Logopedics, Phoniatrics, Vocology, 29,* 84–86.

Globlek, D., Stajner-Katusic, S., Musura, M., Horga, D., & Liker, M. (2004). Comparison of alaryngeal voice and speech. *Logopedics, Phoniatrics, Vocology, 29,* 87–91.

Goberman, A., Coelho, C., & Robb, M. (2002). Phonatory characteristics of Parkinsonian speech before and after morning medication: The ON and OFF states. *Journal of Communication Disorders, 35,* 217–239.

Goberman, A. M., & Robb, M. P. (1999). Acoustic examination of preterm and full-term infant cries: The long-time average spectrum. *Journal of Speech, Language, and Hearing Research, 42,* 850–861.

Goberman, A. M., & Robb, M. P. (2005). Acoustic characteristics of crying in infantile laryngomalacia. *Logopedics Phoniatrics Vocology, 30,* 79–84.

Gobl, C., & Chasaide, A. N. (2003). The role of voice quality in communicating emotion, mood and attitude. *Speech Communication, 40,* 189–212.

Goetz, C. G., Poewe, W., Rascol, O., Sampaio, C., Stebbins, G. T., Counsell, C., . . . Seidl, L. (2004). Movement disorder society task force report on the Hoehn and Yahr staging scale: Status and recommendations. The Movement Disorder Society Task Force on Rating Scales for Parkinson's Disease. *Movement Disorders 19,* 1020–1028.

Gokcan, K. M., & Dursun, G. (2009). Vascular lesions of the vocal fold. *European Archives of Otorhinolaryngology, 266,* 527–533.

Gold, L. (1999). Voice training for the transsexual. Available from www.vasta.org/newsletter/99/summer03.html

Gold, D. R., & Wright, R. (2005). Population disparities in asthma. *Annual Review of Public Health, 26,* 89–113.

Goldman, J., & Muers, M. (1991). Vocal cord dysfunction and wheezing. *Thorax, 46,* 401–404.

Goldstein, E. A., Heaton, J. T., Stepp, C. A., & Hillman, R. E. (2007). Training effects on speech production using a hands-free electromyographically controlled electrolarynx. *Journal of Speech, Language, and Hearing Research, 50,* 335–351.

Golub, J. S., Chen, P.-H., Otto, K. J., Hapner, E., & Johns III, M. M. (2006). Prevalence of perceived dysphonia in a geriatric population. *JAGS, 54,* 1736–1739.

Goncalves, A. J., Bertelli, A. A. T., Malavasi, T. R., Kikuchi, W., Rodrigues, A. N., & Menezes, M. B. (2010). Results after supracricoid horizontal partial laryngectomy. *Auris Nasus Larynx, 37,* 84–88.

Gorham-Rowan, M. M., & Laures-Gore, J. (2006). Acoustic-perceptual correlates of voice quality in elderly men and women. *Journal of Communication Disorders, 39,* 171–184.

Gorham-Rowan, M., & Morris, R. (2006). Aerodynamic analysis of male-to-female transgender voice. *Journal of Voice, 20,* 251–262.

Gracco, C., & Kahane, J. (1989). Age-related changes in the vestibular folds of the human larynx: A histomorphometric study. *Journal of Voice, 3,* 204–212.

Gracely, R. (2001). Dyspnea and pain: Similarities and contrasts between two very unpleasant sensations. *American Pain Society Bulletin, 11.* Available from www.ampainsoc.org/pub/bulletin/mar01/upda1.htm

Graham, M. S. (2006). Strategies for excelling with alaryngeal speech methods. *Perspectives on Voice and Voice Disorders, 16,* 25–32.

Graham, M. S. (2004). Alaryngeal speech rehabilitation in a group setting. *Topics in Language Disorders, 24,* 125–136.

Graville, D. J., Palmer, A. D., Wax, M. K., & Andersen, P. E. (2009). Tracheoesophageal voice restoration after salvage total laryngectomy. *Perspectives on Voice and Voice Disorders, 19*(2), 58–65.

Gregore, D. R. (n.d.). Exercise induced paradoxical vocal cord dysfunction (EI-PVCD). PPT presentation available from www.udel.edu/shs/staff/manuals/technical/VCD.ppt

Gregory, S. W. Jr., Green, B. E., Carrothers, R. M., Dagan, K. A., & Webster, S. W. (2001). Verifying the primacy of voice fundamental frequency in social status accommodation. *Language and Communication, 21,* 37–60.

Groblewski, J. C., Shah, R. K., & Zalzal, G. H. (2009). Microdebrider-assisted supraglottoplasty for laryngomalacia. *Annals of Otology, Rhinology, & Laryngology, 118,* 592–597.

Grosjean, F. (1989). Neurolinguists, beware! The bilingual is not two monolinguals in one person. *Brain and Language, 36,* 3–15.

Gross, M. (1999). Pitch-raising surgery in male-to-female transsexuals. *Journal of Voice, 13,* 246–250.

Gugatschka, M., Kiesler, K., Obermayer-Pietsch, B., Schoekler, B., Schmid, C., Groselj-Strele, A., & Friedrich, G. (2010). Sex hormones and the elderly male voice. *Journal of Voice, 24,* 369–373.

Guimaraes, I., & Abberton, E. (2004). An investigation of the Voice Handicap Index with speakers of Portuguese: Preliminary data. *Journal of Voice, 18,* 71–82.

Gultekin, E., Yelken, K., Garca, M. F., Develioglu, O. N., & Kulekci, M. (2011). Effects of neck dissection and radiotherapy on short-term speech success in voice prosthesis restoration patients. *Journal of Voice, 25,* 245–248.

Gurevich-Uvena, J., Parker, J. M., Fitzpatrick, T. M., Makashay, M. J., Perello, M. M., Blair, E. A., & Solomon, N. P. (2010). Medical comorbidities for paradoxical vocal fold motion (vocal cord dysfunction) in the military population. *Journal of Voice,* 24, 728–731.

Gustafson, L. M., Hartley, B. E., Liu, J. H., Link, D. T., Chadwell, J., Koebbe, C., et al. (2000). Single-stage laryngotracheal reconstruction in children: A review of 200 cases. *Otolaryngology—Head and Neck Surgery, 123,* 430–434.

Hadjikoutis, S., & Wiles, C. M. (2001). Respiratory complications related to bulbar dysfunction in motor neuron disease. *Acta Neurologica Scandinavica, 103,* 207–213.

Hairston, J. A., & Wilson, K. M. (2006). Current trends in head and neck cancer. *Perspectives on Voice and Voice Disorders, 16,* 3–9.

Halum, S. L., & Moberly, A. C. (2010). Patient tolerance of the flexible CO_2 laser for office-based laryngeal surgery. *Journal of Voice, 24,* 750–754.

Hamdan, A.-L., Mahfoud, L., Sibai, A., & Seoud, M. (2009). Effect of pregnancy on the speaking voice. *Journal of Voice, 23,* 490–493.

Hammer, G. P., Windisch, G., Prodinger, P. M., Anderhuber, F., & Friedrich, G. (2010). The cricothyroid joint—functional aspects with regard to different types of its structure. *Journal of Voice, 24,* 140–145.

Hammond, T. H., Zhou, R., Hammond, E. H., Pawlak, A., & Gray, S. D. (1997). The intermediate layer: A morphologic study of the elastin and hyaluronic acid constituents of normal human vocal folds. *Journal of Voice, 11,* 59–66.

Hammoud, D., & El Haddad, B. (2010). Squamous cell carcinoma of the lungs arising in recurrent respiratory papillomatosis. *Respiratory Medicine CME, 3,* 270–272.

Hanamitsu, M., Kataoka, H., Takeuchi, E., & Kitajima, K. (1999). Comparative study of vocal function after near-total laryngectomy. *Laryngoscope, 109,* 1320–1323.

Hans, S., Vaissiere, J., Crevier-Buchman, L., Laccourreye, O., & Brasnu, D. (2000). Aerodynamic and acoustic parameters in CO_2 laser posterior transverse cordotomy for bilateral vocal fold paralysis. *Acta Otolaryngologica, 120,* 330–335.

Hansen, J. K., & Thibeault, S. L. (2006). Current understanding and review of the literature: Vocal fold scarring. *Journal of Voice, 20,* 110–120.

Hanson, D. G., Kamel, P. L., & Kahrilas, P. J. (1995). Outcomes of antireflux therapy for the treatment of chronic laryngitis. *Annals of Otology, Rhinology & Laryngology, 104,* 550–555.

Hapner, E. R., & Johns, M. M. (2007). Recognizing and understanding the limitations of laryngeal videostroboscopy. *Perspectives on Voice and Voice Disorders, 17*(1), 3–7.

Hapner, E. R., & Klein, A. (2009). A synopsis of the management of vocal fold scar. *Perspectives on Voice and Voice Disorders, 19*(1), 15–23.

Hapner, E., Portone-Maira, C., & Johns III, M. M. (2009). A study of voice therapy dropout. *Journal of Voice, 23,* 337–340.

Harel, B. T., Cannizzaro, M. S., Cohen, H., Reilly, N., & Snyder, P. J. (2004). Acoustic characteristics of Parkinsonian speech: A potential biomarker of early disease progression and treatment. *Journal of Neurolinguistics, 17,* 439–453.

Harel, B., Cannizzaro, M., & Snyder, P. J. (2004). Variability in fundamental frequency during speech in prodromal and incipient Parkinson's disease: A longitudinal case study. *Brain and Cognition, 56,* 24–29.

Hargreaves, M. K., Baquet, C., & Gamshadzahi, A. (1989). Diet, nutritional state, and cancer risk in American blacks. *Nutrition and Cancer, 12,* 1–28.

Harman, E. M. (2002). Recurrent respiratory papillomatosis. Available from www.emedicine.com/med/topic2535.htm

Harnsberger, J. D., Brown, W. S., Shrivastav, R., & Rothman, H. (2010). Noise and tremor in the perception of vocal aging in males. *Journal of Voice, 24,* 523–530.

Harnsberger, J. D., Shrivastav, R., Brown, W. S., Rothman, H., & Hollien, H. (2008). Speaking rate and fundamental frequency as speech cues to perceived age. *Journal of Voice, 22,* 58–69.

Harper, B. (2005). Huntington disease. *Journal of the Royal Society of Medicine, 98,* 550.

Hartelius, L., Carlstedt, A., Ytterberg, M., Lillvik, M., & Laakso, K. (2003). Speech disorders in mild and moderate Huntington disease: Results of dysarthria assessments of 19 individuals. *Journal of Medical Speech-Language Pathology, 11,* 1–14.

Hartet, T. V., Wheeler, A. P., & Sheller, J. R. (1999). Use of pulse oximetry to recognize severity of airflow obstruction in obstructive airway disease. *Chest, 115,* 475–481.

Hartl, D. M., de Mones, E., Hans, S., Janot, F., & Brasnu, D. (2007). Treatment of early stage glottic cancer by transoral laser resection. *Annals of Otology, Rhinology & Laryngology, 116,* 832–836.

Hartl, D. M., Hans, S., Crevier-Buchman, L., Vaissiere, J., & Brasnu, D. F. (2009). Long-term acoustic comparison of thyroplasty versus autologous fat injection. *Annals of Otology, Rhinology, & Laryngology, 118,* 827–832.

Hartl, D. M., Leboulleux, S., Klap, P., & Schlumberger, M. (2007). Myasthenia gravis mimicking unilateral vocal fold paralysis at presentation. *The Journal of Laryngology & Otology, 121,* 174–178.

Hartnick, C. J. (2002). Validation of a pediatric voice quality of life instrument. *Archives of Otolaryngology—Head and Neck Surgery, 128,* 919–922.

Hartnick, C. J., Boseley, M. E., Franco, R. A., Cunningham, M. J., & Pransky, S. (2007). Efficacy of treating children with anterior commissure and true vocal fold respiratory papilloma with the 585-nm pulsed-dye laser. *Archives of Otolaryngology—Head and Neck Surgery, 133,* 127–130.

Hartnick, C. J., Volk, M., & Cunningham, M. (2003). Establishing normative voice related quality of life scores within the pediatric otolaryngology population. *Archives of Otolaryngology—Head and Neck Surgery, 129,* 1090–1093.

Hartnick, C. J., & Zeitels, S. M. (2005). Pediatric video laryngo-stroboscopy. *International Journal of Pediatric Otorhinolaryngology, 69,* 215–219.

Harvey, P. L. (1997). The three ages of voice: The young adult patient. *Journal of Voice, 11,* 144–152.

Hay, I., Oates, J., Giannini, A., Berkowitz, R., & Totenberg, B. (2009). Pain perception of children undergoing nasoendoscopy for investigation of voice and resonance disorders. *Journal of Voice. 23,* 380–388.

Hedbom, E., Heinegard, D. (1993). Binding of fibromodulin and decorin to separate sites on fibrillar collagens. *Journal of Biological Chemistry, 268,* 27307–27312.

Heinegard, D., Lidgren, L., & Saxne, T. (2003). Recent developments and future research in the bone and joint decade 2000–2010. *Bulletin of the World Health Organization, 81,* 686–688.

Helidoni, M. E., Murry, T., Moschandreas, J., Lionis, C., Printza, A., & Velegrakis, G. A. (2010). Cross-cultural adaptation and validation of the Voice Handicap Index into Greek. *Journal of Voice, 24,* 221–227.

Heman-Ackah, Y. D., & Barr, A. (2006). Mild vocal fold paresis: Understanding clinical presentation and electromyographic findings. *Journal of Voice, 20,* 269–281.

Heman-Ackah, Y.D., & Barr, A. (2006). The value of laryngeal electromyography in the evaluation of laryngeal motion abnormalities. *Journal of Voice, 20,* 452–460.

Herbst, C., & Ternstrom, S. (2006). A comparison of different methods to measure the EGG contact quotient. *Logopedics, Phoniatrics, Vocology, 31,* 126–138.

Herbst, C. T., Howard, D., & Schlomicher-Thier, J. (2010). Using electroglottographic real-time feedback to control posterior glottal adduction during phonation. *Journal of Voice, 24,* 72–85.

Hertegard, S., Hallen, L., Laurent, C., Linstrom, E., Olofsson, K., Testad, P., & Dahqvist, A. (2004). Long-term effects of vocal fold function post-injection with Hylan B gel versus Bovine cross-linked collagen. *Acta Otolaryngologica, 124,* 1208–1214.

Hickman, C. P., Roberts, L. S., & Larson, A. L. (2003). *Integrated principles of zoology.* Dubuque, IA: McGraw-Hill.

Hicks, M., Brugman, S. M., & Katial, R. (2008). Vocal cord dysfunction/paradoxical vocal fold motion. *Primary Care and Clinical Office Practice, 35,* 81–103.

Hilgers, F. J., & Schouwenburg, P. F. (1990). A new low-resistance, self-retaining prosthesis (Provox) for voice rehabilitation after total laryngectomy. *Laryngoscope, 100,* 1202–1207.

Hilgers, F. J. M., & Ackerstaff, A. H. (2006). Development and evaluation of a novel tracheostoma button and fixation system (Provox LaryButton and LaryClip adhesive) to facilitate hands-free tracheoesophageal speech. *Acta Oto-Laryngologica, 126,* 1218–1224.

Hilgers, F. J. M., & Ackerstaff, A. H. (2005). Respiratory consequences of total laryngectomy and the need for pulmonary protection and rehabilitation. In P. C. Doyle & R. L. Keith (Eds.), *Contemporary considerations in the treatment and rehabilitation of head and neck cancer: Voice, speech, and swallowing* (pp. 503–520). Austin, TX: Pro-Ed.

Hilgers, F. J. M., Ackerstaff, A. H., Van Rossum, M., Jacobi, I., Balm, A. J. M., Tan, I. B., Van den Brekel, M. W. M. (2010). Clinical phase I/feasibility study of the next generation indwelling Provox voice prosthesis (Provox Vega). *Acta Oto-Laryngologica, 130,* 511–519.

Hillel, A. D., Benninger, M., Blitzer, A., Crumley, R., Flint, P., Kashima, H. K., . . . Schaefer, S. (1999). Evaluation and management of bilateral vocal cord immobility. *Otolaryngology—Head and Neck Surgery, 121,* 760–765.

Hillman, R. E., Walsh, M. L., Wolf, F. T., Fisher, S. G., & Hong, W. K. (1998). Functional outcomes following treatment for advanced laryngeal cancer: Part I—Voice preservation in advanced laryngeal cancer; Part II—Laryngectomy rehabilitation: The state of the art in the VA system. *Annals of Otology, Rhinology, & Laryngology, 107,* 1–17.

Hinds, M. W., Thomas, D. B., & O'Reilly, H. P. (1979). Asbestos, dental x-rays, tobacco, and alcohol in the epidemiology of laryngeal cancer. *Cancer, 44,* 1114–1120.

Hirano, M. (1974). Morphological structure of the vocal cord as a vibrator and its variations. *Folia Phoniatrica, 26,* 89–94.

Hirano, M. (1977). Structure and vibratory behavior of the vocal folds. In M. Sawashima & F. S. Cooper (Eds.), *Dynamic aspects of speech production* (pp. 13–27). University of Tokyo.

Hirano, M. (1981). *Clinical examination of voice.* New York: Springer-Verlag.

Hirano, S., Bless, D. M., Massey, R. J., Hartig, G. K., & Ford, C. N. (2003). Morphological and functional changes of human vocal fibroblasts with hepatocyte growth factor. *Annals of Otology, Rhinology, & Laryngology, 112,* 1026–1033.

Hirano, M., Kurita, S., & Nakashima, T. (1981). The structure of the vocal folds. In K. Stevens & M. Hirano (Eds.), *Vocal fold physiology* (pp. 33–41). University of Tokyo.

Hirano, M., Kurita, S., & Sakaguchi, S. (1989). Ageing of the vibratory tissue of human vocal folds. *Acta Otolaryngologica, 107,* 428–433.

Hirano, S., Minamiguchi, S., Yamashita, M., Ohno, T., Kanemaru, S., & Kitamura, M. (2009). Histologic characterization of human scarred vocal folds. *Journal of Voice 23,* 399–407.

Hirsch, S. (2006). Resonance. In R. K. Adler, S. Hirsch, & M. Mordaunt (Eds.), *Voice and communication therapy for the transgender/transsexual client* (pp. 209–224). San Diego, CA: Plural Publishing.

Hirschberg, J. (1999). Dysphonia in infants. *International Journal of Pediatric Otorhinolaryngology, 49* (Suppl. 1), 293–296.

Hirschi, S. D., Gray, S. D., & Thibeault, S. L. (2002). Fibronectin: An interesting vocal fold protein. *Journal of Voice, 16,* 310–316.

Hitchings, A., Crampsey, D., & Kubba, H. (2007). A variant of laryngomalacia in the neurologically normal older child. *International Journal of Pediatric Otorhinolaryngology, 71,* 571–574.

Hixon, T. J., & Hoit, J. D. (2005). *Evaluation and management of speech breathing disorders.* Tucson, AZ: Redington Brown.

Hocevar-Boltezar, I., Zargi, M., & Strojan, P. (2009). Risk factors for voice quality after radiotherapy for early glottic cancer. *Radiotherapy and Oncology, 93,* 524–529.

Hochman, I., Sataloff, R. T., Hillman, R. E., & Zeitels, S. M. (1999). Ectasias and varices of the vocal fold: Clearing the striking zone. *Annals of Otology, Rhinology, & Laryngology, 108,* 10–16.

Hodge, F. S., Colton, R. H., & Kelley, R. T. (2001). Vocal intensity characteristics in normal and elderly speakers. *Journal of Voice, 15,* 503–511.

Hoehn, M., & Yahr, M. (1967). Parkinsonism: Onset, progression and mortality. *Neurology, 17,* 427–442.

Hoff, S. R., Schroeder Jr., J. W., Rastatter, J. C., & Holinger, L. D. (2010). Supraglottoplasty outcomes in relation to age and comorbid conditions. *International Journal of Pediatric Otorhinolaryngology, 74,* 245–249.

Hogikyan, N. D., Wodchis, W. P., Terrell, J. E., Bradford, C. R., & Esclamado, R. M. (2000). Voice-Related Quality of Life (V-RQOL) following type I thyroplasty for unilateral vocal fold paralysis. *Journal of Voice, 14,* 378–386.

Hogikyan, N. D., Wodchis, W. P., Spak, C., & Kileny, P. R. (2001). Longitudinal effects of botulinum toxin injections on Voice-Related Quality of Life (V-RQOL) for patients with adductory spasmodic dysphonia. *Journal of Voice, 15,* 576–586.

Hoh, J. F. Y. (2005). Laryngeal muscle fibre types. *Acta Physiological Scandinavia, 183,* 133–149.

Hoit, J. D., & Hixon, T. J. (1987). Age and speech breathing. *Journal of Speech and Hearing Research, 30,* 351–366.

Hoit, J. D., Hixon, T. J., Altman, M. E., & Morgan, W. J. (1989). Speech breathing in women. *Journal of Speech and Hearing Research, 32,* 353–365.

Hoit, J., Hixon, T., Watson, P., & Morgan, W. (1990). Speech breathing in children and adolescents. *Journal of Speech and Hearing Research, 33,* 51–69.

Hoit, J. D., Lansing, R. W., & Perona, K. E. (2007). Speaking-related dyspnea in healthy adults. *Journal of Speech, Language, and Hearing Research, 50,* 361–374.

Holden, P. K., Vokes, D. E., Taylor, M. B., Till, J. A., & Crumley, R. L. (2007). Long-term botulinum toxin dose consistency for treatment of adductor spasmodic dysphonia. *The Annals of Otology, Rhinology & Laryngology, 116,* 891–896.

Holinger, L. D. (1998). Evaluation of stridor and wheezing. Available from www.childsdoc.org/spring98/stridor/stridor.asp

Holland, B. W., Koufman, J. A., Postma, G. N., & McGuirt Jr., W. F. (2009). Laryngopharyngeal reflux and laryngeal web formation in patients with pediatric recurrent respiratory papillomas. *Laryngoscope, 112,* 1926–1929.

Holland, R. W., & DeJarnette, G. (2002). Voice and voice disorders. In D. E. Battle (Ed.), *Communication disorders in multicultural populations* (3rd ed., pp. 299–333). Boston, MA: Butterworth Heinemann.

Holler, T., Allegro, J., Chadha, N. K., Hawkes, M., Harrison, R. V., Forte, V., & Campisi, P. (2009). Voice outcomes following repeated surgical resection of laryngeal papillomata in children. *Otolaryngology—Head and Neck Surgery, 141,* 522–526.

Hollien, H. (1960). Vocal pitch variation related to changes in vocal fold length. *Journal of Speech and Hearing Research, 3,* 150–156.

Hollien, H. (1974). On vocal registers. *Journal of Phonetics, 2,* 25–43.

Hollien, H., & Curtis, J. F. (1960). A laminagraphic study of vocal pitch. *Journal of Speech and Hearing Research, 3,* 362–371.

Hollien, H., Green, R., & Massey, K. (1994). Longitudinal research on adolescent voice change in males. *Journal of the Acoustical Society of America, 96,* 2646–2654.

Hollien, H., & Michel, J. F. (1968). Vocal fry as a phonational register. *Journal of Speech and Hearing Research, 11,* 600–604.

Hollien, H., & Moore, P. (1960). Measurements of the vocal folds during changes in pitch. *Journal of Speech and Hearing Research, 3,* 157–165.

Hollien, H., Moore, P., Wendahl, R. W., & Michel, J. F. (1966). On the nature of vocal fry. *Journal of Speech and Hearing Research, 9,* 245–247.

Hollien, H., & Shipp, T. (1972). Speaking fundamental frequency and chronologic age in males. *Journal of Speech and Hearing Research, 15,* 150–160.

Holmberg, E. B., Doyle, P., Perkell, J. S., Hammarberg, B., & Hillman, R. E. (2003). Aerodynamic and acoustic voice measurements of patients with vocal nodules: Variation in baseline and changes across voice therapy. *Journal of Voice, 3,* 269–282.

Holmberg, E. B., Hillman, R. E., Hammarberg, B., Sodersten, M., & Doyle, P. (2001). Efficacy of a behaviorally-based voice therapy protocol for vocal nodules. *Journal of Voice, 15,* 395–412.

Holmberg, E. B., Ihre, E., & Sodersten, M. (2007). Phonetograms as a tool in the voice clinic: Changes across voice therapy for patients with vocal fatigue. *Logopedics Phoniatrics Vocology, 32,* 113–127.

Holmberg, E. B., Oates, J., Dacakis, G., & Grant, C. (2010). Phonetograms, aerodynamic measurements, self-evaluations, and auditory perceptual ratings of male-to-female transsexual voice. *Journal of Voice. 24,* 511–522.

Holmes, R. L., & Fadden, C. T. (2004). Evaluation of the patient with chronic cough. Downloaded from the American Family Physician Web site at www.aafp.org/afp

Holmes, R. J., Oates, J. M., Phyland, D. J., & Hughes, A. J. (2000). Voice characteristics in the progression of Parkinson's disease. *International Journal of Language & Communication Disorders, 35,* 407–418.

Holsinger, F. C., Howard, N. S., & McWhorter, A. (2008). Practical tips for laser resection of laryngeal cancer. In C. R. Cernea, F. L. Dias, D. Fliss, R. A. Lima, E. N. Myers, & W. Wei (Eds.), *Pearls and pitfalls in head and neck surgery* (pp. 72–73). Basel: Karger.

Holstege, G. (1998). The organization of vocalization in mammals and the relation with vocalization and speech in humans. Invited symposium: Neural Mechanism of Mammalian Vocalization, INABIS. Retrieved from www.mcmaster.ca/inabis98/brudzynski/holstege0261/two.html

Holzki, J., Laschat, M., & Stratmann, C. (1998). Stridor in the neonate and infant: Implications for the paediatric anaesthetist. Prospective description of 155 patients with congenital and acquired stridor in early infancy. *Paediatric Anaesthesia, 8,* 221–227.

Hong, K. H., & Jung, K. S. (2001). Arytenoid appearance and vertical level difference between the paralyzed and innervated vocal cords. *The Laryngoscope, 111,* 227–232.

Hong, K. H., Kim, H. K., & Kim, Y. H. (2001). The role of the pars recta and pars oblique of cricothyroid muscle in speech production. *Journal of Voice, 15,* 512–518.

Hong, K. H., Ye, M., Kim, Y. M., Kevorkian, K. F., Kreiman, J., & Berke, G. S. (1998). Functional differences between the two bellies of the cricothyroid muscle. *Otolaryngology—Head and Neck Surgery, 118,* 714–722.

Honjo, I., & Isshiki, N. (1980). Laryngoscopic and voice characteristics of aged persons. *Archives of Otolaryngology, 106,* 149–150.

Hooper, C. R. (2004). Treatment of voice disorders in children. *Language, Speech, and Hearing Services in Schools, 35,* 320–326.

Horiuchi, M., & Sasaki, C. T. (1978). Cricothyroid muscle in respiration. *Annals of Otology, Rhinology, and Laryngology, 87,* 386–391.

Hornig, J. D., Wilhoit, C. S. T., Sonne, J. E., & Schaefer, S. D. (2008). Supraglottic cancer: Treatment. Available from http://emedicine.medscape.com/article/852908-treatment

House, A. O., & Andrews, H. B. (1987). The psychiatric and social characteristics of patients with functional dysphonia. *Journal of Psychosomatic Research, 31,* 483–490.

Howell, S., Tripoliti, E., & Pring, T. (2009). Delivering the Lee Silverman Voice Treatment (LSVT) by web camera: A feasibility study. *International Journal of Language & Communication Disorders, 44,* 287–300.

Hsiao, T. Y. (2011). Prolonged ulcerative laryngitis: A new disease entity. *Journal of Voice 25,* 230–235.

Hsiung, M. W., Kang, B. H., Pai, L., Su, W. F., & Lan, Y. H. (2004). Combination of fascia transplantation and fat injection into the vocal fold for sulcus vocalis: Long-term results. *Annals of Otology, Rhinology, Laryngology, 113,* 359–366.

Hsiung, M. W., & Pai, L. (2006). Autogenous fat injection for glottic insufficiency: Analysis of 101 cases and correlation with patients' self-assessment. *Acta Oto-Laryngologica, 126,* 191–196.

Huber, J. E. (2008). Effects of utterance length and vocal loudness on speech breathing in older adults. *Respiratory Physiology and Neurobiology, 164,* 323–330.

Huber, J. E., & Spruill III, J. (2008). Age-related changes to speech breathing with increased vocal loudness. *Journal of Speech, Language, and Hearing Research, 51,* 651–668.

Hudson, A. I., & Holbrook, A. (1981). A study of the reading fundamental vocal frequency of young black adults. *Journal of Speech and Hearing Research, 24,* 18–29.

Huer, M. B., & Saenz, T. I. (2003). Challenges and strategies for conducting survey and focus group research with culturally diverse groups. *American Journal of Speech-Language Pathology, 12,* 209–220.

Hughes, R. G., & Morrison, M. (2005). Vocal cord medialization by transcutaneous injection of calcium hydroxylapatite. *Journal of Voice, 19,* 674–678.

Hunt, V. P., & Walker, F. O. (1989). Dysphagia in Huntington's disease. *Journal of Neuroscience Nursing, 21,* 92–95.

Hunter, E. J., & Titze, I. R. (2009). Quantifying vocal fatigue recovery. Dynamic vocal recovery trajectories after a vocal loading exercise. *Annals of Otology, Rhinology, & Laryngology, 118,* 440–460.

Husein, O. F., Husein, T. N., Gardner, R., Chiang, T., Larson, D. G., Obert, K., . . . Forrest, L. A. (2008). Formal psychological testing in patients with paradoxical vocal fold dysfunction. *Laryngoscope, 118,* 740–747.

Hussain, A., & Shakeel, M. (2010). Selective lateral laser thyroarytenoid myotomy for adductor spasmodic dysphonia. *The Journal of Laryngology & Otology, 124,* 886–891.

Ihre, E., Zetterstrom, O., Ihre, E., & Hammarberg, B. (2004). Voice problems as side effects of inhaled corticosteroids in asthma patients—A prevalence study. *Journal of Voice, 18,* 403–414.

Ilomaki, I., Maki, E., & Laukkanen, A-M. (2005). Vocal symptoms among teachers with and without voice education. *Logopedics Phoniatrics Vocology, 30,* 171–174.

Imhof, M. (2010). Listening to voices and judging people. *The International Journal of Listening, 24,* 19–33.

Inagi, K., Ford, C. N., Bless, D. M., & Heisey, D. (1996). Analysis of factors affecting botulinum toxin results in spasmodic dysphonia. *Journal of Voice, 10,* 306–313.

Isenberg, J. S., Crozier, D. L., & Dailey, S. H. (2008). Institutional and comprehensive review of laryngeal leukoplakia. *Annals of Otology, Rhinology & Laryngology, 117,* 74–79.

Ishikawa, K., & Thibeault, S. (2010). Voice rest versus exercise: A review of the literature. *Journal of Voice, 24,* 379–387.

Isshiki, N., & Sanuki, T. (2010). Surgical tips for type II thyroplasty for adductor spasmodic dysphonia: Modified technique after reviewing unsatisfactory cases. *Acta Oto-Laryngologica, 130,* 275–280.

Iwarsson, J., & Sundberg, J. (1999). Breathing behaviors during speech in healthy females and patients with vocal fold nodules. *Logopedics, Phoniatrics, Vocology, 24,* 154–169.

Iwata, S., Nakamura, A., Nakamura, N., Sakashita, I., & Fukunaga, H. (1988). 2 cases of Creutzfeldt-Jacob disease with bilateral vocal cord paralysis. *Clinical Neurology, 28,* 333–337.

Izadi, F., Delarestaghi, M. M., Memari, F., Mohseni, R., Pousti, B., & Mir, P. (2010). The butterfly procedure: A new technique and review of the literature for treating anterior laryngeal webs. *Journal of Voice, 24,* 742–749.

Jacobson, B. J., Johnson, A., Grywalski, C., Silbergleit, A., Jacobson, G., Benninger, M. S., & Newman, C. W. (1997). The Voice Handicap Index (VHI): Development and validation. *American Journal of Speech-Language Pathology, 6,* 66–70.

Jaryszak, E. M., & Collins, W. O. (2009). Microdebrider resection of bilateral subglottic cysts in a pre-term infant: A novel approach. *International Journal of Pediatric Otorhinolaryngology, 73,* 139–142.

Jaworowska, E., Serrano-Fernandez, P., Tarnowska, C., Lubinksi, J., Kram, A., Masojc, B., . . . Lubinski, J. (2007). Clinical and epidemiological features of familial laryngeal cancer in Poland. *Cancer Detection and Prevention, 31,* 270–275.

Jaywant, A., & Pell, M. D. (2010). Listener impressions of speakers with Parkinson's disease. *Journal of the International Neuropsychological Society, 16,* 49–57.

Jenkins, M. E., Adams, S., Dykstra, A. D., & Jog, M. S. (2006). Effects of topiramate on essential tremor of the voice, jaw, and upper limbs. *Journal of Medical Speech-Language Pathology, 14,* 43–51.

Jiang, J., O'Mara, T., Chen, H-J., Stern, J. I., Vlagos, D., & Hanson, D. (1999). Aerodynamic measurements of patients with Parkinson's disease. *Journal of Voice, 13,* 583–591.

Jiang, J., O'Mara, T., Conley, D., & Hanson, D. (1999). Phonation threshold pressure measurements during phonation by airflow interruption. *The Laryngoscope, 109,* 425–432.

Jines, N., & Drummond, S. (2006). The diagnosis of vocal cord dysfunction: A case study. Presented at the annual convention of the American Speech-Language-Hearing Association, Miami, November.

Johansson, M., Ryden, A., & Finizia, C. (2008). Self evaluation of communication experiences after laryngeal cancer—A longitudinal questionnaire study in patients with laryngeal cancer. *BMC Cancer, 8,* doi:10.1186/1471-2407-8-80

John, A., Enderby, P., & Hughes, A. (2005). Comparing outcomes of voice therapy: A benchmarking study using the Therapy Outcome Measure. *Journal of Voice, 19,* 114–123.

Johnson, K., & Derkay, C. (2009). Palliative aspects of recurrent respiratory papillomatosis. *Otolaryngologic Clinics of North America, 42,* 57–70.

Johnson, R. F., Rutter, M., Cotton, R., Vijayasekeran, S., & White, D. (2008). Cricotracheal resection in children 2 years of age and younger. *Annals of Otology, Rhinology, & Laryngology, 117,* 110–112.

Johnson, T. (2008). Transgender communication therapy 101: Working with an underserved population. Paper presented at the American Speech-Language-Hearing Association Annual Convention, Chicago.

Jongmans, P., Hilgers, F. J. M., Pols, L. C. W., & Van As-Brooks, C. J. (2006). The intelligibility of tracheoesophageal speech, with an emphasis on the voiced-voiceless distinction. *Logopedics, Phoniatrics, Vocology, 31,* 172–181.

Jongmans, P., Wempe, T. G., van Tinferen, H., Hilgers, F. J. M., Pols, L. C. W., & van As-Brooks, C. J. (2010). Acoustic analysis of the voiced-voiceless distinction in Dutch tracheoesophageal speech. *Journal of Speech, Language, and Hearing Research, 53,* 284–297.

Joniau, S., Bradshaw, A., Esterman, A., & Carney, A. S. (2007). Reflux and laryngitis: A systematic review. *Otolaryngology—Head and Neck Surgery, 136,* 686–692.

Jotz, G. P., de Campos, D., Rodrigues, M. F., & Xavier, L. L. (2011). Histological asymmetry of the human recurrent laryngeal nerve. *Journal of Voice, 25,* 8–14.

Jovanovic, M. B., Mulutinovic, Z., Perovic, J., Grubor, A., Milenkovic, S., & Malobabic, S. (2007). Contact telescopy reveals blood vessel alterations of vocal fold mucosa in Reinke's edema. *Journal of Voice, 21,* 355–360.

Jovanovic, M. B., Mulutinovic, Z., Perovic, J., Grubor, A., Milenkovic, S., & Malobabic, S. (2009). Vocal fold mucosa "blue lines" observed on contact telescopy at Reinke's edema. *Journal of Voice. 23,* 512–515.

Juel, V. C., & Massey, J. M. (2007). Myasthenia gravis. *Orphanet Journal of Rare Diseases, 2,* 44–62.

Justice, L. M., & Fey, M. E. (2004, Sept. 21). Evidence-based practice in schools: Integrating craft and theory with science and data. *The ASHA Leader,* pp. 4–5, 30–32.

Kagel, M. C., & Leopold, N. A. (1992). Dysphagia in Huntington's disease: A 16-year retrospective. *Dysphagia, 7,* 106–114.

Kahane, J. (1982). Growth of the human prepubertal and pubertal larynx. *Journal of Speech and Hearing Research, 25,* 446–455.

Kahane, J. (1990). Age-related changes in the peripheral speech mechanism: Structural and physiological changes. Proceedings of the research symposium on communication sciences and disorders and aging. ASHA Reports, No. 19 (pp. 75–87). Rockville, MD: American Speech-Language-Hearing Association.

Kahane, J. C., & Mayo, R. (1989). The need for aggressive pursuit of healthy childhood voices. *Language, Speech, and Hearing Services in Schools, 20,* 102–107.

Kahn, A. R., & Kahane, J. C. (1986). India ink pinprick assessment of age-related changes in the cricoarytenoid joint (CAJ) articular surfaces. *Journal of Speech and Hearing Research, 29,* 536–543.

Kahrilas, P. J. (2000). Maximizing outcome of extraesophageal reflux disease. *The American Journal of Managed Care, 6* (Suppl), S876–S882.

Kalliakosta, G., Mandros, C., & Tzelepis, G. E. (2007). Chest wall motion during speech production in patients with advanced ankylosing spondylitis. *Journal of Speech, Language, and Hearing Research, 50,* 109–118.

Kaltenbach, T., Crockett, S., & Gerson, L. B. (2006). Are lifestyle measures effective in patients with gastroesophageal reflux disease? An evidence-based approach. *Archives of Internal Medicine, 166,* 965–971.

Kamel, P. L., Hanson, D., & Kahrilas, P. J. (1994). Omeprazole for the treatment of posterior laryngitis. *American Journal of Medicine, 96,* 321–326.

Kanagalingam, J., Georgalas, C., Wood, G. R., Ahluwalia, S., Sandhu, G., & Cheesman, A. D. (2005). Cricothyroid approximation and subluxation in 21 male-to-female transsexuals. *Laryngoscope, 115,* 611–618.

Kanaparthi, L. K., Lessnau, K-D., & Sharma, S. (2009). Restrictive lung disease. Available from http://emedicine.medscape.com/article/301760-overview

Kandogan, T., & Sanal, A. (2005). Quality of life, functional outcome, and voice handicap index in partial laryngectomy patients for early glottic cancer. *BMC Ear, Nose and Throat Disorders, 5,* 3. doi:10.1186/1472-6815-5-3

Kandogan, T., & Ziya, O. M. (2007). Role of thyroplasty in the management of sulcus vocalis. *Internet Journal of Head and Neck Surgery, 1.* Available from www.ispub.com/ostia/index.php?xmlFilePath=journals/ijhns/vol1n2/vocalis.xml

Kanemaru, S. I., Fukushima, H., Kojima, H., Kaneko, K. I., Yamashita, M., & Ito, J. (2007). A case report of myasthenia gravis localized to the larynx. *Auris Nasus Larynx, 34,* 401–403.

Kapstein, A. A., Hughes, B. M., Scharloo, M., Hondebrink, N., & Langeveld, T. P. M. (2010). Psychological aspects of adductor spasmodic dysphonia: A prospective population controlled questionnaire study. *Clinical Otolaryngology, 35,* 31–38.

Karkos, P. D., Leong, S. C., Apostolidou, M. T., & Apostolidis, T. (2006). Laryngeal manifestations and pediatric laryngopharyngeal reflux. *American Journal of Otolaryngology—Head and Neck Medicine and Surgery, 27,* 200–203.

Karkos, P. D., Yates, P. D., Carding, P. N., & Wilson, J. A. (2007). Is laryngopharyngeal reflux related to functional dysphonia? *Annals of Otology, Rhinology, & Laryngology, 116,* 24–29.

Karnell, M. P., Melton, S. D., Childes, J. M., Coleman, T. C., Dailey, S. A., & Hoffman, H. T. (2007). Reliability of clinician-based (GRBAS and CAPE-V) and patient-based (V_RQOL and IPVI) documentation of voice disorders. *Journal of Voice, 21,* 576–590.

Karpenko, A. N., Dworkin, J. P., Meleca, R. J., & Stachler, R. (2003). Cymetra injection for unilateral vocal fold paralysis. *Annals of Otology, Rhinology, and Laryngology, 112,* 927–934.

Kasperbauer, J. L., & Thomas, J. E. (2004). Voice rehabilitation after near total laryngectomy. *Otolaryngologic Clinics of North America, 37,* 655–677.

Kavabata, N. K., Neto, A. L. S., Goncalves, A. J., Alcadipani, F. A. M. C., & Menezes, M. B. (2004). A nine-year institutional experience with near-total laryngectomy. *The American Journal of Surgery, 188,* 111–114.

Kazi, R., De Cordova, J., Singh, A., Venkitaraman, R., Nutting, C. M., Clarke, P., . . . Harrington, K. J. (2007). Voice-related quality of life in laryngectomees: Assessment using the VHI and V-RQOL symptom scales. Journal of Voice, 21, 728–734.

Kazi, R., Kanagalingam, J., Venkitaraman, R., Prasad, V., Clarke, P., Nutting, C. M., . . . Harrington, K. J. (2009). Electroglottographic and perceptual evaluation of tracheoesophageal speech. *Journal of Voice, 23,* 247–254.

Kazi, R., Kiverniti, E., Prasad, V., Venkitaraman, R., Nutting, C. M., Clarke, P., . . . Harrington, K. J. (2006). Multidimensional assessment of female tracheoesophageal prosthetic speech. *Clinical Otolaryngology, 31,* 511–517.

Kazi, R., Singh, A., Al-Mutairy, A., De Cordova, J., O'Leary, L., Nutting, C., . . . Harrington, K. (2008). Electroglottographic analysis of valved speech following total laryngectomy. *Logopedics, Phoniatrics, Vocology, 33,* 12–21.

Kazi, R., Singh, A., De Cordova, J., Al-Mutairy, A., Clarke, P., Nutting, C., . . . Harrington, K. (2006). Validation of a voice prosthesis questionnaire to assess valved speech and its related issues in patients following total laryngectomy. *Clinical Otolaryngology, 31,* 404–410.

Kazi, R., Venkitaraman, R., Johnson, C., Prasad, V., Clarke, P., Newbold, K., . . . Harrington, K. (2008). Prospective, longitudinal electroglottographic study of voice recovery following accelerated hypofractionated radiotherapy for T1/T2 larynx cancer. *Radiotherapy and Oncology, 87,* 230–236.

Kelchner, L., de Alarcon, A., Weinrich, B., & Brehm, S. B. (2009). Special considerations in the management of the pediatric voice and airway patient. *Perspectives on Voice and Voice Disorders, 19,* 96–104.

Kelchner, L., Weinrich, B., & Baker, S. (2007). Use of stroboscopic laryngeal imaging in children. *Perspectives on Voice and Voice Disorders, 17*(1), 8–11.

Kelchner, L. N., Brehm, S. B., Weinrich, B., Middendorf, J., de Alarcon, A., Levin, L., & Elluru, R. (2010). Perceptual evaluation of severe pediatric voice disorders: Rater reliability using the Consensus Auditory Perceptual Evaluation of Voice. *Journal of Voice, 24,* 441–449.

Kelchner, L. N., Brehm, S. B., Weinrich, B., Middendorf, J., de Alarcon, A., Levin, L., & Elluru, R. (2010). Perceptual evaluation of severe pediatric voice disorders: Rater reliability using the Consensus Auditory-Perceptual Evaluation of Voice. *Journal of Voice, 24,* 441–449.

Kelchner, L. N., Horne, J., Lee, L., Klaben, B., Stemple, J. C., Adam, S., . . . Levin, L. (2007). Reliability of speech-language pathologist and otolaryngologist ratings of laryngeal signs of reflux in an asymptomatic population using the reflux finding score. *Journal of Voice, 21,* 92–100.

Kempster, G. B. (2005). Recent advances in conservation laryngectomy procedures. In P. C. Doyle & R. L. Keith (Eds.), *Contemporary considerations in the treatment and rehabilitation of head and neck cancer: Voice, speech, and swallowing* (pp. 225–235). Austin, TX: Pro-Ed.

Kempster, G. B., Gerratt, B. R., Verdolini Abbott, K., Barkmeier-Kraemer, J., & Hillman, R. E. (2009). Consensus Auditory-Perceptual Evaluation of Voice: Development of a standardized clinical protocol. *American Journal of Speech-Language Pathology, 18,* 124–132.

Kendall, K. A., & Leonard, R. J. (2011). Interarytenoid muscle Botox injection for treatment of adductor spasmodic dysphonia with vocal tremor. *Journal of Voice, 25,* 114–119.

Kent, R. D. (1994). *Reference manual for communicative sciences and disorders: Speech and language.* Austin, TX: Pro-Ed.

Kent, R. D. (2006). Evidence-based practice in communication disorders: Progress not perfection. *Language, Speech, and Hearing Services in Schools, 37,* 268–270.

Kent, R. D., Sufit, R. L., Rosenbek, J. C., Kent, J. F., Weismer, G., Martin, R. E., & Brooks, B. R. (1991). Speech deterioration in amyotrophic lateral sclerosis: A case study. *Journal of Speech and Hearing Research, 34,* 1269–1275.

Kent, J. F., Kent, R. D., Rosenbek, J. C., Weismer, G., Martin, R., Sufit, R., & Brooks, B. R. (1992). Quantitative description of the dysarthria in women with amyotrophic lateral sclerosis. *Journal of Speech and Hearing Research, 35,* 723–733.

Kent, R. D., Vorperian, H. K., Kent, J. F., & Duffy, J. R. (2003). Voice dysfunction in dysarthria: Application of the Multi-Dimensional Voice Program. *Journal of Communication Disorders, 36,* 281–306.

Kersing, W., & Jennekens, F. G. I. (2004). Age-related changes in human thyroarytenoid muscles: A histological and histochemical study. *European Archives of Oto-Rhino-Laryngology, 261,* 386–392.

Khan, A. M., Hashmi, S. R., Elahi, F., Tariq, M., & Ingrams, D. R. (2006). Laryngopharyngeal reflux: A literature review. *Surgeon, 4,* 221–225.

Khidr, A. (2003). Effects of the "Smith Accent Technique" of voice therapy on the laryngeal functions and voice quality of patients with unilateral vocal fold paralysis. *International Congress Series, 1240,* 1235–1241.

Khidr, A. (2010). The Smith accent technique of voice therapy; Clinical Manual. Presented at the Annual Convention of the American Speech-Language-Hearing Association, Philadelphia.

Kieff, D., & Zeitels, S. (1996). Phonosurgery. *Comprehensive Therapy, 22,* 222–230.

Kilic, M. A., Okur, E., Yildirim, I., & Guzelsoy, S. (2004). The prevalence of vocal fold nodules in school-age children. *International Journal of Pediatric Otorhinolaryngology, 68,* 409–412.

Kim, H. S., Moon, J. W., Chung, S. M., & Lee, J. H. (2011). A short-term investigation of dysphonia in asthmatic patients using inhaled budesonide. *Journal of Voice, 25,* 88–93.

Kim, H-T., & Auo, H-J. (2008). Office-based 585 nm pulsed dye laser treatment for vocal polyps. *Acta Oto-Laryngologica, 128,* 1043–1047.

Kimball, J. (2004). The extracellular matrix (ECM). Retrieved from http://home.comcast.net/john.kimball1/Biology/Pages/E/ECM.html

Kimberlin, D. W. (2004). Current status of antiviral therapy for juvenile onset recurrent respiratory papillomatosis. *Antiviral Research, 63,* 141–151.

Kimura, M., Nito, T., Imagawa, H., Sakakibara, K.-I., Chan, R. W., & Tayama, N. (2010). Collagen injection for correcting vocal fold asymmetry. High-speed imaging. *Annals of Otology, Rhinology, & Laryngology, 119,* 359–368.

Kimura, M., Nito, T., Imagawa, H., Tayama, N., & Chan, R. W. (2008). Collagen injection as a supplement to arytenoid adduction for vocal fold paralysis. *Annals of Otology, Rhinology, & Laryngology, 117,* 430–436.

King, J. B., Lindstedt, D. E., & Jensen, M. (1999). Transgender voice: Considerations in case history management. *Logopedics, Phoniatrics, Vocology, 24,* 14–18.

Kishimoto, Y., Hirano, S., Kojima, T., Kanemaru, S., & Ito, J. (2009). Implantation of an atelocollagen sheet for the treatment of vocal fold scarring and sulcus vocalis. *Annals of Otology, Rhinology, & Laryngology, 119,* 613–620.

Klaben, B. K. (2006). Voicing problems of tracheoesophageal speakers. *Perspectives on Voice and Voice Disorders, 16*(2), 32–34.

Klein, A. M., Stong, B. C., Wise, J., DelGaudio, J. M., Hapner, E. R., & Johns III, M. M. (2008). Vocal outcome measures after bilateral posterior cricoarytenoid muscle botulinum toxin injections for abductor spasmodic dysphonia. *Otolaryngology—Head and Neck Surgery, 139,* 421–423.

Knowlton, G. E., & Larkin, K. T. (2006). The influence of voice volume, pitch, and speech rate on progressive relaxation training: Application of methods from speech pathology and audiology. *Applied Psychophysiology and Biofeedback, 31,* 173–185.

Kocak, I., Akpinar, M. E., Cakir, A., Dogan, M., Bengisu, S., & Celikoyar, M. M. (2010). Laser reduction glottoplasty for managing androphonia after failed cricothyroid approximation surgery. *Journal of Voice, 24,* 758–764.

Kohnert, K., Kennedy, M. R. T., Glaze, L., Kan, P. F., & Carney, E. (2003). Breadth and depth of diversity in Minnesota: Challenges to clinical competency. *American Journal of Speech-Language Pathology, 12,* 259–272.

Koltai, P. J., Ellis, B., Chan, J., & Calabro, A. (2006). Anterior and posterior cartilage graft dimensions in successful laryngotracheal reconstruction. *Archives of Otolaryngology Head and Neck Surgery, 132,* 631–634.

Konnai, R. M., Jayaram, M., & Scherer, R. C. (2010). Development and validation of a voice disorder outcome profile for an Indian population. *Journal of Voice, 24,* 206–220.

Kooijman, P. G. C., Thomas, G., Graamans, K., & De Jong, F. I. C. R. S. (2007). Psychosocial impact of the teacher's voice throughout the career. *Journal of Voice, 21,* 316–324.

Koschkee, D. L., & Rammage, L. (1997). *Voice care in the medical setting.* San Diego, CA: Singular Publishers.

Kotby, M. N., El-Sady, S., Abou-Rass, Y., & Hegazi, M. (1991). Efficacy of the Accent Method of voice therapy. *Journal of Voice, 5,* 316–320.

Kotby, M. N., & Fex, B. (1998). The Accent method: Behavior readjustment voice therapy. *Logopedics, Phoniatrics, Vocology, 23,* 39–43.

Koufman, J. A. (1991). The otolaryngologic manifestations of gastroesophageal reflux disease: a clinical investigation of 225 patients using ambulatory 24-hour pH monitoring and an experimental investigation of the role of acid and pepsin in the development of laryngeal injury. *Laryngoscope, 101* (Suppl. 53), 1–78.

Koufman, J. A. (1994). Paradoxical vocal cord movement. *The Visible Voice, 3,* 49–53, 70–71.

Koufman, J. A. (1995). Evaluation of laryngeal biomechanics by fiberoptic laryngoscopy. In J. S. Rubin, R. T. Sataloff, G. S. Korovin, & W. J. Gould (Eds.), *Diagnosis and treatment of voice disorders* (pp. 359–365). New York: Igaku-Shoin.

Koufman, J. A. (1995). Gastroesophageal reflux and voice disorders. In J. S. Rubin (Ed.), *Diagnosis and treatment of voice disorders*. New York: Igaku-Shoin.

Koufman, J. A. (1996). Infectious and inflammatory diseases of the larynx. In J. J. Ballenger & J. B. Snow (Eds.), *Otorhinolaryngology* (15th ed., pp. 535–555). Philadelphia: Williams and Wilkins.

Koufman, J. A., Aviv, J. E., Casiano, R. R., & Shaw, G. Y. (2002). Laryngopharyngeal reflux: Position statement of the Committee on Speech, Voice, and Swallowing Disorders of the American Academy of Otolaryngology—Head and Neck Surgery. *Otolaryngology—Head and Neck Surgery, 127,* 32–35.

Koufman, J. A., & Blalock, P. D. (1988). Vocal fatigue and dysphonia in the professional voice user: Bogart-Bacall syndrome. *Laryngoscope, 98,* 493–498.

Koufman, J. A., & Block, C. (2008). Differential diagnosis of paradoxical vocal fold movement. *American Journal of Speech-Language Pathology, 17,* 327–334.

Koufman, J. A., Rees, C. J., Frazier, W. D., Kilpatrick, L. A., Wright, S. C., Halum, S. L., & Postma, G. N. (2007). Office-based laryngeal laser surgery: A review of 443 cases using three wavelengths. *Otolaryngology—Head and Neck Surgery, 137,* 146–151.

Kozlakowski, L. (2003). The aging voice and differentiating diseases. Available from msu.edu/. . ./2003%20Powerpoint%20Presentations/Differentiating%20the%20Aging%20Voice%20from%20Disease.ppt

Krause, E., Hempel, J.-M., & Gurkov, R. (2009). Botulinum toxin A prolongs functional durability of voice prostheses in laryngectomees with pharyngoesophageal spasm. *American Journal of Otolaryngology—Head and Neck Medicine and Surgery, 30,* 371–375.

Krecicki, T., Liebhart, J., Morawska-Kochman, M., Liebhart, E., Zatonski, M., & Zalesska-Krecicka, M. (2006). Corticosteroid-induced laryngeal disorders in asthma. *Medical Science Monitor, 12,* 351–354.

Krengli, M., Policarpo, M., Manfredda, I., Aluffi, P., Gambaro, G., Panella, M., & Pia, F. (2004). Voice quality after treatment to T1a glottic carcinoma. *Acta Oncologica, 43,* 284–289.

Krischke, S., Weigelt, S., Hoppe, U., Kollner, V., Klotz, M., Eysholdt, U., & Rosanowski, F. (2005). Quality of life in dysphonic patients. *Journal of Voice, 19,* 132–137.

Krival, K., Kelchner, L. N., Weinrich, B., Baker, S. E., Lee, L., Middendorf, J. H., & Zur, K. B. (2007). Vibratory source, vocal quality and fundamental frequency following pediatric laryngotracheal reconstruction. *International Journal of Pediatric Otorhinolaryngology, 71,* 1261–1269.

Kuhn, J., Toohill, R. J., Ulualp, S. O., Kulpa, J., Hofmann, C., Arndorfer, R., & Shaker, R. (1998). Pharyngeal acid reflux events in patients with vocal cord nodules. *The Laryngoscope, 108,* 1146–1149.

Kumai, Y., Murukami, D., Masuda, M., & Yumoto, E. (2007). Arytenoid adduction to treat impaired adduction of the vocal fold due to rheumatoid arthritis. *Auris Nasus Larynx, 34,* 545–548.

Kummer, A. W. (2007). Resonance disorders and velopharyngeal dysfunction: Simple low tech and no-tech procedures for evaluation and treatment. Available from www.speechpathology.com/articles/article_detail.asp?article_id=332

Kuo-Sheng, L., Bo-Nien, C., Cheng-Chien, Y., & Yu-Chun, C. (2007). CO_2 laser supraglottoplasty for severe laryngomalacia: A study of symptomatic improvement. *International Journal of Pediatric Otorhinolaryngology, 71,* 889–895.

Kwon, T-K., Rosen, C. A., & Gartner-Schmidt, J. (2005). Preliminary results of a new temporary vocal fold injection material. *Journal of Voice, 19,* 668–673.

Lacomblez, L., Bensimon, G., Leigh, P. N., & Meininger, V. (1996). Dose-ranging study of Riluzole in amyotrophic lateral sclerosis. *Lancet, 347,* 1425–1431.

Lagier, A., Nicollas, R., Sanjuan, M., Benoit, L., & Triglia, J. M. (2009). Laser cordotomy for the treatment of bilateral vocal cord paralysis in infants. *International Journal of Pediatric Otorhinolaryngology, 73,* 9–13.

Lai, S. Y., & Weinstein, G. S. (2009). Conservation laryngeal surgery, supracricoid laryngectomy. Available from http://emedicine.medscape.com/article/851248-overview

Lam, P. K. Y., Chan, K. M., Ho, W. K., Kwong, E., Yiu, E. M., & Wei, W. I. (2006). Cross-cultural adaptation and validation of the Chinese Voice Handicap Index-10. *Laryngoscope, 116,* 1192–1198.

Lam, P., Wei, W. I., Hui, Y., & Ho, W.-K. (2006). Prevalence of pH-documented laryngopharyngeal reflux in Chinese patients with clinically suspected reflux laryngitis. *American Journal of Otolaryngology—Head and Neck Medicine and Surgery, 27,* 186–189.

Lam, P. K.-Y., Ho, W.-K., Ho, A. C.-W., Ng, R. W.-M., Yuen, A. P. W., & Wei, W. I. (2005). Long-term performance of indwelling tracheoesophageal speaking valves in Chinese patients undergoing laryngectomy. *Archives of Otolaryngology—Head and Neck Surgery, 131.* Retrieved from www.archoto.com

Larson, C. R. (1985). The midbrain periaqueductal grey: A brainstem structure involved in vocalization. *Journal of Speech and Hearing Research, 28,* 241–249.

Larson, C. R., Altman, K. W., Liu, H., & Hain, T. C. (2008). Interactions between auditory and somatosensory feedback for voice F0 control. *Experimental Brain Research, 187,* 613–621.

Lauri, E.-R., Alku, P., Vilkman, E., Sala, E., & Sihvo, M. (1997). Effects of prolonged oral reading on time-based glottal flow waveform parameters with special reference to gender differences. *Folia Phoniatrica et Logopedica, 49,* 234–246.

Lavy, J. A., Wood, G., Rubin, J. S., & Harried, M. (2000). Dysphonia associated with inhaled steroids. *Journal of Voice, 14,* 581–588.

Lawrence, V. L. (1987). Common medications with laryngeal effects. *Ear, Nose and Throat Journal, 66,* 318–322.

Le Bihan, D., Mangin, J.-F., Poupon, C., Clark, C. A., Pappatas, S., Molko, N., & Chabriat, H. (2001). Diffusion tensor imaging: Concepts and applications. *Journal of Magnetic Resonance Imaging, 13,* 534–546.

Leder, S. B., Acton, L. M., Kmiecik, J., Ganz, C., & Blom, E. D. (2005). Voice restoration with the Advantage tracheoesophageal voice prosthesis. *Otolaryngology—Head and Neck Surgery, 133,* 681–684.

Lee, A. S., & Rosen, C. A. (2004). Efficacy of cidofovir injection for the treatment of recurrent respiratory papillomatosis. *Journal of Voice, 18,* 551–556.

Lee, B., & Woo, P. (2005). Chronic cough as a sign of laryngeal sensory neuropathy: Diagnosis and treatment. *Annals of Otology, Rhinology, & Laryngology, 114,* 253–257.

Lee, E.-K., & Son, Y.-I. (2005). Muscle tension dysphonia in children: Voice characteristics and outcome of voice therapy. *International Journal of Pediatric Otorhinolaryngology, 69,* 911–917.

Lee, H. M., Mazloff, D., & Henry, C. (1999). Vocal characteristics of older adults and stereotyping. *Journal of Nonverbal Behavior, 2,* 111–132.

Lee, K. H., & Rutter, M. J. (2008). Role of balloon dilation in the management of adult idiopathic subglottic stenosis. *Annals of Otology, Rhinology, & Laryngology, 117,* 81–84.

Lee, L., Friesen, M., Lambert, I. R., & Loudon, R. G. (1998). Evaluation of dyspnea during physical and speech activities in patients with pulmonary diseases. *Chest, 113,* 625–632.

Lee, M. S., & Marsden, C. D. (1994). Movement disorders following lesions of the thalamus or subthalamic region. *Movement Disorders, 9,* 493–507.

Lee, S., Potamianos, A., & Narayanan, S. (1999). Acoustics of children's speech: Developmental changes of temporal and spectral parameters. *Journal of the Acoustical Society of America, 105,* 1455–1468.

Lee, V. S., Zhou, X. P., Rahn III, D. A., Wang, E. Q., & Jiang, J. J. (2008). Perturbation and nonlinear dynamic analysis of acoustic phonatory signal in Parkinsonian patients receiving deep brain stimulation. *Journal of Communication Disorders, 41,* 485–500.

Leeper, H. A., Parsa, V., Jamieson, D. G., & Heeneman, H. (2002). Acoustical aspects of vocal function following radiotherapy for early T1a laryngeal cancer. *Journal of Voice, 16,* 289–302.

Lemos, E. M., Sennes, L. U., Imamura, R., & Tsuji, D. H. (2005). Vocal process granuloma: clinical characterization, treatment and evolution. *Brazilian Journal of Otorhinolaryngology, 71,* 494–498.

Lenderking, W. R., Hillson, E., Crawley, J. A., Moore, D., Berzon, R., & Pashos, C. L. (2003). The clinical characteristics and impact of laryngopharyngeal reflux disease on health-related quality of life. *Value in Health, 6,* 560–565.

Leonard, R., Dworkin, J. P., Meleca, R. J., Colton, R. H., Leeper, H. A., & Till, J. A. (2002). Assessment of the disordered voice: A roundtable discussion. *Journal of Medical Speech-Language Pathology, 10,* 111–131.

Leonard, R., & Kendall, K. (2005). Effects of voice therapy on vocal process granuloma: A phonoscopic approach. *American Journal of Otolaryngology—Head and Neck Medicine and Surgery, 26,* 101–107.

Leopold, N. A., & Kagel, M. C. (1985). Dysphagia in Huntington's disease. *Archives of Neurology, 42,* 57–60.

Letson, J. A., & Tatchell, R. (2005). Arytenoid movement. In R. T. Sataloff (Ed.), *Voice science* (pp. 89–103). San Diego, CA: Plural Publishing.

Leung, A. K. C., & Cho, H. (1999). Diagnosis of stridor in children. *American Family Physician, 60.* Available from www.aafp.org/afp/991115ap/2289.html

Leung, R., & Berkowitz, R. G. (2007). Incidence of severe acquired subglottic stenosis in newborns. *International Journal of Pediatric Otorhinolaryngology, 71,* 763–768.

Leung, R., Hawkes, M., & Campisi, P. (2007). Severity of juvenile onset recurrent respiratory papillomatosis is not associated with socioeconomic status in a setting of universal health care. *International Journal of Pediatric Otorhinolaryngology, 71,* 965–972.

Levy, D. (2000). Two transsexuals reflect on university's pioneering gender dysphoria program. Available from http://news-service.stanford.edu/news/2000/may3/sexchange-53.html

Lewin, J. S., Bishop-Leone, J. K., Forman, A. D., & Diaz Jr., E. M. (2001). Further experience with Botox injection for tracheoesophageal speech failure. *Head Neck, 23,* 456–460.

Lewis, A. F., Carron, J. D., & Vedanarayanan, V. (2010). Congenital bilateral vocal fold paralysis and Charcot-Marie-Tooth disease. *Annals of Otology, Rhinology, & Laryngology, 119,* 47–49.

Leydon, C., Bielamowicz, S., & Stager, S. V. (2005). Perceptual ratings of vocal characteristics and voicing features in untreated patients with unilateral vocal fold paralysis. *Journal of Communication Disorders, 38,* 163–185.

Leydon, C., Wroblewski, M., Eichorn, N., & Sivasankar, M. (2010). A meta-analysis of outcomes of hydration intervention on phonation threshold pressure. *Journal of Voice, 24,* 637–643.

Li, A. J., Johns, M. M., Jackson-Menaldi, C., Dailey, S., Heman-Ackah, Y., Merati, A., & Rubin, A. D. (2011). Glottic closure patterns: Type I thyroplasty versus Type I thyroplasty with arytenoid adduction. *Journal of Voice, 25,* 259–264.

Li, L., Saigusa, H., Nagayama, H., Nakamura, T., Aino, I., Komachi, T., & Yamaguchi, S. (2009). A case of Creutzfeldt-Jacob disease with bilateral vocal fold abductor paralysis. *Journal of Voice, 23,* 635–638.

Liberman, M., & Mathisen, D. J. (2009). Treatment of idiopathic laryngotracheal stenosis. *Seminars in Thoracic and Cardiovascular Surgery, 21,* 278–283.

Liew, L., Blaney, S. P. A., & Morrison, G. A. J. (2003). Surgical selection and outcomes in laryngotracheal reconstruction for subglottic stenosis. *International Congress Series, 1254,* 147–150.

Lim, J.-Y., Choi, J.-N., Kim, K.-M., & Choi, H.-S. (2006). Voice analysis of patients with diverse types of Reinke's edema and clinical use of electroglottographic measurements. *Acta Oto-Laryngologica, 126,* 62–69.

Lim, J.-Y., Lim, S. E., Choi, S. H., Kim, J. H., Kim, K.-M., & Choi, H.-S. (2007). Clinical characteristics and voice analysis of patients with mutational dysphonia: Clinical significance of diplophonia and closed quotients. *Journal of Voice, 21,* 12–19.

Lim, X., Tateya, I., Tateya, T., Munoz-del-Rio, A., & Bless, D. M. (2006). Immediate inflammatory response and scar formation in wounded vocal folds. *Annals of Otology, Rhinology & Laryngology, 115,* 921–929.

Lin, H. W., Richmon, J. D., Emerick, K. S., de Venecia, R. K., Zeitels, S. M., Faquin, W. C., & Lin, D. T. (2010). Malignant transformation of a highly aggressive human papillomavirus type 11-associated recurrent respiratory papillomatosis. *American Journal of Otolaryngology—Head and Neck Medicine and Surgery, 31,* 291–296.

Lind, K., & Wermke, K. (2002). Development of the vocal fundamental frequency of spontaneous cries during the first 3 months. *International Journal of Pediatric Otorhinolaryngology, 64,* 97–104.

Lindholm, P., Vilkman, E., Raudaskoski, T., Suvanto-Luukkonen, E., & Kauppila, A. (1997). The effect of postmenopause and postmenopausal HRT on measured voice values and vocal symptoms. *Maturitas, 28,* 47–53.

Lindsay, F., Bloom, D., Pransky, S., Stabley, R., & Shick, P. (2008). Histologic review of cidofovir-treated recurrent respiratory papillomatosis. *Annals of Otology, Rhinology & Laryngology, 117,* 113–117.

Linville, S. E. (1992). Glottal gap configuration in two age groups of women. *Journal of Speech and Hearing Research, 35,* 1209–1215.

Linville, S. E. (2001). *Vocal aging.* San Diego, CA: Singular/Thomson Learning.

Linville, S. E., & Fisher, H. (1985). Acoustic characteristics of perceived versus actual vocal age in controlled phonation by adult females. *Journal of the Acoustical Society of America, 78,* 40–48.

Liotti, M., Brannan, S., Egan, G., Shade, R., Madden, L., Abplanalp, B., . . . Denton, D. (2001). Brain responses associated with consciousness of breathlessness (air hunger). *PNAS, 98,* 2035–2040.

Little, M. A., McSharry, P. E., Hunter, E. J., Spielman, J., & Ramig, L. O. (2009). Suitability of dysphonia measurements for telemonitoring of Parkinson's disease. *IEEE Transactions on Biomedical Engineering, 56,* 1015–1022.

Liu, B. P., Bove, M. J., & Nemeth, A. J. (2010). Posterior glottic stenosis with a calcified interarytenoid scar band: CT and laryngoscopic correlation. *American Journal of Neuroradiology.* doi:10.3174/ajnr.A1980

Liu, H., & Ng, M. L. (2007). Electrolarynx in voice rehabilitation. *Auris Nasus Larynx, 34,* 327–332.

Liu, W.-B., Xia, Q., Men, L.-N., Wu, Z.-K., & Huang, R.-X. (2007). Dysphonia as a primary manifestation in myasthenia gravis (MG): A retrospective review of 7 cases among 1520 MG patients. *Journal of the Neurological Sciences, 260,* 16–22.

Llewellyn, C. D., McGurk, M., & Weinman, J. (2005). Are psychosocial and behavioural factors related to health-related quality of life in patients with head and neck cancer? A systematic review. *Oral Oncology, 41,* 440–454.

Lo, H.-I., Ho, H. C., & Hwang, J.-H. (2005). Paradoxical vocal cord motion—A case report. *Auris Nasus Larynx, 32,* 427–430.

Logemann, J. A., Pauloski, B. R., Rademaker, A. W., Lazarus, C. L., Gaziano, J., Stachowiak, L., . . . Mittal, B. (2008). Swallowing disorders in the first year after radiation and chemoradiation. *Head Neck, 30,* 148–158.

Lombard, L. E., & Popovich, A. A. (2008). Laryngectomy rehabilitation. Available from http://emedicine.medscape.com/article/883689-overview

Lorenz, R. R., Esclamado, R. M., Teker, A. M., Strome, M., Scharpf, J., Hicks, D., . . . Lee, W. T. (2008). Ansa cervicalis-to-recurrent laryngeal nerve anastomosis for unilateral vocal fold paralysis: Experience of a single institution. *Annals of Otology, Rhinology, & Laryngology, 117,* 40–45.

Loucks, T. M. J., Poletto, C. J., Simonyan, K., Reynolds, C. L., & Ludlow, C. L. (2007). Human brain activation during phonation and exhalation: Common volitional control for two upper airway functions. *NeuroImage, 36,* 131–143.

Loughran, S., Calder, N., MacGregor, F. B., Carding, P., & MacKenzie, K. (2005). Quality of life and voice following endoscopic resection or radiotherapy for early glottic cancer. *Clinical Otolaryngology, 30,* 42–47.

Lowell, S. Y., Barkmeier-Kraemer, J. M., Hoit, J. D., & Story, B. H. (2008). Respiratory and laryngeal function during spontaneous speaking in teachers with voice disorders. *Journal of Speech, Language, and Hearing Research, 51,* 333–349.

Lublin, F. D., & Reingold, S. C. (1996). Defining the clinical course of multiple sclerosis: Results of an international survey. National Multiple Sclerosis Society (USA) Advisory Committee on Clinical Trials of New Agents in Multiple Sclerosis. *Neurology, 46,* 907–911.

Ludlow, C. L. (2005). Central nervous system control of the laryngeal muscles in humans. *Respiratory Physiology and Neurobiology, 147,* 205–222.

Ludlow, C. L., Adler, C. H., Berke, G. S., Bielamowicz, S. A., Blitzer, A., Bressman, S. B., . . . Woodson, G. E. (2008). Research priorities in spasmodic dysphonia. *Otolaryngology—Head and Neck Surgery, 139,* 495–505.

Ludlow, C. L., & Connor, N. P. (1987). Dynamic aspects of phonatory control in spasmodic dysphonia. *Journal of Speech and Hearing Research, 30,* 197–206.

Luff, D. A., Izzat, S., & Farrington, W. T. (1999). Viscoaugmentation as a treatment for leakage around the Provox2 voice rehabilitation system. *Journal of Laryngology and Otology, 113,* 847–848.

Luna-Ortiz, K., Pasche, P., Tamez-Velarde, M., & Villavicencio-Valencia, V. (2009). Supracricoid partial laryngectomy with cricohyoidoepiglottopexy in patients with radiation therapy failure. *World Journal of Surgical Oncology, 7,* doi:10.1186/1477-7819-7-101

Lundstrom, E., & Hammarberg, B. (2004). High-speed imaging of the voicing source in laryngectomees during production of voiced-voiceless distinctions for stop consonants. *Logopedics, Phoniatrics, Vocology, 29,* 31–40.

Lundstrom, E., Hammarberg, B., Munck-Wikland, E., & Edsborg, N. (2008). The pharyngoesophageal segment in laryngectomees—videoradiographic, acoustic, and voice quality perceptual data. *Logopedics, Phoniatrics, Vocology, 33,* 115–125.

Lundy, D. S., Roy, S., Xue, J. W., Casiano, R. R., & Jassir, D. (2004). Spastic/spasmodic vs. tremulous vocal quality: Motor speech profile analysis. *Journal of Voice, 18,* 146–152.

Lunn, W. W., & Sheller, J. R. (1995). Flow volume loops in the evaluation of upper airway obstruction. *Otolaryngology Clinics of North America, 28,* 721–729.

Luschei, E. S., Ramig, L. O., Baker, K. L., & Smith, M. E. (1999). Discharge characteristics of laryngeal single motor units during phonation in young and older adults and in persons with Parkinson's disease. Downloaded from jn.physiology.org on January 26, 2007, pp. 2131–2139.

Luscher, M. S., Pedersen, U., & Johansen, L. V. (2001). Treatment outcome after laser excision of early glottic squamous cell carcinoma. *Acta Oncologica, 7,* 796–800.

Luu, Q., Tsai, V., Mangunta, V., Berke, G. S., & Chhetri, D. K. (2007). Safety of percutaneous injection of bovine dermal crosslinked collagen for glottic insufficiency. *Otolaryngology—Head and Neck Surgery, 136,* 445–449.

Ma, E. P. M., & Love, A. L. (2010). Electroglottographic evaluation of age and gender effects during sustained phonation and connected speech. *Journal of Voice, 24,* 146–152.

Ma, E., Roberson, J., Radford, C., Vagne, S., El-Halabi, R., & Yiu, E. (2007). Reliability of speaking and maximum voice range measures in screening for dysphonia. *Journal of Voice, 21,* 397–406.

Ma, E. P. M., & Yiu, E. M. L. (2001). Voice activity and participation profile: Assessing the impact of voice disorders on daily activities. *Journal of Speech, Language and Hearing Research, 44,* 511–524.

Ma, E. P. M., Yiu, E. M. L., & Abbott, K. V. (2007). Application of the ICF in voice disorders. *Seminars in Speech and Language, 28,* 343–350.

MacArthur, C. J., Kearns, G. H., & Healy, G. B. (1994). Voice quality after laryngotracheal reconstruction. *Archives of Otolaryngology—Head and Neck Surgery, 120,* 641–647.

Mahendra, N., Battle, D., & Payne, J. (2006). Cultural competence in action: A framework and practical strategies for clinicians. Paper presented at the American Speech-Language-Hearing Association annual convention, Miami.

Makeieff, M., Giovanni, A., & Guerrier, B. (2007). Laryngostroboscopic evaluation after supracricoid partial laryngectomy. *Journal of Voice, 21,* 508–515.

Makitie, A. A., Aaltonen, L-M., Niemensivu, R., Back, L., Juvas, A., & Lehtonen, H. (2003). Postlaryngectomy voice restoration using a voice prosthesis: A single institution's ten-year experience. *Annals of Otology, Rhinology & Laryngology, 112,* 1007–1010.

Maloney, E. M., Unger, E. R., Tucker, R. A., Swan, D., Karem, K., Todd, W., & Reeves, W. C. (2006). Longitudinal measures of human papilloma virus 6 and 11 viral loads and antibody response in children with recurrent respiratory papillomatosis. *Archives of Otolaryngology—Head and Neck Surgery, 132,* 711–715.

Mankekar, G., Eaton, D. A., & Murray, A. D. (2009). Glottic stenosis. Available from http://emedicine.medscape.com/article/864439-overview

Mann, E. A., McClean, M. D., Gurevich-Uvena, J., Barkmeier, J., McKenzie-Garner, P., Paffrath, J., &

Patow, C. (1999). The effects of excessive vocalization on acoustic and videostroboscopic measures of vocal fold condition. *Journal of Voice, 13,* 294–302.

Manning, S. C., Inglis, A. F., Mouzakes, J., Carron, J., & Perkins, J. A. (2005). Laryngeal anatomic differences in pediatric patients with severe laryngomalacia. *Archives of Otolaryngology—Head and Neck Surgery, 131,* 340–343.

Manor, Y., Balas, M., Giladi, N., Mootanah, R., & Cohen, J. T. (2008). Anxiety, depression and swallowing disorders in patients with Parkinson's disease. *Parkinsonism and Related Disorders, 15,* 453–456.

Manor, Y., Posen, J., Amir, O., Dori, N., & Giladi, N. (2005). A group intervention model for speech and communication skills in patients with Parkinson's disease. *Communication Disorders Quarterly, 26,* 94–101.

Mao, V. H., Abaza, M., Spiegel, J. R., Mandel, S., Hawkshaw, M., Heuer, R. J., & Sataloff, R. T. (2001). Laryngeal myasthenia gravis: Report of 40 cases. *Journal of Voice, 15,* 122–130.

Marcelino, F. C., & Oliveira, D. T. (2005). Histopathological changes of vocal folds induced by chronic pollutant exposure: An experimental study. *Journal of Voice, 19,* 529–533.

Marchese-Ragona, R., Marioni, G., Chiarello, G., Staffieri, A., & Pastore, A. (2005). Supracricoid laryngectomy with cricohyoidopexy for recurrence of early-stage glottic carcinoma after irradiation: Long-term oncological and functional results. *Acta Oto-Laryngologica, 125,* 91–95.

Marge, M. (1984). The prevention of communication disorders. *ASHA, 26,* 35–38.

Marom, T., Roth, Y., & Cinamon, U. (2010). Laryngocele: A rare long-term complication following neck surgery? *Journal of Voice.* doi:10.1016/j.voice.2010.01.011

Martinez, F. D. (2007). Genes, environments, development and asthma: A reappraisal. *European Respiratory Journal, 29,* 179–184.

Martins, R. H. G., Defaveri, J., Domingues, M. A. C., & Silva, R. D. A. E. (2011). Vocal polyps: Clinical, morphological, and immunohistochemical aspects. *Journal of Voice, 25,* 98–106.

Martins, R. H. G., Defaveri, J., Domingues, M. A. C., Silva, R. D. A. E., & Fabro, A. (2010). Vocal fold nodules: Morphological and immunohistochemical investigations. *Journal of Voice, 24,* 531–539.

Martins, R. H. G., Fabro, A. T., Domingues, M. A. C., Chi, A. P., & Gregorio, E. A. (2009). Is Reinke's edema a precancerous lesion? Histological and electron microscope aspects. *Journal of Voice, 23,* 721–725.

Martins, R. H. G., Santana, M. F., & Tavares, E. L. M. (2011). Vocal cysts: Clinical, endoscopic, and surgical aspects. *Journal of Voice. 25,* 107–110.

Maryn, Y., Corthals, P., Van Cauwenberge, P., Roy, N., & De Bodt, M. (2010). Toward improved ecological validity in the acoustic measurement of overall voice quality: Combining continuous speech and sustained vowels. *Journal of Voice, 24,* 540–555.

Maryn, Y., De Bodt, M., & Van Cauwenberge, P. (2006). Effects of biofeedback in phonatory disorders and phonatory performance: A systematic literature review. *Applied Psychophysiology and Biofeedback, 31,* 65–83.

Mastrovich, J. D., & Greenberger, P. A. (2002). Psychogenic cough in adults: A report of two cases and review of the literature. *Allergy and Asthma Proceedings, 23,* 27–33.

Masuda, T., Ikeda, Y., Manako, H., & Komiyama, S. (1993). Analysis of vocal abuse: Fluctuations in phonation time and intensity in 4 groups of speakers. *Acta Otolaryngologica, 113,* 547–552.

Matal, V., Cheesman, D., & Clarke, P. M. (2003). Cricothyroid approximation and thyroid chondroplasty: A patient survey. *Otolaryngology—Head and Neck Surgery, 128,* 841–847.

Mathers-Schmidt, B. A. (2001). Paradoxical vocal fold motion: A tutorial on a complex disorder and the speech-language pathologist's role. *American Journal of Speech-Language Pathology, 10,* 111–125.

Mathers-Schmidt, B. A., & Brilla, L. R. (2005). Inspiratory muscle training in exercise-induced paradoxical vocal fold motion. *Journal of Voice, 19,* 635–644.

Mathers-Schmidt, B., Brilla, L., Jamieson, A., & Parsons, S. (n.d.). Inspiratory muscle training in three athletes with exercise-induced PVFM. Available from www.ac.wwu.edu/~csd/IMT%20in%203%20PVFM%20athletes%20handout.pdf

Mathieson, L. (2001). *Greene and Mathieson's the voice and its disorders* (6th ed.). Philadelphia, PA: Whurr Publications.

Mathieson, L., Hirani, S. P., Epstein, R., Baken, R. J., Wood, G., & Rubin, J. S. (2009). Laryngeal manual therapy: A preliminary study to examine its treatment effects in the management of muscle tension dysphonia. *Journal of Voice, 23,* 353–366.

Maue, W. M., & Dickson, D. R. (1971). Cartilages and ligaments of the adult human larynx. *Archives of Otolaryngology, 94,* 432–439.

Mayer, R. M., & Gelfer, M. P. (2008). Outcomes of voice therapy for male-to-female transgendered individuals. Paper presented at the American Speech-Language-Hearing Association Annual Convention, Chicago.

McAllister, A., Sederholm, E., Sundberg, J., & Gramming, P. (1994). Relations between voice range profile and physiological and perceptual voice characteristics in 10-year-old children. *Journal of Voice, 8,* 230–239.

McCabe, D. J., & Titze, I. R. (2002). Chant therapy for treating vocal fatigue among public school teachers: A preliminary study. *American Journal of Speech-Language Pathology, 11,* 356–369.

McCarthy, K., & Dweik, R. A. (2010). Pulmonary function testing. Available from http://emedicine.medscape.com/article/303239-overview

McClay, J. E. (2001). Recurrent respiratory papillomatosis surgery. Available from www.emedicine.com/ent/topic594.htm

McColl, D. A. (2006). Intelligibility of tracheoesophageal speech in noise. *Journal of Voice, 20,* 605–615.

McCoy, J. M., Wicks, J. R., & Audoly, L. P. (2002). The role of prostaglandin E2 receptors in the pathogenesis of rheumatoid arthritis. *Journal of Clinical Investigation, 110,* 651–658.

McElhinney, D. B., Jacobs, I., McDonald-McGinn, D. M., Zackai, E. H., & Goldmuntz, E. (2002). Chromosomal and cardiovascular anomalies associated with congenital laryngeal web. *International Journal of Pediatric Otorhinolaryngology, 66,* 23–27.

McFadden, E. R., & Zawadski, D. K. (1996). Vocal cord dysfunction masquerading as exercise-induced asthma: A physiologic cause for "choking" during athletic activities. *American Journal of Respiratory Critical Care Medicine, 153,* 942–947.

McGarvey, L. P. A. (2005). Idiopathic chronic cough: A real disease or a failure of diagnosis? *Cough, 1,* 9–13.

McGarvey, L. P. A., & Elder, J. (2010). Future directions in treating cough. *Otolaryngology Clinics of North America, 43,* 199–211.

McGarvey, L., McKeagney, P., Polley, L., MacMahon, J., Costello, R. W. (2009). Are there clinical features of a sensitized cough reflex? *Pulmonary Pharmacology & Therapeutics, 22,* 59–64.

McGlone, R. E., & Shipp, T. (1971). Some physiologic correlates of vocal fry phonation. *Journal of Speech and Hearing Research, 14,* 769–775.

McHenry, M. A., Kuna, S. T., Minton, J. T., Vanoye, C. R., & Calhoun, K. (1997). Differential activity of the pars recta and pars oblique in fundamental frequency control. *Journal of Voice, 11,* 48–58.

McHenry, M., Reich, A., & Minifie, F. (1982). Acoustic characteristics of intended syllabic stress in excellent esophageal speakers. *Journal of Speech and Hearing Research, 25,* 554–564.

McHenry, M., Whatman, J., & Pou, A. (2002). The effect of botulinum toxin A on the vocal symptoms of spastic dysarthria: A case study. *Journal of Voice, 16,* 124–131.

McKenna, M., & Brodsky, L. (2005). Extraesophageal acid reflux and recurrent respiratory papilloma in children. *International Journal of Pediatric Otorhinolaryngology, 69,* 597–605.

McKinney, J. (1994). *The diagnosis and correction of vocal faults* (2nd ed.). Nashville, TN: Genevox Music Group.

McNeill, E. J. M., Wilson, J. A., Clark, S., & Deakin, J. (2008). Perception of voice in the transgender client. *Journal of Voice, 22,* 727–733.

McQuestion, M., Fitch, M., & Howell, D. (2011). The changed meaning of food: Physical, social and emotional loss for patients having received radiation treatment for head and neck cancer. *European Journal of Oncology Nursing,* 15, 145–151.

McWhorter, A. J., & Hoffman, H. T. (2005). Transoral laser microsurgery for laryngeal malignancies. *Current Problems in Cancer, 29,* 180–189.

Megale, S. R. M. C. L., Scanavini, A. B. A., Andrade, E. C., Fernandes, M. I. M., & Anselmo-Lima, W. T. (2006). Gastroesophageal reflux disease: Its importance in ear, nose, and throat practice. *International Journal of Pediatric Otorhinolaryngology, 70,* 81–88.

Mehta, D., & Hillman, R. E. (2007). Use of aerodynamic measures in clinical voice assessment. *Perspectives in Voice and Voice Disorders, 17,* 14–18.

Meining, A., & Classen, M. (2004). The role of diet and lifestyle measures in the pathogenesis and treatment of gastroesophageal reflux disease. *The American Journal of Gastroenterology, 95,* 2692–2697.

Melcon, M. C., Hoit, J. D., & Hixon, T. J. (1989). Age and laryngeal airway resistance during vowel production. *Journal of Speech and Hearing Disorders, 54,* 282–286.

Meleca, R. J., Dworkin, J. P., Zormeier, M. M., Simpson, M. L., Shibuya, T., & Mathog, R. H. (2000). Videostroboscopy of the pharyngoesophageal segment in laryngectomy patients treated with botulinum toxin. *Otolaryngology—Head and Neck Surgery, 123,* 38–43.

Meline, T., & Paradiso, T. (2003). Evidence-based practice in schools: Evaluating research and reducing barriers. *Language, Speech, and Hearing Services in Schools, 34,* 273–283.

Meltzner, G. S., & Hillman, R. E. (2005). Impact of aberrant acoustic properties on the perception of sound quality in electrolarynx speech. *Journal of Speech, Language and Hearing Research, 48,* 766–777.

Meltzner, G., Hillman, R. E., Heaton, J., Houston, K., Kobler, J., & Qi, Y. (2005). Electrolarynx speech: The state-of-the-art and future directions. In P. Doyle (Ed.), *Contemporary considerations in the treatment and rehabilitation of head and neck cancer* (pp. 571–590). Austin, TX: Pro-Ed.

Men, S., Ikis, A. O., Topcu, I., Cakmakci, H., & Ecevit, C. (2006). CT and virtual endoscopy findings in congenital laryngeal web. *International Journal of Pediatric Otorhinolaryngology, 70,* 1125–1127.

Mendes-Laureano, J., Sa, M. F. S., Ferriani, R. A., Reis, R. M., Aguiar-Ricz, L. N., Valera, F. C. P., . . . Romao, G. S. (2006).

Comparison of fundamental voice frequency between menopausal women and women at menacme. *Maturitas, 55,* 195–199.

Mendes-Laureano, J., Sa, M. F. S., Reis, R. M., Ferriani, R. A., Romao, G. S., Aguiar-Ricz, L. N., . . . Kupper, D. S. (2007). Impact of menopause and hormonal replacement therapy on harmonics-to-noise ratio of the voice. *Maturitas, 56,* 223–224.

Merati, A. L., Shemirani, N., Smith, T. L., & Toohill, R. J. (2006). Changing trends in the nature of vocal fold motion impairment. *American Journal of Otolaryngology—Head and Neck Medicine and Surgery, 27,* 106–108.

Merson, R. M., & Rolnick, M. (1998). Speech-language pathology and dysphagia in multiple sclerosis. *Physical and Medical Rehabilitation Clinics of North America, 9,* 631–641.

Mesallam, T. A., Stemple, J. C., Sobeih, T. M., & Elluru, R. G. (2007). Reflux Symptom Index versus Reflux Finding Score. *Annals of Otology, Rhinology, & Laryngology, 116,* 436–440.

Meurer, E. M., Garcez, V., Corleta, H. v. E., & Capp, E. (2009). Menstrual cycle influences on voice and speech in adolescent females. *Journal of Voice, 23,* 109–113.

Michelsson, K., & Michelsson, O. (1999). Phonation in the newborn, infant cry. *International Journal of Pediatric Otorhinolaryngology, 49* (Suppl. 1), 297–301.

Middendorf, J. H. (2007, Nov. 6). Phonotrauma in children: Management and treatment. *The ASHA Leader,* 14–17.

Mikita, J. A., & Mikita, C. P. (2006). Vocal cord dysfunction. *Allergy and Asthma Proceedings, 27,* 411–414.

Milbrath, R. L., & Solomon, N. P. (2003). Do vocal warm-up exercises alleviate vocal fatigue? *Journal of Speech, Language, and Hearing Research, 46,* 422–436.

Milgrom, H., Corsello, P., Freedman, M., Blager, F., & Wood, R. (1990). Differential diagnosis and management of chronic cough. *Comprehensive Therapy, 16,* 46–53.

Miller, A. (2006). Pseudobulbar affect in multiple sclerosis: Toward the development of innovative therapeutic strategies. *Journal of the Neurological Sciences, 245,* 153–159.

Miller, N., Noble, E., Jones, D., Allcock, L., & Burn, D. J. (2008). How do I sound to me? Perceived changes in communication in Parkinson's disease. *Clinical Rehabilitation, 22,* 14–22.

Miller, Q., & Kline, A. L. (2007). Thymoma. Available from http://emedicine.medscape.com/article/193809-overview

Mirasola, K. L., Braun, N., Blumin, J. H., Kerschner, J. E., & Merati, A. L. (2008). Self-reported voice-related quality of life in adolescents with paradoxical vocal fold dysfunction. *Journal of Voice, 22,* 373–378.

Mirza, N., Kasper Schwartz, S., & Antin-Ozerkis, D. (2004). Laryngeal findings in users of combination corticosteroid and bronchodilator therapy. *Laryngoscope, 114,* 1566–1569.

Mirza, N., Ruiz, C., Baum, E. D., & Staab, J. P. (2003). The prevalence of major psychiatric pathologies in patients with voice disorders. *Ear, Nose and Throat Journal, 82,* 808–814.

Mitchell, J. L. (2002). Cross-cultural issues in the disclosure of cancer. *Cancer Practice, 6,* 153–160.

Molassiotis, A., Bryan, G., Caress, A., Bailey, C., & Smith, J. (2010). Pharmacological and non-pharmacological interventions for cough in adults with respiratory and non-respiratory diseases: A systematic review of the literature. *Respiratory Medicine, 104,* 934–944.

Molina, M. A., Cheung, M. C., Perez, E. A., Byme, M. M., Franceschi, D., Moffat, F. L., . . . Koniaris, L. G. (2008). African American and poor patients have a dramatically worse prognosis for head and neck cancer: An examination of 20,915 patients. *Cancer,* doi:10.1002/cncr.23889

Monnier, P., Ikonomidis, C., Jaquet, Y., & George, M. (2009). Proposal of a new classification for optimizing outcome assessment following partial cricotracheal resections in severe pediatric subglottic stenosis. *International Journal of Pediatric Otorhinolaryngology, 73,* 1217–1221.

Moore, B. A., Holsinger, C., Diaz, E. M., & Weber, R. S. (2005). Organ-preservation laryngeal surgery in the era of chemoradiation. *Current Problems in Cancer, 29,* 169–179.

Moran, M. J., Hague, D., & Roper, L. (2008). SLP and Theatre: A collaborative approach for a transsexual client. Paper presented at the American Speech-Language-Hearing Association Annual Convention, Chicago.

Mordaunt, M. (2006). Pitch and intonation. In R. K. Adler, S. Hirsch, & M. Mordaunt (Eds.), *Voice and communication therapy for the transgender/transsexual client* (pp. 169–207). San Diego, CA: Plural Publishing.

Morgan, M., Triana, M., & Hertel, M. (2006). Longitudinal case study of treatment for adult onset laryngeal papillomatosis. Paper presented at the annual convention of the American Speech-Language-Hearing Association, Philadelphia.

Morgan, E. E., & Rastatter, M. (1986). Variability of voice fundamental frequency in elderly female speakers. *Perceptual and Motor Skills, 63,* 215–218.

Morris, M. J. (2006). Vocal cord dysfunction and asthma. Business Briefing: US Respiratory Care.

Morris, M. J., Perkins, P. J., & Allan, P. F. (2006). Vocal cord dysfunction: Etiologies and treatment. *Clinical Pulmonary Medicine, 13,* 73–86.

Morris, R. J. (1997). Speaking fundamental frequency characteristics of 8- through 10-year-old white and African-American boys. *Journal of Communication Disorders, 30,* 101–116.

Morris, R. J., Gorham-Rowan, M. M., & Harmon, A. B. (2011). The effect of initiating oral contraceptive use on voice: A case study. *Journal of Voice. 25,* 223–229.

Morrison, M. (1997). Pattern recognition in muscle misuse voice disorders: How I do it. *Journal of Voice, 11,* 108–114.

Morrison, M., Rammage, L., & Emami, A. J. (1999). The irritable larynx syndrome. *Journal of Voice, 13,* 447–455.

Mortensen, M., & Woo, P. (2008). High-speed imaging used to detect vocal fold paresis: A case report. *Annals of Otology, Rhinology, & Laryngology, 117,* 684–687.

Most, T., Tobin, Y., & Mimran, R. C. (2000). Acoustic and perceptual characteristics of esophageal and tracheoesophageal speech production. *Journal of Communication Disorders, 33,* 165–181.

Mouadeb, D. A., & Belafsky, P. C. (2007). In-office laryngeal surgery with the 585 nm pulsed dye laser (PDL). *Otolaryngology—Head and Neck Surgery, 137,* 477–481.

Mount, K. H., & Salmon, S. J. (1988). Changing the vocal characteristics of a postoperative transsexual patient: A longitudinal study. *Journal of Communication Disorders, 21,* 229–238.

Mu, L., & Sanders, I. (2009). The human cricothyroid muscle: Three muscle bellies and their innervation patterns. *Journal of Voice, 23,* 21–28.

Mundt, J. C., Snyder, P. J., Cannizzaro, M. S., Chappie, K., & Geralts, D. S. (2007). Voice acoustic measures of depression severity and treatment response collected via interactive voice response (IVR) technology. *Journal of Neurolinguistics, 20,* 50–64.

Mupparapu, M., & Vuppalapati, A. (2005). Ossification of laryngeal cartilages on lateral cephalometric radiographs. *Angle Orthodontics, 75,* 196–201.

Murdoch, B. E., Pitt, G., Theodoros, D. G., & Ward, E. C. (1999). Real-time continuous visual biofeedback in the treatment of speech breathing disorders following childhood traumatic brain injury: Report of one case. *Pediatric Rehabilitation, 3,* 5–20.

Murphy, K., Corfield, D. R., Guz, A., Fink, G. R., Wise, R. J. S., Harrison, J., & Adams, L. (1997). Cerebral areas associated with motor control of speech in humans. *Journal of Applied Physiology, 83,* 1438–1447.

Murphy, T. D., & Ren, C. L. (2009). Congenital stridor. Emedicine.

Murry, T., Abitbol, J., & Hersan, R. (1999). Quantitative assessment of voice quality following laser surgery for Reinke's edema. *Journal of Voice, 13,* 257–264.

Murry, T., McRoy, D. M., & Parhizkar, N. (2007). Common medications and their effects on the voice. *Journal of Singing, 63,* 293–297.

Murry, T., Medrado, R., Hogikyan, N. D., & Aviv, J. E. (2004). The relationship between ratings of voice quality and quality of life measures. *Journal of Voice, 18,* 183–192.

Murry, T., & Sapienza, C. (2010). The role of voice therapy in the management of paradoxical vocal fold motion, chronic cough, and laryngospasm. *Otolaryngology Clinics of North America, 43,* 73–83.

Murry, T., Tabaee, A., & Aviv, J. E. (2004). Respiratory retraining of refractory cough in laryngopharyngeal reflux in patients with paradoxical vocal fold movement. *Laryngoscope, 114,* 1341–1345.

Murry, T., & Woodson, G. E. (1992). A comparison of three methods for the management of vocal fold nodules. *Journal of Voice, 3,* 271–276.

Muscat, J. E., & Wynder, E. L. (1992). Tobacco, alcohol, asbestos, and occupational risk factors for laryngeal cancer. *Cancer, 69,* 2244–2251.

Musser, J., Kelchner, L., Neils-Strunjas, J., & Montrose, M. (2011). A comparison of rating scales used in the diagnosis of extraesophageal reflux. *Journal of Voice, 25,* 293–300.

Myer, C. M., O'Connor, D. M., & Cotton, R. T. (1994). Proposed grading system for subglottic stenosis based on endotracheal tube sizes. *Annals of Otology, Rhinology, Laryngology, 103,* 310–323.

Naiman, A. N., Abedipour, D., Ayari, S., Fresnel, E., Coulombeau, B., Bour, J.-B., & Froelich, P. (2006a). Natural history of adult-onset laryngeal papillomatosis following multiple cidofovir injections. *Annals of Otology, Rhinology & Laryngology, 115,* 175–181.

Naiman, A. N., Ayari, S., Nicollas, R., Landry, G., Colombeau, B., & Froelich, P. (2006b). Intermediate-term and long-term results after treatment by cidofovir and excision in juvenile laryngeal papillomatosis. *Annals of Otology, Rhinology & Laryngology, 115,* 667–672.

Nair, G. (1999). *Voice-tradition and technology: A state-of-the-art studio.* San Diego, CA: Singular.

Nakamura, K., Muta, H., Watanabe, Y., Mochizuki, R., Yoshida, T., & Suzuki, M. (2008). Surgical treatment for adductor spasmodic dysphonia-efficacy of bilateral thyroarytenoid myectomy under microlaryngoscopy. *Acta Oto-Laryngologica, 128,* 1348–1353.

Nakashima, T., Tomita, H., & Chitose, S. (2005). Radiotherapy of the neck influences the distribution of laryngeal secretory glands. *Journal of Laryngology & Otology, 119,* 976–980.

Nakayama, M., Okamoto, M., Miyamoto, S., Takeda, M., Yokobori, S., Masaki, T., & Seino, Y. (2008). Supracricoid laryngectomy with cricohyoidoepiglotto-pexy or cricohyoido-pexy: Experience on 32 patients. *Auris Nasus Larynx, 35,* 77–82.

Narayana, S., Jacks, A., Robin, D. A., Poizner, H., Zhang, W., Franklin, C., . . . Fox, P. T. (2009). A noninvasive imaging approach to understanding speech changes following deep brain stimulation in Parkinson's disease. *American Journal of Speech-Language Pathology, 18,* 146–161.

Nasri, S., Sercarz, J. A., Mcalpin, T., & Berke, G. S. (1995). Treatment of vocal fold granuloma using botulinum toxin type A. *Laryngoscope, 105,* 585–588.

National Cancer Institute. (2005). Head and neck cancer: Questions and answers. Available from www.cancer.gov/cancertopics/factsheet/sites-types/head-and-neck

Neely., J. L., & Rosen, C. (2000). Vocal fold hemorrhage associated with coumadin therapy in an opera singer. *Journal of Voice, 14,* 272–277.

Neuenschwander, M., & Dollar, J. (2005). Vocal fold hemorrhage. *Ear Nose Throat Journal, 84,* 756–757.

Neuenschwander, M. C., Sataloff, R. T., Abaza, M. M., Hawkshaw, M. J., Reiter, D., & Spiegel, J. R. (2001). Management of vocal fold scar with autologous fat implantation: Perceptual results. *Journal of Voice, 15,* 295–304.

Neumann, K., Welzel, C., & Berghaus, A. (2002). Cricothyroidopexy in male-to-female transsexuals—modification of thyroplasty type IV. *International Journal of Transgenderism, 6,* 1–14.

Neumann, K., & Welzel, C. (2004). The importance of the voice in male-to-female transsexualism. *Journal of Voice, 18,* 153–167.

Newcombe, P. A., Sheffield, J. K., Juniper, E. F., Marchant, J. M., Halsted, R. A., Masters, I. B., & Chang, A. B. (2008). Development of a parent-proxy quality-of-life chronic cough-specific questionnaire. *Chest, 133,* 386–395.

Newman, D., & Ramadan, N. (1998). Neurologic disorders: An orientation and overview. In A. Johnson & B. Jacobson (Eds.), *Medical speech-language pathology: A practitioner's guide* (pp. 211–242). New York: Thieme Medical.

Newman, K. B., Mason, III, U. G., & Schmaling, K. B. (1995). Clinical features of vocal cord dysfunction. *American Journal of Respiratory Critical Care Medicine, 152,* 1382–1386.

Newsom, J., & Robbins, R. (2010). Voice personality is a powerful lever to motivate health behavior. HealthLeaders Media. Retrieved from http://healthplans.hcpro.com/HEP-247427/Voice-Personality-is-a-Powerful-Lever-to-Motivate-Health-Behavior

Nguyen, D. D., & Kenny, D. T. (2009). Effects of muscle tension dysphonia on tone phonation: Acoustic and perceptual studies in Vietnamese female teachers. *Journal of Voice, 23,* 446–459.

Nguyen, D. D., & Kenny, D. T. (2009). Impact of muscle tension dysphonia on tonal pitch target implementation in Vietnamese female teachers. *Journal of Voice, 23,* 690–698

Nguyen, D. D., Kenny, D. T., Tran, N. D., & Livesey, J. R. (2008). Muscle tension dysphonia in Vietnamese female teachers. *Journal of Voice, 23,* 195–208.

Nicollas, R., Garrel, R., Ouaknine, M., Giovanni, A., Nazarian, B., & Triglia, J.-M. (2008). Normal voice in children between 6 and 12 years of age: Database and nonlinear analysis. *Journal of Voice, 22,* 671–675.

Nicollas, R., & Triglia, J. M. (2008). The anterior laryngeal webs. *Otolaryngologic Clinics of North America, 41,* 877–888.

Niedzielska, G. (2001). Acoustic analysis in the diagnosis of voice disorders in children. *International Journal of Pediatric Otorhinolaryngology, 57,* 189–193.

Nielson, D. W., Heldt, G. P., & Tooley, W. H. (1990). Stridor and gastroesophageal reflux in infants. *Pediatrics, 85,* 1034–1039.

Nienkerke-Springer, A., McAllister, A., & Sundberg, J. (2005). Effects of family therapy on children's voices. *Journal of Voice, 19,* 103–113.

Nierengarten, M. B. (2009). Vocal fold paresis: A well recognized condition of ambiguous significance. *ENT Today, 4,* 6–7.

Nilson, H., & Schneiderman, C. R. (1983). Classroom program for the prevention of vocal abuse in elementary school children. *Language, Speech, and Hearing Services in Schools, 14,* 172–178.

Noyes, B. E., & Kemp, J. S. (2007). Vocal cord dysfunction in children. *Paediatric Respiratory Reviews, 8,* 155–163.

Nunez, R. A., & Rosen, C. A. (2005). Dynamic voice evaluation using flexible endoscopy. Available from www.emedicine.com/ent/topic685.htm

Oates, J. (2004). The evidence base for the management of individuals with voice disorders. In S. Reilly, J. Douglas, & J. Oates (Eds.), *Evidence-based practice in speech pathology* (pp. 110–139). Philadelphia: Whurr.

Oates, J. (2006). Evidence based practice in voice therapy for transgender/transsexual clients. In R. K. Adler, S. Hirsch, & M. Mordaunt (Eds.). *Voice and communication therapy for the transgender/transsexual client: A comprehensive clinical guide* (pp. 23–43). San Diego, CA: Plural Publishing, Inc.

Ochs, M., Nyengaard, J. R., Jung, A., Knudsen, L., Voigt, M., Wahlers, T., . . . Gundersen, H. J. G. (2004). The number of alveoli in the human lung. *American Journal of Respiratory and Critical Care Medicine, 169,* 120–124.

O'Connell, M. A., Sklarew, P. R., & Goodman, D. L. (1995). Spectrum of presentation of paradoxical vocal cord motion in ambulatory patients. *Annals of Allergy Asthma Immunology, 74,* 341–344.

O'Donnell, S., Murphy, J., Bew, S., & Knight, L. C. (2007). Aryepiglottoplasty for laryngomalacia: Results and recommendations following a case series of 84. *International Journal of Pediatric Otorhinolaryngology, 71,* 1271–1275.

Oeken, J., Hansch, U., Thiel, S., & Bootz, F. (2001). Swallowing function after endoscopic resection of supraglottic carcinoma with the carbon dioxide laser. *European Archives of Otorhinolaryngology, 258,* 250–254.

Ohala, J. J. (1972). How is pitch lowered? Paper presented at the 83rd meeting of the Acoustical Society of America, Buffalo, NY. Retrieved 5/1/2010 from www.linguistics.berkeley.edu/phonlab/users/ohala/papers/how-whole.pdf

O'Hollaren, M. T. (n.d.). Dyspnea due to vocal cord dysfunction: Diagnosis of VCD. Available from www.medscape.com/viewarticle/440355_5

Olthoff, A., Zeiss, D., Laskawi, R., Kruse, E., & Steiner, W. (2005). Laser microsurgical bilateral posterior cordectomy for the treatment of bilateral vocal fold paralysis. *Annals of Otology, Rhinology, & Laryngology, 114,* 599–604.

Op de Coul, B. M. R., Hilgers, F. J. M., Balm, A. J. M., Tan, I. B., van den Hoogen, F. J. A., & van Tinteren, H. (2000). A decade of postlaryngectomy vocal rehabilitation in 318 patients. *Archives of Otolaryngology—Head and Neck Surgery, 126,* 1320–1328.

Oreggia, F., De Stefani, E., Boffetta, P., Brennan, P., Deneo-Pellegrini, H., & Ronco, A. L. (2001). Meat, fat and risk of laryngeal cancer: A case-control study in Uruguay. *Oral Oncology, 37,* 141–145.

Orenstein, S. R., Orenstein, D. M., & Whittington, P. F. (1983). Gastroesophageal reflux causing stridor. *Chest, 84,* 301–302.

Orlikoff, R. F. (1990). The relationship of age and cardiovascular health to certain acoustic characteristics of male voices. *Journal of Speech and Hearing Research, 33,* 450–457.

Orlikoff, R. F., & Kraus, D. H. (1996). Dysphonia following nonsurgical management of advanced laryngeal carcinoma. *American Journal of Speech Language Pathology, 5,* 47–52.

Orloff, L. A., & Goldman, S. N. (1999). Vocal fold granuloma: Successful treatment with botulinum toxin. *Otolaryngology—Head and Neck Surgery, 121,* 410–413.

Osman, M., Hansell, A., Simpson, C. R., Hollowell, J., & Helms, P. J. (2007). Gender specific presentations for asthma, allergic rhinitis and eczema to primary care. *Primary Care Respiratory Journal, 16,* 28–35.

Ossoff, R. H., Sisson, G. A., Moselle, H. I., Duncavage, J. A., Andrews, P. E., & Mcmillan, W. G. (1984). Endoscopic laser arytenoidectomy for the treatment of bilateral vocal cord paralysis. *Laryngoscope, 94,* 1293–1297.

Owaki, S., Kataoka, H., & Shimizu, T. (2010). Relationship between transglottal pressure and fundamental frequency of phonation—study using a rubber model. *Journal of Voice, 24,* 127–132.

Ozcan, K. M., Bahar, S., Ozcan, I., Pasaoglu, L., Sennaroglu, E., Karaaslan, Y., & Dere, H. (2007). Laryngeal involvement in systemic lupus erythematosus: Report of two cases. *Journal of Clinical Rheumatology, 13,* 278–279.

Paiva, L. S., Silva, H. C. A., Mansur, L. L., Callegaro, D., Scaff, M., & Marchior, P. E. (2001). Identification and analysis of the motor systems at work on oral language production in amyotrophic lateral sclerosis. *ALS and Other Motor Neuron Disorders, Suppl. 161, 2,* 88–96.

Paleri, V., Wight, R. G., Owen, S., Hurren, A., & Stafford, F. W. (2006). Defining the stenotic post-laryngectomy tracheostoma and its impact on the quality of life in laryngectomees: Development and validation of a stoma function questionnaire. *Clinical Otolaryngology, 31,* 418–424.

Palombini, B. C., Villanova, C. A. C., Araujo, E., Gastal, O. L., Alt, D. C., Stolz, D. P., & Palombini, C. O. (1999). A pathogenic triad in chronic cough. *Chest, 116,* 279–284.

Paniello, R. C., Edgar, J. D., & Perlmutter, J. S. (2009). Vocal exercise versus voice rest following botulinum toxin injections: A randomized crossover trial. *Annals of Otology, Rhinology, & Laryngology, 118,* 759–763.

Pannbacker, M. (1998). Voice treatment techniques: A review and recommendations for outcome studies. *American Journal of Speech-Language Pathology, 7,* 49–64.

Pannbacker, M. (1999). Treatment of vocal nodules: Options and outcomes. *American Journal of Speech-Language Pathology, 8,* 209–217.

Panzarino, P. J. (n.d.). Stress. Available from www.medicinenet.com/stress/article.htm#what

Papsin, B. C., Abel, S. M., & Leighton, S. E. J. (1999). Diagnostic value of infantile stridor: A perceptual test. *International Journal of Pediatric Otorhinolaryngology, 51,* 33–39.

Park, J.-B., Simpson, L. L., Anderson, T. D., & Sataloff, R. (2003). Immunologic characterization of spasmodic dysphonia patients who develop resistance to botulinim toxin. *Journal of Voice, 17,* 255–264.

Parker, A. J. (2008). Aspects of transgender laryngeal surgery. *Sexologies, 17,* 277–282.

Parsons, J. P., Benninger, C., Hawley, M. P., Philips, G., Forrest, L. A., & Mastronarde, J. G. (2010). Vocal cord dysfunction: Beyond severe asthma. *Respiratory Medicine, 104,* 504–509.

Pasa , G., Oates, J., & Dacakis, G. (2007). The relative effectiveness of vocal hygiene training and vocal function exercises in preventing voice disorders in primary school teachers. *Logopedics Phoniatrics Vocology, 32,* 128–140.

Pasricha, N., Dacakis, G., & Oates, J. (2008). Communicative satisfaction of male-to-female transsexuals. *Logopedics Phoniatrics Vocology, 33,* 25–34.

Patel, N. J., Jorgensen, C., Kuhn, J., & Merati, A. L. (2004). Concurrent laryngeal abnormalities in patients with paradoxical vocal fold dysfunction. *Otolaryngology—Head and Neck Surgery, 130,* 686–689.

Patel, R., Dailey, S., & Bless, D. (2008). Comparison of high-speed digital imaging with stroboscopy for laryngeal imaging of glottal disorders. *Annals of Otology, Rhinology, and Laryngology, 117,* 413–424.

Patel, R. R., Bless, D. M., & Thibeault, S. L. (2010). Boot camp: A novel intensive approach to voice therapy. *Journal of Voice,* doi:10.1016/j.jvoice.2010.01.010

Pauloski, B. R. (2008). Rehabilitation of dysphagia following head and neck cancer. *Physical Medicine and Rehabilitation Clinics of North America, 19,* 889–928.

Paulsen, F. P., Bernhard, N., & Tillmann, B. N. (1998). Degenerative changes in the human cricoarytenoid joint. *Archives of Otolaryngology—Head and Neck Surgery, 124,* 903–906.

Pavord, I. D., & Chung, K. F. (2008). Management of chronic cough. *Lancet, 371,* 1375–1384.

Pawar, P. V., Sayed, S. I., Kazi, R., & Jagade, M. V. (2008). Current status and future prospects in prosthetic voice rehabilitation following laryngectomy, *Journal of Cancer Research and Therapy, 4,* 186–191.

Pawlak, A. S., Hammond, T., Hammond, E., & Gray, S. D. (1996). Immunocytochemical study of proteoglycans in vocal folds. Annals of *Otology, Rhinology, and Laryngology, 105,* 6–11.

Pearson, B. W., DeSanto, L., Olsen, K. D., & Salassa, J. R. (1998). Results of near-total-laryngectomy. *Annals of Otology, Rhinology, & Laryngology, 107,* 820–825.

Pedersen, T., Hovhannisyan, K., & Moller, A. M. (2009). Pulse oximetry for perioperative monitoring. Cochrane Database of Systematic Reviews, Issue 4. Art. No.: CD002013.DOS:10.1002/14651858.CD002013.pubz

Pederson, M. F., Moller, S., Krabbe, S., Bennett, O., & Svenstrup, B. (1990). Fundamental voice frequency in female puberty measured with Electroglottography during continuous speech as a secondary sex characteristic: A comparison between voice, pubertal stages, oestrogens, and androgens. *Journal of Pediatric Otorhinolaryngology, 20,* 16–23.

Pegoraro-Krook, M. I. (1988). Speaking fundamental frequency characteristics of normal Swedish subjects obtained by glottal frequency analysis. *Folia Phoniatrica et Logopedica, 40,* 82–90.

Penner, J. L. (2009). Psychosocial care of patients with head and neck cancer. *Seminars in Oncology Nursing, 25,* 231–241.

Perazzo, P. S. L., Duprat, A. D. C., & Lancellotti, C. L. P. (2009). Histological behavior of the vocal fold after hyaluronic acid injection. *Journal of Voice, 23,* 95–98.

Peretti, G., Piazza, C., Cattaneo, A., De Benedetto, L., Martin, E., & Nicolai, P. (2006). Comparison of functional outcomes after endoscopic versus open-neck supraglottic laryngectomees. *Annals of Otology, Rhinology & Laryngology, 115,* 827–832.

Perie, S., Ming, X., Dewolf, E., St. Guily, J. L. (2002). Autologous fat injection to treat leakage around tracheoesophageal puncture. *American Journal of Otolaryngology, 23,* 345–350.

Perkner, J. J., Fennelly, K. P., Balkissoon, R., Bartelson, B. B., Ruttenber, A. J., Wood, R. P., et al. (1998). Irritant-associated vocal cord dysfunction. *Journal of Occupational and Environmental Medicine, 40,* 136–143.

Petrovic-Lazic, M., Babac, S., Vukovic, M., Kosanovic, R., & Ivankovic, Z. (2009). Acoustic voice analysis of patients with vocal fold polyp. *Journal of Voice.* doi:10.1016/j.jvoice.2009.04.002

Petty, B. E., & Dailey, S. H. (2009). The collaborative medical and behavioral management of chronic cough. *Perspectives on Voice and Voice Disorders, 19,* 49–57.

Pfuetzenreiter, E. G., Dedivitus, R. A., Queija, D. S., Bohn, N. P, & Barros, A. P. B. (2010). The relationship between the glottic configuration after frontolateral laryngectomy and the acoustic voice analysis. *Journal of Voice, 24,* 499–502.

Pickuth, D., Brandt, S., Neumann, K., Berghaus, A., Spielmann, R. P., & Heywang-Köbrunner, S. H. (2000). Spiral computed tomography before and after cricothyroid approximation. *Clinical Otolaryngology & Allied Sciences, 25,* 311–314.

Pinto, J. A., Freitas, M. L. A. D. S., Carpes, A. F., Zimath, P., Marquis, V., & Godoy, L. (2007). Autologous grafts for treatment of vocal sulcus and atrophy. *Otolaryngology—Head and Neck Surgery, 137,* 785–791.

Plant, R. L., & Younger, R. M. (2000). The interrelationship of subglottic air pressure, fundamental frequency, and vocal intensity during speech. *Journal of Voice, 14,* 170–177.

Plante, E. (2004). Evidence-based practice in communication sciences and disorders. *Journal of Communication Disorders, 37,* 389–390.

Plowman-Prine, E. K., Okun, M. S., Sapienza, C. M., Shrivastav, R., Fernandez, H. H., Foote, K. D., . . . Rosenbek, J. C. (2009). Perceptual characteristics of Parkinsonian speech: A comparison of the pharmacological effects of levadopa across speech and non-speech motor systems. *NeuroRehabilitation, 24,* 131–144.

Poburka, B. J. (1999). A new stroboscopy rating form. *Journal of Voice, 13,* 403–413.

Poletto, C. J., Verdun, L. P., Strominger, R., & Ludlow, C. L. (2004). Correspondence between laryngeal vocal fold movement and muscle activity during speech and nonspeech gestures. *Journal of Applied Physiology, 97,* 858–866.

Pontes, P., Avelino, M., Pignatari, S., & Weckx, L. L. M. (2006). Effect of local application of cidofovir on the control of recurrences in recurrent laryngeal papillomatosis. *Otolaryngology—Head and Neck Surgery, 135,* 22–27.

Pontes, P., Brasolotto, A., & Behlau, M. (2005). Glottic characteristics and voice complaint in the elderly. *Journal of Voice, 19,* 84–94.

Pontes, P., Kyrillos, L., Behlau, M., De Biase, N., & Pontes, A. (2002). Vocal nodules and laryngeal morphology. *Journal of Voice, 16,* 408–414.

Portas, J. G., Queija, D. D. S., Arine, L. P., Ferreira, A. S., Dedivitis, R. A., Lehn, C. N., & Barros, A. P. B. (2009). Voice and swallowing disorders: Functional results and quality of life following supracricoid laryngectomy with cricohyoidoepiglottopexy. *Ear, Nose & Throat Journal,* (Suppl.), 8–28.

Porter, S. R., Scully, C., & Hegarty, A. M. (2004). An update of the etiology and management of xerostomia. *Oral Surgery, Oral Medicine, Oral Pathology, 97,* 28–46.

Portone, C., Johns, III, M. M., & Hapner, E. R. (2008). A review of patient adherence to the recommendations for voice therapy. *Journal of Voice, 22,* 192–196.

Postma, G., Blalock, P., & Koufman, J. (1998). Bilateral medialization laryngoplasty. *Laryngoscope, 108,* 1429–1434.

Postma, G. N., Courey, M. S., & Ossoff, R. H (1998). Microvascular lesions of the true vocal fold. *Annals of Otology, Rhinology, & Laryngology, 107,* 472–476.

Powell, D. W., Miffli, R. C., Valentich, J. D., Crowe, S. E., Saada, J. I., & West, A. B. (1999). Myofibroblasts. I. Paracrine cells important in health and disease. *American Journal of Cell Physiology, 277,* C1–C19.

Preciado-Lopez, J., Perez-Fernandez, C., Calzada-Uriondo, M., & Preciado-Ruiz, P. (2007). Epidemiological study of voice disorders among teaching professionals of La Rioja, Spain. *Journal of Voice.*

Preuss, S. F., Klussmann, J. P., Jungehulsing, M., Eckel, H. E., Guntinas-Lichius, O., & Damm, M. (2007). Long-term results of surgical treatment for recurrent respiratory papillomatosis. *Acta Oto-Laryngologica, 127,* 1196–1201.

Pribuisiene, R., Uloza, V., Kupcinskas, L., & Jonaitis, L. (2006). Perceptual and acoustic characteristics of voice changes in reflux laryngitis patients. *Journal of Voice, 20,* 128–136.

Prochaska, J. O., & Velicer, W. F. (1997). The transtheoretical model of health behavior change. *American Journal of Health Promotion, 12,* 38–48.

Pruett, S. B. (2003). Stress and the immune system. *Pathophysiology, 9,* 133–153.

Puts, D. A., Hodges, C. R., Cardenas, R. A., & Gaulin, S. J. C. (2007). Men's' voices as dominance signals: Vocal fundamental and formant frequencies influence dominance attributions among men. *Evolution and Human Behavior, 28,* 340–344.

Putzer, M., Barry, W. J., & Moringlane, J. R. (2007). Effect of deep brain stimulation on different speech subsystems in patients with multiple sclerosis. *Journal of Voice, 21,* 741–753.

Putzer, M., Barry, W. J., & Moringlane, J. R. (2008). Effect of bilateral stimulation of the subthalamic nucleus on different speech subsystems in patients with Parkinson's disease. *Clinical Linguistics and Phonetics, 22,* 957–973.

Qadeer, M. A., Colabianchi, N., Strome, M., Vaezi, M. F., & Sepi, M. (2006). Gastroesophageal reflux and laryngeal cancer: Causation or association? A critical review. *American Journal of Otolaryngology—Head and Neck Medicine and Surgery, 27,* 119–128.

Rahbar, R., Valdez, T. A., & Shapsay, S. M. (2000). Preliminary results of intraoperative mitomycin-C in the treatment and prevention of glottic and subglottic stenosis. *Journal of Voice, 14,* 282–286.

Raitiola, H., Pukander, J. (2000). Symptoms of laryngeal carcinoma and their prognostic significance. *Acta Oncologica, 39,* 213–216.

Raj, A., Gupta, B., Chowdhury, A., & Chadha, S. (2010). A study of voice changes in various phases of menstrual cycle and in postmenopausal women. *Journal of Voice. 24,* 363–368.

Raj, A. A., & Birring, S. S. (2007). Clinical assessment of chronic cough severity. *Pulmonary Pharmacology & Therapeutics, 20,* 334–337.

Ramig, L. O., Countryman, S., Thompson, L. L., & Horii, Y. (1995). A comparison of two forms of intensive speech treatment in Parkinson disease. *Journal of Speech & Hearing Research, 38,* 1232–1251.

Ramig, L. O., Sapir, S., & Fox, C. (2001). Changes in vocal loudness following intensive voice treatment (LSVT) in individuals with Parkinson's disease: A comparison with untreated patients and normal age-matched controls. *Movement Disorders, 16,* 79–83.

Ramig, L. A., Scherer, R. C., Titze, I. R., & Ringel, S. P. (1988). Acoustic analysis of voices of patients with neurologic disease: A rationale and preliminary data. *Annals of Otology and Rhinology, 97,* 164–172.

Ramig, L. A., Scherer, R. C., Klasner, E. R., Titze, I.R., & Horii, Y. (1990). Acoustic analysis of voice in amyotrophic lateral sclerosis: A longitudinal study. *Journal of Speech and Hearing Disorders, 55,* 2–14.

Ramig, L. O., & Verdolini, K. (1998). Treatment efficacy: Voice disorders. *Journal of Speech, Language, and Hearing Research, 41,* S101–S116.

Ramig, L. O., & Verdolini, K. (n.d.). Treatment efficacy summary. Available from www.asha.org/UploadedFiles/public/TESLaryngealBasedVoiceDisorders.pdf

Rammage, L., Morrison, M., & Nichol, H. (2001). *Management of the voice and its disorders* (2nd ed.). Vancouver, Canada: Singular/Thomson Learning.

Ransom, E. R., Antunes, M. B., Smith, L. P., & Jacobs, I. N. (2009). Microdebrider resection of acquired subglottic cysts: Case series and review of the literature. *International Journal of Pediatric Otorhinolaryngology, 73,* 1833–1836.

Rantala, L., Vilkman, E., & Bloigu, R. (2002). Voice changes during work: Subjective complaints and objective measurements for female primary and secondary schoolteachers. *Journal of Voice, 16,* 344–355.

Rattenbury, H. J., Carding, P. N., & Finn, P. (2004). Evaluating the effectiveness and efficiency of voice therapy using transnasal flexible laryngoscopy: A randomized controlled trial. *Journal of Voice, 18,* 522–533.

Rawlings, B. A., Derkay, C. S., Chu, M. W., & John, J. (2009). Surgical treatment of laryngomalacia. *Operative Techniques in Otolaryngology, 20,* 222–228.

Rees, C. J., Blalock, P. D., Kemp, S. E., Halum, S. L., & Koufman, J. A. (2007). Differentiation of adductor-type spasmodic dysphonia from muscle tension dysphonia by spectral analysis. *Otolaryngology—Head and Neck Surgery, 137,* 576–581.

Reichel, O., Dressel, H., Wiederanders, K., & Issing, W. J. (2008). Double-blind, placebo-controlled trial with esomeprazole for symptoms and signs associated with laryngopharyngeal reflux. *Otolaryngology—Head and Neck Surgery, 139,* 414–420.

Remacle, M., Lawson, G., Hantzakos, A., & Jamart, J. (2009). Endoscopic partial supraglottic laryngectomies: Techniques and results. *Otolaryngology—Head and Neck Surgery, 141,* 374–381.

Remacle, M., Matar, N., Morsomme, C., Verduyckt, I., & Lawson, G. (2011). Glottoplasty for male-to-female transsexualism: Voice results. *Journal of Voice, 25,* 120–123.

Remacle, M., Matar, N., Verduyckt, I., & Lawson, G. (2010). Relaxation thyroplasty for mutational falsetto treatment. *Annals of Otology, Rhinology, & Laryngology, 119,* 105–109.

Remacle, M. J., & Declaye, X. J. (1988). Gax-collagen injection to correct an enlarged tracheoesophageal fistula for a vocal prosthesis. *Laryngoscope, 98,* 1350–1352.

Remacle, M., Lawson, G., Keghian, J., & Jamart, J. (1999). Use of injectable autologous collagen for correcting glottic gaps: Initial results. *Journal of Voice, 13,* 280–288.

Reubold, U., Harrington, J., & Kleber, F. (2010). Vocal aging effects on F0 and the first formant: A longitudinal analysis in adult speakers. *Speech Communication, 52,* 638–651.

Reulbach, T. R., Belafsky, P. C., Blalock, P. D., Koufman, J. A., & Postma, G. N. (2001). Occult laryngeal pathology in a community-based cohort. *Otolaryngology—Head and Neck Surgery, 124,* 448–450.

Reveiz, Ll, Cardona, A. F., & Ospina, E. G. (2007). Antibiotics for acute laryngitis in adults. Cochrane Database of Systematic Reviews, Issue 2. Art. No.: CD004783. DOI: 10.1002/14651858.CD004783.pub3

Richter, G. T., & Thompson, D. M. (2008). The surgical management of laryngomalacia. *Otolaryngologic Clinics of North America, 41,* 837–864.

Richter, G. T., Wootten, C. T., Rutter, M. J., & Thompson, D. M. (2009). Impact of supraglottoplasty on aspiration in severe laryngomalacia. *Annals of Otology, Rhinology, & Laryngology, 118,* 259–266.

Riede, T., & Zuberbuhle, K. (2003). Pulse register phonation in Diana monkey alarm calls. *Journal of the Acoustical Society of America, 113,* 2919–2926.

Rieder, A. A., Conley, S. F., & Rowe, L. (2004). Pediatric myasthenia gravis and velopharyngeal incompetence. *International Journal of Pediatric Otorhinolaryngology, 68,* 747–752.

Riegel, B., Warmouth, J. E., Middaugh, S. J., Kee, W. G., Nicholson, L. C., Melton, M., . . . Rosenberg, J. C. (1995). Psychogenic cough treated with biofeedback and psychotherapy: A review and case report. *American Journal of Physical Medicine and Psychotherapy, 74.*

Rieves, A. L., Regner, M. F., & Jiang, J. J. (2009). Phonation threshold pressure estimation using electroglottography in an airflow redirection system. *Laryngoscope, 119,* 2378–2383.

Ringel, R. L., & Chodzko-Zajko, W.J. (1987). Vocal indices of biological age. *Journal of Voice, 1,* 31–37.

Risberg-Berlin, B., Ryden, A., Moller, R. Y., & Finizia, C. (2009). Effects of total laryngectomy on olfactory function, health-related quality of life, and communication: A 3-year follow-up study. *BMC Ear, Nose and Throat Disorders, 9,* doi: 10.1186/1472-6815-9-8

Rizzi, M. D., Thorne, M. C., Zur, K. B., Jacobs, I. N. (2009). Laryngotracheal reconstruction with posterior costal cartilage grafts: Outcomes at a single institution. *Otolaryngology—Head and Neck Surgery, 140,* 348–353.

Robb, M. P., Crowell, D. H., & Dunn-Rankin, P. (2007). Cry analysis in infants resuscitated for apnea of infancy. *International Journal of Pediatric Otorhinolaryngology, 71,* 1117–1123.

Robb, M., & Saxman, J. (1985). Developmental trends in vocal fundamental frequency of young children. *Journal of Speech and Hearing Research, 28,* 420–429.

Robert, D., Pouget, J., Giovanni, A., Azulay, J.-P., & Triglia, J.-M. (1999). Quantitative voice analysis in the assessment of bulbar involvement in amyotrophic lateral sclerosis. *Acta Oto-Laryngologica, 119,* 724–731.

Robinson, J. L., Mandel, S., & Sataloff, R. T. (2005). Objective voice measures in nonsinging patients with unilateral superior laryngeal nerve paresis. *Journal of Voice, 19,* 665–667.

Robitschek, J., Peck, J. J., Klem, C., & Rassekh, C. H. (2009). Conservation laryngeal surgery: Vertical partial laryngectomy. Emedicine Specialties, Otolaryngology and Facial Plastic Surgery, Head and Neck Surgery. Available from www.medscape.com/article/853246-overview

Rodero, E. (2011). Intonation and emotion: Influence of pitch levels and contour type on creating emotions. *Journal of Voice, 25,* 25–34.

Rodriguez-Parra, M. J., Adrian, J. A., & Casado, J. C. (2009). Voice therapy used to test a basic protocol for multidimensional assessment of dysphonia. *Journal of Voice, 23,* 304–318.

Roh, J. L., Kim, H. S., & Kim, A. Y. (2008). The effect of acute xerostomia on vocal function. *Archives of Otolaryngology—Head and Neck Surgery, 132,* 542–546.

Roland, N. J., Bhalla, R. K., & Earis, J. (2004). The local side effects of inhaled corticosteroids. *Chest, 126,* 213–219.

Rollnick, S., & Miller, W. R. (1995). What is motivational interviewing? *Behavioural and Cognitive Psychotherapy, 23,* 325–334.

Rontal, E., & Rontal, M. (2003). Permanent medialization of the paralyzed vocal fold utilizing botulinim toxin and Gelfoam. *Journal of Voice, 17,* 434–441.

Rosati, G. (2001). The prevalence of multiple sclerosis in the world: An update. *Neurological Sciences, 22,* 117–139.

Rosen, C. A. (2000). Vocal fold scar: Evaluation and treatment. *Otolaryngologic Clinics of North America, 33,* 1081–1086.

Rosen, C. A. (2002). Vocal fold paralysis, unilateral. *eMedicine Journal, 3,* www.emedicine.com/ent/topic347.htm

Rosen, C. A., & Bryson, P. C. (2004). Indole-3-carbinol for recurrent respiratory papillomatosis: Long-term results. *Journal of Voice, 18,* 248–253.

Rosen, C. A., & Thekdi, A. A. (2004). Vocal fold augmentation with injectable calcium hydroxylapatite: Short-term results. *Journal of Voice, 18,* 387–391.

Rosen, E. J., & Pou, A. M. (2000). Supraglottic laryngectomy. Grand Rounds Presentation, UTMB, Dept. of Otolaryngology. Available from www.otohns.net/default.asp?id=13093

Rosen, C. A., & Simpson, C. B. (2008). *Operative techniques in laryngology.* Berlin: Springer-Verlag.

Rosenblatt, A., Ranen, N. G., Nance, M. A., & Paulsen, J. S. (1999). *A physician's guide to the management of Huntington's disease* (2nd ed.). Huntington's Disease Society of America.

Rosenfield, D. (1991). Pharmacologic approaches to speech motor disorders. In D. Vogel & M. Cannito (Eds.), *Treating disordered speech motor control.* Austin, Texas: Pro-Ed.

Ross, J., Noordzji, J. P., & Woo, P. (1998). Voice disorders in patients with suspected laryngo-pharyngeal reflux disease. *Journal of Voice, 12,* 84–88.

Rotenberg, B. W., & Berkowitz, R. G. (2006). Changing trends in the success rate of anterior cricoid split. *Annals of Otology, Rhinology and Laryngology, 115,* 833–836.

Rothstein, J. D., Martin, L. J., & Kuncl, R. W. (1992). Decreased glutamate transport by the brain and spinal cord in amyotrophic lateral sclerosis. *The New England Journal of Medicine, 326,* 1464–1468.

Roubeau, B., Henrich, N., & Castellengo, M. (2009). Laryngeal vibratory mechanisms: The notion of vocal register revisited. *Journal of Voice, 23,* 425–438.

Rousseau, B., Sohn, J., Montequin, D. W., Tateya, I., & Bless, D. M. (2004). Functional outcomes of reduced hyaluronan in acute vocal fold scar. *Annals of Otology, Rhinology, & Laryngology, 113,* 767–776.

Rousseau, B., Tateya, I., Lim, X. H., Munoz-del-Rio, A., & Bless, D. M. (2006). Investigation of anti-hyaluronidase treatment on vocal fold wound healing. *Journal of Voice, 20,* 443–451.

Roxburgh, J., & Perry, A. (2004). Use of a "hands-free" tracheostoma valve in patients with laryngectomy and tracheoesophageal puncture. *Annals of Otology Rhinology & Laryngology, 113,* 565–570.

Roy, N., Bless, D. M., & Heisey, D. (2000). Personality and voice disorders: A multitrait-multidisorder analysis. *Journal of Voice, 14,* 521–547.

Roy, N., Gray, S. D., Simon, M., Dove, H., Corbin-Lewis, K., & Stemple, J. C. (2001). An evaluation of the effects of two treatment approaches for teachers with voice disorders: A prospective randomized clinical trial. *Journal of Speech, Language, and Hearing Research, 44,* 286–296.

Roy, N., & Hendarto, H. (2005). Revisiting the pitch controversy: Changes in speaking fundamental frequency (SFF) after management of functional dysphonia. *Journal of Voice, 19,* 582–591.

Roy, N., Holt, K. I., Redmond, S., & Muntz, H. (2007). Behavioral characteristics of children with vocal fold nodules. *Journal of Voice, 21,* 157–168.

Roy, N., Smith, M. E., Allen, B., & Merrill, R. M. (2007). Adductor spasmodic dysphonia versus muscle tension dysphonia: Examining the diagnostic value of recurrent laryngeal nerve lidocaine block. *Annals of Otology, Rhinology, & Laryngology, 116,* 161–168.

Roy, N., Weinrich, B., Gray, S. D., Tanner, K., Stemple, J. C., & Sapienza, C. M. (2003). Three treatments for teachers with voice disorders: A randomized clinical trial. *Journal of Speech, Language, and Hearing Research, 46,* 670–688.

Roy, N., Weinrich, B., Gray, S. D., Tanner, K., Toledo, S. W., Dove, H., . . . Stemple, J. (2002). Voice amplification versus vocal hygiene instruction for teachers with voice disorders: A treatment outcomes study. *Journal of Speech, Language, and Hearing Research, 45,* 625–638.

Roy, N. R., & Ferguson, N. A. (2001). Formant frequency changes following manual circumlaryngeal therapy for functional dysphonia: Evidence of laryngeal lowering? *Journal of Medical Speech-Language Pathology, 3,* 169–175.

Roy, S., & Vivero, R. J. (2008). Recurrent respiratory papillomatosis. *Ear, Nose and Throat Journal, 87,* 18–19.

Rubak, S., Sandbaek, A., Lauritzen, T., & Christensen, B. (2005). Motivational interviewing: A systematic review and meta-analysis. *British Journal of General Practice, 55,* 305–312.

Rubin, A. D., Praneetvatakul, V., Heman-Ackah, Y., Moyer, C. A., Mandel, S., & Sataloff, R. T. (2005). Repetitive phonatory tasks for identifying vocal fold paresis. *Journal of Voice, 19,* 679–686.

Rubin, A. D., Wodchis, W. P., Spak, C., Kileny, P. R., & Hogikyan, N. D. (2004). Longitudinal effects of Botox injections on voice-related quality of life (V-RQOL) for patients with adductory spasmodic dysphonia. *Archives of Otolaryngology—Head and Neck Surgery, 130,* 415–420.

Rubin, J. S., Blake, E., & Mathieson, L. (2007). Musculoskeletal patterns in patients with voice disorders. *Journal of Voice, 21,* 477–484.

Rubin, J. S., & Greenberg, M. (2002). Psychogenic voice disorders in performers: A psychodynamic model. *Journal of Voice, 16,* 544–548.

Ruddy, B. H., & Sapienza, C. M. (2004). Treating voice disorders in the school-based setting: Working within the framework of IDEA. *Language, Speech, and Hearing Services in Schools, 35,* 327–332.

Rudman, D. T., Elmaraghy, C. A., Shiels, W. E., & Wiet, G. J. (2003). The role of airway fluoroscopy in the evaluation of stridor in children. *Archives of Otolaryngology—Head and Neck Surgery, 129,* 305–309.

Ruiz, D. M. C. F., Pontes, P., Behlau, M., & Richieri-Costa, A. (2006). Laryngeal microweb and vocal nodules. *Folia Phoniatrica et Logopaedica, 68,* 392–399.

Russell, A., Oates, J., & Greenwood, K. M. (1998). Prevalence of voice problems in teachers. *Journal of Voice, 12,* 467–479.

Russell, B. (2008). Using manual tension reduction techniques to treat pediatric functional dysphonia. Poster presented at the annual convention of the American Speech-Language-Hearing Association, Chicago.

Russell, J. A., Ciucci, M. R., Connor, N. P., & Schallert, T. (2010). Targeted exercise therapy for voice and swallow in persons with Parkinson's disease. *Brain Research, 1341,* 3–11.

Russell, A., Penny, L., & Pemberton, C. (1995). Speaking fundamental frequency changes over time in women: A longitudinal study. *Journal of Speech and Hearing Research, 38,* 101–109.

Rutter, M. J. (2006). Evaluation and management of upper airway disorders in children. *Seminars in Pediatric Surgery, 15,* 116–123.

Ryan, W. J., & Capadano, H. L. (1978). Age perceptions and evaluative reactions toward adult speakers. *Journal of Gerontology, 33,* 98–102.

Ryan, M., & Kenny, D. T. (2009). Perceived effects of the menstrual cycle on young female singers in the Western classical tradition. *Journal of Voice, 23,* 99–108.

Ryan, N. M., & Gibson, P. G. (2009). Characterization of laryngeal dysfunction in chronic persistent cough. *Laryngoscope, 119,* 640–645.

Ryan, N. M., Vertigan, A. E., Bone, S., & Gibson, P. G. (2010). Cough reflex sensitivity improves with speech language pathology management of refractory chronic cough. *Cough, 6,* 5–12.

Ryan, N. M., Vertigan, A. E., & Gibson, P. G. (2009). Chronic cough and laryngeal dysfunction improve with specific treatment of cough and paradoxical vocal fold movement. *Cough, 5,* 4–11.

Sabol, L., Lee, L., & Stemple, J. C. (1995). The value of vocal function exercises in the practice regime of singers. *Journal of Voice, 9,* 27–36.

Sachin, S., Shukia, G., Goyal, V., Singh, S., Aggarwal, V., Gureshkumar, & Behari, M. (2008). Clinical speech impairment in Parkinson's disease, progressive supranuclear palsy, and multiple system atrophy. *Neurology India, 56,* 122–126.

Saito, K., Araki, K., Ogawa, K., & Shiotani, A. (2009). Laryngeal function after supracricoid laryngectomy. *Otolaryngology—Head and Neck Surgery, 140,* 487–492.

Saito, R., Onodera, H., Tago, H., Suzuki, Y., Shimizu, M., Matsumura, Y., . . . Itoyama, Y. J. (2005). Altered expression of chemokine receptor CXCR5 on T cells of myasthenia gravis patients. *Journal of Neuroimmunology, 170,* 172–178.

Sakakura, K., Chikamatsu, K., Toyoda, M., Kaai, M., Yasuoka, Y., & Furuya, N. (2008). Congenital laryngeal anomalies presenting as chronic stridor: A retrospective study of 55 patients. *Auris Nasus Larynx, 35,* 527–533.

Sala, E., Laine, A., Simberg, S., Pentti, J., & Suonpää, J. (2001). The prevalence of voice disorders among day care center teachers compared with nurses: A questionnaire and clinical study. *Journal of Voice, 15,* 413–423.

Salas-Provance, M. B., Erickson, J. G., & Reed, J. (2002). Disabilities as viewed by four generations of one Hispanic family. *American Journal of Speech-Language Pathology, 11,* 151–162.

Salmon S. (2005). Commonalities among alaryngeal speech methods. In P.C. Doyle & R. L. Keith (Eds.), *Contemporary considerations in the treatment and rehabilitation of head and neck cancer: Voice, speech, and swallowing* (pp. 59–74). Austin, TX: Pro-Ed.

Samlan, R., & Webster, K. (2002). Swallowing and speech therapy after definitive treatment for laryngeal cancer. *Otolaryngology Clinics of North America, 35,* 1115–1133.

Sandage, M. (2006, July 11). Sniffs, gasps, and coughs: Irritable larynx syndrome across the lifespan. *The ASHA Leader.*

Sandage, M. J., & Zelazny, S. K. (2004). Paradoxical vocal fold motion in children and adolescents. *Language, Speech, and Hearing Services in Schools, 35,* 353–362.

Sandulache, V. C., Dohar, J. E., & Hebda, P. A. (2005). Fibroblast transplantation in the airway. *Archives of Otolaryngology—Head and Neck Surgery, 131,* 1090–1096.

Sandyk, R. (1997). Speech impairment in Parkinson's disease is improved by transcranial application of electromagnetic fields. *International Journal of Neuroscience, 92,* 63–72.

Sant'Anna, G. D., & Mauri, M. (2010). Use of the microdebrider for Reinke's edema surgery. *Laryngoscope, 110,* 2114–2116.

Sanuki, T., Yumoto, E., Minoda, R., & Kodama, N. (2010). Effects of type II thyroplasty on adductor spasmodic dysphonia. *Otolaryngology—Head and Neck Surgery, 142,* 540–546.

Sapienza, C., & Ruddy, B. H. (2009). *Management of head and neck cancer* (pp. 395–442). San Diego, CA: Plural Publishing.

Sapienza, C. M., Ruddy, B. H., & Baker, S. (2004). Laryngeal structure and function in the pediatric larynx: Clinical applications. *Language, Speech, and Hearing Services in Schools, 35,* 299–307.

Sapienza, C. M., Walton, S., & Murry, T. (2000). Adductor spasmodic dysphonia and muscular tension dysphonia: Acoustic analysis of sustained phonation and reading. *Journal of Voice, 14,* 502–520.

Sapir, S., Baker, K. K., Larson, C. R., & Ramig, L. O. (2000). Short-latency changes in voice F0 and neck surface EMG induced by mechanical perturbations of the larynx during sustained vowel phonation. *Journal of Speech, Language, and Hearing Research, 43,* 268–276.

Sapir, S., Keidat, A., & Mathers-Schmidt, B. (1993). Vocal attrition in teachers: Survey findings. *International Journal of Language and Communication Disorders, 28,* 177–185.

Sapir, S., Pawlas, A. A., Ramig, L. O., Countryman, S., O'Brien, C., Hoehn, M. M., & Thompson, L. A. (2001). Voice and speech abnormalities in Parkinson disease: Relation to severity of motor impairment, duration of disease, medication, depression, gender, and age. *Journal of Medical Speech-Language Pathology, 9,* 213–226.

Sapir, S., Pawlas, A. A., Ramig, L. O., Seeley, E., Fox, C., & Corboy, J. (2001). Effects of intensive phonatory-respiratory treatment (LSVT) on voice in two individuals with multiple sclerosis. *Journal of Medical Speech-Language Pathology, 9,* 141–151.

Sapir, S., Spielman, J., Ramig, L. O., Hinds, S. L., Countryman, S., Fox, C., & Story, B. (2003). Effects of intensive voice treatment (the Lee Silverman Voice Treatment [LSVT]) on ataxic dysarthria: A case study. *American Journal of Speech-Language Pathology, 12,* 387–399.

Sasaki, C. T., Leder, S. B., Acton, L. M., & Maune, S. (2006). Comparison of the glottic closure reflex in traditional "open" versus endoscopic laser supraglottic laryngectomy. *Annals of Otology, Rhinology, & Laryngology, 115,* 93–96.

Sataloff, R. T. (2005). *Voice science.* San Diego, CA: Plural Publishing.

Sataloff, R. T., Castell, D. O., Katz, P. O., & Sataloff, D. M. (2006). *Reflux laryngitis and related disorders* (3rd ed.). San Diego, CA: Plural Publishing.

Sataloff, R. T., Hawkshaw, M., & Anticaglia, J. (2005). Medications and the voice. In R.T. Sataloff, *The science and art of clinical care* (3rd ed., pp. 905–924). San Diego, CA: Plural Publishing.

Sataloff, R. T., Hawkshaw, M., & Caputo Rosen, D. (1998). Medications: Effects and side effects in professional voice users. In R. T. Sataloff (Ed.), *Vocal health and pedagogy* (pp. 223–235). San Diego, CA: Singular Publishing Group.

Sataloff, R. T., Heuer, R. J., Munz, M., Yoon, M. S., & Spiegel, J. R. (2002). Vocal tremor reduction with deep brain stimulation: A preliminary report. *Journal of Voice, 16,* 132–135.

Sataloff, R. T., Praneevatakul, P., Heuer, R. J., Hawkshaw, M. J., Heman-Ackah, Y. D., Schneider, S. M., & Mandel, S. (2010). Laryngeal electromyography: Clinical application. *Journal of Voice, 24,* 228–238.

Sataloff, R. T., Spiegel, J. R., & Caputo Rosen, D. (1998). The effects of age on the voice. In R. T. Sataloff (Ed.), *Vocal health and pedagogy* (pp. 123–131). San Diego, CA: Singular Publishing Group.

Sato, K., & Hirano, M. (1997). Age-related changes of elastic fibers in the superficial layer of the lamina propria of vocal folds. *Annals of Otology, Rhinology, and Laryngology, 104,* 839–844.

Sauder, C., Roy, N., Tanner, K., Houtz, D. R., & Smith, M. E. (2010). Vocal function exercises for presbylaryngis: A multidimensional assessment of treatment outcomes. *Annals of Otology, Rhinology, & Laryngology, 119,* 460–467.

Saunders, R. (2005). Asthma. In H. A. Boushey, P. B. Corry, J. V. Fahey, E. G. Burchard, & P. G. Wood (Eds.), *Mason, Murray and Nadel's textbook of respiratory medicine* (4th ed.). Philadelphia, PA: Elsevier.

Saunders, M. W., Thirlwall, A., Jacob, A., & Albert, D. M. (1999). Single or two-stage laryngotracheal reconstruction: Comparison of outcomes. *International Journal of Pediatric Otorhinolaryngology, 50,* 51–54.

Sayed, S. I., Elmiyeh, B., Rhys-Evans, P., Syrigos, K. N., Nutting, C. M., Harrington, K. J., & Kazi, R. (2009). Quality of life and outcomes research in head and neck cancer: A review of the state of the discipline and likely future directions. *Cancer Treatment Reviews, 35,* 397–402.

Schaeffer, N., Cavallo, S. A., Wall, M., & Diakow, C. (2002). Speech breathing behavior in normal and moderately to severely dysphonic subjects during connected speech. *Journal of Medical Speech-Language Pathology,* Available from www.highbeam.com/doc/1G1-94207642.html

Schaeffer, N., & Sidavi, A. (2010). Toward a more quantitative measure to assess severity of dysphonia: Preliminary observations. *Journal of Voice, 24,* 556–563.

Schalling, E., Hammarberg, B., & Hartelius, L. (2007). Perceptual and acoustic analysis of speech in individuals with spinocerebellar ataxia (SCA). *Logopedics, Phoniatrics, Vocology, 32,* 31–46.

Scheenstra, R. J., Muller, S. H., Vincent, A., Sinaasappel, M., Zuur, J. K., & Hilgers, F. J. M. (2009). Endotracheal temperature and humidity measurements in laryngectomized patients: Intra- and inter-patient variability. *Medical Biological Engineering and Computing, 47,* 773–782.

Scheff, J. D., Calvano, S. E., Lowry, S. F., & Androulakis, I. P. (2010). Modeling the influence of circadian rhythms on the acute inflammatory response. *Journal of Theoretical Biology, 264,* 1068–1076.

Scheiner, E., Hammerschmidt, K., Jurgens, U., & Zwirner, P. (2002). Acoustic analyses of developmental changes and emotional expression in the preverbal vocalizations of infants. *Journal of Voice, 16,* 509–529.

Scheinfeld, N. S., & Goodwin, J. E. (2010). Intravenous immunoglobulin. Available from http://emedicine .medscape.com/article/210367-overview

Scherer, R. C. (2005). Laryngeal function during phonation. In R. T. Sataloff, *Voice Science* (pp. 167–184). San Diego, CA: Plural Publishing.

Schindler, A., Bottero, A., Capaccio, P., Ginocchio, D., Adorni, F., & Ottaviani, F. (2008). Vocal improvement after voice therapy in unilateral vocal fold paralysis. *Journal of Voice, 22,* 113–118.

Schindler, A., Palonta, F., Preti, G., Ottaviani, F., Schindler, O., & Cavalot, A. L. (2004). Voice quality after carbon dioxide laser and conventional surgery for T1A glottic carcinoma. *Journal of Voice, 18,* 545–550.

Schmidt, M. V., Scharf, S. H., Sterlemann, V., Ganea, K., Liebl, C., Holsboer, F., & Muller, M. B, (2010). High susceptibility to chronic social stress is associated with a depression-like phenotype. *Psychoneuroendocrinology, 35,* 635–643.

Schnapp, L. M., & Cohen, N. H. (1990). Pulse oximetry: Uses and abuses. *Chest, 98,* 1244–1250.

Schneider, B., & Bigenzahn, W. (2003a). Influence of glottal closure configuration on vocal efficacy in young normal-speaking women. *Journal of Voice, 17,* 468–480.

Schneider, B., Denk, D. M., & Bigenzahn, W. (2003). Functional results after external vocal fold medialization thyroplasty with the titanium vocal fold medialization implant. *Laryngoscope, 113,* 628–634.

Schneider, B., Denk, D. M., & Bigenzahn, W. (2003b). Acoustic assessment of the voice quality before and after medialization thyroplasty using the titanium vocal fold medialization implant (TVFMI). *Otolaryngology—Head and Neck Surgery, 128,* 815–822.

Schraff, S., Derkay, C. S., Burke, B., & Lawson, L. (2004). American Society of Pediatric Otolaryngology members' experience with recurrent respiratory papillomatosis and the use of adjuvant therapy. *Archives of Otolaryngology—Head and Neck Surgery, 130,* 1039–1042.

Schubert, C., Lambertz, M., Nelesen, R. A., Bardwell, W., Choi, J-B., & Dimsdale, J. E. (2009). Effects of stress on heart rate complexity: A comparison between short-term and chronic stress. *Biological Psychology, 80,* 325–332.

Schulz, G. M., & Grant, M. K. (2000). Effects of speech therapy and pharmacologic and surgical treatments on voice and speech in Parkinson's disease: A review of the literature. *Journal of Communication Disorders, 33,* 59–88.

Schulz, G. M., Greer, M., & Friedman, W. (2000). Changes in vocal intensity in Parkinson's disease following pallidotomy surgery. *Journal of Voice, 14,* 589–606.

Schwartz, I. S., & Grishman, E. (1980). Rheumatoid nodules of the vocal cords as the initial manifestation of systemic lupus erythematosus. *Journal of the American Medical Association, 244,* 2751–2752.

Schweinfurth, J., & Ossoff, R. (2006). Iatrogenic vocal fold scar. Available from www.emedicine.com/ent/topic607 .htm

Schweinfurth, J., & Ossoff, R. (2008). Vascular lesions of the vocal fold. Available from www.emedicine.com/ article607.htm

Searl, J. (2006). Technological advances in alaryngeal speech rehabilitation. *Perspectives on Voice and Voice Disorders, 16,* 12–18.

Searl, J. (2007). Bilabial contact pressure and oral air pressure during tracheoesophageal speech. *Annals of Otology, Rhinology & Laryngology, 116,* 304–311.

Searl, J. P., & Carpenter, M. A. (2002). Acoustic cues to the voicing feature in tracheoesophageal speech. *Journal of Speech, Language and Hearing Research, 45,* 282–294.

Searl, J. P., Carpenter, M. A., & Banta, C. L. (2001). Intelligibility of stops and fricatives in tracheoesophageal speech. *Journal of Communication Disorders, 34,* 305–321.

Searl, J., & Ousley, T. (2004). Phonation offset in tracheoesophageal speech. *Journal of Communication Disorders, 37,* 371–387.

Sedlacek, T. V., Lindheim, S., Eder, C., Hasty, L., Woodland, M., Ludomirsky, A., & Rando, R. F. (1989). Mechanism for human papillomavirus transmission at birth. *American Journal of Obstetrics & Gynecology, 161,* 55–59.

Seedat, R. Y., Thukane, M., Jansen, A. C., Rossouw, I., Goedhals, D., & Burt, F. J. (2010). HPV types causing juvenile recurrent laryngeal papillomatosis in South Africa. *International Journal of Pediatric Otorhinolaryngology, 74,* 255–259.

Segas, J., Stavroulakis, P., Manolopoulos, L., Yiotakis, J., & Adamopoulos, G. (2001). Management of bilateral vocal fold paralysis: Experience at the University of Athens. *Otolaryngology—Head and Neck Surgery, 124,* 68–71.

Segebarth, P. B., & Limbird, T. J. (2007). Perioperative acute upper airway obstruction secondary to severe rheumatoid arthritis. *Journal of Arthroplasty, 22,* 916–919.

Seifert, E., & Kollbrunner, J. (2005). Stress and distress in non-organic voice disorders. *Swiss Medical Weekly, 135,* 387–397.

Seifert, E., & Kollbrunner, J. (2006). An update in thinking about nonorganic voice disorders. *Archives of Otolaryngology—Head and Neck Surgery, 132,* 1128–1132.

Selber, J., Sataloff, R., Spiegel, J., & Heman-Ackah, Y. (2003). Gore-Tex medialization thyroplasty: Objective and subjective evaluation. *Journal of Voice, 17,* 88–95.

Selby, J. C., Gilbert, H. R., & Lerman, J. W. (2003). Perceptual and acoustic evaluation of individuals with laryngopharyngeal reflux pre- and post-treatment. *Journal of Voice, 17,* 557–570.

Seneviratne, J. K., & Ross, M. A. (2008). Neuromuscular diseases of the older adult. In J. I. Sirven, & B. L. Malamut (Eds.) *Clinical neurology of the older adult* (2nd ed., pp. 420–432). Wolters Kluwer/Lippincott Williams & Wilkins.

Sesterhenn, A. M., Zimmermann, A. P., Bernhard, M., Kussin, A., Timmesfeld, N., Stiller, S., . . . Werner, J. A. (2009). Polysomnography outcomes following transoral CO_2 laser microsurgery in pediatric patients with laryngomalacia. *International Journal of Pediatric Otorhinolaryngology, 73,* 1339–1343.

Sewnaik, A., Hakkesteegt, M. M., Meeuwis, C. A., De Gier, H. H. W., & Kerrebijn, J. D. F. (2006). Supracricoid partial laryngectomy with cricohyoidoepiglottopexy for recurrent laryngeal cancer. *Annals of Otology, Rhinology, & Laryngology, 115,* 419–424.

Shah, A. K. (2009). Myasthenia gravis. *eMedicine Neurology*. Available from http://emedicine.medscape.com/article/1171206-overview

Shah, R. K., Engel, S. H., & Choi, S. S. (2008). Relationship between voice quality and vocal nodule size. *Otolaryngology—Head and Neck Surgery, 139,* 723–726.

Shah, R. K., Feldman, H. A., & Nuss, R. C. (2007). A grading scale for pediatric vocal fold nodules. *Otolaryngology—Head and Neck Surgery, 136,* 193–197.

Shah, R. K., & Shapshay, S. (2006). Acute laryngitis. www.emedicine.com/ent/topic353.htm

Shah, R. K., Woodnorth, G. H., Glynn, A., & Nuss, R. C. (2005). Pediatric vocal nodules: Correlation with perceptual voice analysis. *International Journal of Pediatric Otorhinolaryngology, 69,* 903–909.

Shanks, J. C. (1995). Coping with laryngeal cancer. *Seminars in Speech and Language, 16,* 180–190.

Sharma, D., Nagarkar, A. N., Jindal, P., Kaur, R., & Gupta, A. (2008). Personality changes and the role of counseling in the rehabilitation of patients with laryngeal cancer. *Ear, Nose & Throat Journal,* (Suppl.), 3–12.

Shirley, W. P., & Wiatrak, B. (2004). Is cydofovir a useful adjunctive therapy for recurrent respiratory papillomatosis in children? *International Journal of Pediatric Otorhinolaryngology, 68,* 413–418.

Sidell, D., Shamouelian, D., Erman, A., Gerratt, B. R., & Chhetri, D. (2010). Improved tracheoesophageal prosthesis sizing in office-based tracheoesophageal puncture. *Annals of Otology, Rhinology, & Laryngology, 119,* 37–41.

Silbergleit, A. K., Johnson, A. F., & Jacobson, B. H. (1997). Acoustic analysis of voice in individuals with amyotrophic lateral sclerosis and perceptually normal voice quality. *Journal of Voice, 11,* 222–231.

Simberg, S., & Laine, A. (2007). The resonance tube method in voice therapy: Description and practical implementations. *Logopedics, Phoniatrics, Vocology, 32,* 165–170.

Simberg, S., Sala, E., & Ronnemaa, A-M. (2004). A comparison of the prevalence of vocal symptoms among teacher students and other university students. *Journal of Voice, 18,* 363–368.

Simonelli, M., Ruoppolo, G., de Vincentiis, M., Di Mario, M., Calcagno, P., Vitiello, C., . . . Gallo, A. (2010). Swallowing ability and chronic aspiration after supracricoid partial laryngectomy. *Otolaryngology—Head and Neck Surgery, 142,* 873–878.

Simons, J. P., Rosen, C. A., Casselbrant, M. I., Chi, D. H., Schaitkin, B. M., Rubinstein, E. J., & Mandell, D. L. (2008). Comparison of Pediatric Voice Outcome Survey, Reflux Symptom Index, Reflux Finding Score, and esophageal biopsy results. *Archives of Otolaryngology—Head and Neck Surgery, 134,* 837–841.

Simonyan, K., & Jurgens, U. (2003). Efferent subcortical projections of the laryngeal motor cortex in the rhesus monkey. *Brain Research, 974,* 45–59.

Simonyan, K., Tovar-Moll, F., Ostuni, J., Hallett, M., Kalasinsky, V. F., Lewin-Smith, M. R., Rushing, E. J., Vortmeyer, A. O., & Ludlow, C. L. (2008). Focal white matter changes in spasmodic dysphonia: a combined DTI and neuropathological study. *Brain, 131,* 447–459.

Simpson, C. B., Archilla, A. S., Velazquez, R. A., & McGuff, H. S. (2006). Resolution of vocal fold leukoplakia with proton-pump inhibitor therapy. *Ear, Nose and Throat Journal,* 362–364.

Simpson, C. B., Cheung, E. J., & Jackson, C. J. (2009). Vocal fold paresis: Clinical and electrophysiologic features in a tertiary laryngology practice. *Journal of Voice, 23,* 396–398.

Sims, H. S., Smith, B. E., & Johnson, B. C. (2007). The predictive value of the Voice Handicap Index-30 for compliance with voice restorative therapy. Presented at the 36th Annual Symposium: Care of the Professional Voice, Philadelphia, PA.

Singer, S., Merbach, M., Dictz, A., & Schwarz, R. (2007). Psychosocial determinants of successful voice rehabilitation after laryngectomy. *Journal of the Chinese Medical Association, 70,* 407–423.

Singh, A., Kazi, R., De Cordova, J., Nutting, C. M., Clarke, P., & Harrington, K. J. (2008). Multidimensional assessment of voice after vertical partial laryngectomy: A comparison with normal and total laryngectomy voice. *Journal of Voice, 22,* 740–745.

Sittel, C., Friedrich, G., Zorowka, P., & Eckel, H.-E. (2002). Surgical voice rehabilitation after laser surgery for glottic carcinoma. *Annals of Otology, Rhinology, & Laryngology, 111,* 493–499.

Sivasankar, M., Erickson, E., Schneider, S., & Howes, A. (2008). Phonatory effects of airway dehydration: Preliminary evidence for impaired compensation to oral breathing in individuals with a history of vocal fatigue. *Journal of Speech, Language, and Hearing Research, 51,* 1494–1506.

Sivasankar, M., & Fisher, K. V. (2002). Oral breathing increases Pth and vocal effort by superficial drying of vocal fold mucosa. *Journal of Voice, 16,* 172–181.

Skodda, S., Visser, W., & Schlegel, U. (2011). Gender-related patterns of dysprosody in Parkinson disease and correlations between speech variables and motor symptoms. *Journal of Voice, 25,* 76–82.

Skodda, S., Visser, W., & Schlegel, U. (2010). Acoustical analysis of speech in progressive supranuclear palsy. *Journal of Voice,* doi:10.1016/j.voice.2010.01.002

Skodda, S., Visser, W., & Schlegel, U. (2010). Short- and long-term dopaminergic effects on dysarthria in early Parkinson's disease. *Journal of Neural Transmission, 117,* 197–205.

Slavin, D. C. (1997). Alaryngeal speech rehabilitation. In C. T. Ferrand & R. L. Bloom (Eds.), *Introduction to organic and neurogenic disorders of communication: Current scope of practice* (pp. 273–300). Needham Heights, MA: Allyn and Bacon.

Slavin, D. C., & Ferrand, C. T. (1995). Factor analysis of proficient esophageal speech: Toward a multidimensional model. *Journal of Speech and Hearing Research, 38,* 1224–1231.

Slavit, D. (1999). Phonosurgery in the elderly: A review. *Ear, Nose and Throat Journal, 78,* 505–512.

Smart, J. F., & Smart, D. W. (1997). The racial/ethnic demography of disability. *Journal of Rehabilitation, 63,* 73–82.

Smith, A. D., Cowan, J. O., Filsell, S., McLachlan, C., Monti-Sheehan, G., Jackson, P., & Taylor, D. R. (2004). Diagnosing asthma: Comparisons between exhaled nitric oxide measurements and conventional tests. *Respiratory and Critical Care Medicine, 169,* 473–478.

Smith, B. E., Kempster, G. B., & Sims, H. S. (2010). Patient factors related to voice therapy attendance and outcomes. *Journal of Voice, 24,* 694–701.

Smith, C. G., Finnegan, E. M., & Karnell, M. P. (2005). Resonant voice: Spectral and nasendoscopic analysis. *Journal of Voice, 19,* 607–622.

Smith, E., Verdolini, K., Gray, S., Nichols, S., Lemke, J., Barkmeier, J., . . . Hoffman, H. (1996). Effect of voice disorders on quality of life. *Journal of Medical Speech-Language Pathology, 4,* 223–244.

Smith, E. M., Summersgill, K. F., Allen, J., Hoffman, H. T., McCulloch, T., Turek, L. P., & Haugen, T. H. (2000). Human papillomavirus and risk of laryngeal cancer. *Annals of Otology, Rhinology, & Laryngology, 109,* 1069–1076.

Smith, G. A., Ward, P. A., & Berci, G. (1978). Laryngeal lupus erythematosus. *Journal of Laryngology & Otology, 92,* 67–73.

Smith, M. E., Marsh, J. H., Cotton, R. T., & Myer, C. M. (1993). Voice problems after pediatric laryngotracheal reconstruction: Videolaryngostroboscopic, acoustic, and perceptual assessment. *International Journal of Pediatric Otorhinolaryngology, 25,* 173–181.

Smith, M. E., Roy, N., & Stoddard, K. (2008). Ansa-RLN reinnervation for unilateral vocal fold paralysis in adolescents and young adults. *International Journal of Pediatric Otorhinolaryngology, 72,* 1311–1316.

Smith, M. E., & Sauder, C. (2009). Pediatric vocal fold paralysis/immobility. *Perspectives on Voice and Voice Disorders, 19,* 113–121.

Smith, S., & Thyme, K. (1976). Statistic research on changes in speech due to pedagologic treatment (the accent method). *Folia Phoniatrica, 28,* 98–103.

Smits, I., Ceuppens, P., & De Bodt, M. S. (2005). A comparative study of acoustic voice measurements by means of Dr. Speech and Computerized Speech Lab. *Journal of Voice, 19,* 187–196.

So, Y. K., Yun, Y.-S., Baek, C. H., Jeong, H.-S., & Son, Y.-I. (2009). Speech outcome of supracricoid partial laryngectomy: Comparison with total laryngectomy and anatomic considerations. *Otolaryngology—Head and Neck Surgery, 141,* 770–775.

Soderpalm, E., Larsson, A. K., & Almquist, S.-A. (2004). Evaluation of a consecutive group of transsexual individuals referred for vocal intervention in the west of Sweden. *Logopedics, Phoniatrics, Vocology, 29,* 18–30.

Sodersten, M., Granqvist, S., Hammarberg, B., & Szabo, A. (2002). Vocal behavior and vocal loading factors for preschool teachers at work studied with binaural DAT recordings. *Journal of Voice, 16,* 356–371.

Sodersten, M., Hertegard, S., & Hammarberg, B. (1995). Glottal closure, transglottal airflow, and voice quality in healthy middle-aged women. *Journal of Voice, 9,* 182–197.

Sodersten, M., & Lindestad, P. A. (1990). Glottal closure and perceived breathiness during phonation in normally speaking subjects. *Journal of Speech and Hearing Research, 33,* 601–611.

Solomon, N. P. (2008). Vocal fatigue and its relation to vocal hyperfunction. *International Journal of Speech-Language Pathology, 10,* 254–266.

Solomon, N. P., & Charron, S. (1998). Speech breathing in able-bodied children and children with cerebral palsy: A review of the literature and implications for clinical intervention. *American Journal of Speech-Language Pathology, 7,* 61–78.

Solomon, N. P., & Di Mattia, M. S. (2000). Effects of a vocally fatiguing task and systemic hydration on phonation threshold pressure. *Journal of Voice, 14,* 341–359.

Solomon, N. P., Glaze, L. E., Arnold, R. R., & van Mersbergen, M. (2003). Effects of a vocally fatiguing task and systemic hydration on men's voices. *Journal of Voice, 17,* 31–46.

Solomon, N. P., Helou, L. B., & Stojadinovic, A. (2011). Clinical versus laboratory ratings of voice using the CAPE-V. *Journal of Voice, 25,* 7–14.

Solomon, N. P., McKee, A. S., & Garcia-Barry, S. (2001). Intensive voice treatment and respiration treatment for hypokinetic-spastic dysarthria after traumatic brain injury. *American Journal of Speech-Language Pathology, 10,* 51–64.

Solomon, N. P., McKee, A. S., Larson, K. J., Nawrocki, M. D., Tuite, P. J., Eriksen, S., . . . Maxwell, R. E. (2000). Effects of pallidal stimulation on speech in three men with severe Parkinson's disease. *American Journal of Speech-Language Pathology, 9,* 241–256.

Solomon, N. P., Ramanathan, P., & Makashay, M. J. (2007). Phonation threshold pressure across the pitch range: Preliminary test of a model. *Journal of Voice, 21,* 541–550.

Sorenson, D. N. (1989). A FO investigation of children ages 6–10 years old. *Journal of Communication Disorders, 22,* 115–123.

Spector, S. (2009). Use of mannitol inhalation challenge in assessment of cough. *Lung,* doi:10.1007/s00408-009-9174-2

Spencer, K. A., Yorkston, K. M., & Duffy, J. R. (2003). Behavioral management of respiratory/phonatory dysfunction from dysarthria: A flowchart for guidance in clinical decision making. *Journal of Medical Speech-Language Pathology, 11,* xxxix–lxi.

Sperry, E. E., & Klich, R. J. (1992). Speech breathing in senescent and younger women during oral reading. *Journal of Speech and Hearing Research, 35,* 1246–1255.

Speyer, R., Bogaardt, H. C. A., Lima Passos, V., Roodenburg, N. P. H. D., Zumach, A., Heijnen, M. A. M., . . . Brunings, J. W. (2010). Maximum phonation time: Variability and reliability. *Journal of Voice, 24,* 281–284.

Speyer, R., Wieneke, G. H., van Wijck-Warnaar, I., & Dejonckere, P. H. (2003). Effects of voice therapy on the voice range profiles of dysphonic patients. *Journal of Voice, 17,* 544–556.

Spiegel, J. H. (2006). Phonosurgery for pitch alteration: Feminization and masculinization of the voice. *Otolaryngology Clinics of North America, 39,* 77–86.

Spielman, J., Ramig, L. O., Mahler, L., Halpern, A., & Gavin, W. J. (2007). Effects of an extended version of the Lee Silverman Voice Treatment on voice and speech in Parkinson's disease. *American Journal of Speech-Language Pathology, 16,* 95–107.

Sridhara, S. R., Ashok, K. G., Raghunathan, M., & Mann, S. G. S. (2003). To study voice quality before and after thyroplasty type I in patients with symptomatic unilateral vocal cord paralysis. *American Journal of Otolaryngology, 24,* 361–365.

Stager, S. V., & Bielamowicz, S. A. (2010). Using laryngeal electromyography to differentiate presbylarynges from paresis. *Journal of Speech, Language, and Hearing Research, 53,* 100–113.

Stager, S., Bielamowicz, S. A., Gupta, A., Marullo, S., Regnell, J. R., & Barkmeier, J. M. (2001). Quantification of static and dynamic supraglottic activity. *Journal of Speech, Language, and Hearing Research, 44,* 1245–1256.

Stager, S., Bielamowicz, S. A., Regnell, J. R., Gupta, A., & Barkmeier, J. M. (2000). Supraglottic activity: Evidence of vocal hyperfunction or laryngeal articulation? *Journal of Speech, Language, and Hearing Research, 43,* 229–238.

Stajner-Katusic, S., Horga, D., Musura, M., & Globlek, D. (2006). Voice and speech after laryngectomy. *Clinical Linguistics and Phonetics, 20,* 195–203.

Stanton, A. E., Sellars, C., MacKenzie, K., McConnachie, A., & Bucknall, C. E. (2009). Perceived vocal morbidity in a problem asthma clinic. *The Journal of Laryngology and Otology, 123,* 96–102.

Starmer, H. M., Tippett, D. C., & Webster, K. T. (2008). Effects of laryngeal cancer on voice and swallowing. *Otolaryngology Clinics of North America, 41,* 793–818.

Stathopoulos, E. (1986). Relationship between intraoral air pressure and vocal intensity in children and adults. *Journal of Speech and Hearing Research, 29,* 71–74.

Stavroulaki, P. (2006). Diagnostic and management problems of laryngopharyngeal reflux disease in children. *International Journal of Pediatric Otorhinolaryngology, 70,* 579–590.

Stemple, J. C. (2000). Successful voice therapy. In J. Stemple (Ed.), *Voice therapy: Clinical studies* (2nd ed.). San Diego, CA: Singular Publishing Group.

Stemple, J. C. (2005). A holistic approach to voice therapy. *Seminars in Speech and Language, 26,* 131–137.

Stemple, J., Glaze, L., & Klaben, B. (2000). *Clinical voice pathology: Theory and management* (3rd ed). Clifton Park, NJ: Delmar Learning.

Stemple, J. C., Lee, L., D'Amico, B., & Pickup, B. (1994). Efficacy of vocal function exercises as a method of improving voice production. *Journal of Voice, 8,* 271–289.

Stenton, C. (2008). The MRC breathlessness scale. *Occupational Medicine, 58,* 226–227.

Stepp, C. E., Heaton, J. T., & Hillman, R. E. (2008). Postlaryngectomy speech respiration patterns. *Annals of Otology, Rhinology, & Laryngology, 117,* 557–563.

Stern, Y., Felipovich, A., Cotton, R. T., & Segal, K. (2007). Immunocompetency in children with recurrent respiratory papillomatosis: Prospective study. *Annals of Otology, Rhinology, & Laryngology, 116,* 169–171.

Stewart, C. F., Brin, M. F., & Blitzer, A. (1997). Spasmodic dysphonia. In C. T. Ferrand & R. L. Bloom (Eds.), *Introduction to organic and neurogenic disorders of communication: Current scope of practice* (pp. 301–318). Needham Heights, MA: Allyn and Bacon.

Stolz, D., Anderson, S., Gysin, C., Miedinger, D., Surber, C., Tamm, H., & Leuppi, J. D. (2009). Airway reactivity to inhaled mannitol in cigarette smokers: A longitudinal study. *Respiratory Medicine, 101,* 1470–1476.

Stong, B. C., DelGaudio, J. M., Hapner, E. R., & Johns III, M. M. (2005). Safety of simultaneous bilateral botulinim toxin injections for abductor spasmodic dysphonia. *Archives of Otolaryngology—Head and Neck Surgery, 131,* 793–795.

Strand, E. A., Buder, E. H., Yorkston, K. M., & Ramig, L. O. (1994). Differential phonatory characteristics of four women with amyotrophic lateral sclerosis. *Journal of Voice, 8,* 327–339.

Strauss, S. (2000). Sonographic appearance of cricoid cartilage calcification in healthy children. *American Journal of Radiology, 174,* 223–228.

Sudhir, P. M., Chandra, P. S., Shivashankar, N., & Yamini, B. K. (2009). Comprehensive management of psychogenic dysphonia: A case illustration. *Journal of Communication Disorders, 42,* 305–312.

Suehiro, A., Hirano, S., Kishimoto, Y., Tanaka, S., & Ford, C. N. (2009). Comparative study of vocal outcomes with silicone versus Gore-Tex thyroplasty. *Annals of Otology, Rhinology, & Laryngology, 118,* 405–408.

Suhr, J., Anderson, S., & Tranel, D. (1999). Progressive muscle relaxation in the management of behavioural disturbance in Alzheimer's disease. *Neuropsychological Rehabilitation,* 31–44.

Sulica, L., & Behrman, A. (2003). Management of benign vocal fold lesions: A survey of current opinion and practice. *Annals of Otology, Rhinology, Laryngology, 113,* 827–833.

Sulter, A. M., Schutte, H. K., & Miller, D. G. (1995). Differences in phonetogram features between male and female subjects with and without vocal training. *Journal of Voice, 9,* 363–377.

Syal, R., Tyagi, I., & Goyal, A. (2006). Traumatic laryngotracheal stenosis—An alternative surgical technique. *International Journal of Pediatric Otorhinolaryngology, 70,* 353–357.

Takahashi, H., Nakao, M., Kikuchi, Y., & Kaga, K. (2008). Intra-oral pressure-based voicing control of electrolaryngeal speech with intra-oral vibrator. *Journal of Voice, 22,* 420–429.

Tamura, Y., Tanaka, S., Asato, R., Hirano, S., Yamashita, M., Tamaki, H., & Ito, J. (2007). Therapeutic outcomes of laryngeal cancer at Kyoto University Hospital for 10 years. *Acta Oto-Laryngologica, 127,* 62–65.

Tanner, K., Roy, N., Merrill, R. M., Kimber, K., Sauder, C., Houtz, D. R., . . . Smith, M. E. (2011). Risk and protective factors for spasmodic dysphonia: A case-control investigation. *Journal of Voice, 25,* 35–46.

Tanoue, L. T. (1998). Pulmonary manifestations of rheumatoid arthritis. *Clinics in Chest Medicine, 19,* 667–685.

Tantawy, A. (2003). Long-term results of Provox voice prosthesis for voice rehabilitation after total laryngectomy: "A seven years experience." *International Congress Series, 1240,* 871–877.

Tarin, T. T., Martinez, J. A., & Shapiro, N. L. (2005). Familial bilateral abductor vocal cord paralysis. *International Journal of Pediatric Otorhinolaryngology, 69,* 1693–1696.

Tasca, R. A., McCormick, M., & Clarke, R. W. (2006). British Association of Paediatric Otorhinolaryngology members' experience with recurrent respiratory papillomatosis. *International Journal of Pediatric Otorhinolaryngology, 70,* 1183–1187.

Tavares, E. L. M., & Martins, R. H. G. (2007). Vocal evaluation in teachers with or without symptoms. *Journal of Voice, 21,* 407–414.

Teitel, A. D., Mackenzie, C. R., Stern, R., & Paget, S. A. (1992). Laryngeal involvement in systemic lupuserythematosus. *Seminars in Arthritis and Rheumatism, 22,* 203–214.

Teles-Magalhaes, L. C., Pegoraro-Krook, M. I., & Pegoraro, R. (2000). Study of the elderly females' voice by phonetography. *Journal of Voice, 14,* 310–321.

Terada, T., Saeki, N., Toh, K., Uwa, N., Sagawa, K., Takayasu, S., & Sakagami, M. (2007). Voice rehabilitation with Provox2 TM voice prosthesis following total laryngectomy for laryngeal and hypopharyngeal carcinoma. *Auris Nasus Larynx, 34,* 65–71.

Tervonen, H., Bäck, L., Juvas, A., Räsänen, P., Mäkitie, A. A., Sintonen, H., Roine, R. P., Vilkman, E., & Aaltonen, L. M. (2005). Automatic speaking valve in speech rehabilitation for laryngectomized patients. *European Archives of Otorhinolaryngology, 262,* 816–820.

Terrell, J. E., Fisher, S. G., & Wolf, G. T. (1998). Long-term quality of life after treatment of laryngeal cancer. *Archives of Otolaryngology—Head and Neck Surgery, 124,* 964–971.

Teshigawara, M., Amir, N., Amir, O., Wlosko, E. M., & Avivi, M. (2007). Effects of random splicing on listeners' perceptions. *ICPHS, XVI,* 2101–2104.

Tezcaner, C. Z., Ozgursoy, S. K., Sati, I., & Dursun, G. (2009). Changes after voice therapy in objective and subjective voice measurements of pediatric patients with vocal nodules. *European Archives of Otorhinolaryngology, 266,* 1923–1927.

Theis, S. M., Connor, N. P., & McMurray, J. S. (2006). Pediatric laryngotracheal reconstruction: Case studies. *Perspectives on Voice and Voice Disorders, 16*(3), 20–23.

Theis, S. M., & Heatley, D. G. (2009). Evaluation and treatment of pediatric gastroesophageal reflux and its effects on voice. *Perspectives on Voice and Voice Disorders, 19,* 90–95.

The Merck Manual. (2005). www.merck.com/pubs/mmanual/section5/chapter50/50d.htm

Thibeault, S. (2006). International focus on voice—introduction. *The ASHA Leader, 11,* 3.

Thibeault, S. L., & Duflo, S. (2008). Inflammatory cytokine responses to synthetic extracellular matrix injection to the vocal fold lamina propria. *Annals of Otology, Rhinology, & Laryngology, 117,* 221–226.

Thibeault, S. L., & Gray, S. (2004). Response of the vocal mechanism to trauma. In C. M. Sapienza & J. Casper (Eds.), *Vocal rehabilitation for medical speech-language pathology* (pp. 11–28). Austin, TX: Pro-Ed.

Thibeault, S. L., & Gray, S.D. (2005).Vocal fold injury and repair. In R. T. Sataloff, *Voice science* (pp. 105–113). San Diego, CA: Plural Publishing.

Thibeault, S. L., Merrill, R. M., Roy, N., Gray, S. D., & Smith, E. M. (2004). Occupational risk factors associated with voice disorders among teachers. *Annals of Epidemiology, 14,* 786–792.

Thomas, G., Kooijman, P. G. C., Donders, A. R. T., Cremers, C. W. R. J., & De Jong, F. I. C. R. S. (2007). The voice handicap of student-teacher and risk factors perceived to have a negative influence on the voice. *Journal of Voice, 21,* 325–336.

Thomas, L. B., Harrison, A. L., & Stemple, J. C. (2008). Aging thyroarytenoid and limb skeletal muscle: lessons in contrast. *Journal of Voice, 22,* 430–450.

Thomas, L. B., & Stemple, J. C. (2007). The aging voice: From clinical symptoms to biological realities. Retrieved from [1137-2012Thomas_Lisa_089594_Oct04_2007_Time_072146AM]

Thomas, L. B., & Stemple, J. C. (2007). Voice therapy: Does science support the art? *Communication Disorders Review, 1,* 49–77.

Thome, R., Thome, D. C., & De La Cortina, R. A. C. (2000). Lateral thyrotomy approach on the paraglottic space for laryngocele resection. *Laryngoscope, 110,* 447–450.

Thompson, A. R. (1995). Pharmacological agents with effects on voice. *American Journal of Otolaryngology, 16,* 12–18.

Thornton, J. (2008). Working with the transgender voice: The role of the speech and language therapist. *Sexologies, 17,* 271–276.

Threats, T. T. (2006). Towards an international framework for communication disorders: Use of the ICF. *Journal of Communication Disorders, 39,* 251–265.

Tiago, R., Pontes, P., & Campones do Brasil, O. (2007). Age-related changes in human laryngeal nerves. *Otolaryngology—Head and Neck Surgery, 136,* 747–751.

Tillmann, B., Pietzsch-Rohrschneider, I., & Huenges, H. L. (1977). The human vocal cord surface. *Cell and Tissue Research, 185,* 279–283.

Timmermans, B., De Bodt, M. S., Wuyts, F. L., & Van de Heyning, P. H. (2005). Analysis and evaluation of a voice-training program in future professional voice users. *Journal of Voice, 19,* 202–210.

Timms, M. S., Bruce, I. A., & Patel, N. K. (2007). Radiofrequency ablation (coblation): A promising new technique for laryngeal papillomata. *The Journal of Laryngology and Otology, 121,* 28–30.

Tindall, L. R., Huebner, R. A., Stemple, J. C., & Kleinert, H. L. (2008). Videophone-delivered voice therapy: A comparative analysis of outcomes to traditional delivery for adults with Parkinson's disease. *Telemedicine and eHealth, 14,* 1070–1077.

Titze, I. R. (1994). *Principles of Voice Production.* Englewood Cliffs, NJ: Prentice Hall.

Titze, I. R. (1999). Toward occupational safety criteria for vocalization. *Logopedics Phoniatrics Vocology, 24,* 49–54.

Titze, I. R. (2001). Acoustic interpretation of resonant voice. *Journal of Voice, 15,* 519–528.

Titze, I. R. (2006). Voice training and therapy with a semi-occluded vocal tract: Rationale and scientific underpinnings. *Journal of Speech, Language, and Hearing Research, 49,* 448–459.

Titze, I. R. (2011). Vocal fold mass is not a useful quantity for describing fundamental frequency in vocalization. *Journal of Speech, Language and Hearing Research, 54,* 520–522.

Titze, I. R., & Sundberg, J. (1992). Vocal intensity in speakers and singers. *Journal of the Acoustical Society of America, 91,* 2936–2946.

Torrejano, G., & Guimaraes, I. (2009). Voice quality after supracricoid laryngectomy and total laryngectomy with insertion of voice prosthesis. *Journal of Voice, 23,* 240–246.

Torrente, M. C., & Ojeda, J. M. (2007). Exploring the relation between human papilloma virus and larynx cancer. *Acta Oto-Laryngologica, 127,* 900–906.

Trani, M., Ghidini, A., Bergamini, G., & Presutti, L. (2007). Voice therapy in pediatric functional dysphonia: A prospective study. *International Journal of Pediatric Otorhinolaryngology, 71,* 379–384.

Treasure, J. (2004). Motivational interviewing. *Advances in Psychiatric Treatment, 10,* 331–337.

Treole, K., Trudeau, M. D., & Forrest, L. A. (1999). Endoscopic and stroboscopic description of adults with paradoxical vocal fold dysfunction. *Journal of Voice, 13,* 143–152.

Tsunoda, K., & Soda, Y. (1996). Hoarseness as the initial manifestation of systemic lupus erythematosus. *Journal of Laryngology & Otology, 110,* 478–479.

Tucker, H. M. (1999). Long-term preservation of voice improvement following surgical medialization and reinnervation for unilateral vocal fold paralysis. *Journal of Voice, 13,* 251–256.

Turley, R., & Cohen, S. (2009). Impact of voice and swallowing problems in the elderly. *Otolaryngology—Head and Neck Surgery, 140,* 33–36.

Turner, C. (2007). A review of myasthenia gravis: Pathogenesis, clinical features and treatment. *Current Anesthesia & Critical Care, 18,* 15–23.

Umeno, H., Chitose, S., Sato, K., & Nakashima, T. (2008). Efficacy of additional injection laryngoplasty after framework surgery. *Annals of Otology, Rhinology, & Laryngology, 117,* 5–10.

Umeno, H., Chitose, S., Sato, K., & Nakashima, T. (2009). Comparative study of framework surgery and fat injection laryngoplasty. *The Journal of Laryngology & Otology, 123* (Suppl. S31), 35–41.

Unal, E., Oran, B., Baysal, T., Baspinar, O., Keser, M., Karaarslan, S., & Arbag, H. (2006). Pulmonary arterial pressure in infants with laryngomalacia. *International Journal of Pediatric Otorhinolaryngology, 70,* 2067–2071.

U.S. Bureau of the Census. (2000). *Statistical abstract of the United States* (120th ed.). Washington, DC: Author.

U.S. Department of Labor, Bureau of Labor Statistics. (2006). Occupational employment and wages, 2006 [Data file]. Retrieved from http:\\www.bls.gov/oes

Urquhart, A. C., & St. Louis, E. (2005). Idiopathic vocal cord palsies and associated neurological conditions. *Archives of Otolaryngology—Head and Neck Surgery, 131,* 1086–1089.

Valdez, T. A., & Shapshay, S. M. (2002). Idiopathic subglottic stenosis revisited. *Annals of Otology, Rhinology, & Laryngology, 111,* 690–695.

Valera, F. C. P., Tamashiro, E., De Araujo, M. M., Sander, H. H., & Kupper, D. S. (2006). Evaluation of the efficacy of supraglottoplasty in obstructive sleep apnea syndrome associated with severe laryngomalacia. *Archives of Otolaryngology—Head and Neck Surgery, 132,* 489–493.

Van As, C. J., Koopmans-van Beinum, F. J., & Hilgers, F. J. M. (2003). Perceptual evaluation of tracheoesophageal speech by naïve and experienced judges through the use of semantic differential scales. *Journal of Speech, Language, and Hearing Research, 46,* 947–959.

Van As-Brooks, C. J., Koopmans-van Beinum, F. J., Pols, L. C. W., Hilgers F. J. M. (2006). Acoustic signal typing for evaluation of voice quality in tracheoesophageal speech. Journal of Voice, 20, 355–368.

Van Beurden, H. E., Von den Hoff, J. W., Torensma, R., Maltha, J. C., & Kuijpers-Jagtman, A. M. (2005). Myofibroblasts in palatal wound healing: Prospects for the reduction of wound contraction after cleft palate repair. *Journal of Dental Research, 84,* 871–880.

Van Borsel, J., De Cuypere, G., & den Berghe, H. (2001). Physical appearance and voice in male-to-female transsexuals. *Journal of Voice, 15,* 570–575.

Van Borsel, J., De Pot, K., & De Cuypere, G. (2009). Voice and physical appearance in female-to-male transsexuals. *Journal of Voice, 23,* 494–497.

Van Borsel, J., Van Eynde, E., De Cuypere, G., & Bonte, K. (2008). Feminine after cricothyroid approximation? *Journal of Voice, 22,* 379–384.

Van den Berg, J. (1958). Myoelastic aerodynamic theory of voice production. *Journal of Speech and Hearing Research, 1,* 227–243.

Van der Merwe, A. (2004). The Voice Use Reduction Program. *American Journal of Speech-Language Pathology, 13,* 208–218.

Van der Torn, M., Verdonck-de Leeuw, I. M., Kuik, D. J., & Mahieu, H. F. (2002). Communicative suitability of voice following radiotherapy for T1 glottic carcinoma: Testing the reliability of a rating instrument. *Journal of Voice, 16,* 398–407.

Vance, C., Rogelj, B., Hortobágyi, T., De Vos, K. J., Nishimura A. L., Sreedharan, J., Hu, X., Smith, B., Ruddy, D., Wright, P., Ganesalingam, J., Williams, K. L., Tripathi, V., Al-Saraj, S., Al-Chalabi, A., Leigh, P. N., Blair, I. P., Nicholson, G., de Belleroche, J., Gallo, J. M., Miller, C. C., & Shaw, C. E. (2009). Mutations in FUS, an RNA processing protein, cause familial amyotrophic lateral sclerosis type 6. *Science, 323,* 1208–1211.

Van Gogh, C. D. L., Verdonck-de Leeuw, I. M., Boon-Kamma, B. A., Rinkel, R. N. P. M., de Bruin, M. D., Langendijk, J. A., . . . Mahieu, H. F. (2006). The efficacy of voice therapy in patients after treatment for early glottic carcinoma. *Cancer, 106,* 95–105.

Van Houtte, E., Claeys, S., Wuyts, F., & Van Lierde, K. (2010). The impact of voice disorders among teachers: Vocal complaints, treatment-seeking behavior, knowledge of vocal care, and voice-related absenteeism. *Journal of Voice.* doi:10.1016/j.voice.2010.04.008

Van Houtte, E., Van Lierde, K., & Claeys, S. (2011). Pathophysiology and treatment of muscle tension dysphonia: A review of the current knowledge. *Journal of Voice, 25,* 202–207.

Van Leer, E., & Connor, N. P. (2010). Patient perceptions of voice therapy adherence. *Journal of Voice, 24,* 458–469.

Van Leer, E., Hapner, E. R., & Connor, N. P. (2008). Transtheoretical model of health behavior change applied to voice therapy. *Journal of Voice, 22,* 688–698.

Van Lierde, K. M., De Bodt, M., D'haeseleer, E., Wuyts, F., & Claeys, S. (2010). The treatment of muscle tension dysphonia: A comparison of two treatment techniques by means of an objective multiparameter approach. *Journal of Voice, 24,* 294–301.

Van Lierde, K. M., De Ley, S., Clement, G., De Bodt, M., & Van Cauwenberge, P. (2004). Outcome of laryngeal manual therapy in four Dutch adults with persistent moderate-to-severe vocal hyperfunction: A pilot study. *Journal of Voice, 18,* 467–474.

Van Mersbergen, M., Patrick, C., & Glaze, L. (2008). Functional dysphonia during mental imagery: Testing the trait theory of voice disorders. *Journal of Speech, Language, and Hearing Disorders, 51,* 1405–1423.

Van Rossum, M. A., Quene, H., & Nooteboom, S. G. (2008). Prosodic boundaries in alaryngeal speech. *Clinical Linguistics & Phonetics, 22,* 215–231.

Vegas, A., Cobeta, I., Mico, A., & Rivera, T. (2010). Pedunculated polyp removal by means of larynx fiberendoscopic surgery. *European Archives of Otorhinolaryngology, 267,* 1255–1260.

Verdolini, K. (1998). National Center for Voice and Speech's guide to vocology. National Center for Voice and Speech.

Verdolini, K., & Ramig, L. O. (2001). Review: Occupational risks for voice problems. *Logopedics Phoniatrics Vocology, 26,* 37–46.

Verdolini, K., Rosen, C. A., & Branski, R. C. (Eds.) (2006). *Classification manual for voice disorders-I.* Mahwah, NJ: Lawrence Erlbaum Associates, Inc.

Verdolini-Marston, K., Burke, M. K., Lessac, A., Glaze, L., & Caldwell, E. (1995). Preliminary study of two methods of treatment for laryngeal nodules. *Journal of Voice, 9,* 74–85.

Verdolini-Marston, K., Titze, I., & Druker, D. (1991). Changes in phonation threshold pressure with induced conditions of hydration. *Journal of Voice, 4,* 142–151.

Verdolini-Marston, K., Sandage, M., & Titze, I. R. (1994). Effect of hydration treatments on laryngeal nodules and polyps and related voice measures. *Journal of Voice, 8,* 30–47.

Verduyckt, I., Remacle, M., Jamart, J., Benderitter, C., & Morsomme, D. (2011). Voice-related complaints in the pediatric population. *Journal of Voice, 25,* 373–380.

Vernon, M., Leidy, N. K., Nacson, A., & Nelsen, L. (2009). Measuring cough severity: Perspectives from the literature and from patients with chronic cough. *Cough, 5,* 5–12.

Vertigan, A. E., Theodoros, D. G., Gibson, P. G., & Winkworth, A. L. (2006). Efficacy of speech pathology management for chronic cough: A randomized placebo controlled trial of treatment efficacy. *Thorax, 61,* 1065–1069.

Vertigan, A. E., Theodoros, D. G., Gibson, P. G., & Winkworth, A. L. (2007). Voice and upper airway symptoms in people with chronic cough and paradoxical vocal fold movement. *Journal of Voice, 21,* 361–383.

Vertigan, A. E., Theodoros, D. G., Winkworth, A. L., & Gibson, P. G. (2007b). Perceptual voice characteristics in chronic cough and paradoxical vocal fold movement. *Folia Phoniatrica et Logopedica, 59,* 256–267.

Vertigan, A. E., Theodoros, D. G., Winkworth, A. L., & Gibson, P. G. (2008). A comparison of two approaches to the treatment of chronic cough: Perceptual, acoustic, and electroglottographic outcomes. *Journal of Voice, 22,* 581–589.

Vipperla, R., Renals, S., & Frankel, J. (2010). Ageing voices: The effect of changes in voice parameters on ASR performance. *EURASIP Journal on Audio, Speech, and Music Processing.* doi:10.1155/2010/525783

Vlahakis, N. E., Patel, M. A., Maragos, N. E., & Beck, K. C. (2002). Diagnosis of vocal cord dysfunction: The utility of spirometry and plethysmography. *Chest, 122,* 2246–2249.

Vodovotz, V., Constantine, G., Rubin, J., Csete, M., Voit, E. O., & An, G. (2009). Mechanistic simulations of inflammation: Current state and future prospects. *Mathematical Biosciences, 217,* 1–10.

Vogel, K. G., Paulsson, M., & Heingard, D. (1984). Specific inhibition of type I and type II collagen fibrillogenesis by the small proteoglycans of tendon. *Biochemistry Journal, 223,* 587–597.

Von Leden, H., & Alessi, D. M. (1994). The aging voice. In M. S. Benninger, B. H. Jacobson, & A. F. Johnson (Eds.). *Vocal arts medicine: The care and prevention of professional voice disorders* (pp. 269–286). New York: Thieme Medical Publishers, Inc.

Wagner, I., Fugain, C., Monneron-Girard, L., et al (2003). Pitch-raising surgery in fourteen male-to-female transsexuals. *Laryngoscope, 113,* 1157–1165.

Walker, M., & Messing, B. (2006). Stroboscopic interpretation: Inter-rater reliability among professionals. Presented at the Annual Convention of the American Speech-Language-Hearing Association, Miami.

Walling, A. D. (1999). Amyotrophic lateral sclerosis: Lou Gehrig's disease. Available from www.aafp.org/afp/990315ap/1489.html

Wallis, L., Jackson-Menaldi, C., Holland, W., & Giraldo, A. (2004). Vocal fold nodule vs. vocal fold polyp: Answer from surgical pathologist and voice pathologist point of view. *Journal of Voice, 18,* 125–129.

Walton, J. H., & Orlikoff, R. F. (1994). Speaker race identification from acoustic cues in the vocal signal. *Journal of Speech and Hearing Research, 37,* 738–745.

Wang, C.-P., Ko, J.-Y., Wang, Y.-H., Hu, Y.-L., & Hsiao, T.-Y. (2009). Vocal process granuloma—A result of long-term observation in 53 patients. *Oral Oncology, 45,* 821–825.

Wang, T.-G., Shau, Y.-W., & Hsiao, T.-Y. (2010). Effects of surgery on the phonation threshold pressure in patients with vocal fold polyps. *Formosa Medical Association, 109,* 62–68.

Wang, Y-T., Kent, R. D., Kent, J. F., Duffy, J. R., & Thomas, J. E. (2009). Acoustic analysis of voice in dysarthria following stroke. *Clinical Linguistics and Phonetics, 23,* 335–347.

Wanger, J., Clausen, J. L., Coates, A., Pedersen, O. F., Brusasco, V., Burgos, F., . . . Viegi, G. (2005). Standardisation of the measurement of lung volumes. *European Respiratory Journal, 26,* 511–522.

Ward, P. D., Thibeault, S. L., & Gray, S. D. (2002). Hyaluronic acid: Its role in voice. *Journal of Voice, 16,* 303–309.

Watson, G. J., Malik, T. H., Khan, N. A., Sheehan, P. Z., & Rothera, M. P. (2007). Acquired paediatric subglottic cysts: A series from Manchester. *International Journal of Pediatric Otorhinolaryngology, 71,* 533–538.

Watson, P. J., & Hughes, D. (2006). The relationship of vocal loudness manipulation to prosodic F0 and durational variables in healthy adults. *Journal of Speech, Language, and Hearing Research, 49,* 636–644.

Watson, P. J., & Hixon, T. J. (2001). Effects of abdominal trussing on breathing and speech in men with cervical spinal cord injury. *Journal of Speech, Language, and Hearing Research, 44,* 751–762.

Watson, P. J., & Schlauch, R. S. (2009). Fundamental frequency variation with an electrolarynx improves speech understanding: A case study. *American Journal of Speech-Language Pathology, 18,* 162–167.

Watts, C., Nye, C., & Whurr, R. (2006). Botulinum toxin for treating spasmodic dysphonia (laryngeal dystonia): A systematic Cochrane review. *Clinical Rehabilitation, 20,* 2112–2122.

Watts, C. R., & Vanryckeghem, M. (2001). Laryngeal dysfunction in amyotrophic lateral sclerosis: A review and case report. *BMC Ear, Nose and Throat Disorders.* Available at: www.biomedcentral.com/1472-6815/1/1

Webster, K. T., Samlan, R. A., Jones, B., Bunton, K., & Tufano, R. P. (2010). Supracricoid partial laryngectomy: Swallowing, voice, and speech outcomes. *Annals of Otology, Rhinology, & Laryngology, 119,* 10–16.

Weiler, J. M., Layton, T., & Hunt, M. (1998). Asthma in United States Olympic athletes who participated in the 1996 Summer Games. *Journal of Allergy and Clinical Immunology, 102,* 722–726.

Wein, R. O., & Weber, R. S. (2005). The current role of vertical partial laryngectomy and open supraglottic laryngectomy. *Current Problems in Cancer, 29,* 201–214.

Weinberg, B., & Bennett, S. (1971). Speaker sex recognition of five & six-year-old children's voices. *Journal of the Acoustical Society of America, 50,* 1210–1213.

Weinrich, B., Baker, S., Kelchner, L., Middendorf, J., Krival, K., Elluru, R., & Zur, K. B. (2007). Examination of aerodynamic measures and strain by vibratory source. *Otolaryngology—Head and Neck Surgery, 136,* 455–458.

Weinrich, B., Salz, B., & Hughes, M. (2005). Aerodynamic measurements: Normative data for children ages 6:0 to 10:11 years. *Journal of Voice, 19,* 326–339.

Welham, N. V., Dailey, S. H., Ford, C. N., & Bless, D. M. (2007). Voice handicap evaluation of patients with pathologic sulcus vocalis. *Annals of Otology, Rhinology, & Laryngology, 116,* 411–417.

Welham, N. V., Lim, X., Tateya, I., & Bless, D. M. (2008). Inflammatory factor profiles one hour following vocal fold injury. *Annals of Otology, Rhinology, & Laryngology, 117,* 145–152.

Welham, N. V., & Maclagan, M. A. (2003). Vocal fatigue: Current knowledge and future directions. *Journal of Voice, 17,* 21–30.

Welham, N. V., Rousseau, B., Ford, C. N., & Bless, D. M. (2003). Tracking outcomes after phonosurgery for sulcus vocalis: A case report. *Journal of Voice, 17,* 571–578.

Westcott, C. J., Hopkins, M. B., Bach, K., Postma, G. N., Belafsky, P. C., & Koufman, J. A. (2004). Fundoplication for laryngopharyngeal reflux disease. *Journal of the American College of Surgeons, 199,* 23–30.

Westerblad, H., & Allen, D. G. (2002). Recent advances in the understanding of skeletal muscle fatigue. *Current Opinion in Rheumatology.*

Wheat, M. C., & Hudson, A. I. (1988). Spontaneous speaking fundamental frequency of 6-year-old black children. *Journal of Speech and Hearing Research, 31,* 723–725.

Wheeler, K. M., Collins, S. P., & Sapienza, C. M. (2006). The relationship between VHI scores and specific acoustic measures of mildly disordered voice production. *Journal of Voice, 20,* 308–317.

Wheeler, K. M., & Sapienza, C. M. (2005). Swallowing and respiration: Shared neural substrates. Retrieved 4/18/10 from www.speechpathology.com/articles/pf_article_detail.asp?article_id=283

White, D. R., Cotton, R. T., Bean, J. A., & Rutter, M. J. (2005). Pediatric cricotracheal resection. *Archives of Otolaryngology, 131,* 896–899.

Whiteside, S. P., & Hodgson, C. (2000). Some acoustic characteristics in the voices of 6- to 10-year old children and adults: A comparative sex and developmental perspective. *Logopedics, Phoniatrics, Vocology, 25,* 122–132.

Whiteside, S. P., Hodgson, C., & Tapster, C. (2002). Vocal characteristics in pre-adolescent and adolescent children: A longitudinal study. *Logopedics, Phoniatrics, Vocology, 27,* 12–20.

Whurr, R., Nye, C., & Lorch, M. (1998). Meta-analysis of botulinum toxin treatment of spasmodic dysphonia: A review of 22 studies. *International Journal of Language & Communication Disorders, 33,* 327–329.

Whymark, A. D., Clement, W. A., Kubba, H., & Geddes, N. K. (2006). Laser epiglottopexy for laryngomalacia. *Archives of Otolaryngology—Head and Neck Surgery, 132,* 978–982.

Williams, R. A. (1975). *Textbook of black-related diseases.* New York: McGraw-Hill.

Williams, S.L., & Deem, J.F. (2000). Likelihood of classroom teachers incorporating vocal hygiene practices into daily routines. *Paper presented at the American Speech-Language-Hearing Association Annual Convention,* Washington, DC.

Williamson, I. J., Matusiewicz, S. P., Brown, P. H., Greening, A. P., & Crompton, G. K. (1995). Frequency of voice problems and cough in patients using pressurized aerosol inhaled steroid preparations. *European Respiratory Journal, 8,* 590–592.

Willinger, U., & Aschauer, H. N. (2005). Personality, anxiety and functional dysphonia. *Personality and Individual Differences, 39,* 1441–1449.

Willinger, U., Volkl-Kernstock, S., & Aschauer, H. N. (2005). Marked depression and anxiety in patients with functional dysphonia. *Psychiatry Research, 134,* 85–91.

Witt, R. E., Hoffman, M. R., Friedrich, G., Rieves, A. L., Schoepke, B. J., & Jiang, J. J. (2010). Multiparameter analysis of titanium vocal fold medializing implant in an excised larynx model. *Annals of Otology, Rhinology, & Laryngology, 119,* 125–132.

Witt, R. L. (2005). Recurrent laryngeal nerve electrophysiologic monitoring in thyroid surgery: The standard of care? *Journal of Voice, 19,* 497–500.

Wo, J. M., Goudy, S., Winstead, W., & Mohiuddin, Z. (2003). Lifestyle and dietary modification as the primary therapy for laryngopharyngeal reflux. *Gastroenterology, 124* (Suppl. 1), A540.

Wolf, M., Primov-Fever, A., Talmi, Y., & Kronenberg, J. (2007). Posterior glottic stenosis in adults. *Israeli Medical Association Journal, 9,* 597–599.

Wolfe, V. I., Ratusnik, D. L., Smith, F. H., & Northrop, G. E. (1990). Intonation and fundamental frequency in male-to-female transsexuals. *Journal of Speech and Hearing Disorders, 55,* 43–50.

Wong, A. Y.-H., Ma, E. P.-M., & Yiu, E. M.-L. (2011). Effects of practice variability on learning of relaxed phonation in vocally hyperfunctional speakers. *Journal of Voice, 25,* 103–113.

Woo, P. (1999). Phonosurgery techniques after partial laryngectomy. *Operative Techniques in Otolaryngology—Head and Neck Surgery, 10,* 53–60.

Woo, P., & Carroll, L. M. (2009). Management of adult vocal fold nerve injury. *Perspectives on Voice and Voice Disorders, 19*(1), 24–33.

Woo, P., Mendelsohn, J., & Humphrey, D. (1995). Rheumatoid nodules of the larynx. *Otolaryngology—Head and Neck Surgery, 113,* 147–150.

Woodnorth, G. H. (2006). Children with upper airway pathology: Behavioral management of voice. *Perspectives on Voice and Voice Disorders, 16*(3), 2006.

Woodson, G. (2008). Management of neurologic disorders of the larynx. *Annals of Otology, Rhinology, & Laryngology, 117,* 317–326.

Woodson, G., Hochstetler, H., & Murry, T. (2006). Botulinum toxin therapy for abductor spasmodic dysphonia. *Journal of Voice, 20,* 137–143.

Woodson, G. E., & Murry, T. (1994). Botulinum toxin in the treatment of recalcitrant mutational falsetto. *Journal of Voice, 8,* 347–351.

World Health Organization. (2001). International Classification of Functioning, Disability, and Health (ICIDH-2), final draft. Available at www.who.int/icidh

Worley, G., Bajaj, Y., Cavalli, L., & Hartley, B. (2007). Laser arytenoidectomy in children with bilateral vocal fold immobility. *The Journal of Laryngology & Otology, 121,* 25–27.

Worrall, L. E., & Bennett, S. (2001). Evidence-based practice: Barriers and facilitators for speech-language pathologists. *Journal of Medical Speech-Language Pathology, 9,* xi–xvi.

Wright, C. (2007). Laser surgery for laryngeal cancer. Retrieved 10/23/2010 from www.utmb.edu/otoref/grnds/laryngeal-ca-071128/laryngeal-ca-071128.pdf

Wright, C. D. (2008). Surgical management of subglottic stenosis. *Operative Techniques in Thoracic and Cardiovascular Surgery,* 53–65. doi:10.1053/j.optechstcvs.2008.01.003

Wyatt, M. E., & Hartley, B. E. J. (2005). Laryngotracheal reconstruction in congenital laryngeal webs and atresias. *Otolaryngology—Head and Neck Surgery, 132,* 232–238.

Xu, J. H., Ikeda, Y., & Komiyama, S. (1993). Biofeedback and the yawning breath pattern in voice therapy. *Journal of Voice, 7,* 75–80.

Xu, J. J., Chen, X., Lu, M. P., & Qiao, M. Z. (2009). Perceptual evaluation and acoustic analysis of pneumatic artificial larynx. *Otolaryngology—Head and Neck Surgery, 141,* 776–780.

Xu, W., Han, D., Hou, L., Hu, R., & Wang, L. (2009). Clinical and electrophysiological characteristics of larynx in myasthenia gravis. *Annals of Otology, Rhinology, & Laryngology, 18,* 656–661.

Xue, A., & Mueller, P. B. (1997). Acoustic and perceptual characteristics of the voices of sedentary and physically active elderly speakers. *Logopedics, Phoniatrics, Vocology, 22,* 51–60.

Xue, S. A., & Deliyski, D. (2001). Effects of aging on selected acoustic voice parameters: Preliminary normative data and educational implications. *Educational Gerontology, 27,* 159–168.

Xue, S. A., & Hao, J. G. (2006). Normative standards for vocal tract dimensions by race as measured by acoustic pharyngometry. *Journal of Voice, 20,* 391–400.

Yamaguchi, H., Yotsukure, Y., Sata, H., Wotanabe, Y., Hirose, H., Kabayashi, N., & Bless, D. M. (1993). Pushing exercise program to correct glottal incompetencies. *Journal of Voice, 7,* 250–256.

Yan, Y., Damrose, E., & Bless, D. (2007). Functional analysis of voice using simultaneous high-speech imaging and acoustic recordings. *Journal of Voice, 21,* 604–616.

Yan, Y., Olszewski, A. E., Hoffman, M. R., Zhuang, P., Ford, C. N., Dailey, S. H., & Jiang, J. J. (2010). Use of lasers in laryngeal surgery. *Journal of Voice, 24,* 102–109.

Yang, C. Y., Palmer, A. D., Murray, K. D., Meltzer, T. R., & Cohen, J. I. (2002). Cricothyroid approximation to elevate vocal pitch in male-to-female transsexuals: Results of surgery. *Annals of Otology, Rhinology, Laryngology, 111,* 477–485.

Yeager, V. L., Lawson, C., & Archer, C. R. (1982). Ossification of the laryngeal cartilages as it relates to computed tomography. *Investigative Radiology, 17.*

Yelken, K., Gultekin, E., Guven, M., Eyibilen, A., & Aladag, I. (2010). Impairment of voice quality in paradoxical vocal fold motion dysfunction. *Journal of Voice, 24,* 724–727.

Yilmaz, S., Yildizbas, S., Yaman, H., Guclu, E., & Ozturk, O. (2010). Stridor in a newborn caused by a congenital laryngocele and bifid epiglottis: A case report and review of the literature. *International Journal of Pediatric Otorhinolaryngology Extra, 5,* 28–31.

Yiotakis, J., Stavroulaki, P., Nikolopoulos, T., Manalopoulos, L., Kandiloros, D., Ferekidis, E., & Adamopoulos, G. (2003). Partial laryngectomy after irradiation failure. *Otolaryngology—Head and Neck Surgery, 128,* 200–209.

Yiu, E. M. (2002). Impact and prevention of voice problems in the teaching profession: Embracing the consumers' view. *Journal of Voice, 16,* 215–228.

Yiu, E. M. L., & Chan, R. M. M. (2003). Effect of hydration and vocal rest on vocal fatigue in amateur karaoke singers. *Journal of Voice, 17,* 216–227.

Yiu, E. M-L., Ho, E. M., Ma, E. P-M., Abbott, K. V., & Branski, R. (2011). Possible cross-cultural differences in the perception of impact of voice disorders. *Journal of Voice, 25,* 348–353.

Ylitalo, R. (2006). Helicobacter pylori infection and its correlation to extraesophageal and esophageal reflux in contact granuloma patients. *Logopedics Phoniatrics Vocology, 31,* 57–60.

Ylvisaker, M., Coelho, C., Kennedy, M., Moore Sohlberg, M., Turkstra, L., Avery, J., & Yorkston, K. (2002). Reflections on evidence-based practice and rational clinical decision making. *Journal of Medical Speech-Language Pathology, 10,* xxv–xxxiii.

Yonekawa, H. (1988). A clinical study of Reinke's edema. *Auris Nasus Larynx, 15,* 57–78.

Yorkston, K. M., Spencer, K. A., & Duffy, J. R. (2003). Behavioral management of respiratory/phonatory dysfunction from dysarthria: A systematic review of the evidence. *Journal of Medical Speech-Language Pathology, 11,* xiii–xxxviii.

Yorkston, K. M., Spencer, K., Duffy, J., Beukelman, D., Golper, L. A., Miller, R., . . . Sullivan, M. (2001). Evidence-based medicine and practice guidelines: Application to the field of speech-language pathology. *Journal of Medical Speech-Language Pathology, 9,* 243–256.

Young, B., Lowe, J. S., Stevens, A., & Heath, J. W. (2006). *Wheater's functional histology* (5th ed., pp. 207–233). Philadelphia, PA: Elsevier Limited.

Ysunza, A., Landeros, L., Pamplona, C., Prado, H., Arrieta, J., & Fajardo, G. (2007). The role of laryngeal electromyography in the diagnosis of vocal fold immobility in children. *International Journal of Pediatric Otorhinolaryngology, 71,* 949–958.

Yun, K. I., Lee, J. A., & Park, J. U. (2008). Intubation granuloma: Report of a case. *Journal of Oral and Maxillofacial Surgery, 66,* 1263–1265.

Yun, Y-S., Kim, M-B., & Son, Y-I. (2007). The effect of vocal hygiene education for patients with vocal polyp. *Otolaryngology—Head and Neck Surgery, 137,* 569–575.

Zagolski, O. (2009). Electroglottography in elderly patients with vocal fold palsy. *Journal of Voice, 23,* 567–571.

Zagolski, O., & Carlson, E. (2002). Electroglottographic measurements of glottal function in vocal fold paralysis in women. *Clinical Otolaryngology, 27,* 246–253.

Zalzal, G. H. (1999). Posterior glottic stenosis. *International Journal of Pediatric Otorhinolaryngology, 49* (Suppl. 1), S279–S282.

Zalzal, G. H., Loomis, S. R., Derkay, C. S., Murray, S. L., & Thomsen, J. (1991). Vocal quality of decannulated children following laryngeal reconstruction. *Laryngoscope, 101,* 425–429.

Zawadzka-Glos, L., & Chmielik, M. (2006). Acquired laryngotracheal stenosis in children. *New Medicine, 3,* 56–57.

Zeitels, S., Hillman, R., Desloge, R., & Bunting, G. (1999). Cricothyroid subluxation: A new innovation for enhancing the voice with laryngoplastic phonosurgery. *Annals of Otology, Rhinology and Laryngology, 108,* 1126–1131.

Zeitels, S., Hochman, I., & Hillman, R. (1998). Adduction arytenopexy: A new procedure for paralytic dysphonia with implications for implant medialization. *Annals of Otology, Rhinology and Laryngology, 173* (Suppl.), 224.

Zeitels, S. M. (2004). Optimizing voice after endoscopic partial laryngectomy. *Otolaryngology Clinics of North America, 37,* 627–636.

Zeitels, S. M., Akst, L. M., Burns, J. A., Hillman, R. E., Broadhurst, M. S., & Anderson, R. R. (2006). Pulsed angiolytic laser treatment of ectasias and varices in singers. *Annals of Otology, Rhinology, & Laryngology, 115,* 571–580.

Zeitels, S. M., Blitzer, A., Hillman, R. E., & Anderson, R. R. (2007). Foresight in laryngology and laryngeal surgery: A 2020 vision. *Annals of Otology, Rhinology, & Laryngology, 116* (Suppl. 198), 1–16.

Zeitels, S. M., & Hillman, R. E. (2009). Laryngeal laser surgery for recurrent respiratory papillomatosis, cancer and dysplasia: Operating room and office. *Perspectives on Voice and Voice Disorders, 19,* 74–83.

Zeitels, S. M., Mauri, M., & Dailey, S. H. (2003). Medialization laryngoplasty with Gore-tex for voice restoration secondary to glottal incompetence: Indications and observations. *Annals of Otology, Rhinology, Laryngology, 112,* 180–184.

Zemlin, W. (1998). *Speech and hearing science: Anatomy and physiology* (4th ed.). Boston, MA: Allyn & Bacon.

Zhang, F., Sprecher, A. J., Wei, C., & Jiang, J. J. (2010). Implantation of gelatin sponge combined with injection of autologous fat for sulcus vocalis. *Otolaryngology—Head and Neck Surgery, 143,* 198–203.

Zhang, W., & Davenport, P. W. (2005). Neural control of breathing. *Perspectives on Voice and Voice Disorders, 15*(1), 20–24.

Zinman, L., Ng, E., & Bril, V. (2007). IV immunoglobulin in patients with myasthenia gravis: A randomized controlled trial. *Neurology, 68,* 837–841.

Zipoli, R. P., & Kennedy, M. (2005). Evidence-based practice among speech-language pathologists: Attitudes, utilization, and barriers. *American Journal of Speech-Language Pathology, 14,* 208–220.

Zormeier, M. M., Meleca, R. J., Simpson, M. L., Dworkin, J. P., Klein, R., Gross, M., & Mathog, R. H. (1999). Botulinum toxin injection to improve tracheoesophageal speech after total laryngectomy. *Otolaryngology—Head and Neck Surgery, 120,* 314–319.

Zoumalan, R., Maddalozzo, J., & Holinger, L. D. (2007). Etiology of stridor in infants. *Annals of Otology, Rhinology & Laryngology, 116,* 329–334.

Zraick, R. I., & Jacobson, B. H. (2008). Quality of life in persons with voice disorders. Presented at the Annual Convention of the American Speech-Language-Hearing Association, Chicago.

Zraick, R. I., Kempster, G. B., Connor, N. P., Thibeault, S., Klaben, B. K., Bursac, Z., . . . Glaze, L. E. (2011). Establishing validity of the Consensus Auditory Perceptual Evaluation of Voice (CAPE-V). *American Journal of Speech Language Pathology, 20,* 14–22.

Zraick, R. I., Risner, B. Y., Smith-Olinde, L., Gregg, B. A., Johnson, F. L., & McWeeny, E. K. (2007). Patient versus partner perception of voice handicap. *Journal of Voice, 21,* 485–494.

Zur, K. B. (2006). Pediatric upper airway pathologies. *Perspectives on Voice and Voice Disorders, 16*(3), 11–14.

Zur, K. B., Cotton, S., Kelchner, L., Baker, S., Weinrich, B., & Lee, L. (2007). Pediatric Voice Handicap Index (pVHI): A new tool for evaluating pediatric dysphonia. *International Journal of Pediatric Otorhinolaryngology, 71,* 77–82.

Zuur, J. K., Muller, S. H., de Jongh, F. H. C., van Zandwijk, N., & Hilgers, F. J. M. (2006). The physiological rationale of heat and moisture exchangers in post-laryngectomy pulmonary rehabilitation: A review. *European Archives of Otorhinolaryngology, 263,* 1–8.

Zuur, J. K., Muller, S. H., Vincent, A., Sinaasappel, M., de Jongh, F. H. C., & Hilgers, F. J. M. (2009). The influence of a heat and moisture exchanger on tracheal climate in a cold environment. *Medical Engineering & Physics, 31,* 852–857.

Name Index

Note: Page numbers followed by *f* indicate figures; page numbers followed by *t* indicate tables.

Abaza, M. M., 98, 99, 101, 102
Abberton, E., 125
Abbott, G. C., 6
Abbott, K. V., 98, 102
Abel, S. M., 387
Abitbol, B., 76
Abitbol, J., 76, 77, 286
Abitbol, P., 76
Abouchahine, S., 397*t*
Abou-Rass, Y., 184
Abrahams, J. J., 197
Abramson, A. L., 356
Ackermann, H., 317, 318
Ackerstaff, A. H., 439, 441, 454
Acton, L., 434, 441, 452
Adamopoulos, G., 203
Adams, S., 151, 337
Adams, T. M., 413, 414*t*
Adler, C. H., 333*t*
Adler, R. K., 175, 180
Adrian, J. A., 151
Agada, F. O., 264
Agarwal, J. P., 430
Agarwal, M., 27–28
Agrawal, N., 255
Aguiar-Ricz, L., 447, 449
Ahmad, S. M., 285, 286
Ahn, S-H., 256
Akst, L. M., 273
Aladag, I., 396
Albert, D. M., 255, 256
Alcadipani, F. A. M. C., 436
Alessi, D., 78–79, 219*t*
Alexander, R. A., 270, 271
Ali, S. O., 328
Alku, P., 296
Allan, P. F., 396, 397*t*
Allcock, L., 324
Allen, D. G., 293
Allen, K. D., 179
Allison, R., 366
Almquist, S-A., 373
Alonso-Navarro, H., 151
Alpert, M., 351
Altenberg, E. P., 103, 105, 107, 108*t*
Altieri, A., 426
Altman, K. W., 319, 356, 357, 398, 401, 403, 405, 406, 407, 408, 409
Altman, M. E., 67
Alvarez-Neri, H., 256
American Cancer Society, 106, 421, 422, 423
American Joint Committee on Cancer, 423
American Psychiatric Association, 360
American Society of Pediatric Otolaryngology (ASPO), 271
American Speech-Language-Hearing Association (ASHA), 87, 93, 94–95, 95*t*, 98, 103, 104*t*, 109, 111, 116, 138, 140*t*, 165, 169, 213
American Thoracic Society, 384, 385
Amin, M. R., 230
Amir, N., 81
Amir, O., 76, 81, 125, 174, 325
Amirlak, B., 228
Andersen, P. E., 436
Anderson, R. R., 195
Anderson, S., 176
Anderson, T. D., 206*t*, 207, 335
Andersson, K., 359, 361, 363, 363*t*
Andrade, D. F., 356
Andrade, E. C., 229
Andrews, B. T., 311
Andrews, H. B., 361
Andrews, M. L., 189*t*, 246, 260, 306, 317, 337, 339, 340, 426, 434
Andrews, S., 177
Andrianopoulos, M. V., 107, 108*t*, 396, 397*t*, 401
Androulakis, I. P., 215
Andrus, J. G., 198
Angsuwarangsee, T., 357, 359
Anselmo-Lima, W. T., 229
Anticaglia, J., 101
Antin-Ozerkis, D., 394*t*
Antunes, M. B., 265
Apostolidis, T., 228
Apostolidou, M. T., 228
Araki, K., 435
Archer, C. R., 78
Archer, S., 219*t*
Archilla, A. S., 287
Argiris, A., 421
Arnold, R. R., 293
Aronson A. E., 4, 303, 304*t*
Arsura, E. L., 316
Aschauer, H. N., 353, 362
Ashok, K. G., 151
Ashraf, V. V., 313, 314
Asmundson, G. J. G., 354
Assuncao, A. A., 294
Atkins, J. P., 319
Atkinson, C., 356
Aubry, K., 199, 311
Auo, H-J., 284, 286
Avelino, M., 273
Aviv, J. E., 57, 96, 237
Avivi, M., 81
Awan, S. N., 108*t*, 134, 146, 363
Axon, P. R., 256
Ayad, T., 292
Azadarmaki, R., 307, 308, 309
Aziz, L., 311
Azulay, J.-P., 339

Babac, S., 151
Bach, K. K., 133, 133*t*
Badillo, A., 330
Baeck, H. E., 70
Baek, C-H., 435
Bailey, C., 256, 416
Bailey, E. F., 15
Bajaj, Y., 201
Baken, R. J., 51, 59, 60, 154, 178*t*
Baker, J., 361, 362
Baker, K. K., 51–52, 81
Baker, K. L., 59
Baker, S., 67, 249, 250, 251, 252, 253, 255, 256
Bakthavachalam, S., 253
Balas, M., 324
Balm, A. J. M., 450
Balter, M. S., 151, 393, 394*t*

Bandi, V., 240
Bandler, R., 56
Banta, C. L., 455
Banzett, R. B., 384
Baquet, C., 106
Baredes, S., 385
Barer, T., 76
Barkmeier, J. M., 330, 331, 332*t*, 356
Barkmeier-Kraemer, J., 131, 181
Barr, A., 135, 158, 304, 305
Barreto, S. M., 294
Barrett, L. F., 351
Barrichelo-Lindstrom, V., 184–185
Barros, A. P. B., 151, 433
Barry, W. J., 323
Bass, H., 389
Bassiouny, S., 184
Bastian, R., 219*t*
Batory, M., 304, 305
Battle, D., 103
Baudonck, N., 75–76
Baum, E. D., 353
Baylor, C. R., 195, 198*t*, 199, 308, 310, 311, 335
Baz, R., 267
Bean, J. A., 256
Beaudin, P. G., 455
Beck, K. C., 398
Beckenham, E. J., 258, 259
Beden, A. B., 246
Behlau, M., 70, 79, 96, 125, 184–185, 260, 280
Behrman, A., 174, 176, 188, 189*t*, 190, 191*t*, 192, 279, 283, 356, 357
Belafsky, P. C., 133, 203, 204, 230, 232, 233, 356
Bell, J., 264
Bellandese, M. H., 423, 447, 455, 456, 458*t*, 459
Bellomo, A., 151
Bender, B., 335
Benderitter, C., 128
Bennett, S., 110, 111, 146
Benninger, M. S., 218, 219*t*, 222, 283, 432
Benoit, L., 200
Bensimon, G., 339
Benson, B. E., 385
Bent III, J., 256
Berardelli, A., 328
Berci, G., 239
Bergamini, G., 194, 209, 310
Berghaus, A., 374
Berjawi, G., 240, 241
Berke, G. S., 207, 290, 304, 333*t*
Berkowitz, R., 137, 251, 255
Berliti, S., 226
Bernaldez, R., 436
Bernhard, N., 78, 255
Bernstein Ratner, N., 110
Berry, D. A., 21
Bertino, G., 151, 429*t*, 432
Bestall, J. C., 385
Bew, S., 248
Bhalla, R. K., 391, 393, 394
Bhuta, T., 152
Biary, N., 323
Bidus, K., 330
Bielamowicz, S., 158, 175–176, 308, 330, 333*t*, 334, 356
Bielecki, I., 273
Bien, S., 439, 440, 440*t*, 441
Biever, D. M., 77, 79–80, 81
Bigenzahn, W., 75–76, 80*t*, 197
Billante, C. R., 198
Birkent, H., 334, 335
Biron-Shental, T., 76
Birring, S. S., 411
Bisetti, M. S., 282
Bishop-Leone, J. K., 455
Bitar, M., 267, 272, 273
Blager, F., 409–410
Blager, F. B., 406
Blake, E., 356
Blalock, P., 183, 195, 230, 330, 356, 357
Blaney, S. P. A., 255
Blaugrund, S. M., 195–197
Bleecker, E. R., 391
Bless, D., 33, 74, 77, 79–80, 81, 144, 151, 177, 188, 207–208, 216, 221, 230, 334, 356, 357, 362
Bliss-Moreau, E., 351
Blitzer, A., 195, 328, 329, 333*t*, 334
Block, B. B., 230, 235
Block, C., 397*t*, 398, 400, 402*t*
Bloigu, R., 292
Blom, E. D., 450, 452
Blomgren, M., 59, 60
Bloom, D., 266
Bloom, R. L., 73*t*, 146, 373
Bluestone, C. D., 251
Blumin, J. H., 126, 304, 310, 311, 319, 398
Boers, J., 56
Bohn, N. P., 151, 433
Bohnenkamp, T. A., 445, 455
Boliek, C. A., 63–64, 66
Bone, S., 409
Bonelli, R. M., 327
Bo-Nien, C., 246
Bonner, J. A., 430
Boone, D., 181, 182
Bootz, F., 434
Borg, G. A., 385, 386*t*
Bosch, D., 290
Boscolo-Rizzo, P., 428, 429*t*, 450
Boseley, M. E., 124*t*, 126, 271
Bosetti, C., 426
Boshoff, P., 107
Bosley, B., 199, 201, 311
Bothe, A. C., 125
Boucher, V. J., 292
Boutsen, F., 335
Bove, M. J., 260
Bovo, R., 93, 295, 295*t*, 296, 298
Boynukalin, S., 209, 262
Braden, M. N., 335
Bradford, C. R., 125
Bradshaw, A., 230
Braman, S. S., 240, 391
Bramlett, R. E., 125
Branco, A., 70, 71
Brandon, C. A., 38
Branski, R., 1, 2, 33, 102, 129, 170, 171, 208, 216, 218, 219, 280, 284, 360
Branton, C., 391
Brasnu, D., 201, 208
Brasolotto, A., 79
Braun, N., 126, 398
Breatnach, E., 6
Brehm, S. B., 252
Breiss, B., 186
Bressman, S. B., 333*t*
Brigger, M. T., 251, 256
Bril, V., 316
Brilia, L., 406
Brilla, L. R., 397*t*, 400
Brin, M. F., 329
Bristol, L. A., 339
Brodsky, L., 230, 235, 274
Brondbo, K., 432
Brooks, B. R., 339, 340
Brown, D. H., 450, 452
Brown, J. R., 4, 303, 304*t*
Brown, M., 366, 369*t*, 370, 372, 374, 375*t*
Brown, P. H., 393
Brown, S., 52, 53
Brown, W. S., 79, 81, 147
Bruce, I. A., 270
Brugman, S., 390*f*, 395, 398
Brunner, H., 240
Brunner, N. G., 316
Bryan, G., 416
Bryson, P. C., 197, 268, 272
Buckmire, R. A., 197, 198*t*, 199, 201, 240, 241
Bucknall, C. E., 393
Buddiga, P., 397*t*, 403, 407*t*
Buder, E. H., 71, 339
Bunting, G., 195
Burke, B., 266, 270, 270*t*
Burke, M. K., 185
Burn, D. J., 324
Burns, J. A., 423, 429, 432

Caceres, C., 197
Cady, J., 440*t*, 441, 442
Cakmakci, H., 258
Calder, N., 432
Caldwell, E., 185
Calhoun K., 42
Calvano, S. E., 215
Calzada-Uriondo, M., 294
Camphina-Bacote, J., 103
Campisi, P., 270
Campones do Brasil, O., 78

Cannito, M. P., 330, 331, 334, 335, 337
Cannizzaro, M. S., 148, 351
Cantu, E., 450, 454
Capadano, H. L., 82
Caputo Rosen, D., 67, 354, 355, 361
Cardenas, R. A., 74
Carding, P., 111, 129, 170, 229, 298, 359, 362, 432
Cardona, A. F., 226
Caress, A., 416
Carew, L., 373, 375*t*
Carleton, R. N., 354
Carlson, E., 129, 156
Carlstedt, A., 326
Carney, A. S., 230, 428, 429, 429*t*, 432, 433
Carney, E., 102
Carney, I. K., 407, 408, 409, 411
Carpene, S., 428
Carpenter, M. A., 455
Carr, M. M., 457
Carrau, R. L., 229*t*, 232, 234*t*, 235
Carroll, L. M., 308, 309, 310
Carroll, T. L., 204
Carron, J., 246, 266, 270*t*, 311
Carrothers, R. M., 351
Casado, J. C., 151
Case, J. L., 77, 134, 137, 210, 330, 332*t*, 354
Casiano, R. R., 78, 237, 330
Casper, J. K., 68, 148, 149, 183
Casper, M. A., 318
Castell, D. O., 227
Castellengo, M., 59
Castillo, M., 78
Catten, M., 33, 218
Cavalli, L., 201
Cavallo, S. A., 181
Cellucci, T., 413
Cervera-Paz, F. J., 280
Ceuppens, P., 151
Chadha, S., 74, 77
Chan, R. M. M., 175–176
Chan, R. W., 21, 206
Chandra, P. S., 359
Chang, A., 176, 293
Chang, C. Y., 274, 334, 336
Chang, C-H., 314
Chapman, K. R., 151
Chappie, K., 351
Charron, S., 15, 66
Chasaide, A. N., 351
Chastang, C., 316
Chatham, M., 391
Chawla, S., 428, 429, 429*t*, 432, 433
Chay, O. M., 401
Cheang, H. S., 319
Cheesman, A. D., 370, 372
Cheesman, D., 376
Chen, A., 338, 339, 340
Chen, J., 107, 260
Chen, J-J., 411
Chen, P-H., 83
Chen, S. H., 184–185, 294, 296, 297*t*, 298
Chen, Y., 59, 73*t*
Cheng, A. T. L., 258, 259
Cheng-Chien, Y., 246
Chernobelsky, S., 154, 156, 364, 365
Cheung, Y. L., 176
Chevret, S., 316
Chhetri, D. K., 207, 209, 219, 331, 450
Chi, A. P., 285
Chiang, S-C., 184–185, 294
Chiang, W. C., 401, 403
Chiarello, G., 435
Chirayath, J., 240
Chitose, S., 208, 260, 261, 311, 429*t*
Chmielik, M., 250, 251, 252, 253
Cho, H., 386, 387
Chodzko-Zajko, W.J., 82
Choi, S. S., 282
Chone, C. T., 449, 450, 455
Chowdhury, A., 74, 77
Christensen, B., 190, 191
Christopher, K. L., 395, 396, 398, 399*t*, 403, 404
Chu, M. W., 247
Chun, J. Y., 434
Chung, B. J., 273
Chung, J. H., 229*t*, 280
Chung, K. F., 408, 410, 411, 413
Chung, S. M., 393
Chung, Y-M., 184–185, 294
Cinamon, U., 262
Ciucci, M. R., 324
Claeys, S., 75–76, 76, 177, 296, 355
Clair, B., 316
Clark, S., 376
Clarke, P. M., 376
Clarke, R. W., 270
Clary, J., 198
Clary, R. A., 256
Classen, M., 235
Clement, G., 177
Clement, W. A., 193, 248
Cobeta, I., 151, 286
Cockroft, D. W., 393
Coelho, C., 321
Cofala, M., 273
Cohen, A. P., 258
Cohen, H., 148
Cohen, J. I., 376
Cohen, J. T., 324
Cohen, N. H., 391
Cohen, S., 83
Cohen, S. B., 230
Cohen, S. M., 284, 285, 286, 432
Cohen-Kettenis, P. T., 366, 367
Cohn, J. R., 391
Colabianchi, N., 228
Collimore, K. C., 354
Collins, S. P., 96
Collins, W. O., 264, 265
Colton, R. H., 68, 78, 81, 148, 149, 183
Comar, M., 267
Comins, R., 294
Conley, S. F., 313
Connaghan, K. P., 15
Connelly, A., 193
Connor, N. P., 128, 188, 190, 192, 194, 230, 232, 258, 324, 329
Constantinescu, G. A., 325
Cooksey, J. M., 75
Coppens, P., 315
Corbin-Lewis, K., 174, 174*t*, 187
Cornwell, P. L., 317, 318
Corrao, W. M., 391
Corsello, P., 409–410
Corthais, P., 151
Coruh, I., 209, 262
Corvo, M. A., 284
Costa, D. J., 258
Costello, R. W., 408
Cotton, R., 249, 251, 256, 258, 267
Countryman, S., 324
Courey, M. S., 21
Craig, S., 271, 272
Crampsey, D., 247
Crawley, J. A., 234*t*
Cremers, C. W. R. J., 297
Crevier-Buchman, L., 201, 208
Crockett, S., 235
Crompton, G. K., 393
Crowell, D. H., 70
Crozier, D. L., 287
Crumley, R. L., 328
Cummings, 56
Cunningham, M. J., 126, 271
Curtis, J. F., 59

Dacakis, G., 157, 174, 369, 369*t*, 370, 373, 375*t*, 376
Dagan, K. A., 351
Dagli, M., 365
Dahl, L. D., 356
Dailey, S., 144, 206, 220, 221, 222, 287, 410, 415
D'Alatri, L., 323
D'Amico, B., 183
Da Mosto, M. C., 428
Damrose, E., 76, 151, 249
Damrose, J. F., 334
Damste, H., 59
Daneshi, A., 255
Daniilidou, P., 359, 362, 363
Darley, F. L., 4, 303, 304*t*
Darrow, D. H., 266, 270, 272
Darrow, K. N., 107
Davenport, P. W., 15, 408
Davis, J. K., 234*t*
Davis, P. J., 56–57
Davis, R. K., 433
Deakin, J., 376
Deal, L. V., 82
De Alarcon, A., 252, 256
De Araujo, M. M., 246
Deary, I. J., 124*t*, 362, 363*t*
Deary, V., 359
De Biase, N., 280
Debnath, I., 211
De Bodt, M., 149, 151, 177, 179, 281, 297

Debruyne, F., 81, 374
de Campos, D., 57
de Carvalho, E. C., 176
Declaye, X. J., 452
Decoster, W., 81
De Cuypere, G., 377
Dedivitis, R. A., 151, 433, 434
Deem, J. F., 174, 317, 323, 337, 338, 340, 341, 361, 372, 397*t*, 404, 440, 444, 454
Defaveri, J., 280, 284
De Gier, H. H. W., 431
DeJarnette, G., 93–94, 106, 107
Dejonckere, P. H., 150, 353, 354
De Jong, F. I. C. R. S., 296, 297, 374
de Jongh, F. H. C., 440
De Krijger, R. R., 251
De La Cortina, R. A. C., 262
DeLeo LeBorgne, W., 149, 150
De Letter, M., 322
De Ley, S., 177
DelGaudio, J. M., 335, 393, 394*t*
Deliyski, D., 79, 80*t*, 138, 144, 144*t*, 151, 152
De Medeiros, A. M., 294, 296, 297*t*
De Menezes, L. N., 81
Demmink-Geertman, L., 353, 354
den Berghe, H., 377
Denk, D. M., 197
Denny, D., 365, 366, 367
de Paula, A. A. D., 176
De Peuter, S., 384, 385
De Pinto, O., 147
Depondt, J., 423, 440*t*, 441, 442
Depypere, H., 75–76, 76
Derkay, C. S., 247, 256, 266, 267, 268, 270, 270*t*, 271, 272, 273, 274
DeSanto, L., 436
Deschler, D. G., 439
Desloge, R., 195
de Souza, M. N., 70
De Stefani, E., 426
Dettmar, P. W., 408
Devaney, K. O., 290
Develioglu, O. N., 450
Devesa, P. M., 262, 263
Devlieger, P. J., 104
de Weerd, H., 56
Dewolf, E., 452
D'haeseleer, E., 75–76, 77, 80*t*, 177
Diakow, C., 181
Diaz, E. M., 431, 455
Dictz, A., 456
Dietrich, M., 356
Dikkers, F. G., 280
Di Mattia, M. S., 50, 60, 175–176, 293
Di Nicola, V., 435
Docherty, G. J., 111, 170
Dogan, M., 341, 394*t*
Dollar, J., 291
Domingues, M. A. C., 280, 284, 285
Donders, A. R. T., 297
Donne, A. J., 266, 273
Donzelli, G., 71
Dori, N., 325
Doshi, D. R., 395, 400, 403
dos Santos, C. B., 176
Dove, H., 174, 174*t*, 187
Doyle, P., 174, 280
Doyle, P. C., 151, 152, 153, 444, 449, 454, 455, 458, 458*t*, 459
Draganov, P., 266, 267
Dressel, H., 230
Drinnan, M., 298, 359
Dromey, C., 52, 177, 324, 337, 338, 356, 359
Druker, D., 50
Drummond, S., 405
DSM-IV-TR, 365
Duff, M. C., 2
Duffy, J., 151–152, 179, 180, 195, 310, 316, 317, 318, 326, 328, 360, 361, 363
Duflo, S., 208, 216
Duguay, M. J., 448, 449
Dukas, M., 174
Dumont, A., 256
Duncan, F., 458, 458*t*, 459
Duncan, N. O., 387
Dunn-Rankin, P., 70
Duprat, A. D. C., 207, 284
Dursun, G., 209, 262, 263, 282, 290, 291, 292, 365
Duynstee, M. L. G., 251
Dweik, R. A., 388, 389
Dworkin, J. P., 198, 198*t*, 210, 216, 226, 230, 306, 309, 310, 317, 356, 430, 435, 436
Dykstra, A. D., 337

Eadie, T. L., 97, 98, 129, 151, 152, 153, 195, 310, 331, 335, 449, 454, 455, 456, 457, 458, 458*t*, 459
Earis, J., 393
Eaton, D. A., 249, 250, 253, 255, 258, 260, 261
Ecevit, C., 258
Echternach, M., 59
Eckel, H-E., 433
Eckley, C. A., 228, 284, 285
Edgar, J. D., 330, 334
Edmondson, N. E., 256
Edmunds, A. L., 228, 237, 239
Edsborg, N., 447
Eerenstein, S. E. J., 452
Eguchi, S., 146
Eitnier, C. M., 264
Ejnell, H., 311
Eksteen, E. C., 435
Elahi, F., 236*t*
Elder, J., 408
El Haddad, B., 266
El-Hakim, H., 311
Eller, R., 221
Elluru, R. G., 230
Elmaraghy, C. A., 387
Elmiyeh, B., 334, 454, 455
El-Serag, H. B., 426
El Sharkawi, A., 324
Emami, A. J., 290, 398
Emerick, K. S., 450
Enderby, P., 111
Engel, S. H., 282
Enright, P. L., 393
Epstein, R., 124*t*, 126, 127*t*, 129, 178*t*, 354
Erickson, E., 293, 393, 394*t*
Erickson, J. G., 102, 104–105, 106
Erman, A., 450
Eryilmaz, A., 365
Esclamado, R. M., 125
Esterman, A., 230
Ettema, S. L., 250
Eustace, C. S., 293
Evans, M. K., 151
Evans, S., 79
Everett, C. F., 408, 410, 411
Everts, E. C., 258
Evitts, P. M., 455, 456
Eyibilen, A., 396

Fabro, A. T., 285
Fadden, C. T., 407, 408, 409
Fajdiga, I., 246, 247
Fanta, C. H., 391
Farrand, P., 458*t*, 459
Farrell, A., 323
Farrington, W. T., 452
Fasyh, N. A., 395–396
Fatterpekar, G. M., 78
Fayoux, P., 255
Feehery, J. M., 311
Feijo, A. V., 340, 341
Fekete, S. M. W., 71
Feldman, H. A., 282
Felipovich, A., 267
Ferguson, N. A., 359
Ferlito, A., 151, 290, 422, 423, 435, 436
Fernandas, M. I. M., 229
Ferrand, C. T., 73*t*, 74, 79, 80*t*, 81, 98, 103, 105, 107, 108*t*, 146, 148, 373, 447, 458
Ferrero, F. E., 151
Ferris, R., 421
Fex, B., 183, 184
Fex, S., 184
Fey, M. E., 110
Filho, P. A. A., 313
Finck, C. L., 151, 207
Finizia, C., 441–442
Finn, P., 170
Finnegan, E. M., 51, 184
Fiorella, M. L., 435
Fiorella, R., 435
Fischer, S., 79
Fisher, K. V., 99
Fisher, S. G., 443, 457

Fitch, M., 147, 430
Fletcher, K. E., 413, 414*t*
Flynn, P. T., 93, 94
Fong Kan, P., 102
Ford, C. N., 177, 197, 206, 207, 219*t*, 220, 221, 222, 230, 334, 356, 357
Forman, A. D., 455
Forrest, L. A., 400
Forte, V., 264
Fox, C. M., 319, 324
Franco, R. A., 198, 271, 287, 288
Francois, M., 256
Franic, D., 125
Frankel, J., 81
Fraser, R. G., 6
Freed, G. L., 267, 268, 274
Freedman, M., 409–410
French, C. T., 413, 414*t*
Fried, M. P., 270, 271
Friedman, E. M., 387
Friedman, W., 323
Friedrich, G., 197, 433
Fritzell, B., 294
Froeschels, E., 181, 182
Froud, K., 52
Fuchs, M., 75
Fujimura, M., 391
Fulcher, R., 413
Fuleihan, N., 267
Fuller, D., 439, 440, 440*t*, 441, 442
Fung, F., 105
Fung, K., 429
Fuocco, G., 264

Gaafar, A. H., 395–396
Gabel, R., 456
Gajdos, P., 316
Galceran, M., 93
Galgano, J., 52, 199
Gallena S. K., 412, 415*t*
Gallivan, G. J., 264, 394, 394*t*, 396
Gallivan, H. K., 264, 394
Gallivan, K. H., 394, 396
Gallus, S., 426
Gamboa, J., 148
Gamshadzahi, A., 106
Gandour, J., 449
Ganz, C., 452
Garabedian, E-N., 256
Garavello, W., 426
Garca, M. F., 450
Garcia, M. J. V., 151, 326
Garcia-Barry, S., 316
Garfield, I., 356
Garnett, J. D., 152, 250, 251, 288, 289, 290
Garrett, C. G., 284, 285, 286, 338, 339, 340
Gartner-Schmidt, J., 116, 199, 205, 209, 311, 356
Gasparini, G., 96, 125
Gaulin, S. J. C., 74
Gavin, L. A., 398
Gavin, W. J., 324
Gay, M., 409, 410
Gay, T., 50
Geddes, N. K., 248
Gehanno, P., 423, 440*t*, 441, 442
Geibel, J. M., 318
Gelfer, M. P., 129, 366, 369, 369*t*, 370, 371, 372, 373, 374, 375*t*
Gelman, J., 443
George, M., 249, 250, 258
Geralts, D. S., 351
Gerber, M. E., 260
Gerein, J., 272
Gerein, V., 266, 267, 268, 272
Gerratt, B. R., 131, 133, 450
Gerson, L. B., 235
Ghafari, S., 176
Ghidini, A., 137, 194
Ghufoor, K., 262
Giannoni, C., 387
Gibson, P. G., 404, 408, 409, 410, 411, 413, 414, 415, 416
Giladi, N., 324, 325
Gilbert, H. R., 59, 237, 455
Gilchrist, K. W., 221
Gildea, T. R., 383, 387, 388, 389, 391
Gillivan-Murphy, P., 298
Gilman, F., 122
Gilman, M., 180
Giovanni, A., 339, 435
Giraldo, A., 280
Glaze, L., 67, 68, 74, 102, 185, 293, 363, 443
Gliklich, R. E., 124*t*
Globlek, D., 436, 447, 449
Glynn, A., 235
Goberman, A. M., 71, 248, 321, 322
Gobl, C., 351
Godlewski, A., 330
Goetz, C. G., 320*t*
Goh, A., 401
Gokcan, K. M., 290, 291, 292
Gold, D. R., 367, 374, 391
Goldman, J., 405
Goldman, S. N., 290, 334
Goldmuntz, E., 258
Goldstein, E. A., 446
Goldstein, W., 78
Golub, J. S., 83
Goncalves, A. J., 435, 436
Goodman, D. L., 400
Goodwin, J. E., 316
Gorham-Rowan, M., 76, 80, 81, 372, 373
Goudy, S., 235
Goyal, A., 253
Graamans, K., 296
Gracco, C., 79
Gracely, R., 384
Graham, M. S., 442, 443, 444, 445, 448, 456, 457, 458*t*, 459
Gramming, P., 74
Granqvist, S., 294–295
Grant, C., 157
Grant, M. K., 318, 319, 321, 322, 323, 324
Graville, D. J., 436
Gray, S., 31, 33, 174, 174*t*, 187, 216, 218, 294
Green, B. E., 351
Green, R., 74–75
Greenberg, M., 353, 359
Greenberger, P. A., 409
Greening, A. P., 393
Greenwood, K. M., 294
Greer, M., 323
Gregore, D. R., 403, 405, 406
Gregorio, E. A., 285
Gregory, S. W. Jr., 351
Grishman, E., 239
Grob, D., 316
Groblewski, J. C., 248
Groessl, E. J., 334
Grosjean, F., 102
Gross, M., 374, 375, 375*t*
Guclu, E., 263
Guerrier, B., 435
Gugatschka, M., 74, 79
Guimaraes, I., 125, 435
Gultekin, E., 396, 429*t*, 450
Gupta, A., 356, 457
Gupta, B., 74, 77
Gurevich-Uvena, J., 395, 400
Gurkov, R., 449
Gustafson, L. M., 251
Guven, M., 396
Guzelsoy, S., 280–281

Hadjikoutis, S., 339
Hadley, K., 433
Hague, D., 370
Hain, T. C., 319
Hairston, J. A., 422, 423, 427, 429*t*, 430
Hakkesteegt, M. M., 431
Hall, B., 323
Hallett, M., 333*t*
Halpern, A., 324
Halum, S. L., 203, 330
Hamdan, A-L., 76
Hamilton, C., 79
Hammarberg, B., 75–76, 174, 280, 294–295, 317, 391, 447, 455, 456
Hammer, G. P., 21, 319
Hammerschmidt, K., 71
Hammond, E., 33, 218
Hammond, T., 33, 218
Hammoud, D., 266
Hampson, L., 266
Han, D., 313
Hanamitsu, M., 436
Hans, S., 201, 208
Hansch, U., 434
Hansell, A., 391
Hansen, J. K., 207, 216, 218, 220
Hansen, K., 455
Hanson, D., 237
Hao, J. G., 107

Hapner, E., 83, 138, 144, 144*t*, 145, 188, 189, 189*t*, 192, 218, 221, 222, 335
Hapner, M., 122
Harel, B. T., 148, 319
Har-El, G., 423
Hargreaves, M. K., 106
Harman, 266, 267, 268, 271, 272, 273
Harmegnies, B., 151
Harmon, A. B., 76
Harnsberger, J. D., 79, 81
Harried, M., 393, 395*t*
Harrington, J., 81
Harris, K. S., 318
Harrison, A. L., 44
Hartelius, L., 317, 326
Hartet, T. V., 391
Hartig, G. K., 207
Hartl, D. M., 208, 314, 432
Hartley, B., 201, 259, 260, 260*t*
Hartley, C., 256
Hartnick, C. J., 124*t*, 126, 144*t*, 145, 251, 256, 271
Harvey, P. L., 189*t*
Harvis, L., 397*t*
Hashmi, S. R., 236*t*
Hassannia, F., 255
Hatzopoulos, S., 93
Hawkes, M., 270
Hawkshaw, M., 98, 101, 221
Hay, I., 137
Healy, G. B., 258
Heath, J. W., 409
Heatley, D. G., 235
Heaton, J. T., 445, 446
Hebda, P. A., 2, 33, 208, 216
Hedbom, E., 33
Heeneman, H., 428–429
Hegarty, A. M., 99
Hegazi, M., 184
Heingard, D., 33
Heisey, D., 334, 362
Heldt, G. P., 387
Helidoni, M. E., 125
Helms, P. J., 391
Helou, L. B., 129
Heman-Ackah, Y. D., 135, 158, 197, 304, 305
Hembree, A., 174
Hempel, J-M., 449
Hendarto, H., 183
Henkel, 318, 321, 322, 323
Henrich, N., 59
Henry, C., 82
Hepworth, E. J., 426
Herbst, C., 153, 155–156
Hersan, R., 286
Hertegard, S., 75–76, 208
Hertel, M., 274
Hertrich, I., 317, 318
Hesse, J., 445
Hester, R. P., 266, 270*t*
Heuer, R. J., 338
Heylen, L., 149
Hickman, C. P., 31
Hicks, M., 390*f*, 395, 397*t*, 398, 401, 402*t*, 403, 406, 407*t*
Higashakawa, M., 15
Higgins, 79
Hilgers, F. J. M., 440, 441, 450, 452, 454, 455, 456
Hillel, A. D., 311, 313
Hillman, R. E., 131, 134, 157, 158, 174, 195, 199, 280, 292, 443, 445, 446
Hillson, E. M., 234*t*
Hinds, M. W., 426
Hirani, S. P., 126, 178*t*
Hirano, M., 35, 79, 131, 184, 216
Hirano, S., 197, 207, 208, 218, 221
Hirose, H., 50
Hirsch, S., 185, 372
Hirschberg, J., 70
Hirschi, S. D., 33
Hirsh, L. J., 146
Hitchings, A., 247
Hixon, T. J., 63–64, 64–65*f*, 66, 67, 81, 180, 384
Ho, E. M., 102
Ho, H. C., 405
Hocevar-Boltezar, I., 430
Hochman, I., 199, 292
Hochstetler, H., 330
Hodge, F. S., 78, 81
Hodges, C. R., 74
Hodgson, C., 73*t*
Hoehn, M., 320*t*
Hoff, S. R., 248
Hoffman, H. T., 21, 51, 432, 433
Hogikyan, N. D., 96, 124*t*, 125, 126*t*, 328, 335
Hoh, J. F. Y., 43
Hoit, J. D., 15, 64–65*f*, 66, 67, 81, 181, 384
Holden, P. K., 328, 334
Holinger, L. D., 248, 385, 386–387
Holland, B. W., 260
Holland, R. W., 93–94, 106, 107
Holland, W., 280
Holler, A., 455
Holler, T., 271
Hollien, H., 27–28, 59, 60, 74–75, 81, 147
Hollowell, J., 391
Holmberg, E. B., 157, 174, 280, 282, 372
Holmes, R. J., 319
Holmes, R. L., 407, 408, 409
Holsinger, C., 431
Holsinger, F. C., 427, 432, 435
Holstege, G., 21, 56
Holt, K. I., 281
Holzki, J., 387
Homer, J. J., 266, 273
Honda, 51
Hondebrink, N., 335
Hong, K. H., 21, 42, 307
Hong, W. K., 443
Honjo, I., 147
Hooper, C. R., 193, 194
Hopkin, R. J., 258
Horga, D., 447
Horii, Y., 324, 339
Horiuchi, M., 43
Hornig, J. D., 434
Horsley, I. A., 111, 170
Hou, L., 313
House, A. O., 361
Houtz, D. R., 188
Hovhannisyan, K., 391
Howard, D., 153, 156
Howard, N. S., 427
Howell, D., 430
Howell, S., 325
Howes, A., 293
Hsiao, L-C., 184–185, 294
Hsiao, T-Y., 184–185, 226, 286, 294
Hsiung, M. W., 220, 221, 222, 224, 225
Hu, R., 313
Huang, R-X., 314
Huber, J. E., 14, 67
Hudson, A. I., 108*t*, 109*t*, 146
Huebner, R. A., 325
Huenges, H. L., 31
Hughes, A., 111, 319
Hughes, B. M., 335
Hughes, D., 51–52
Hughes, R. G., 209
Hulshoff, A. C., 56
Hulstaert, C. E., 280
Humphrey, D., 240
Hunt, M., 391
Hunt, V. P., 326
Hunter, E. J., 293, 325
Hurren, A., 441
Husein, O. F., 395–396, 398
Hussain, A., 335, 336
Hwang, J-H., 405

Ihre, E., 391, 394*t*
Ikeda, Y., 182, 294
Ikis, A. O., 258
Ikonomidis, C., 249, 250
Ilomaki, I., 297
Im, B. S-H., 384
Imagawa, H., 206
Imamura, R., 289
Imhof, M., 81–82
Inagi, K., 221, 334
Inglis, A. F., 246
Ingrams, D. R., 236*t*
Irish, J., 337, 450
Irwin, R. S., 391, 413, 414*t*
Isenberg, J. S., 286, 287
Ishikawa, K., 176
Isshiki, N., 147, 195–197, 336
Issing, W. J., 230
Ito, J., 221
Ivankovic, Z., 151

Iwarsson, J., 280
Izadi, F., 261
Izzat, S., 452

Jackson-Menaldi, C., 280
Jackson-Menaldi, M. C., 329
Jacob, A., 255
Jacobs, I., 255, 258, 265
Jacobson, B. H, 126, 148, 339
Jacobson, B. J., 123, 124*t*, 125, 125*t*
Jagade, M. V., 450
Jailwala, J., 228
Jamart, J., 128, 207
James, A., 264
Jamieson, A., 406
Jamieson, D. G., 428–429
Jaquet, Y., 249, 250
Jaryszak, E. M., 264, 265
Jassir, D., 330
Jaworowska, E., 421, 426
Jayaram, M., 96
Jaywant, A., 324
Jecker, P., 272
Jenkins, M. E., 337, 338
Jensen, M., 368
Jeong, H-S., 435
Jiang, J., 50, 60, 158, 208, 250
Jimenez-Jimenez, F. J., 151
Jindal, P., 457
Jines, N., 405
Jinnah, H. A., 333*t*
Jog, M. S., 337
Johansen, L. V., 422
John, A., 111
John, J., 247
Johns, M. M., 83, 138, 144, 144*t*, 145, 188, 335
Johnson, A. B., 324
Johnson, A. F., 148, 339
Johnson, B. C., 189*t*
Johnson, K., 267
Johnson, R. F., 251, 256
Johnson, T., 367, 368*t*, 369, 369*t*, 370
Johnson Jr., C. S., 450
Jonaitis, L., 229*t*
Jones, A. S., 391
Jones, D., 324
Jones, P. B., 63–64
Jongmans, P., 455
Joniau, S., 230
Jorgensen, C., 396
Jotz, G. P., 57
Jovanovic, M. B., 285
Juel, V. C., 313, 314, 315, 316
Juergens, U., 333*t*
Jung, K. S., 307
Jurgens, U., 56, 71
Justice, L. M., 110

Kaga, K., 446
Kagel, M. C., 326
Kahane, J., 74, 77, 78, 79, 93–94
Kahn, A. R., 78
Kahrilas, P. J., 228, 237
Kalliakosta, G., 15
Kaltenbach, T., 235
Kalvatchev, Z., 266
Kamel, P. L., 237
Kanagalingam, J., 374
Kanaparthi, L. K., 389
Kanemaru, S., 221
Kanemaru, S-I., 313, 314
Kang, B. H., 220
Kapfhammer, H. P., 327
Kapstein, A. A., 335
Karchev, T., 266
Karkos, P. D., 228, 229, 230, 235
Karnell, M. P., 86, 184, 280, 282, 293
Karpenko, A. N., 210
Kasperbauer, J. L., 436
Kasper Schwartz, S., 394*t*
Kastein, S., 181
Kastelik, J. A., 408
Kataoka, H., 50, 436
Katial, R., 390*f*, 395
Katz, P. O., 227
Kauppila, A., 77
Kaur, R., 457
Kavabata, N. K., 436
Kazi, R., 155, 450, 455, 456, 459
Kearns, G. H., 258
Keghian, J., 207
Keidat, A., 297
Kelchner, L., 129, 133, 144*t*, 145, 229*t*, 233, 251, 252
Kelley, R. T., 78, 81
Kellie, S., 317
Kemp, J. S., 398*t*, 399, 403, 404
Kemp, S. E., 330
Kempster, G. B., 131, 132*t*, 134, 189, 431, 433, 434
Kendall, K., 179, 329, 330, 334
Kennedy, M., 102, 110
Kenny, D. T., 76, 296, 356
Kent, J. F., 151–152
Kent, R. D., 110, 147, 149, 151–152, 339
Keppel, K. L., 126
Kerrebijn, J. D. F., 431
Kerschner, J. E., 126, 398
Khan, A. M., 236*t*
Khan, N. A., 264
Khidr, A., 184, 221, 234*t*, 310
Kieff, D., 208
Kikuchi, Y., 446
Kileny, P. R., 328, 335
Kilic, M. A., 280–281
Kim, A. Y., 99
Kim, H. K., 21
Kim, H. S., 99, 393, 394*t*
Kim, H-T., 284, 286
Kim, K. H., 256
Kim, M-B., 284
Kim, Y. H., 21
Kimball, J., 31
Kimberlin, D. W., 274
Kimura, M., 206, 210
King, J. B., 368, 368*t*, 369, 369*t*, 370
Kishimoto, Y., 197, 221, 222
Kitajima, K., 436
Klaben, B., 67, 68, 455
Klap, P., 314
Klasner, E. R., 339
Kleber, F., 81
Klein, A., 218, 221, 222, 285, 286
Kleinert, H. L., 325
Klem, C., 431
Klich, R. J., 67
Kline, A. L., 315
Klop, E. M., 56
Kmiecik, J., 452
Knight, L., 248, 264
Knowlton, G. E., 176
Kobler, J. B., 446
Kocak, I., 374, 375, 375*t*
Kodama, N., 335
Kohnert, K., 102
Kojima, T., 221
Kollbrunner, J., 352, 361, 362, 363, 363*t*
Koltai, P. J., 273
Komiyama, S., 182, 294
Konnai, R. M., 96
Kooijman, P. G. C., 296, 297
Koopmans-van Beinum, F. J., 455, 456
Kosanovic, R., 151
Koschkee, D. L., 145, 157
Kotby, M. N., 183, 184
Koufman, J, 133, 183, 195, 203, 204, 219*t*, 225, 226, 228, 229*t*, 230, 232, 233, 237, 240, 241, 260, 330, 356, 357, 397*t*, 398, 400, 401, 402*t*, 426
Kozlakowski, L., 81
Kraus, D. H., 429, 429*t*, 430
Krause, E., 449, 455
Krecicki, T., 394*t*
Kreiman, J., 133
Krengli, M., 430, 432
Krischke, S., 96
Krishna, P., 208
Krival, K., 252*t*, 255, 256, 258
Krivec, U., 246
Kronenberg, J., 260
Kruse, E., 203
Kubba, H., 193, 247, 248
Kuhn, J., 396
Kuijpers-Jagtman, A. M., 218
Kuik, D. J., 428
Kulekci, M., 450
Kumai, Y., 240
Kumar, M., 385
Kummer, A. W., 88
Kuna, S. T., 42
Kuncl, R. W., 339
Kuo, W-R., 314
Kuo-Sheng, L., 246, 247, 248
Kupcinskas, L., 229*t*
Kupper, D. S., 246

Kurita, S., 35, 79
Kwon, T-K., 205, 206, 209
Kyrillos, L., 280

Laakso, K., 326
Laccourreye, O., 201
Lacomblez, L., 339
Lagier, A., 200, 201, 311
Lai, S. Y., 435
Laine, A., 186, 294
Lam, P. K. Y., 125, 452
Lan, Y. H., 220
Lancellotti, C. L. P., 207
Langenberg, P. W., 323
Langeveld, T. P. M., 335
Lansing, R. W., 384
Larkin, K. T., 176
Larson, A. L., 31
Larson, C. R., 56–57, 319
Larsson, A. K., 373
Laschat, M., 387
Laskawi, R., 203
Laukkanen, A-M., 297
Laures-Gore, J., 80, 81
Lauri, E-R., 296
Lauritzen, T., 190, 191
La Vecchia, C., 426
Lavy, J. A., 393, 394*t*, 395*t*
Lawrence, V. L., 101
Lawson, C., 78
Lawson, G., 207, 374
Lawson, L., 266, 270, 270*t*
Layton, T., 391
Lazarus, C., 356
Le Bihan, D., 329
Leboulleux, S., 314
Lebowitz, M. D., 393
Leder, S. B., 434, 452
Lee, A. S., 273
Lee, E-K., 179, 356, 359
Lee, H. M., 82
Lee, J. A., 288
Lee, J. H., 393
Lee, K. H., 256
Lee, K-W., 314
Lee, L., 183, 188, 293
Lee, M. S., 56
Lee, P., 426
Lee, V. S., 250
Leeper, H. A., 428–429, 429*t*
Lefebvre, J-L., 422
Lefebvre, P., 151
Legezda, A. T. R., 384
Leigh, P. N., 339
Leighton, S. E. J., 387
Lemos, E. M., 289, 290
Lenderking, W. R., 235
Leonard, R., 68, 144, 144*t*, 148, 151, 152, 179, 183, 329, 330, 334
Leong, S. C., 228
Leopold, N. A., 326
Lerman, J. W., 237, 455
Lesperance, 251
Lessac, A., 185
Lessnau, K-D., 389
Letson, J. A., 21
Leung, A. K. C., 386, 387
Leung, R., 251, 270
Leverson, G. E., 230
Levy, S., 98, 367
Lewin, J. S., 455
Lewis, A. F., 311
Leydon, C., 175–176, 308
Li, L., 311
Liberman, M., 249
Lidgren, L., 33
Liew, L., 255
Lillvik, M., 326
Lim, J-Y., 156, 365
Lim, X., 33, 216
Limbird, T. J., 240, 241
Lin, H. W., 266
Lin, Y., 78
Lind, K., 71
Lindestad, P. A., 75–76
Lindholm, P., 77
Lindsay, F., 266, 267, 268, 272
Lindstedt, D. E., 368
Linville, S. E., 75–76, 77, 78, 79, 98, 195, 199, 206
Liotti, M., 52, 384
Little, M. A., 325
Liu, B. P., 260
Liu, H., 319, 444, 445, 446
Liu, W-B., 314, 315, 316
Livesey, J. R., 296, 356
Llewellyn, C. D., 458*t*, 459
Lloyd, S., 262
Lo, H-I., 405
Logemann, J. A., 430
Lombard, L. E., 447, 451, 452
Loomis, S. R., 256
Lorcan, P. A., 408, 409
Lorch, M., 335
Lorenz, R. R., 210, 211, 311
Loucks, T. M. J., 52
Loughran, S., 432
Love, A. L., 79, 80*t*
Lowe, J. S., 409
Lowell, S. Y., 181, 294, 296, 297*t*
Lowry, S. F., 215
Lublin, F. D., 341
Ludlow, C. L., 17, 42, 44, 52, 56–57, 328, 329, 330, 331, 332*t*, 333*t*
Luff, D. A., 452
Luna-Ortiz, K., 435
Lundstrom, E., 447, 454, 455, 456
Lundy, D. S., 330
Lunn, W. W., 389
Luschei, E. S., 51–52, 59
Luscher, M. S., 422, 432
Luu, Q., 207

Ma, E. P-M., 79, 80*t*, 96, 98, 102, 124*t*, 149, 179–180
MacArthur, C. J., 258
MacGregor, F. B., 432
Mackenzie, C. R., 239
MacKenzie, K., 362, 393, 432
Maclagan, M. A., 292, 296
MacMahon, J., 408
Maddalozzo, J., 386–387
Mahendra, N., 103
Mahfoud, L., 76
Mahieu, H. F., 428
Mahler, L., 324
Majaess, L., 457
Makashay, M. J., 50
Makeieff, M., 435
Maki, E., 297
Makitie, A. A., 452
Malik, T. H., 264
Maloney, E. M., 266
Maltha J. C., 218
Manako, H., 294
Mandel, S., 148
Mandros, C., 15
Mangunta, V., 207
Mankekar, G., 260, 261
Mann, E. A., 292
Mann, S. G. S., 151
Manning, S. C., 246, 247, 248
Manolopoulos, L., 203
Manor, Y., 324, 325
Mao, V. H., 313, 314, 315, 316
Maragos, N. E., 398
Marcelino, F. C., 295*t*, 296
Marchese-Ragona, R., 435
Marge, M., 93
Marioni, G, 435
Marom, T., 262
Maronian, N. C., 195, 335
Marsden, C. D., 56
Marsh, J. H., 256
Martin, G., 151
Martin, L. J., 339
Martin, S. B., 333*t*
Martinez, F. D., 391
Martinez, J. A., 311
Martins, R. H. G., 263–264, 280, 284, 285, 296, 297*t*
Maryn, Y., 151, 152, 179
Mason, P., 391
Mason III, U. G., 396
Massey, J. M., 313, 314, 315, 316
Massey, K., 74–75
Massey, R. J., 207
Mastrovich, J. D., 409
Masuda, M., 240
Masuda, T., 294, 295*t*
Matal, V., 376
Matar, N., 374
Mathers-Schmidt, B., 297, 397*t*, 400, 401, 404, 406
Mathieson, L., 68, 122, 123*t*, 129, 131, 137, 177, 178*t*, 179, 289, 290, 317, 337, 340, 353, 356, 361, 426, 429
Mathisen, D. J., 249
Matusiewicz, S. P., 393

Mau, T., 21
Maune, S., 423, 434
Mauri, M., 221, 286
Mayer, R. M., 373, 375*t*
Mayo, R., 93–94
Mazloff, D., 82
McAllister, A., 74, 359
Mcalpin, T., 290
McCabe, D. J., 181, 292, 298
McCarthy, K., 383, 387, 388, 389, 391
McClay, J. E., 251, 253, 266, 267, 268, 270
McColl, D. A., 455, 456
McConnachie, A., 393
McCormick, M., 270
McDonald-McGinn, D. M., 258
McElhinney, D. B., 258
McFadden, E. R., 407
McFarlane, S., 181, 182
McGarvey, L., 408, 409, 411
McGlone, R. E., 146
McGuff, H. S., 287
McGuirt Jr., W. F., 260
McGurk, M., 459
McHenry, M., 42, 317, 449
McKeagney, P., 408
McKee, A. S., 316
McKenna, M., 274
McKinney, J., 59
McMullin, B.T., 199, 311
McMurray, J. S., 258
McNeill, E. J. M., 376
McQuestion, M., 430
McRoy, D. M., 99
McSharry, P. E., 325
McWhorter, A., 427, 432, 433
Medical Research Council (MRC), 385
Medrado, R., 96
Meeuwis, C. A., 431
Megale, S. R. M. C. L., 229
Mehta, D., 134, 157, 158
Meining, A., 235
Meininger, V., 339
Melcon, M. C., 81
Meleca, R. J., 198, 210, 356, 449, 455
Meline, T., 110
Meltzer, T. R., 376
Meltzner, G. S., 445
Men, L-N., 314
Men, S., 258, 261
Mendelsohn, J., 240
Menezes, M. B., 436
Merati, A. L., 126, 250, 307, 310, 311, 396, 398
Merbach, M., 456
Merck Manual, The, 2005, 240
Merrill, R. M., 177, 294
Merrot, O., 255
Merson, R. M., 341
Mertens, F., 149
Mesallam, T. A., 230
Messing, B., 138, 140, 141, 144, 144*t*, 145
Michel, J. F., 59, 79
Michelsson, K., 70, 71
Michelsson, O., 70, 71
Mico, A., 286
Middendorf, J. H., 194
Mikita, C. P., 401, 406
Mikita, J. A., 401, 406
Mikos, V. A., 371
Milbrath, R. L., 292
Milczuk, H. A., 258
Milenkovic, P., 74
Milgrom, H., 409–410
Miller, A., 317
Miller, D. G., 149
Miller, E. G., 339
Miller, L., 317, 323, 337, 338, 340, 341, 361, 372, 397*t*, 404, 440, 444, 454
Miller, N., 324
Miller, Q., 315
Miller, W. R., 190, 191, 191*t*
Mimran, R. C., 447
Ming, X., 452
Minoda, R., 335
Minton, J. T., 42
Mirasola, K. L., 398
Mirza, N., 307, 353, 363, 394*t*
Mitchell, J. L., 459
Miyamoto, R. C., 258
Mniszek, J., 273
Moberly, A. C., 203
Mohammadi, S., 255
Mohiuddin, Z., 235
Molassiotas, A., 176, 416
Molina, M. A., 422
Moller, A. M., 391
Moller, R. Y., 441–442
Monnier, P., 250, 251, 258
Montequin, D. W., 21, 207–208
Montrose, M., 233
Moon, J. W., 393
Moon Sung, J., 104
Moore, B. A., 431, 432, 435
Moore, C. A., 15
Moore, G. P., 59
Moore, P., 59
Moorhead, 262, 263, 264
Mootanah, R., 324
Moran, M. J., 369*t*, 370
Mordaunt, M., 370, 372
Morgan, E. E., 147
Morgan, M., 274
Morgan, W., 64, 67
Morice, A. H., 408, 411
Moringlane, J. R., 323
Morris, M. J., 395, 396, 397*t*, 398, 399*t*, 400, 401, 403, 404, 406
Morris, R., 76, 79, 357, 372, 373
Morrison, C. E., 319
Morrison, G. A. J., 255
Morrison, M., 101, 209, 290, 357, 358, 359, 397*t*, 398
Morsomme, C., 374
Morsomme, D., 128
Mortensen, M., 144, 144*t*, 145, 304, 305
Most, T., 447
Mouadeb, D. A., 203, 204
Mouzakes, J., 246
Mu, L., 42, 43
Muallem, M., 267
Mudd, P. A., 228
Mueller, P. B., 82, 108*t*, 146
Muers, M., 405
Mukherji, S. K., 78
Mullen, R., 110
Muller, S. H., 440
Munck-Wikland, E., 447
Mundt, J. C., 351
Munnur, U., 240
Munoz-del-Rio, A., 33, 216
Muntz, H., 281
Munz, M., 338
Mupparapu, M., 78
Murdoch, B. E., 180, 317
Murphy, J., 248
Murphy, K., 15, 53
Murphy, T. D., 386–387
Murray, A. D., 249, 250, 253, 255, 258, 260, 261
Murray, K. D., 376
Murray, S. L., 256
Murry, T., 59, 96, 99, 102, 170, 283, 286, 330, 365, 397*t*, 409, 410, 412, 413
Murukami, D., 240
Muscat, J. E., 426
Musser, J., 233
Musura, M., 447
Myer, C. M., 249, 256

Nagarkar, A. N., 457
Naiman, A. N., 273
Nair, G., 155
Nakamura, K., 336
Nakao, M., 446
Nakashima, T., 35, 208, 260, 311, 429*t*
Nakayama, M., 435, 436
Nance, M. A., 326
Narayana, S., 323
Narcy, P., 256
Nasri, S., 290
National Cancer Institute, 421, 423–426*t*
National Heart, Lung and Blood Institute, 391
National Institutes of Health, 102, 271
National Multiple Sclerosis Society, 341
Neave, N., 79
Neely. J. L., 291, 292
Neils-Strunjas, J., 233
Nemeth, A. J., 260
Nesbitt, M., 435
Neto, A. L. S., 436
Netterville, J. L., 198
Neuenschwander, M. C., 208, 221, 222, 291
Neumann, K., 374, 375, 375*t*, 376
Newcombe, P. A., 413
Newman, D., 337

Newman, K. B., 396, 400, 401
Newman, S. P., 126
Newsom, J., 82
Ng, E., 316
Ng, M. L., 59, 444, 445, 446
Ngan, E., 52
Nguyen, D. D., 296, 297*t*, 356
Nichol, H., 101
Nicollas, R., 72*t*, 200, 258, 261
Niedzielska, G., 151
Nielson, D. W., 387
Nienkerke-Springer, A., 359, 360
Nierengarten, M. B., 305
Nilson, H., 94
Nishi, K., 391
Nishizawa, Y., 391
Nissen, S. L., 177, 356
Nito, T., 206
Noble, E., 324
Noordzji, J. P., 232
Nooteboom, S. G., 449
Norbart, T. C., 374
Norman, P., 391
Northrop, G. E., 372
Noyes, B. E., 398*t*, 399, 403, 404
Nunez, R. A., 135, 136
Nuss, R. C., 235, 282
Nye, C., 328, 335

Oates, J., 133, 137, 157, 174, 294, 319, 373, 374, 376
Ochs, M., 6
O'Connell, M. A., 400
O'Connor, D. M., 249
O'Donnell, S., 248
O'Dwyer, T. P., 298
Oeken, J., 434
Ogawa, H., 391
Ogawa, K., 435
Ohala, J. J., 50, 51
O'Hollaren, M. T., 403
Ojeda, J. M., 266
Okla, S., 439
Okur, E., 280–281
Oliveira, D. T., 296
Olsen, K. D., 436
Olthoff, A., 203, 311
Omidi, M., 226
Oosterbaan, J. A., 280
Oosterlinck, K., 374
Op De Coul, 452, 454
Oreggia, F., 426
O'Reilly, H. P., 426
Orenstein, D. M., 387
Orenstein, S. R., 387
Orlikoff, R. F., 82, 107, 109*t*, 429, 429*t*, 430
Orloff, L. A., 290, 334
Osman, M., 391
Ospina, E. G., 226
Ossoff, R., 208, 219, 221, 291, 292, 311
Otto, K. J., 83
Ousley, T., 4553
Owaki, S., 50
Owen, S., 441
Owren, M. J., 351
Oxford Public Schools, Massachusetts, 194
Oyer, H. J., 82
Ozcan, K. M., 239
Ozgursoy, S. K., 209, 262, 282
Ozturk, O., 263

Paget, S. A., 239
Pai, L., 220, 222
Paiva, L. S., 339
Palazzi-Churas, K. L. P., 230
Paleri, V., 440*t*, 441
Palmer, A. D., 376, 436
Palombini, B. C., 408
Paniello, R. C., 211, 334
Pannbacker, M., 170, 175, 280
Panzarino, P. J., 353
Papsin, B. C., 387
Paradiso, T., 110
Parhizkar, N., 99
Park, J. U., 288
Park, J-B., 335
Parker, A. J., 371, 374, 375, 376
Parsa, V., 428–429
Parsons, J. P., 395, 400
Parsons, S., 406
Pasa G., 174
Pasche, P., 435
Pashos, C. L., 234*t*
Pasricha, N., 376
Pastore, A., 435
Patel, M. A., 398
Patel, M. R., 197
Patel, N. J., 396
Patel, N. K., 270
Patel, R., 144, 145, 188
Patrick, C., 363
Patrick, L., 152
Pauloski, B. R., 429*t*, 430, 433, 434, 440*t*, 443
Paulsen, F. P., 78
Paulsen, J. S., 326
Paulsson, M., 33
Pavord, I. D., 408, 410, 411
Pawar, P. V., 450, 452
Pawlak, A., 33
Payne, J., 103
Pazera, J. F., 129
Pearson, B. W., 436
Peck, J. J., 431
Pedersen, T., 146, 391
Pedersen, U., 422
Pegorano, R., 79
Pegoraro-Krook, M. I., 79, 147
Pell, M. D., 319, 324
Peluso, D. L., 354
Pengilly, A., 256
Penner, J. L., 457, 458*t*, 459
Pentti, J., 294
Perazzo, P. S. L., 207
Peretti, G., 434
Perez-Fernandez, C., 294
Perie, S., 452
Perkell, J. S., 280
Perkins, J. A., 246
Perkins, P. J., 396
Perkner, J. J., 400
Perlmutter, J. S., 333*t*, 334
Perona, K. E., 384
Perry, A., 370, 372, 454
Petrovic-Lazic, M., 151, 284, 286
Petrucelli, J., 93
Petty, B. E., 410, 415
Pfafflin, F., 366, 367
Pfister, H., 272
Pfuetzenreiter, E. G., 151, 433, 434
Phyland, D. J., 319
Pickup, B., 183
Pickuth, D., 376
Pietzsch-Rohrschneider, I., 31
Pignatari, S., 273
Pimental, P. A., 323
Pinto, J. A., 221
Pitt, G., 180
Plant, R. L., 51–52
Plante, E., 110
Plowman-Prine, E. K., 319, 321
Poburka, B. J., 137, 138, 141, 143*t*
Poletto. C. J., 44, 45, 52
Polley, L., 408
Pols, L. C. W., 455
Pontes, A., 280
Pontes, P., 78, 79, 260, 273, 280
Poolinsky, D. E., 319
Popovich, A. A., 447, 451, 452
Portas, J. G., 435
Porter, S. R., 99
Portone, C., 189, 189*t*
Portone-Maira, C., 188
Portugal, L., 455
Posen, J., 325
Postma, G., 195, 291
Postma, G. N., 133, 230, 232, 233, 260
Pou, A., 317, 434, 449
Pouget, E. R., 351
Pouget, J., 339
Powell, D. W., 218
Pransky, S., 266, 271
Preciado-Lopez, J., 294, 296, 297*t*
Preciado-Ruiz, P., 294
Presutti, L., 194
Preuss, S. F., 267, 270, 271
Pribuisiene, R., 229*t*
Primov-Fever, A., 260
Pring, T., 325, 370, 372
Prochaska, J. O., 192
Proctor, A., 2
Pruett, S. B., 354
Pukander, J., 426–427
Puts, D. A., 74
Putter, M. J., 258
Putzer, M., 323

Qadeer, M. A., 228
Queija, D. S., 151, 433
Quene, H., 449

Raben, D., 421
RadiologyInfo, 271
Raghunathan, M., 151
Rahbar, R., 249
Rahn III, D. A., 250
Raitiola, H., 426–427
Raj, A., 74, 76, 77, 411
Rajgopalan, P., 78
Ramadan, N., 337
Ramanathan, P., 50
Ramig, L. A., 339
Ramig, L. O., 51–52, 59, 106, 111, 298, 319, 324, 325, 339
Rammage, L., 101, 145, 149, 157, 199, 290, 337, 355, 356, 364, 373, 374, 398
Ranen, N. G., 326
Ransom, E. R., 265
Rantala, L., 292, 295
Rao, S., 313
Raphael, L. J., 318
Rassekh, C. H., 431
Rastatter, J. C., 248
Rastatter, M., 147
Rastorguev, E., 272
Rattenbury, H. J., 170, 179
Ratusnik, D. L., 372
Raudaskoski, T., 77
Rawlings, B. A., 247, 248
Redmond, S., 281
Reed, J., 102
Rees, C. J., 330, 331
Regnell, J. R., 356
Rehder, M. I., 70, 71
Reichel, O., 230, 237
Reilly, N., 148
Reingold, S. C., 341
Remacle, A., 151
Remacle, M., 207, 365, 374, 375, 434, 452
Remade, M., 128
Ren, C. L., 386–387
Renals, S., 81
Reubold, U., 81
Reulbach, T. R., 230
Reveiz, L., 226
Reynolds, C. L., 52
Rich, J. T., 211
Richieri-Costa, A., 260
Richter, G. T., 247, 248
Ridha, H., 298
Riede, T., 59, 60
Rieder, A. A., 313
Riegel, B., 409
Rieger, J., 435
Rinaldo, A., 290, 422
Ringel, R. L., 82
Ringel, S. P., 339
Risberg-Berlin, B., 440*t*, 441–442
Rivera, T., 286
Rizzi, M. D., 255, 256, 258
Robb, M., 70, 71, 146, 248, 321
Robbins, R., 82
Robert, D., 339
Roberts, L. S., 31
Robinson, J. L., 148, 151
Robitschek, J., 431, 432, 433
Rodero, E., 351
Rodrigues, M. F., 57
Rodriguez-Parra, M. J., 151, 152
Roehm, P. C., 135, 136, 136*t*
Roesler, T. A., 398
Roh, J. L., 99
Roland, N. J., 391, 393, 394, 394*t*
Rollnick, S., 190, 191, 191*t*
Rolnick, M., 341
Rontal, E., 198, 198*t*, 307, 310
Rontal, M., 198, 198*t*, 307, 310
Rope, A. F., 258
Roper, L., 370
Rosati, G., 340
Roseberry-McKibbin, C., 105
Rosen, C., 2, 33, 116, 135, 136, 136*t*, 170, 197–198, 198*t*, 199, 204, 205, 206, 208, 209, 216, 218, 221, 222, 268, 272, 273, 291, 292, 307, 308, 310, 311, 313, 356, 360
Rosen, E. J., 434
Rosenblatt, A., 326, 327
Rosenfield, D., 326
Ross, J., 232
Ross, M. A, 339
Rotenberg, B. W., 255
Roth, Y., 262
Rothera, M. P., 256, 264, 273
Rothman, H., 81
Rothstein, J. D., 339
Roubeau, B., 59
Rounsley, C. A., 366
Rousseau, B., 33, 207–208
Rowe, L., 313
Roxburgh, J., 454
Roy, N., 1, 151, 174, 174*t*, 175, 177, 183, 187, 188, 189, 189*t*, 211, 281, 294, 330, 356, 359, 362, 363, 363*t*
Roy, S., 271, 330
Rubak, S., 190, 191
Rubin, A. D., 304, 305, 335
Rubin, J. S., 178*t*, 353, 356, 359, 393, 395*t*
Ruddy, B. H., 67, 193, 194, 427–428*t*, 429, 450, 451
Rudman, D. T., 387
Rugolo, L. M. S. S., 71
Ruiz, C., 353
Ruiz, D. M. C. F., 260
Ruiz, P. J., 78
Russell, A., 147, 294, 295*t*, 296
Russell, B., 179
Russell, J. A., 324
Rutledge, J., 174
Rutter, M. J., 247, 251, 256, 262
Ryan, M., 76
Ryan, N. M., 409–410, 416
Ryan, W. J., 82, 450
Ryden, A., 441–442

Sabol, L., 188
Sachin, S., 319
Saito, K., 435, 436
Saito, R., 315
Sakaguchi, S., 79
Sakakura, K., 385, 386–387
Sala, E., 294, 296
Salas-Provance, M. B., 102, 104
Salassa, J. R., 436
Salmon S., 442, 443, 445, 449
Sandage, M., 175–176, 397*t*, 400, 401, 402*t*, 406, 407, 408, 413, 415
Sandbaek, A., 190, 191
Sander, H. H., 246
Sanders, I., 42, 43
Sandulache, V., 33, 216
Sandyk, R., 323
Sanjuan, M., 200
Santana, M. F., 263–264
Sant'Anna, G. D., 286
Sanuki, T., 335, 336
Sapienza, C., 15, 52, 67, 68, 96, 193, 194, 330, 331, 333*t*, 410, 412, 413, 427–428*t*, 429, 450, 451
Sapir, S., 51–52, 57, 297, 298, 318, 319, 324, 341, 356
Sasaki, C. T., 43, 434
Sataloff, D. M., 227
Sataloff, R. T., 20, 25, 27–28, 28, 31, 38, 40, 56, 57, 67, 98, 99, 101, 102, 106, 148, 158, 197, 206*t*, 207, 219*t*, 221, 227, 228, 229*t*, 230, 236, 236*t*, 237, 292, 335, 338, 354, 355, 361, 391
Sati, I., 282
Sato, K., 79, 208, 311
Sauder, C., 188, 309, 310, 311
Saunders, M. W., 255, 391
Sawashima, M. S., 50
Saxman, J., 79, 146
Saxne, T., 33
Sayed, S. I., 450, 457
Scanavini, A. B. A., 229
Schaefer, S. D., 434
Schaeffer, N., 133, 181
Schalen, L., 359, 361, 363, 363*t*
Schallert, T., 324
Schalling, E., 317, 318
Scharloo, M., 335
Scheenstra, R. J., 440, 440*t*, 441
Scheff, J. D., 215, 225
Scheiner, E., 71
Scheinfeld, N. S., 316
Scherer, R. C., 27–28, 47, 50, 51, 96, 339
Schindler A., 310, 428, 429, 432, 435
Schlauch, R. S., 446

Schlegel, U., 316
Schlomicher-Thier, J., 153, 156
Schlotthauer, G., 329, 330
Schlumberger, M., 314
Schmaling, K. B., 396
Schmidbauer, J. A., 457
Schmidt, C. P., 189*t*
Schmidt, M. V., 354
Schnapp, L. M., 391
Schneider, B., 75–76, 80*t*, 197
Schneider, S., 293
Schneiderman, C. R., 94
Schofield, K. J., 372, 373
Schouwenburg, P. F., 452
Schraff, S., 270, 271, 272, 273, 274
Schroeder Jr., J. W., 248
Schubert, C., 354
Schulz, G. M., 318, 319, 321, 322, 323, 324
Schutte, H. K., 149, 356
Schwartz, I. S., 239
Schwartz, R. A., 385
Schwarz, R., 456
Schweinfurth, J., 208, 219, 221, 291, 292
Scully, C., 99
Searl, J., 452, 454, 455, 456
Searl, J. P., 455
Sederholm, E., 74
Sedlacek, T. V., 267
Seedat, R. Y., 266
Segal, K., 267
Segas, J., 203
Segebarth, P. B., 240, 241
Seifert, E., 352, 361, 362, 363, 363*t*
Seikaly, H., 435
Selber, J., 197, 198, 198*t*
Selby, J. C., 237
Sellars, C., 393
Seneviratne, J. K., 339
Sennes, L. U., 289
Seoud, M., 76
Sepi, M., 228
Sercarz, J. A., 290
Sesterhenn, A. M., 246, 247, 248
Sewnaik, A., 431, 435, 436
Shah, A. G., 198
Shah, A. K., 313, 314
Shah, R. K., 226, 235, 248, 281, 282
Shaha, A. R., 422
Shakeel, M., 335, 336
Shaker, R., 228
Shamouelian, D., 450
Shanks, J. C., 449
Shapiro, N. L., 311
Shapshay, S., 226, 249, 423
Sharma, D., 457, 458*t*, 459
Sharma, S., 389
Shau, Y-W., 286
Shaw, G. Y., 237
Shaw, H. S., 151
Sheehan, P. Z., 264
Sheller, J. R., 389, 391
Shemirani, N., 307
Sheridon, S., 174
Shewell, C., 129
Shick, P., 266
Shiels, W. E., 387
Shimizu, T., 50
Shiotani, A., 435
Shipp, T., 146, 147
Shirley, W. P., 240, 272
Shiromoto, O., 184
Shivashankar, N., 359
Shnaps-Baum, R., 174
Shott, S. R., 258
Shrivastav, R., 81
Sibai, A., 76
Sidavi, A., 133
Sidell, D., 450
Sihvo, M., 296
Silbergleit, A. K., 148, 339
Silburn, P., 323
Silva, R. D. A. E., 280, 284
Silva, R. R., 351
Silver, C. E., 422
Simberg, S., 186, 294
Simon, M., 174, 174*t*, 187
Simonelli, M., 436
Simons, J. P., 233
Simonyan, K., 52, 56, 328, 329
Simpson, C. B., 199, 204, 205, 206, 287, 304, 307, 308, 311
Simpson, C. R., 391
Simpson, L. L., 335
Simpson, M. L., 356
Sims, H. S., 189, 189*t*
Singelton, A., 333*t*
Singer, M., 450
Singer, S., 456
Singh, A., 434
Sittel, C., 433
Sivasankar, M., 1, 2, 99, 293, 294, 393, 394*t*
Sklarew, P. R., 400
Skodda, S., 316, 317, 319, 322
Slavin, D. C., 444, 447, 449, 454
Slavit, D., 195
Smart, D. W., 106
Smart, J. F., 106
Smith, A. D., 393
Smith, B. E., 189, 189*t*
Smith, C. G., 184
Smith, E., 96, 294, 426
Smith, F. H., 372
Smith, G. A., 239
Smith, J., 258, 416
Smith, L. P., 265
Smith, M. E., 51–52, 59, 188, 211, 256, 309, 310, 311, 433
Smith, P. L., 391
Smith, R. L., 457
Smith, S., 183
Smith, T. L., 307
Smits, I., 151, 152
Snyder, P. J., 148, 351
So, Y. K., 435
Sobeih, T. M., 230
Soda, Y., 239
Soderpalm, E., 373, 374
Sodersten, M., 75–76, 174, 294–295, 295*t*
Sohn, J., 207–208
Soliman, A. M. S., 285, 286, 307
Solomon, N. P., 15, 50, 60, 66, 129, 175–176, 292, 293, 296, 297*t*, 316, 323
Son, Y-I., 179, 284, 356, 359, 435
Sonne, J. E., 434
Sonnenberg, A., 426
Sorenson, D. N., 146
Spak, C., 328, 335
Spector, S., 391, 410
Spencer, K. A., 179, 180, 181, 182
Sperry, E. E., 67
Speyer, R., 129, 150, 240, 241
Spiegel, J., 67, 197, 219*t*, 338, 374
Spielman, J., 324, 325
Spinelli, D. A., 435
Sprecher, A. J., 208
Spruill III, J., 67
Sridhara, S. R., 151, 198
St. Guily, J. L., 452
St. Louis, E., 306
Staab, J. P., 353
Stabley, R., 266
Stachler, R., 198, 210
Staffieri, A., 435
Stafford, F. W., 441
Stager, S. V., 158, 175–176, 308, 330, 356, 357
Stajner-Katusic, S., 447
Stanley, G. B., 446
Stanton, A. E., 393, 394, 394*t*
Starmer, H. M., 426, 427, 430, 432, 433, 434, 435
Stathopoulos, E., 52, 66
Stavroulaki, P., 229, 232, 236, 237, 239
Stavroulakis, P., 203
Steiner, W., 203
Stemple, J. C., 44, 67, 68, 83, 137, 144*t*, 145, 150, 157, 170, 171, 174, 174*t*, 175–176, 177, 181, 183, 185, 187, 188, 189*t*, 206, 221, 230, 240, 263, 266, 284, 293, 311, 325, 337, 364, 427
Stenton, C., 385, 386*t*
Stepp, C. E., 445
Stern, R., 239
Stern, Y., 267, 272, 273
Stevens, A., 409
Stewart, C. F., 329
Stewart, R., 177
Stith, J. A., 258
Stoddard, K., 211
Stojadinovic, A., 129
Stolz, D., 391
Stone, R. E. Jr., 365
Stong, B. C., 335
Story, B. H., 181
Stowell, T., 445

Strand, E. A., 310, 339
Stratmann, C., 387
Strauss, S., 78
Strojan, P., 430
Strome, M., 50, 228
Strominger, R., 44
Stygall, J., 126
Su, W. F., 220
Sudhir, P. M., 359
Suehiro, A., 197, 198*t*
Suhr, J., 176
Sulck, M., 387
Sulica, L., 176, 283
Sullivan, C., 198
Sulter, A. M., 149
Sundberg, J., 51–52, 74, 280, 359
Sung, M-W., 256
Suonpää, J., 294
Susser, R. D., 74
Suvanto-Luukkonen, E., 77
Swash, M., 339
Swensson, J., 284
Syal, R., 253
Szabo, A., 294–295

Taira, T., 195–197
Takahashi, H., 446
Takeuchi, E., 436
Talmi, Y., 260
Taly, A. B., 313
Tamashiro, E., 246
Tamez-Velarde, M., 435
Tamura, Y., 422
Tanaka, S., 197
Tang, J. P. L., 401
Tanner, C. M., 333*t*
Tanner, K., 188, 329
Tanoue, L. T., 240, 241
Tansey, S., 450
Tantawy, A., 452, 455
Tarin, T. T., 311
Tariq, M., 236*t*
Tasca, R. A., 270, 271, 273
Tatchell, R., 21
Tateya, I., 33, 207–208, 216
Tateya, T., 216
Tavares, E. L. M., 263–264, 296, 297*t*
Tayama, N., 206
Taylor, M. B., 328, 335
Taylor, W., 391
Teitel, A. D., 239
Teles-Magalhaes, L. C., 79
Terada, T., 452
Ternstrom, S., 155–156
Terrell, J. E., 125, 457, 458*t*, 459
Tervonen, H., 454
Teshigawara, M., 81
Tezcaner, C. Z., 282
Theis, S. M., 235, 258
Thekdi, A. A., 206, 209
Theodores, D. G., 180, 323, 404, 413
Thibeault, S. L., 31, 33, 102, 176, 188, 207, 208, 216, 218, 220, 294, 295, 295*t*, 296, 298
Thiel, S., 434
Thielke, R. J., 250
Thirlwall, A., 255
Thomas, D. B., 426
Thomas, G., 296, 297
Thomas, J. E., 151, 436
Thomas, L. B., 38, 44, 78, 83, 170, 171, 174, 175–176, 177, 181, 183, 185
Thome, D. C., 262
Thome, R., 262
Thompson, A. R., 99, 101
Thompson, D. M., 247, 248
Thompson, R. H., 408
Thomsen, J., 256
Thorne, M. C., 255
Thornton, J., 366, 371, 372, 373, 376
Threats, T. T., 97, 98
Thwing, J. I., 384
Thyme, K., 183
Tiago, R., 78
Till, J. A., 328
Tillmann, B., 31, 78
Timmermans, B., 297
Timms, M. S., 270, 271
Tindall, L. R., 325
Tippett, D. C., 426
Titze, I. R., 21, 50, 51–52, 60, 149, 175–176, 181, 183, 186, 292, 293, 298, 339
Tobin, Y., 447
Todorov, I., 266
Todorov, S., 266
Tolejano, C. J., 250
Tomita, H., 429*t*
Toohill, R. J., 250, 307
Tooley, W. H., 387
Topcu, I., 258
Torensma R., 218
Torrejano, G., 435
Torrente, M. C., 266
Torres, M. E., 329
Totenberg, B., 137
Tran, N. D., 296, 356
Tranchant, C., 316
Tranel, D., 176
Trani, M., 194
Treadway, C., 306
Treasure, J., 191, 192
Treole, K., 400
Triana, M., 274
Triglia, J-M., 200, 258, 261, 339
Tripoliti, E., 325
Trudeau, M. D., 400
Tsai, V., 207
Tsuji, D. H., 289
Tsunoda, K., 239
Tucker, H. M., 211
Turley, R., 83
Turner, C., 313, 314
Tyagi, I., 253
Tzelepis, G. E., 15
Tzenker, O., 76

Uglic, C., 246
Uloza, V., 229*t*
Umeno, H., 208, 260, 311
Unal, E., 247
Urquhart, A. C., 306
U.S. Bureau of the Census, 102
U.S. Department of Labor, Bureau of Labor Statistics, 294

Vachin, F., 255
Vaezi, M. F., 228
Vaissiere, J., 201, 208
Valdez, T. A., 249
Valera, F. C. P., 246, 247, 248
Van As, C. J., 456
Van As-Brooks, C. J., 439, 455, 456
Van Beurden, H. E., 218
Van Borsel, J., 76, 180, 375*t*, 377
Van Cauwenberge, P., 151, 177, 179
Vance, C., 338
Van de Heyning, P. H., 149, 297
Van den Berg, J., 45, 60
Van der Merwe, A., 176
Van der Torn, M., 428, 429
Van Dine, A., 455
Van Gogh, C. D. L., 430
Van Houtte, E., 295*t*, 296, 297*t*, 298, 355, 356
Van Leer, E., 188, 189*t*, 190, 192
Van Lierde, K., 76, 296, 355
Van Lierde, K. M., 75–76, 177, 179, 181
van Mersbergen, M., 293, 363, 363*t*
Vanoye, C. R., 42
Van Rossum, M. A., 449
Vanryckeghem, M., 339
van Wijck-Warnaar, I., 150
van Zandwijk, N., 440
Vedanarayanan, V., 311
Veerendrakumar, M., 313
Vegas, A., 286
Velazquez, R. A., 287
Velicer, W. F., 192
Verdolini, K., 2, 33, 106, 111, 177, 183, 185, 186, 216, 279, 298, 359, 360, 367
Verdolini Abbot, K., 131, 356
Verdolini-Marston, K., 50, 175–176, 185–186
Verdonck-de Leeuw, I. M., 428
Verdun, L. P., 44
Verduyckt, I., 128, 194, 374
Vernon, M., 413
Vertigan, A. E., 404, 407, 408, 409–410, 411, 413, 414, 415, 416
Verwoerd, C. D. A., 251
Vicente, L. C. C., 81
Vijayasekeran, S., 251
Vilkman, E., 77, 292
Villavicencio-Valencia, V., 435
Vipperla, R., 81
Visser, W., 316
Vivero, R. J., 271
Vlahakis, N. E., 398, 404, 405
Vodovotz, V., 215
Vogel, K. G., 33
Vokes, D. E., 328
Volk, M. S., 126
Volkl-Kernstock, S., 353

Von Berg, S., 181
Von den Hoff, J. W., 218
Von Leden, H., 78–79
Vorperian, H. K., 151–152
Vukovic, M., 151
Vuppalapati, A., 78

Wagner, I., 376
Wakelin, D., 79
Walker, F. O., 326
Walker, M., 138, 140, 141, 144, 144*t*, 145
Wall, M., 181
Walling, 338, 340
Wallis, L., 280
Walsh, M. L., 443
Walton, J. H., 107, 109*t*
Walton, S., 330
Wamboldt, F., 398
Wamboldt, M., 398
Wang, C-P., 288
Wang, E. Q., 250
Wang, L., 313
Wang, T-G., 286
Wang, Y-T., 151
Wanger, J., 12, 13
Ward, E. C., 180, 317, 323
Ward, P. A., 239
Ward, P. D., 31, 33
Warner, J., 177
Warrick, P., 337
Wasylik, K., 133
Watson, G., 264, 391
Watson, P., 64
Watson, P. J., 51–52, 63–64, 180, 446
Watts, C., 328, 335, 339
Wax, M. K., 436
Weber, R. S., 431, 433, 434
Webster, K. T., 426, 435, 436
Webster, S. W., 351
Weckx, L. L. M., 273
Wei, C., 208
Weiler, J. M., 391
Wein, R. O., 433, 434
Weinberg, B., 449
Weinberger, M. M., 395, 400, 403
Weinman, J., 459
Weinrich, B., 72*t*, 149, 150, 252, 258
Weinstein, G. S., 435
Weiss, D. A., 181
Welham, N. V., 207, 216, 221, 222, 292, 296, 297*t*
Wells, A., 208
Welzel, C., 374, 375, 375*t*, 376
Wendahl, R. W., 59
Wenig, B., 226
Wenning, G. K., 327
Wermke, K., 71
Westcott, C. J., 239
Westerblad, H., 293
Whatman, J., 317, 449
Wheat, M. C., 109*t*, 146
Wheeler, A. P., 391
Wheeler, K. M., 15, 96, 152
White, D., 251, 256
Whiteside, S. P., 72*t*, 73*t*
Whittington, P. F., 387
Whurr, R., 328, 335
Whymark, A. D., 248
Wiatrak, B., 272
Wiederanders, K., 230
Wieneke, G. H., 150
Wiet, G. J., 387
Wight, R. G., 441
Wiles, C. M., 339
Wilhoit, C. S. T., 434
Williams, R. A., 107
Williams, S. L., 174
Williamson, I. J., 393, 394, 394*t*
Willinger, U., 353, 360, 362
Wilson, J., 229, 359, 362, 376
Wilson, K. M., 422, 423, 427, 429*t*, 430
Winkworth, A. L., 404, 413
Winstead, W., 235
Witt, R. E., 197, 198*t*
Witt, R. L., 307, 311
Wlosko, E. M., 81
Wo, J. M., 235
Wodchis, W. P., 125, 328, 335
Wolf, F. T., 443
Wolf, G. T., 457
Wolf, M., 260, 261*t*
Wolfe, V. I., 372, 373
Wong, A. Y-H., 179–180
Woo, P., 144, 144*t*, 145, 232, 240, 304, 305, 308, 309, 310
Wood, G., 178*t*, 393, 395*t*
Wood, R., 409–410
Woodnorth, G. H., 194, 235
Woodson, G., 283, 314, 315, 316, 330, 331, 333*t*, 334, 335, 337, 338, 365
Wootten, C. T., 247
World Health Organization, 96, 97*t*
Worley, G., 201
Worrall, L. E., 110, 111
Wright, C., 249, 422, 423
Wright, R., 391
Wright, S., 445
Wu, Z-K., 314
Wuyts, F., 75–76, 149, 177, 296, 297
Wyatt, M. E., 259, 260*t*
Wynder, E. L., 426

Xavier, L. L., 57
Xia, Q., 314
Xu, J. H., 182
Xu, J. J., 444
Xu, W., 313, 314
Xue, A., 82
Xue, J. W., 330
Xue, S. A., 79, 80*t*, 107

Yahr, M., 320*t*
Yairi, E., 2
Yamaguchi, H., 182
Yaman, H., 263
Yamini, B. K, 359
Yan, Y., 151, 203, 204
Yang, C. Y., 375*t*, 376
Yates, P. D., 229
Yeager, V. L., 78
Yelken, K., 396, 450
Yildirim, I., 280–281
Yildizbas, S., 263
Yilmaz, S., 263
Yiotakis, J., 203, 433
Yiu, E. M-L., 96, 98, 102, 105, 124*t*, 175–176, 179–180, 294
Ylitalo, R., 289
Ylvisaker, M., 110–111
Yonekawa, H., 286
Yoon, M. S., 338
Yorkston, K. M., 110, 179, 180, 195, 310, 328, 335, 339
Yoshimi, R., 284
Young, B., 409
Younger, R. M., 51–52
Ysunza, A., 158
Ytterberg, M., 326
Yu-Chun, C., 246
Yumoto, E., 240, 335
Yun, K. I., 288, 289
Yun, Y-S., 284, 286, 435

Zackai, E. H., 258
Zagolski, O., 156
Zalzal, G. H., 248, 251, 256, 260
Zanetti, F., 428
Zargi, M., 430
Zawadski, D. K., 407
Zawadzka-Glos, L., 250, 251, 252, 253
Zeiss, D., 203
Zeitels, S., 144*t*, 145, 195, 199, 203, 204, 208, 221, 290, 291, 292, 423, 432, 433
Zelazny, S. K., 401, 402*t*, 406, 407
Zemlin, W., 60
Zetterstrom, O., 391
Zhang, F., 208, 221–222
Zhang, S. P., 56
Zhang, W., 15
Zhou, R., 33, 218
Zhou, X. P., 250
Zinman, L., 316
Zipoli, R. P., 110
Zormeier, M. M., 449, 455
Zorowka, P., 433
Zoumalan, R., 386–387, 387
Zraick, R. I., 125, 126, 133, 148
Zuberbuhle, K., 59, 60
Zur, K. B., 124*t*, 126, 128*t*, 252, 255
Zuur, J. K., 439, 440, 440*t*, 441
Zwirner, P., 71

Subject Index

Note: Page numbers followed by *f* indicate figures; page numbers followed by *t* indicate tables; page numbers in **bold** refer to images shown in the color insert.

Abdominal trussing, 180–181
Accountability, and EBP, 110
Acetylcholine (ACh), declines in, 313
  and anticholinesterase agents, 314
Acoustic analysis, 145–153
  advantages/disadvantages of, 151–153, 152*t*
  devices for, 145
Acoustic effects, 79–81, 107
Acoustic instrumentation, 318
Acoustic terms, common, 88–90, 89*t*
Acquired subglottic stenosis (ASS), 251, 253
Activity limitations, defined, 97
Acute supraglottitis, 226
Adaptation period, 66
Adductor laryngeal breathing dystonia, 400
Adherence, defined, 188
Adult onset recurrent respiratory papillomatosis (AORRP), 267–268
Adults, 75–76, 230. *See also* Females; males
Aerodynamic measures, 157–158
Age and the aging voice
  auditory cues for, 81
  factors in, 77
  importance of, 83
  nodules, 281
  parameters of, 77*t*
  physiological changes with, 67
  structural changes in, 78–79
  and vocal production, 76–83
Air hunger, 384
Air intake, techniques of, 447–448
Air klunking, 449
Air pressure, measurement of, 50
Air volume, 157
Airflow rate, measures of, 157
Airways
  normal *vs.* asthmatic, 392*f*
  protection of, 57
  widening procedures for, 199–203
Alcohol
  abuse of, 442
  consumption, and laryngitis, 227, 228
  and laryngeal cancer, 426
Alveolar ducts, 6
Alveolar pressure, 10, 12
Alveolar sacs, 6
Amplitude, 89, 141
Amyotrophic lateral sclerosis, 82, 102, 338–340
Androgens, 74
Ansa cervicalis, 210
Anterior commissure, modification of, 374–375
Anterior cricoid split (ACS), 253, 255
Anterior macula flava, 28
Antihistamines, 99
Aphonia, 82, 87
Apnea of infancy (AOI), 71
Apoptosis, 218
Arthritis, cricoarytenoid, 239
Artificial larynx (AL)
  advantages and disadvantages of, 445–447
  available products, 445–447
  hands-free, 446–447
  intelligibility, 444–445
  types of, 444
  use of, 443
Aryepiglottic folds, 16, 25
Arytenoid cartilages, 21
Arytenoid adduction/arytenopexy, 199, 200*f*
Assessments
  aims of, 116
  auditory-perceptual measurements, 133
  clinical indications for, 164
  clinical processes for, 164
  disadvantages of, 133
  documentation of, 165
  protocols for SD, 331
  safety in, 165
  scales for, 130–134
  setting for, 165
  three-tier for MTD, 357–359
  of voice, 163
Asthma
  and air hunger, 384
  cough variant asthma (CVA), 391, 408–409
  defined, 391
  diagnosis of PVFM as, 396
  evaluation and treatment of, 392–395
  prevalence of, 391
  and PVFM, 398*t*, 400–401
Ataxic dysarthria, 317–318
Athletes, breathing techniques for, 406
Auditory-perceptual evaluations, use of, 91–92
Autoimmune diseases, 239–241, 315
Autologous cellular therapy (ACT), 209
Autologous fat, 208–209, 222

Background noise, effect of, 295–296
Balloon dilation, 256
Basal ganglia, 55–56
Basement membrane zone (BMZ), 31, 293
Basic training gesture, 185
Behavior change, transtheoretical model of, 192
Behavioral voice therapy, 170–188, 190, 365, 371–374
Bernoulli's principle, 46–47
Bilateral vocal fold paralysis, 311–313
Biofeedback, 145, 179–180, 180, 407
Blepharospasm, 210
Blom/Singer technique, 450
Body functions, defined, 96–97
Borg Scale of Perceived Exertion, 386*t*
Bradycardia, 71
Bradykinesia, 319
Brain, postmortem studies of, 328–329
Brain centers in respiration, 15
Breathiness, 75–76, 81, 87
Breathing techniques, 406
Bronchi, 6
Bronchial challenge tests, 391, 392–393, 403
Bronchioles, 6
Bronchitis, eosinophilic, 409
Bronchoprovocation, 391, 392–393
Broyle's ligament, 28

Calcium hydroxylapatite (CaHA), 209
Cancer, **35–36**
demographic factors in, 422–423
diagnosis of, 427
ethnic and demographic factors in, 422
glottal, 422–423, 422*f*
head and neck cancers (HNC), 421
laryngeal
evaluation and staging of, 423–426
five-year survival rate, 422
interdisciplinary team members, 427–428*t*
new cases of, 421
number of, 421
risk factors for, 426
surgical options for, 431–442
symptoms of, 426–427
and laryngeal cysts, 264
medical treatment of, 428–431
multidisciplinary approach to, 427–428
Carbon dioxide (CO_2), and air hunger, 384
Cartilage, 78
Cartilage, maturation of, 67–68
Cartilaginous glottis, 36
Cartilaginous stenosis, 250
Case histories, 116–129
form for adults, 118–120*t*
form for children, 120–122*t*
interview, 122–123
Caseness, defined, 353
Catechol-O-methyltransferase (COMT), 322
Central fatigue, 292
Cerebellum, 56–57, 317–318
Chant therapy, 181
Chemoradiation, 429–430
Chemotherapy, 429–430
Chest wall, 6, 15
Chewing technique, 182
Children. *See also* Infants
and airway widening procedures, 201, 203
breathing of, 66
dysphonia in, 233, 235
and endoscopy, 145
F0 of, 47, 72–73*t*, 72–74
and GERD/LPR, 228–229, 247
grading scale of pediatric nodules, 282*t*
and JORRP, 267
and laryngomalacia, 246–248
and LM, 178*t*
and MTD, 356, 359–360
and proton pump inhibitors, 237
quality of life issues of, 126, 128–129
and subglottic stenosis, 249–258
treatment of, 193–194
vocal maturation of, 72–74
Cholinesterase inhibitors, use of, 315–316
Chorea, 326–327
Cidofovir, 273
Clinical management
strategies for, 170
team for, 166–170
CO_2 lasers, use of, 199, 248, 253, 270–271
Cognitive behavioral therapy, 359, 363
Collagen, 31, 206–207
Compliance, 237
Confidential voice, defined, 185
Conflict, and conversation disorders, 360
Congenital subglottic stenosis (CSS), 250–251
Connective tissue, 31
Consensus Auditory-Perceptual Evaluation of Voice (CAPE-V), 131–133, 132*t*
Contact ulcers, 288–290
Continuous positive air pressure (CPAP), 405
Control, loss of vocal, 79
Conus elasticus, 25
Conversation disorders, 360–362
Conversion disorders, 398–399
Coping, and coping strategies, 126, 442
Corniculate cartilages, 21
Corticospinal pathway, 53–54
Corticobulbar (corticonuclear) pathway, 53–54
Cough bouts, 408
Cough-Specific Quality of Life Questionnaire, 413, 414*t*
Cough variant asthma (CVA), 408–409
Coughing, and speaking valves, 454
Coughs
and ACE inhibitors, 408
acute *vs.* chronic, 408
behavioral treatment for, 413–415
causes of, 408–410, 409*t*
challenges for, 410
chronic, 407–416
complications of, 410, 411
diagnosis and evaluation, 410–413
and larynx function, 16–17
nonspecific/idiopathic chronic, 410
outcomes of interventions for, 416
patient interview protocol for, 412
psychogenic, 409
quantifying, 413
refractory CC, 410
strategies for reduction, 415*t*
symptoms of chronic, 410, 411
treatment of, 413–416
triggers for, 408, 415
Cover-body modes of vocal folds, 35, 35*f*
Cranial nerves, role of, 57
Cricoarytenoid arthritis (CA), 239, 240–241
Cricoarytenoid joint, 21, 24*f*
ankylosed, 241
Cricoid cartilage, 20
and anterior cricoid split (ACS), 253, 255
articular facets of, 22*f*
Cricothyroid (CT) joint, and rheumatoid arthritis, 241
Cricothyroid joints, 21
Cricotracheal membrane, 20
Cross-linked collagen, 207
Croup, 226, 229. *See also* Coughs
Cul de sac resonance, 88
Cultural and linguistic competency, 103–104, 104*t*
Culture
anatomic and acoustic factors related to, 106–107
and management of voice disorders, 106
and vocal health, 102–107
Cuneiform cartilages, 21
Cyanosis, 71
Cysts, **25–27**
congenital *vs.* acquired, 264
epidermoid, 264
marsupialization of, 264–265
retention, 263–264
subglottic, 264
and voice rest, 176
Cytokines, 216

Data, validity of, 151–152
Decibels, 89
Decorin, 33, 216
Deep brain stimulation (DBS), 323, 338
Deep layer of the lamina propria (DLLP), 33
Depression, effect of, 353
Diagnosis, disclosure of, 459
Diagnostic and Statistical Manual of Mental Disorders, 4th edition, 360
Diagnostic reports, 158–162, 159–162*f*
Diaphragm, 6, 10, 10*f*, 180
Diet
and cancer risk, 126
and GERD/LPR, 106, 176
modifications in, 236*t*
and vocal health, 106, 235–236
Dilation, defined, 261
Diplophonia, defined, 87
Diplopia, 314
Disabilities, 96, 104–105
Discrepancy, 192
Dopamine, 318, 320
Double-probe 24-hour ambulatory pH monitoring, 230–232, 231*f*, 233
Down syndrome, and subglottic stenosis, 251
Duty cycle, 47
Dynamic range, 90, 149
Dysarthrias
ataxic, 317–318
classification system for, 304*t*
defined, 99
flaccid, 304–316
hyperkinetic, 326–338
hypokinetic, 318–325
mixed, 338–342
Dysphonias
causes of, 90, 213
childhood, 93–94, 193
defined, 49, 87
functional dysphonia (FD), 183, 362–363
and laryngeal cancer, 426–427
muscle tension dysphonia (MTD), 232, 355–360
comprehensive evaluation protocol for, 358*t*
defined, 135–136, 355–356

diagnosis and evaluation of, 357–359
primary *vs.* secondary, 356
vs. SD, 330, 359
symptoms of, 356–357
muscular tension *vs.* spasmodic dysphonia, 330
mutational, 363
and myasthenia gravis, 314
perceptual terms for, 87–88, 88*t*
relation to self and identity, 352*t*
spasmodic dysphonia (SD), 130, 135, 210, 328–337
abductor spasmodic dysphonia, 210, 329–330
adductor SD (ADSD), 142, 210, 329
cause of, 328–329
defined, 328
diagnosis and evaluation of, 330–332
mixed, 330
vs. MTD, 359
screening questions for, 333*t*
speech exam findings expected for, 333*t*
surgical treatment for, 332, 334
symptoms of, 353
treatment for, 332, 334–337
tremor with, 330
types of, 329–330
treating long-term, 188
and vocal fold scars, 221–222
Dyspnea
contributing factors to, 385
defined, 88, 384
evaluation of, 385
severity scale of, 385*t*
and vocal fold paralysis, 308
Dystonias, 56, 327–328

Easy onset technique, 182
Eating, after total laryngectomy, 441–442
Ecchymosis, 291
Echinacoside, 207–208
Ectasias, defined, 290–291
Education
effect of voice impairment on, 193*t*, 194
and patient outcome, 458–459
Effort closure techniques, 181–182
EGG quotients, 156*f*
Elastic membrane, 25
Elastin fibers, 31
Electrical pacing, of bilateral abductor paralysis, 313
Electroglottography (EGG), 153–156
Electrolaryngology (electroglottography), 153–156
Empathy, expressing, 192
End-expiratory level (EEL), 12
Endoscopy, 134–137
advantages/disadvantages of, 144–145
in evaluation of vocal fold paralysis, 308–309
and nodules, 282
phonatory tasks used in, 135–136, 136*t*
and subglottic stenosis, 252–253
use of in biofeedback, 179
Endotracheal intubation, and subglottic stenosis, 251
Entry and Exit Criteria for School-Based Therapy Services, Oxford Public Schools, Massachusetts, 194
Environmental pollutants, 296
Eosinophils, 409
Epiglottis, 20–21
Epithelium, 28, 30–31, 78–79
Erythematous, defined, 216
Esophageal speech (ES), 443, 447–449
Esophagitis, 227
Essential tremor (ET), 337–338
Essential tremor of the voice (ETV), 337–338
Estrogens, 74, 76
Ethnic and linguistic groups, 106–107
Evaluations
auditory-perceptual, 129–134, 130*t*
process of, 116
Evidence-based practice (EBP), 2, 107, 109–111
Exhalation, 12, 14–15
Expiration, accessory muscles for, 12*t*
Expiratory reserve volume (ERV), 12, 64–65*f*
External laryngoceles, 262
Extracel-LG, 208
Extracellular matrix (ECM), 31, 32*f*, 32*t*, 216, 218
Extrapyramidal tract, 54–55
Extrinsic membranes, 26*f*

False (ventricular) vocal folds, 16, 27–28, 29*f*
Fat, autologous, 208
Fat grafts, 224*f*
Fat injection and fascia transplantation (FIFT), 224–225
Females, 422–423. *See also* Gender
and age-related vocal changes, 77
and conversion disorders, 361
F0 changes with aging, 79–80, 80*t*
F0 of, 47, 185
and myasthenia gravis, 313–314
prescribed medications of, 98
quality of life for laryngectomized, 459
risk of voice disorders, 298
and vascular lesions, 291
voice of, 76
Fetal cell transplantation, 323
Fiberoptic Endoscopic Evaluation of Swallowing (FEES), 309
Fiberoptic Endoscopic Evaluation of Swallowing with Sensory Testing (FEESST), 309
Fibroblasts, 31, 216
Fibronectin (FN), 33
Fibrous proteins, 31
Fistulas, in tracheoesophageal puncture, 450
Fixation of the chest, 17
Flaccid dysarthria, 304–316
Flow-volume loops (FVL), 389, 390*f*, 403, 404*f*
Forced expiratory volume, comparison to forced vital capacity, 389
Forced vital capacity and forced expiratory volume, reductions in, 389*t*
Formant frequencies, raising, 372–373
Frequency measures, 145–148
Frequency variability, 89, 148
Functional residual capacity (FRC), 12, 64–65*f*
Fundamental frequency (F0)
and age, 148
average for different age groups, 146–147*t*
defined, 47, 89
differences in by age and cultural/linguistic groups, 108–109*t*
and esophageal speech, 447
and gender identity, 371–372
and language, 107
measurement of, 146
and pitch, 50
and pitch-raising treatment, 375
standard deviation in, 80–81
and TE speech, 455–456
Fungal infections, from corticosteroids, 394

Gardasil, 274
Gas exchange, 6, 12, 260
Gastroesophageal reflux disease (GERD)
causes of, 106, 176, 227, 228*t*
in children, 247
and contact ulcers/granulomas, 289
and H2 blockers, 236
and laryngitis, 227–229
and laryngomalacia, 247
vs. LES, 227*t*
medications for, 101
and menopause, 77
and nodules, 280
pH findings for, 232
and RRP, 274
and stress, 354
and stridor, 387
treatment of, 235–239
and voice disorders, 90
Gender. *See also* Females; males
and age-related changes, 77
changing of, 366–367
and development of vocal problems, 296
frequency differences in, 372–373
nonverbal markers of, 376–377
and vocal cues, 81–82, 371–372
Gender identity disorder, 365–366, 366*t*, 368*t*
Gestures, facial/bodily, 449
Glossopharyngeal press, 448
Glottal dysplasia/leukoplakia, 204
Glottal Function Index (GFI), 133, 133*t*
Glottic closure, evaluation of, 141
Glottic insufficiency, 204, 206–207
Glottic stenosis. *See* Laryngeal web
Glottis
composition of, 35–36
and respiration, 16
shape of, 36*f*, 47, 48*f*
Glutamate, effect of, 338–339

Glycoproteins, 31
Gore-Tex, use of in thyroplasty, 197
Granulation, 206–207, 289
Granulomas, **22–24**
  defined, 288–289
  illustrated, 288*f*
  laser microsurgery for, 203, 204
  symptoms of, 289
  treatment for, 179
GRBAS voice rating scale, 131*t*, 209, 363

Hanbang, 104–105
Handicap, defined, 96
Harmonics-to-noise ratios (HNR), 74, 150–151
Harry Benjamin International Gender Dysphoria Association (HBIGDA), 367
Harshness, defined, 87
Hawking, Stephen, 338
Head and neck cancers (HNC), 421
Health status
  and age-related vocal diseases, 82
  determining, 122
  and MPFR, 148
  perception of, 106
Heartburn, 227
Heat and moisture exchangers (HME), 440–441
Heat shock protein (HSP), 274
Heliox, use of, 404
Hemisiderosis/hemosiderin, 291
Hemorrhage, **28–30**
Hepatocyte growth factor (HGA), 208
Hernias, 262
High-speed digital imaging (HSDI), 145
Histamine receptor antagonists (H2 blockers), 236–237
Hoarseness, and pregnancy, 76
Hoehn and Yahr Staging of Parkinson's disease (H&Y), 319, 320*t*
Hormones
  effects of, 101–102
  and the female voice, 76
  and growth regulation, 74
  and the male voice, 74–75
  and vocal fold lesions, 291
Human papillomavirus (HPV), 266, 274
Huntington's disease, 151, 326–327, 327*t*
Hyaluronic acid (HA) (hyaluronan), 33, 207–208, 216
Hyoid bone, 18
Hyperalgesia, and cough, 409
Hypercapnia, 248
Hyperkeratosis, 226
Hyperkinetic dysarthria, 326–338, 337
Hypernasality, defined, 88
Hypokinesia, defined, 318
Hypokinetic dysarthria, 318–325
Hypoxia, 248

Images, interpretation of, 145
Imaging, high-speed digital, 145
Imaging of vocal tract, 138–140*t*
Immunoglobulins, 316
Impairments, defined, 96, 97
Implants, vocal fold medialization, 197*f*
Indirect laryngoscopy, 134
Individuals with Disabilities Education Improvement Act (IDEIA), 193
Indole-3-carbinol (I3C), 272–273
Infants. *See also* Children
  apnea of infancy (AOI), 71
  F0 of, 70, 71
  intubation of, 251
  and laryngoceles, 262
  premature, 251
  removal of cysts from, 264–265
  and stridor, 387
  symptoms of subglottic stenosis, 250
  vocalizations of, 70–71
Inflammation, defined, 215, 216
Inhalation, 10, 12
  muscle activity for, 14
Injection augmentation (medialization thyroplasty), 305, 310–311
  outcomes studies for, 311
Injection laryngoplasty/vocal fold augmentation, 204–210, 310
  materials used for, 206*t*
  outcomes studies, 209–210
Injection medialization, after resection, 433
Injections, materials used for, 204–209, 206*t*
Inspiration, 14
Inspiratory capacity (IC), 12, 64–65*f*
Instrumental measures, 134–145
  advantages of, 134
Insufflation, 447
Intelligibility, 444–445, 448
Intensity
  average, 89–90, 149
  in elderly speakers, 81
  levels, 89
  measures of, 149
  regulation of, 52
  variability of, 90
Interferon (IFN), 272, 341–342
Intermediate layer (lamina propria) (ILLP), 33
Internal laryngoceles, 262
International Classification of Functioning, Disability, and Health (ICF), 96–98, 97*t*
Interstitial proteins, 33
Intonation characteristics, 107
  and gender identity, 373
Intravenous immunoglobulin, 316
Intubation
  and granulomas, 289
  and laryngeal webs, 260
Intubation, endotracheal, 251
Inverse phonation, 337

Jaw, muscles in, 314
Jitter
  defined, 90
  measures of, 150, 151
Joints, aging of, 78
Juvenile onset recurrent respiratory papillomatosis (JORRP), 267

Keels, silicon, 261–262
Keratin, in cysts, 263
Korean culture, and disability, 104–105

La belle indifference, 360
Lamina densa, 31
Lamina lucida, 31
Lamina propria
  and ACT, 209
  aging of, 78–79
  composition of, 31, 218
  layers of, 33
  sulci in, 221
Laryngeal atresia, 258
Laryngeal cysts, 263–264, 263*f*
Laryngeal electromyography (LEMG), 158, 159*t*, 179–180, 227, 305, 309
Laryngeal functions, 57, 59, 81
Laryngeal hydration, 1–2, 415
Laryngeal manual therapy (LMT), 177–178, 178*t*
Laryngeal massage (LM), 177–179, 359, 362
Laryngeal reinnervation (LR), 210–211, 311
Laryngeal saccule, 28
Laryngeal structure, changes with aging, 78–79
Laryngeal system, anatomy and physiology of, 17–28
Laryngeal tension, reduction of, 359
Laryngeal ventricle, 28, 29*f*
Laryngeal web/glottic stenosis, 258–262
  acquired, 259–260
  classification of, 260, 260*t*
  congenital, 258–259
  illustrated, 259*f*
  posterior glottic stenosis (PGS), 260–261
  treatment for, 261–262
Laryngectomy bibs, 440
Laryngitis, **6–7**, 215, 225–239
  acute, 226
  causes of, 225, 225*f*, 226
  chronic, 226–227
  from steroid inhalers, 393–395
Laryngoceles, 262–263
  classification of, 262
Laryngofissure, 255
Laryngomalacia
  abnormalities associated with, 246
  cause of, 247
  evaluation and treatment of, 247–248
  illustrated, 246*f*
  and LPR, 229
  and stridor, 385, 386–387
  symptoms of, 247
Laryngopharyngeal reflux (LPR)
  causes of, 106, 176, 228*t*
  in children, 247
  clinical signs and symptoms of, 230

diagnosis and evaluation of, 229–235
vs. GERD, 227–239, 227*t*
and nodules, 280
and pH monitoring, 230–232
problems associated with, 229*t*
and proton pump inhibitors, 236–237
and PVFM, 398
and RRP, 274
vs. steroid inhaler laryngitis, 393
and stridor, 387
treatment of, 235–239
Laryngoscopy
direct, 134
use of, 247, 401–402
Larynx
artificial (AL), 443, 444–447
augmentation procedures for, 255
cartilages of, 19*f*
causes of injuries to, 228
diagnostic manipulation of, 357
folds within, 25–28, 27*f*
framework of, 17–21, 17*t*
functions of, 16–17
in infancy and childhood, 67–70
infant, 68*t*
joints of, 21–22
maturation of, 69*f*
membranes and folds of, 25*t*
membranes of, 22–23, 25
muscles of, 37–45
nervous system control of, 52–59
position in neck, 6, 16*f*, 67
soft tissues of, 22–23, 25
views of, 20*f*
Lasers, types of, 203
Leakage, around TEP site, management of, 452
Lee Silverman Voice Treatment (LSVT), 110, 318, 324–325
Leukoplakia, 203, 286–288, 287*f*
Lifestyle
modifications in, 236*t*
and vocal health, 235–236
and vocal hygiene programs, 175, 176
Loft register, 60
Longitudinal phase difference, 49
Lou Gehrig's disease, 338–340
Loudness, 51–52, 130
Lower esophageal sphincter (LES), 227
Lower motor neurons (LMN), 304, 338
Lumen, defined, 6
Lung volumes and capacities, 12, 13*t*, 64–65*f*, 67, 181
Lungs, 6–7
Lx waveforms, 153–155, 153*f*, 154–155*f*
Lymph nodes, removal of, 439
Lysis, defined, 261

Macrophages, 216
Males. *See also* Gender
and conversion disorders, 361
F0 of, 47, 74
and mutational falsetto, 363–364
voice changes in, 75*t*

Manual circumlaryngeal therapy (MCT), 177–179, 178*t*
Masked facies, 319
Maximum phonation time (MPT), 129, 198, 209
Maximum phonational frequency range (MPFR), 89, 148
Medial thyrohyoid ligament, 23
Medialization thyroplasty (injection augmentation), 305
Medications
for ALS, 340
angiotensin converting enzyme (ACE) inhibitors, and coughs, 408
antianxiety, 405
anticholinergics, 322
antihistamines, 226
antihypertensives, 99, 101
antireflux, 236–239
antisecretory drugs, 101
antispasmodics, 317
antitussives, effect of, 99
and asthma corticosteroids, 394
Botox injections
advantages of, 335
and essential tremor, 338
guidance for, 158
for mutational falsetto, 365
outcomes studies, 335
and PVFM, 405
to reduce spasms, 449
for SD, 334–335
use of, 209, 290, 312–313, 317
COMT inhibitors, 322
corticosteroids
effects of, 101, 226
fungal infections from, 394
inhaled, 393
laryngeal signs and symptoms related to, 394*t*
and MS, 341
use of, 239, 290
effects on hydration, 175
effects on the voice, 98–102, 100–101*t*, 151
for essential tremor (ET), 337–338
expectorants (mucolytics), effect of, 99
and GERD/LPR, 176
H2 blockers (histamine receptor antagonists), 236–237
levodopa (L-dopa) and Parkinson's disease, 320–322
monoamine oxidase inhibitors (MAOIs), 322–323
for MS, 341–342
mucolytics (expectorants), 99, 175, 226
neuroleptics (neurologic medications), 102
for Parkinson's disease, 320–323
Meige's syndrome, 328
Membranous glottis, 36
Membranous stenosis, 250
Menopause, and vocal production, 77
Mentation, Behavior, and Mood (MBM) scales, 319–320

Metastasis, 423
Microdebriders/microdebrider excision, 271
Microsurgery, laser, 203–204
Modal register, 60
Motivational interviewing (MI), 190–192, 191*t*
Mouse units (Us), 210
Movement disorders, causes of, 303
MRC Breathlessness Scale, 386*t*
Mucosal wave, 47, 49
evaluation of, 141
Mucus, function of, 6
Multicultural issues, 2, 102–103
Multiphasic closure, 60
Multiple sclerosis, 102, 340–342, 341
Muscle-nerve-muscle (MNM) neurotization, 211
Muscles
adductor and abductor, 43*f*
aging of, 78
aryepiglottic, 25
cricothyroid (CT), 41–43, 44*f*
dysfunctional activity of, 59
external intercostal, 10
extrinsic laryngeal, 38, 39*f*, 40*t*
infrahyoid, 38, 210
for inspiration, 12*t*
interarytenoid (IA), 40
intrinsic laryngeal, 38, 39–45, 41*f*, 42*t*
of the larynx, 37–45
lateral cricoarytenoid (LCA), 40, 313
posterior cricoarytenoid (PCA), 40–41
of respiration, accessory, 12*t*
skeletal, 37*f*
slow *vs.* fast twitch, 38
strap, 38
thyroarytenoid (TA), 28, 43–45, 45*f*, 78
type I and type II fibers, 38*t*
vocal fold, 33
Mutational falsetto, 183, 193, 363–365
Myasthenia gravis (MG), 102, 313–316
Myer-Cotton system, 249–250
Myoelastic-aerodynamic theory of phonation, 45–52, 46*f*
Myofibroblasts, 216, 218
Myofilaments, 37
Myxomatous material, in polyps, 285

Nasal breathing, 175
Nasal emission, defined, 88
Nasal passageways, air conditioning function of, 439–440
Nasoendoscopy, 135
National Center for Evidence-Based Practice, 100
Nerve damage, and vocal paralysis, 307
Neurologic disorders, and PVFM, 400
Nodules, **13–14**
and accent therapy, 184
causes of, 280
evaluation/treatment of, 282–283
examination of, 134
histology of, 280–281
illustration, 281*f*

Nodules (*continued*)
laser microsurgery for, 203
pediatric grading scale, 282*t*
vs. polyps, 283–284, 284*t*
symptoms of, 282
Noncompliance, reasons for, 189*t*
Nucleus ambiguus (NA), 54
Nucleus retroambiguus (NRA), 56

Obstructive lung diseases, 389
Obstructive sleep apnea, and vocal fold paralysis, 312
Occupational risk of laryngeal disease, 106, 294–298
Odynophagia, 226
Odynophonia, 226
Organ preservation therapy, 428
voice and swallowing following, 430
Oromandibular dystonia, 210
Otolaryngologists, 91–92, 116
Outcome studies, PPIs, 237
Outcomes, expected, 163
Oxford Public Schools, Massachusetts, Entry and Exit Criteria for School-Based Therapy Services, 194

Painkillers, effect on voice of, 99
Papillomas, **10–12,** 144, 170, 265–266
Paradoxical vocal fold motion (PVFM)
acute attacks of, 404–405
alleviating of, 405*t*
and asthma, 400–401
vs. asthma, 398*t*
causes of, 398–400, 399*t*, 400
and chronic cough, 409–410
defined, 395
diagnosis and evaluation of, 401–403
evaluation questions for, 402*t*
examination of, 135
irritant/exercise-induced, 400*t*
long-term treatment of, 405–407
symptoms of, 395–398, 397*t*
terms used for, 396*t*
treatment of, 403–407
triggers for, 397*t*
Paralysis
bilateral, **33–34**
unilateral, **31–32**
Paralysis, adductor, 312
Paresis, 130, 304
Parietal pleura, 9
Parkinson's disease
defined, 318
medications used for, 102, 322*t*
prevalence of, 82
staging of, 319–320
surgical treatment of, 323
treatment of, 320–325
vocal symptoms of, 148, 158, 319
voice therapy for, 323–325
Pars oblique, 41–43
Pars recta, 41–43

Patients
compliance of, 188–192
education of, 175, 406
during endoscopic examinations, 137
establishing relationship with, 368–369
first meeting with, 103
increasing motivation of, 191–192
motivation of, 190–191
support available to, 458–459
Pediatric Voice Handicap Index, 127–128*t*
Perceived phonatory effort, 293
Periodicity/regularity, evaluation of, 141
Peripheral fatigue, 293
Periaqueductal grey (PAG), 56
Personality
and conversion disorders, 361
and functional dysphonia, 362–363, 363*t*
and nodules, 281
pH monitoring, 230–232, 231*f*, 233
Phase closure, 141
Phase symmetry, evaluation of, 141
Phonation
cerebellum and subcortical areas involved in, 55*f*
cortical areas involved in, 54*f*
in infants, 71
and the larynx, 17
nervous system structures involved in, 53*t*
neural control of, 199
time of, 294–295
Phonation threshold pressure (PTP), 49–50, 49*f*, 293–294
Phonosurgery, 195–211
Phonotrauma, 279, 280
Phonotraumatic behaviors, 93, 171–172
Physical appearance, and gender perception, 377
Physiological sulcus (Type I), 221
Pitch, 50
assessment of, 130
contributors to, 51*f*
control of, 22
differences in production of, 60
establishing new, 182–183
modification of, 50–51, 372
optimum, 182–183
for trans speakers, 371–372
Pitch breaks, during puberty, 74
Pitch glides, 186, 188
Plasmaphoresis (plasma exchange), 316
Pleural fluid, 9
Pleural linkage, 8–9, 9*f*
Pleural space, 9
Polyps, **15–18**
classification of, 284–285
defined, 283–284
examination of, 134
fibrotic/hyaline, 284–285
hemorrhagic, 284–285
histology of, 284–285
illustration of, 283*f*
importance of treating, 95
vs. nodules, 283–284, 284*t*
symptoms of, 285

translucent, 284
treatment of, 285–286
"Position Statement on Evidence-Based Practice" (ASHA), 109
Posterior glottic stenosis (PGS), 260–261
Posterior macula flava, 28
Posttraumatic stress syndrome, 361
Posture, 180, 183, 357
Preferred practice patterns, 163–165
Pregnancy, 76, 267–268
Premenstrual vocal syndrome, 76
Prepubertal voice change, 74–75
Presbyphonia, 83
Prevention
activities for, 94–95
primary, 93
secondary, 95
terminology of, 94*t*
tertiary, 95
Primary progressive MS, 341
Principles of Ethics, ASHA, 367
Procedures
for acute CA rheumatoid arthritis, 241
anterior commissure, 374–375
arytenoidectomy, 199, 201*f*
cordectomy (resection), 432–433
cordotomy, transverse, 200–201
cricoarytenoid approximation (CTA), 374
cricohyoidoepiglottopexy (CHEP), 435
cricohyoidopexy (CHP), 435
cricotracheal resection (CTR), 256, 257*f*
endoscopic techniques, 239
endoscopic vocal fold shortening, 374
epiglottopexy, 248
fundoplication, 238*f*, 239
for GERD/LPR, 239
glottoplasty, 374–375
for granulomas, 290
for laryngeal webs, 261–262
laryngectomies, 151, 431, 431*t*
laryngotracheal reconstruction (LTR), 253–256, 254*f*, 254*t*
larynx, augmentation for, 255
laser microsurgery, 203–204
585-nm pulsed dye laser (PDL), 271
advantages/disadvantages of, 204
office-based, 203
laser resection, 432
lateral thyrotomy, 264–265
and leukoplakia, 288
for mutational falsetto, 365
near total laryngectomy (NTL), 435, 436
nerve grafts, 211
Nissen fundoplication, 239
for nodules, 283
office-based, 203
pallidotomy, 323
and polyps, 286
problems related to, 439–442
pulsed dye laser, 204
pulsed dye laser procedures, 204
to raise F0, 374–376
relaxation thyroplasty, 365
and RRP, 268, 270–271

sex reassignment (SRS), 367
single stage *vs.* staged, 255
supracricoid laryngectomy (SCL), 435–436
thymectomies, 316, 338
thyroplasty
advantages/disadvantages of, 197–198, 198*t*
implant materials used for, 197
outcomes studies for, 198–199, 311
Type I (medialization), 195–199, 196*f*
Type III (relaxation thyroplasty), 365
total laryngectomy, 436–439, 436*f*
consequences of, 439–440*t*
tracheoesophageal puncture (TEP), 450
advantages of, 454
and intelligibility and quality of speech, 455–456
patient selection for, 454
primary *vs.* secondary, 450
problems with, 455
prosthesis insertion for, 451–452
transplants, for fascia, 222, 224–225
as treatment for sulcus vocalis, 222–225
for UVFP, 310–311
for vocal fold lesions, 292
and vocal fold paralysis, 306–307
and vocal fold scaring, 219–220
voice quality following, 256, 258
Progesterone, 76
Progressive muscle relaxation (PMR), 176–177, 359
Progressive-relapsing MS, 341
Prokinetics, 237, 239
Prolonged intubation, 251
Prosthesis, indwelling, 452
Prosthesis, voice, 453*f*
Proteoglycans, 31
Proton pump inhibitors (PPIs), 101, 236–237
and children, 237
outcome studies for, 237
Ptosis, eyelid, 313, 314
Puberphonia, 363
Puberty, vocal changes during, 74–75
Pulmonary function testing (PFT), 387–391, 403*t*
Pulmonary stretch receptors (PSRs), 15
Pulse oximetry, 391, 403
Pulse register, 60
Pyramidal tract, 53–54

Quadrangular membrane, 25
Quadrate lamina, 20
Quality of life (QOL)
and acoustic measures, 152–153
after Botox injections, 335–336
after surgery, 457–459
after total laryngectomy, 458*t*, 459
assessment of, 123–129
for children, 126, 128–129
and communication, 459
defined, 96
instruments for, 124*t*, 413, 414*t*
and LPR, 234*t*, 235

Radiation therapy (RT), 428–429, 429*t*
Radiofrequency ablation, 271
Rapidly adapting receptors (RARs), 15
Reciting tones, 181
Recurrent respiratory papillomatosis (RRP), 203
adult onset (AORRP), 267–268
assessment scale for, 269–270*t*
cost of, 270
diagnosis and evaluation, 268
and HPV, 266
illustrated, 265*f*
juvenile onset (JORRP), 267
nonsurgical adjuvant therapies for, 271–273, 272*t*
support groups for, 274
symptoms of, 268
treatment of, 268, 274
Reflexes, and laryngeal functions, 57, 59
Reflux, **8–9,** 253
Reflux finding score (RFS), 232–235, 232*t*
Reflux Symptom Index (RSI), 233–235, 233*t*
Registers, 59*t*, 60
Reinke's edema, **19–21**
condition of, 284, 285
laser microsurgery for, 203
symptoms of, 156, 285
Reinke's space, 33
Relapsing polychondritis (RP), 240
Relapsing-remitting MS, 341
Relaxation techniques, 176–177
Relaxed throat breathing, 406, 407*t*
Religion, influence of, 104–105
Repetitive stimulation test (RST), 314
Resection (cordectomy), 432–433
Residual volume (RV), 12, 64–65*f*
Resistance, rolling with, 192
Resonance, 52
Resonant voice, defined, 184
Respiration
accessory muscles for, 11*f*, 12*t*
and the CT muscle, 43
cycle of, 10–12
nervous system control of, 15
ratio of time for inhalation and exhalation, 14
Respiratory-phonatory coordination, 180–181
Respiratory support, increasing, 180–181
Respiratory system, 6–15
Resting expiratory level (REL), 12, 15
Resting tidal breathing, rib cage contribution to, 66*t*
Resting tidal volume (RTV), 64–65*f*
Revised El Escorial Criteria, 339, 340*t*
Rheumatoid arthritis (RA), 240–241
diagnosis and evaluation of, 241
treatment of, 241
Rib cage, and speech breathing, 15
Risk factors, occupational, 294–296

S/z ratio, 129
Safety in assessments, 165
Scales, patient self-perception, 133–134
Scanning speech, 318
Scar remodeling, 218
Scarring
vocal fold, 218–220, 219*t*
vocal fold injections for, 223*f*
Scars, 135
vocal fold, 170
Scars/scarring, 204, 207, 218
and autologous fat injections, 208
causes of, 219*t*
and surgery, 261
Sebum, in cysts, 263
Secondary progressive MS, 341
Self-concept, and voice, 351
Self-efficacy, 192
Semioccluded vocal tracts, 186
Sex reassignment surgery (SRS), 367
Sexual orientation, terminology related to, 368*t*
Shimmer
defined, 90
measures of, 150, 151
Signal-to-noise ratio (SNR), 90, 150–151
Silastic, use of in thyroplasty, 197
Singing, vocal registers in, 59
Smell, loss of, 442
Smith accent method, 184*t*
Smoking
and laryngeal cancer, 423, 426
and laryngitis, 225, 226, 227, 228
and Reinke's edema, 285
vocal health, 235
Somatic compliance, 361
Somatoform disorders, defined, 360
Sonorants, production of, 448
Sounds, high *vs.* low pressure, 448
Spastic dysarthria, 316–317
Speaking fundamental frequency (SFF), 89, 146, 183
Speaking valves, 452, 454
Speech
after surgery, 457*t*
cultural norms of, 102–103, 105
and dyspnea, 384
esophageal, 447–449
rate of, 81, 447, 448, 456
of TE speech, 455–456
tracheoesophageal, 450–456
variability in, 148
Speech breathing
and artificial larynxes, 445
development and maturation of, 63–67
facilitating efficient, 181
vs. life breathing, 13–15, 14*t*
Speech-language pathologists, 442–443
and endoscopic imaging, 138
role of, 116
Speech production, registers in, 59
Speech symptom assessment protocol for ADSD, ABSD, and vocal tremor, 332*t*
Spirometry/spirometers, use of, 388

Spirometric measures and definitions, 388*t*
Sputum, defined, 440
Stenosis
  defined, 248–249
  membranous *vs.* cartilaginous, 250
  staging of, 249–250
  subglottic, 387
Stents, use of, 255
Stiffness *vs.* compliance, 35
Stoma blasts, 449
Stoma covers/guards, 440
Stomas, size and care of, 441
Stress
  and conversation disorders, 360
  defined, 353
  and dysphonia, 353
  effects of, 352, 353–355
  factors related to, 354*t*
  and MTD, 356
  and PVFM, 398
  signs and symptoms of, 355*t*
  tests for, 314
  and voice disorders, 90
Stress response, 354
Stridor
  biphasic, 385
  causes of, 386–387
  defined, 88, 385
  evaluation of, 387
  expiratory, 385
  in infants, 387
  and laryngomalacia, 247
  strategies for, 248
Stroboscopic Rating Form, 142–143*t*
Stroboscopy, 137–138, 144–145, 330
Stroma, in polyps, 285
Student teachers, 296–297
Studies, and EBP, 110
Subglottal air pressure (Ps), 46, 157–158
Subglottic stenosis, 248–258, 250*t*
  acquired (ASS), 251, 253
  in children, 69–70
  congenital (CSS), 250–251, 253
  evaluation of, 252–253
  illustrated, 249*f*
  laser treatment for, 254*f*
  and supraglottic compression, 252*t*
  surgical treatment for, 253–258
  symptoms of, 250
Substantia nigra, 56
Sulci, **5**, 221
Sulcus vergeture (Type II), 221
Sulcus vocalis
  cause of, 221
  fat grafts for, 224*f*
  symptoms and signs of, 221–222
  treatment for, 207, 222–225
  Type III, 221
  view of, 220*f*
Superficial lamina propria (SLP), 33, 290
Support groups
  for laryngectomized speakers, 459
  and RRP, 274
Supraglottal pressures, 47
Supraglottic activity, evaluation of, 142
Supraglottic laryngectomy (SGL), 434–435
Supraglottis, 28
Supraglottitis, 226
Supraglottoplasty, 248
Suprahyoids, 38
Surgeries. *See* Procedures
Swallowing
  after resection, 432–433
  after total laryngectomy, 441–442
  following resection, 432–433
  following VPL, 433–434
  and larynx function, 16
Syllables, accents on, 318
Synechias, 248
Synkinesis, 307
Synovial joint, 21
Systemic lupus erythematosus (SLE), 239

Tachypnea, 250
Teachers
  and background noise, 295–296
  experience of, 296–297
  and resonant voice therapy, 185
  risk factors for, 295*t*
  student, 297
  symptoms reported by, 296–297, 297*t*
  and vocal hygiene programs, 174–175
  and voice disorders, 294
Technology, advances in, 195
Telemedicine Satisfaction Questionnaire, 325
Telepractice, 325
Tensilon tests, 314
Terminology
  consistency in, 352
  to describe variations in gender, 366
  importance of, 368
  importance of consistent, 87
  for sexual orientation and gender identity disorder, 368*t*
Thalamotomy, 323
Thalamus, 56
Therapists, feedback for, 191
Therapy, dropout rate, 188–189
Therapy techniques
  accent method of, 183–184
  barriers to, 190
  breathing management, 405
  confidential voice, 185–186, 317
  direct, 179–183, 194
  direct *vs.* indirect, 170–171, 171*t*
  dropout rate, 188–189
  group therapy, 325
  holistic approaches to, 183–188, 359
  indirect, 171–179, 194
  individual *vs.* group, 456–457
  photodynamic therapy (PDT), 287–288
  resonant voice, 184–185
  resonant voice therapy, 184–185, 372
  semioccluded vocal tract, 186
  success rate of, 189
  vocal function exercises (VFE), 186–188, 187*t*
  voice therapy boot camp, 188
Thoracic cavity, defined, 6
Thymomas, 315
Thymus gland, hyperplastic, 315
Thyroarytenoid myectomy/myotomy, 336
Thyroid cartilage, 18
  effect of tilting, 24*f*
Thyrohyoid membrane, 18, 23, 25
Tidal volume (TV), 12, 157
Titanium, use of in thyroplasty, 197
TNM classification, 423–426*t*
Tongue, 18, 373
Tongue pump, 448
Total laryngectomy, 436–439, 436*f*, 439–440*t*, 442, 458*t*
Total lung capacity (TLC), 12, 64–65*f*
Trachea, 6, 8*f*
Tracheobronchial tree, 6–8, 7*f*
Tracheoesophageal puncture prostheses, 451*t*
Tracheoesophageal speech (TES), 443, 450–456
Tracheomalacia, 247
Tracheostomas, 436, 438*f*, 440
Trans speakers, feminizing strategies for, 371*t*
Transexuals, male-to-female, 366
Transgender, defined, 365–366
Transgendered individuals
  case history questions for, 369*t*
  evaluation of, 368–370
  voice treatment for, 370–376
Transsexual, defined, 365, 366
Transsexual voice, male-to-female, 183, 368–376
Transtheoretical Model of behavior change (TTM), 192, 192*t*
Transverse cordotomy, 200–201
Treatment efficacy, 111, 127–128*t*
"Treatment Efficacy Summary" (ASHA), 111
Treatments
  appropriateness of, 110–111
  efficiency of, 213
  eligibility for, 193–194
  goals for, 213, 370
  remotely delivered, 325
  tracking effectiveness, 129
  types of, 98
  use of acoustic measures with, 151
Triggers, awareness of, 407
True vocal folds, 16, 28–34, 29*f*
Trussing, abdominal, 180–181

Ulcers, 288–290
Unified Parkinson Disease Rating Scale (UPDRS), 319–320, 321*t*
Unilateral vocal fold paralysis (UVFP), 306–311
Upper motor neurons (UMN), 338
U.S. population, cultures in, 102

Vaccines, for HPV, 274
Vagus nerve, 58*f*, 316
Vallecula, 20–21
Varices, defined, 290–291
Vasoconstriction, 216

Ventilation, defined, 383
Ventricular obliteration, 230
Vertical partial laryngectomy (VPL), 433–434
Videoconferencing, use of in LSVT, 325
Videolaryngostroboscopy, 264, 308
Videostroboscopy, 137–138, 140–142, 140*t*
Visceral pleura, 9
Viscosity, and hyaluronic acid, 207
Vital capacity (VC), 12, 13, 64–65*f*, 157
Vocal amplification (VA) devices, use of, 175
Vocal development, verbal stages of, 71
Vocal disability coping questionnaire, 127*t*
Vocal fatigue
  central, 292
  peripheral, 292
  and phonation threshold pressure (PTP), 293–294
  and pregnancy, 76
  recovery from, 293
Vocal fold injections, 205*f*, 223*f*
Vocal fold paralysis (VFP)
  and arthritis, 241
  bilateral, 311–313
  causes of, 306–307, 312
  diagnosis, 309*t*
  diagnosis and evaluation of, 308–309
  and disability, 96
  effect of position of, 308*t*
  evaluation and treatment of, 312–313
  evaluation of, 157, 309*t*
  factors influencing, 307*t*
  idiopathic, 306
  symptoms of, 307–308, 312
  treatment of, 199, 309
  unilateral, 306–311
  voice therapy for, 310
Vocal fold paresis, 304–305
Vocal fold stripping, 286
Vocal folds
  adduction of, 82
  aging, 2
  aspects evaluated by videostroboscopy, 140–142, 140*t*
  assessment of, 142, 153–156
  atrophy of, 305
  augmentation of, 204–210
  changes in with age, 78
  cover-body models of, 35, 35*f*
  cycle of vibration, 48*f*
  edges of, 141
  extent of opening, 141
  fat grafts for, 224*f*
  hemorrhage of, 99
  hydration of, 50, 175–176, 293–294
  illuminated by stroboscopy, 137*f*
  infant *vs.* adult, 70*f*
  and laryngofissure, 255
  layers of, 34*f*
  length of, 33, 68
  lubrication of, 79, 99
  maturation of, 68–70
  microcirculation in, 290
  normal, **1**
  optimal position of, 199
  and Parkinson's disease, 319
  scarring of, **3–4**, 218–220, 219*t*, 226
  shortening of, 374–375
  vascular lesions of, 290–292
Vocal function exercises (VFE), 186–188, 187*t*
Vocal health, cultural factors in, 106
Vocal hygiene programs
  after surgery, 258
  discussed, 171–175
  example of, 172–174*t*
  and MG, 315
  and PVFM, 407
  for teachers, 188
  use of, 222, 286
Vocal hyperfunction, 175, 280
Vocal intensity, and aging, 77
Vocal registers, 59–61
Vocal tract
  defined, 52
  discomfort scale, 122, 123*t*
  raising formant frequencies, 372–373
Vocal training, importance of for teachers, 297–298
Vocal tremor, and aging, 81
Vocalization, neural pathways for, 53–56
Voice
  aperiodic, 151
  attitude toward elderly, 82
  esophageal, 449
  feminizing strategies for, 371*t*, 375
  following organ-preservation therapy, 430
  following resection, 432–433
  following VPL, 433–434
  and gender identity, 367
  normal, 86, 86*t*, 87*t*
  perceptions of, 331, 375
  restoration of, 442–459, 443*t*
  and self-concept, 351
  stereotyping by, 82
  transgender, 365–377
  variables associated with, 115
Voice and swallowing
  after near total laryngectomy, 436
  after supracricoid laryngectomy (SCL), 435–436
Voice arrests, defined, 87
Voice disorders
  causes of, 90, 91*t*
  perception of, 105
  prevention of, 93–95, 298
  and psychiatric caseness, 353
  related to self and identity, 352–353
  team approach to diagnosis and treatment, 90–93
  teams for, 92*t*
Voice evaluation, 116, 117*t*
Voice Handicap Index (VHI), 123–125, 124–125*t*, 331
Voice production, 5
  cortical areas important for, 52–53
  and health status, 82
Voice quality, 88
  following surgery, 256, 258
  and Parkinson's disease, 323–324
  for trans speakers, 372
Voice range profile (VRP), 149–150, 150*f*
Voice-Related Quality of Life (V-RQOL), 125, 126*t*
Voice rest, 2, 176
Voice restoration, 456–459
Voice therapy
  after organ preservation therapy, 430
  for ALS, 340
  behavioral, 310
  for contact ulcers, 290
  for conversion disorders, 362
  following surgery, 258, 262
  for Huntington's disease, 327
  for MTD, 359–360
  for mutational falsetto, 364
  for nodules, 282–283
  outcomes studies for, 311
  and Parkinson's disease, 323–325
  for patients with RRP, 274
  for polyps, 286
  for SD, 336–337
  for sulcus vocalis, 222
  for transgendered individuals, 371–374, 376–377
  for vocal fold lesions, 291–292
Voice therapy boot camp, 188
Voice treatments, behavioral, 111
Voice Use Reduction Program, 176

World Professional Association for Transgender Health, 367
Wound healing, 216, 217*f*

Xerostomia, 98–99

Yawn-sigh technique, 182, 317